Clinical Radiology
The Essentials

Clinical Radiology
The Essentials

FOURTH EDITION

Richard H. Daffner, MD, FACR
Professor of Radiologic Sciences
Drexel University College of Medicine
Department of Diagnostic Radiology
Allegheny General Hospital
Clinical Professor of Radiology
Temple University College of Medicine,
Allegheny Campus
Pittsburgh, Pennsylvania

Matthew S. Hartman, MD
Assistant Professor, Radiologic Sciences
Drexel University College of Medicine
Residency Program Director
Allegheny General Hospital
Forbes Regional Hospital
The Western Pennsylvania Hospital
Adjunct Assistant Professor, Radiology/Diagnostic Imaging
Temple University School of Medicine,
Allegheny Campus
Pittsburgh, Pennsylvania

 Wolters Kluwer | Lippincott Williams & Wilkins
Health
Philadelphia • Baltimore • New York • London
Buenos Aires • Hong Kong • Sydney • Tokyo

Acquisitions Editor: Susan Rhyner
Product Manager: Angela Collins
Marketing: Joy Fisher-Williams, Laura Harrington
Vendor Manager: Alicia Jackson
Design & Art Direction: Joan Wendt, Doug Smock
Compositor: Integra Software Services Pvt. Ltd.

First Edition, 1993
Second Edition, 1999
Third Edition, 2007

Library of Congress Cataloging-in-Publication Data

Daffner, Richard H., 1941- author.
  Clinical radiology : the essentials / Richard H. Daffner, Matthew S. Hartman.
-- 4th edition.
       p. ; cm.
  Includes bibliographical references and index.
  ISBN 978-1-4511-4250-1
  I. Hartman, Matthew S., author. II. Title.
  [DNLM: 1. Diagnostic Imaging--methods--Atlases. WN 17]
  RC78.7.D53
  616.07′54--dc23

                                        2013007058

DISCLAIMER
Care has been taken to confirm the accuracy of the information present and to describe generally accepted practices. However, the authors, editors, and publisher are not responsible for errors or omissions or for any consequences from application of the information in this book and make no warranty, expressed or implied, with respect to the currency, completeness, or accuracy of the contents of the publication. Application of this information in a particular situation remains the professional responsibility of the practitioner; the clinical treatments described and recommended may not be considered absolute and universal recommendations.

       The authors, editors, and publisher have exerted every effort to ensure that drug selection and dosage set forth in this text are in accordance with the current recommendations and practice at the time of publication. However, in view of ongoing research, changes in government regulations, and the constant flow of information relating to drug therapy and drug reactions, the reader is urged to check the package insert for each drug for any change in indications and dosage and for added warnings and precautions. This is particularly important when the recommended agent is a new or infrequently employed drug.

       Some drugs and medical devices presented in this publication have Food and Drug Administration (FDA) clearance for limited use in restricted research settings. It is the responsibility of the health care provider to ascertain the FDA status of each drug or device planned for use in their clinical practice.

To purchase additional copies of this book, call our customer service department at (800) 638-3030 or fax orders to (301) 223-2320.
International customers should call (301) 223-2300.
Visit Lippincott Williams & Wilkins on the Internet: http://www.lww.com. Lippincott Williams & Wilkins customer service representatives are available from 8:30 am to 6:00 pm, EST.
1 2 3 4 5 6 7 8 9 10

To

Morris M. Daffner, PhG; William F. Barry, Jr, MD;
George J. Baylin, MD; and Lawrence A. Davis, MD,
of blessed memories.

And

Carl Furhman, MD, and David Hartman.

Teachers, scholars, friends.

Thank you for all you taught us.

November 1995 marked the centennial of the discovery of x-rays by Roentgen. During those first 100 years, diagnostic imaging, through a variety of modalities, has greatly influenced medical diagnosis and treatment. In 1940, the management of approximately 1 in 10 patients was influenced by a radiographic study. By 1980, virtually all patients underwent some sort of diagnostic imaging study. Now, in the new millennium, imaging is used to guide many therapeutic procedures that previously would have required surgical exposure and prolonged hospitalization.

Diagnostic radiology has undergone dramatic changes in the past four decades. Prior to 1970, the specialty relied primarily on radiographs that were often supplemented by various contrast examinations for clinical problem solving. A revolution in diagnostic imaging began in the early 1970s with the development of cross-sectional and longitudinal imaging using ultrasound. Almost concomitantly, computed tomography (CT) followed, and soon rapid improvements in technology afforded us the ability to directly image areas of the body that previously were accessible only to the surgeon's knife. Magnetic resonance imaging (MRI) joined the diagnostic armamentarium in the early 1980s and added a new dimension for the diagnosis of disorders of the central nervous system, musculoskeletal system, the heart, and the gastrointestinal tract. Now, molecular imaging has emerged as a method of identifying specific tissues in the body. In the next decade, this new imaging technique should move rapidly from the laboratory to practical applications in improving cancer diagnosis and treatment.

Improvements in imaging have also changed the diagnostic approach to many conditions. Invasive procedures such as bronchography, cholecystography, cholangiography, cisternography, laryngography, lymphangiography, pneumoencephalography, and conventional tomography are, thankfully, no longer performed and have all been replaced by CT and/or MRI. Many other procedures such as intravenous urography, sinus radiography, and endoscopic retrograde cholangiopancreatography are on an "endangered species" list of studies and have been largely replaced by CT and/or MRI.

Refinements in existing technology facilitated whole new fields of endeavor for radiologists—interventional and invasive radiology. Radiologists are no longer limited in their abilities to simply make diagnoses. They have now developed the tools and skills to treat many conditions such as aneurysms, gastrointestinal bleeding, tumors, recurrent pulmonary emboli, and certain posttraumatic joint instabilities. Furthermore, using CT guidance, radiologists are now able to safely perform biopsies, drainages, excision, tumor ablation procedures, and surgical screw placements.

Our specialty is in a constantly evolving state. Improvements in computer technology have produced highly detailed multiplanar and three-dimensional imaging, as well as digital imaging. Digital processing of data is now the norm and picture archiving and computer storage is now the standard method of viewing and storing imaging studies, having replaced the conventional film radiography. This new format now allows images to be rapidly sent electronically from the source of origin to the physicians who need to see them.

In the 1990s, the general awareness of the cost of health care led us to seek alternative methods for making diagnoses and treating patients. While there is now an exciting new field of minimally invasive surgery, radiologic-guided intervention is now replacing many surgical procedures. At the beginning of the new millennium, there are more demands for accountability on the part of the medical profession. Diagnostic radiology is ready to answer the call. In addition, while the cost of health care is foremost in everyone's minds, there is also a growing awareness of the dangers of exposure to radiation from diagnostic studies, particularly CT scans. The American College of Radiology (ACR) has responded to these two challenges by developing programs to guide clinicians to ordering the right study for the right reasons, and for radiologists to perform them the right way. The ACR Appropriateness Criteria® attempt to recommend appropriate imaging for a large variety of clinical conditions. Their recommendations are based on reviews of current literature by panels of experts in radiology in consultation with applicable clinicians.

This book is intended for the medical student who is beginning his or her clinical rotations. It is a thorough revision of the third edition and includes the state-of-the-art changes that have occurred in the field. There have been a number of significant changes to the book. The previous editions were a solo effort by myself. In writing the chapters out of my particular area of expertise (musculoskeletal and spine imaging), I relied on my colleagues at Allegheny Radiology Associates for expert advice. For this edition, I enlisted the services of my colleague Matthew S. Hartman, MD, as coauthor/coeditor. In addition, each chapter was revised by a colleague who was, in our estimate, an expert in his/her field. Furthermore, there will be web-based additional material that will include selective case studies. These case studies will be updated on a periodic basis, whereas the main text will have to wait for a new edition for updates.

Significant new material includes discussions on newer interventional techniques and cardiac imaging the reader is likely to encounter. As before, disorders of the pediatric age group are integrated into each chapter rather than considered separately to avoid duplication of material. Other significant changes include the addition of nearly 300 new figure parts and the replacement of many older figures with those that reflect state-of-the-art imaging.

In writing the original edition of this book as well as in its revisions, we have kept the orientation based on clinical problem solving, rather than listing the radiographic signs of various conditions as isolated facts without attempting to correlate them with the pathophysiology that produces them. Diagnostic imaging is true detective work. The image represents the patient at that particular point in time. By knowing one's anatomy, and by observing the changes that the disease has produced to that anatomy, it is possible to identify the pathologic process(es) that produced those changes. It is our goal to show that by recognizing a radiographic *pattern*, it is possible to define the pathophysiologic process producing that pattern.

The first chapter provides an overview of diagnostic imaging, listing the "menu" of imaging options available to help solve clinical problems. The physical basis for each type of imaging is briefly stated. The second chapter discusses radiographic contrast agents, with attention to contrast-induced nephritis. The third chapter is devoted to interventional or invasive radiology. The remainder of the book consists of individual chapters describing imaging of the lungs, heart, breast, abdomen, gastrointestinal tract, urinary tract, obstetrics and gynecology, the musculoskeletal system, and the brain and spinal cord.

Each of the clinical chapters is divided into three sections: technical considerations, anatomic considerations, and pathologic considerations. The *technical considerations* portion of each chapter discusses the types of examinations performed for that area, the use of special imaging, and a description of how each particular examination may be of help in clinical problem solving.

The *anatomic considerations* portion reviews pertinent anatomy of the region being studied. No attempt is made to be encyclopedic; rather, the approach is very brief but covers all of the essentials. It is important for you, the reader, to recognize that the images that you are viewing are two-dimensional representations of three-dimensional structures. You must remember the adage that if you know the gross appearance of a structure, you can easily predict its radiographic or other imaging appearance.

The *pathologic considerations* include those pathophysiologic alterations of normal anatomic structures that produce the abnormalities shown on the images. Logic tells us that there are a limited number of ways for a disease to affect an organ. Similarly, there are limitations in the way an organ responds to that disease process. For example, in the gastrointestinal tract, a mucosal tumor appears the same whether it is located in the esophagus, stomach, small intestine, or colon. The same holds true for other lesions of this system. Furthermore, an extrapolation may be made to other tubular structures in the body—airways, urinary tract, and blood vessels. Once the reader recognizes the *pattern* of a lesion, he/she will recognize it anywhere in the body, even if it is in an unusual location.

Throughout the text, the reader is reminded that there are a large variety of imaging studies that may be performed on a patient. The choice of study should be based on the analysis of the history, physical findings, economics, and good judgment. Any diagnostic study should be *appropriate* for the patient's signs and symptoms. Please remember that these studies are expensive. We have tried to cite examples where duplicative imaging may be performed. It is not necessary to perform a study just because you can ("dog's balls principle").

The reader will find that the text emphasizes certain types of imaging examinations and makes little or no mention of others. The authors' goal is to provide you, the reader, with state-of-the-art imaging information. This revision reflects changes that have occurred in imaging protocols. However, since this text is also used in parts of the world where the most sophisticated imaging techniques are not available, some of the older studies that are still performed are mentioned and are illustrated.

There is a list of suggested additional readings at the end of each chapter. The majority of these are of current textbooks in the various subspecialties of diagnostic radiology. The reader is referred to them for a more in-depth discussion of individual topics. Most of these books should be available in the medical school library, hospital library, or radiology departmental library or as e-books. Furthermore, as previously mentioned, the ACR has published a number of documents on technical standards for diagnostic and therapeutic radiologic studies as well as on appropriateness of imaging studies. These may be accessed without cost from the ACR web site: www.acr.org.

Previous editions of this book included an appendix of diagnostic pearls. We have eliminated this from the end of the book. Instead, we now include these pearls as inserts in the appropriate section of the text. In addition, there are more bulleted lists.

Finally, it is our hope that the book will be easily read and understood. Learning should be fun. It has been our intent to keep it that way in each of the editions of this book.

RICHARD H. DAFFNER, MD, FACR

MATTHEW S. HARTMAN, MD
Pittsburgh, Pennsylvania

Acknowledgments

No book of this nature may be produced without the cooperation of a large number of contributors. The authors wish to acknowledge the following colleagues in addition to my coauthors for their help in producing this book: Jordan Caplan, MD; David Epstein, MD; Melanie Fukui, MD; and Michael Spearman from the Department of Diagnostic Radiology at Allegheny General Hospital, who provided case material and consultation in their areas of expertise.

H. Scott Beasley, MD, and Carl Fuhrman, MD, of the Department of Radiology, University of Pittsburgh School of Medicine; Donna Blankenbaker, MD, of the Department of Radiology, University of Wisconsin School of Medicine; Mihra Taljanovic, MD, of the Department of Radiology, University of Arizona; Leonard E. Swischuk, MD, of the University of Texas Medical Branch at Galveston; Sinda B. Dianzumba, MD, of the Division of Cardiology, Allegheny General Hospital; and John J. Crowley, MD, of the Department of Pediatric Imaging, Children's Hospital of Pittsburgh, also provided case material for this text.

We appreciate the contributions of Patricia Prince, RT, RDMS, formerly of the Department of Obstetrics and Gynecology, Allegheny General Hospital, for the obstetrics/gynecology ultrasound cases.

We would like to thank Donna Spillane of the Department of Communications, Allegheny General Hospital, for photographic assistance and Randall S. McKenzie of McKenzie Illustrations for his superb artwork.

We would also like to thank Maggie Cauley, Department of Diagnostic Radiology, Allegheny General Hospital, for secretarial and editorial assistance in the preparation of the manuscript.

Finally, we especially thank our wives, Alva Daffner and Amy Hartman, for their encouragement and support during the long months of preparation of this work.

From Matthew Hartman: on a personal note, being asked by Dr. Daffner to contribute to this newest edition is a special honor for me as I used an earlier edition of the Daffner textbook as a medical student 10 years ago. The clear images and the pragmatic text inspired me to learn more. In addition, I was very fortunate to have some great radiology educators during my medical school, residency, and fellowship experiences including Dr. Carl Fuhrman at my *alma mater*, the University of Pittsburgh School of Medicine, and my father, Dr. David Hartman, at the Penn State University Medical Center. I hope that future generations of students will continue to be inspired.

Contents

chapter 1

Overview and Principles of Diagnostic Imaging

Richard H. Daffner

Historical Perspectives

The science of radiology had its birth in November 1895 when Wilhelm Conrad Roentgen, a Dutch physicist, discovered a form of radiation that now bears his name, the Roentgen ray. He called this new form of unknown radiation—which was invisible, could penetrate objects, and caused fluorescence—*X-strahlung* (x-ray) because initially he did not understand its nature. Roentgen was experimenting with cathode ray tubes, studying their behavior in a completely darkened room. He noticed that when the tube was operating, a faint glow appeared on his laboratory table. That glow, he discovered, was caused by a fluorescent plate that he had inadvertently left on the bench. When he reached for the plate, he was shocked to see the image of the bones of his hand cast onto the plate. His meticulous work investigating his discovery provided the world with an understanding of this new form of radiation. For his monumental work, Roentgen was awarded the Nobel Prize in physics in 1901.

X-Rays for Diagnosis

The first recorded diagnostic use of x-rays was in 1896. In the first decade of the discovery of the roentgen ray, the physical effects of x-rays on patients were also observed. It was not long before a new medical specialty, radiology, was born. Traditionally, radiology was divided into two distinct branches: diagnostic and therapeutic. The only common area between these disciplines was the use of ionizing radiation. As each field continued to develop and grow in complexity, it became apparent that separation of the two specialties was needed. Specialists now train in either diagnostic radiology or radiation oncology (therapy). A third pathway, interventional radiology, is being developed at the present time.

Developments in Diagnostic Radiology

The last quarter of the twentieth century brought changes in diagnostic radiology that far surpassed those made in the previous 75 years. Developments made in recent decades have revolutionized medical diagnosis, making areas of the body previously inaccessible to nonsurgical examination clearly visible. Furthermore, the ability to precisely image all areas of the body made biopsy procedures and numerous interventional techniques possible using newer methods of diagnostic imaging for guidance. Previously, these procedures would have required surgical exploration. From a personal perspective, I have had the privilege of being part of the "imaging revolution" that has occurred since I began my radiology residency in 1970. Image intensification, electronic imaging, and the use of computers in radiology are taken for granted today. Unfortunately, that was not always the case. The following personal anecdotes epitomize the state of radiology 50 years ago.

I was a third-year medical student serving on my medicine rotation at the county hospital in Buffalo when we scheduled one of my patients for a fluoroscopic examination of his suspected paralyzed right hemidiaphragm. At the appointed hour of the exam, I was summoned to the radiology department in the basement of the old hospital. I was given a heavy, semirigid lead apron and a pair of red goggles, which they told me to put on. I followed the technologist into the fluoroscopy suite, where several other house staff were similarly attired in apron and goggles. As soon as the door closed, the lights were turned off, and I was suddenly blind in the pitch-blackness. I could hear the radiologist, the late Dr. George Alker, talking to the patient. He was asking the patient to breathe and to turn in various directions. At one point he asked, "Does everybody see that?"

"Uh huh," was the reply from everyone in the room but me.

"What about you, Dr. Daffner? Did you see it?"

"Dr. Alker," I replied, "I can't see squat!"

"Good Lord, son. Take off your goggles!"

Nobody had told me that the goggles were only for helping my eyes adapt to the dark. I thought they were needed to see the fluoroscopic screen. Before image intensification became standard in radiology departments, however, that was the state of fluoroscopy.

Fortunately, the department in which I trained was state of the art, and we had image intensification. However, even in the early 1970s, not all departments were so equipped. As a senior resident doing locum tenens work at a small hospital in eastern North Carolina, I was told to provide coverage at the private office of the radiologist, for whom I was filling in. I walked across the parking lot to his office to do an upper gastro-intestinal series. I was somewhat taken aback when I learned that his office did not have image intensification and I would have to use old-fashioned "red goggle" fluoroscopy. I donned my goggles and worked with them on for about a half hour, the prescribed period for dark adaptation, before going into the fluoroscopy suite, where I removed them. I stepped on the foot pedal and looked at the screen and saw nothing but a faint green glow. I decided my eyes were not completely dark adapted, so I put the goggles back on and waited another half hour. Again, the result was the same. I have always believed in "three times is the charm" and decided to give it one more try. This time, when I stepped on the foot pedal, I could actually see something! I had the patient drink some barium and was actually able to follow it down the esophagus, where I lost it in the denser abdomen. After the patient drank some more barium, I moved the fluoroscopic screen around and saw a curvilinear structure. "Aha! The duodenal bulb," I thought to myself. I took four spot films and then instructed the technologist to give the patient more barium and take overhead films. Fifteen minutes later the technologist came into the reading room holding a dripping wet film in a metal frame.* (The hospital had no automatic processing either.) It was my spot film. I held it up to the light box and saw four perfect views of the right femoral head! How far radiology has come since then. Table 1.1, a historic timeline for diagnostic radiology, shows the progress made in the century since Roentgen's discovery.

Five Imaging Modalities

The realm of diagnostic radiology encompasses various modalities of imaging that may be used individually or, more commonly, in combination to provide the clinician with enough information to aid in making a diagnosis. These include radiography, computed tomography (CT), magnetic resonance (MR) imaging, diagnostic ultrasound, and nuclear imaging. Radiography and CT use x-rays. Nuclear imaging is also associated with radiation and involves the detection of emissions from radioactive isotopes in various parts of the body; MR imaging and ultrasound do not use ionizing radiation. The newest frontier in diagnostic imaging, molecular imaging, makes possible the identification of certain molecules within cell structures. Although much of the work is still experimental, molecular imaging promises to be a boon for the diagnosis of malignancies. A brief introduction to each type of examination will help you to understand how these modalities are used in clinical problem solving.

---

* The origin of the term "wet read" relates to the days before automatic film processing when films were placed on metal racks and were developed by hand. If the referring physician needed an immediate interpretation, the wet film was brought to the radiologist before it had been allowed to dry.

Table 1.1 DIAGNOSTIC RADIOLOGY TIMELINE

Year	Development
1895	Roentgen discovers x-rays
1896	First clinical x-ray made
1897	Bismuth used as contrast for stomach x-rays
1901	Dangers of x-rays first reported by William Rollins
1906	First retrograde pyelogram using colloidal silver nitrate
1910	Barium used as contrast agent in GI tract
1911	First double contrast of upper GI
1913	Modern x-ray tube invented by William Coolidge Stationary grid invented by Gustav Bucky X-ray film of nitrocellulose developed
1914	World War I begins
1915	Bucky's grid motorized by Hollis Potter
1919	First pneumoencephalogram
1921	Intensifying screens developed by Carl Patterson First air myelogram
1922	Iodized oil used for myelography
1923	First double-contrast barium enema
1927	First cerebral angiogram
1929	Great Depression begins First excretory urogram
1932	Nephrotomography developed
1937	First angiocardiogram
1938	First successful mammogram
1939	World War II begins
1941	First A-mode ultrasound of the skull
1942	Automatic processor for film developed (no pun intended)
1945	Atom bombs dropped on Hiroshima and Nagasaki
1948	First coronary artery angiogram
1949	Xerography developed
1953	Sven Seldinger introduces technique for vascular puncture
1953	Image intensifier used in radiology
1954	Diatrizoate introduced as a safer contrast medium Echocardiography developed
1957	Whole-body nuclear scanner developed by Hal Anger Space Age begins with the Soviet launch of Sputnik
1962	B-mode ultrasound developed
1963	President Kennedy assassinated
1964	SPECT scanning
1968	First men on the moon
1972	CT developed
1974	PET scan
1978	First brain MR image
1980	First commercial MR scanner
1985	Digital radiography, PACS
1989	Soviet Union collapses; Cold War ends
1990	Helical (spiral) CT

(Continued)

Table 1.1 DIAGNOSTIC RADIOLOGY TIMELINE (*Continued*)

Year	Development
1998	Multislice CT
2000	Molecular imaging
2001	World Trade Towers destroyed

CT, computed tomography; GI, gastrointestinal; MR, magnetic resonance; PACS, picture archiving and communications system; PET, positron emission tomography; SPECT, single photon emission computed tomography.

REALM OF DIAGNOSTIC RADIOLOGY

▶ Radiography
▶ Fluoroscopy
▶ Computed Tomography
▶ Magnetic Resonance Imaging
▶ Ultrasound
▶ Nuclear Imaging
▶ Interventional Radiology

Radiography

Definition

X-rays, or *roentgen rays*, are a form of electromagnetic radiation or energy of extremely short wavelength. The spectrum of electromagnetic radiation is illustrated in Figure 1.1. X-rays in the diagnostic range (shaded area) are near the end of the spectrum of short wavelengths. The shorter the wavelength of an electromagnetic radiation form, the greater its energy and, as a rule, the greater its ability to penetrate various materials.

X-rays are described in terms of particles or packets of energy called *quanta* or *photons*, which travel at the speed of light. The amount of energy carried by each photon depends on the wavelength of the radiation. This is measured in electron volts. An electron volt is the amount of energy an electron gains as it is accelerated through a potential of 1V.

An atom is ionized when it loses an electron. Any photon with approximately 15 or more electron volts of energy is capable of producing ionization in atoms and molecules *(ionizing radiation)*. X-rays, γ-rays, and certain types of ultraviolet radiation are all typical ionizing radiation forms.

Production of X-Rays

X-rays used in diagnostic radiology require a vacuum and the presence of a high potential difference between a cathode and an anode. In the basic x-ray tube, a much more potent version of the incandescent light bulb, electrons are boiled off the cathode (filament) by heating it to a very high temperature. Moving these electrons toward the anode at an energy level sufficient to produce x-rays requires a high potential—up to 125,000 V (125 kV). When the accelerated electrons strike the tungsten anode, x-rays are produced. X-rays follow the same physical laws as light, and as such, will darken photographic (or, in the past x-ray) film. *For the purpose of this discussion, the word "film" is used interchangeably with any type of recording medium (digital receptor plates).*

Production of Images

Image production by x-rays results from *attenuation* of those x-rays by the material through which they pass. Attenuation is the process by which x-rays are removed from a beam through absorption and scatter. In general, the greater the material's density—that is, the number of grams per cubic centimeter—the greater its ability to absorb or scatter x-rays (Fig. 1.2). Absorption is also influenced by the atomic number of the structure. The denser

Electromagnetic Radiation

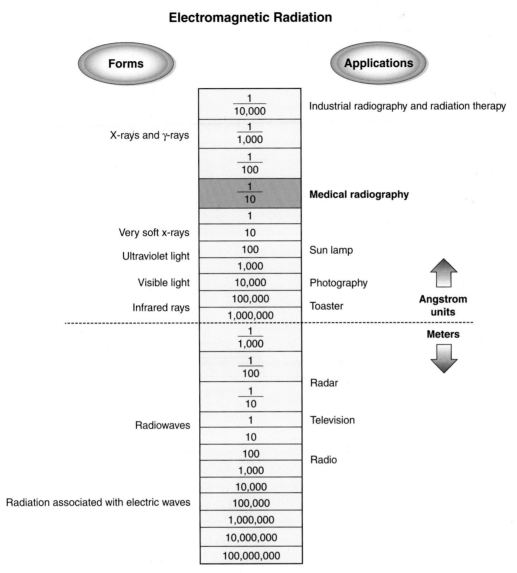

Figure 1.1 Spectrum of electromagnetic radiation. The numbers represent the wavelength of the particular radiation. The shorter the wavelength, the greater the energy associated with that radiation.

the structure, the greater the attenuation, which results in less blackening of the "film" (fewer x-rays strike the "film"). Less-dense structures attenuate the beam to a lesser degree and result in more blackening of the "film" (more x-rays strike the "film"; Fig. 1.3).

Radiographic Density

It is important to differentiate between two types of *densities* that you will hear mentioned when discussing radiographs with radiologists or other colleagues: physical density and radiographic density. *Physical density* is the type of density just described. *Radiographic density* refers to the degree of blackness of a film. *Radiographic contrast* is the difference in radiographic densities on a film. The radiographic density of a substance is related to its physical density. The effect on film or other recording media occurs paradoxically: structures of high physical density produce less radiodensity and vice versa. Structures that produce more blackening on film are referred to as being *radiolucent*; those that produce less blackening are called *radiopaque* or *radiodense*. There are four types of radiographic densities; in increasing order of physical density, these are gas (air), fat, soft tissue (water), and bone (metal). Radiographically, these appear as black, gray-black, gray, and white, respectively. Contrast material containing either barium or iodine molecules, used in conjunction with radiographic studies, is of high radiodensity, above that of water and lower than that of bone. CT has the ability to detect minute differences in the densities of tissues and portray them in varying shades of gray. These CT densities are measured in Hounsfield units, after Godfrey Hounsfield, the father of CT. Distilled water at a standard pressure is

Figure 1.2   **Relationship between density and absorption of x-rays.**   The denser a particular material, the greater its ability to absorb x-rays. Greater absorption produces less darkening on the final image; less absorption produces more darkening.

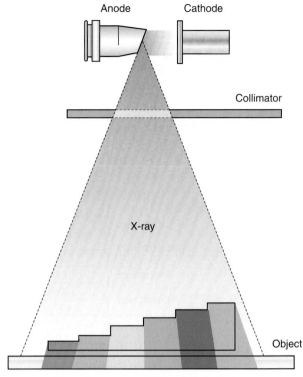

Figure 1.3   **The level of absorption of x-rays depends on the composition of the tissue.** Denser tissue absorbs more x-rays; less-dense tissue transmits more x-rays. The resulting radiographic image is essentially a "shadowgram."

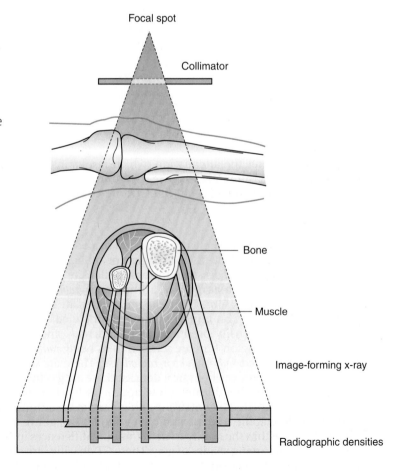

Table 1.2 HOUNSFIELD UNITS (HU) FOR VARIOUS TISSUES

Bone	1,000
Liver	40–60
Brain, white matter	20–30
Brain, gray matter	37–45
Blood	40
Muscle	10–40
Kidney	30
Cerebrospinal fluid	15
Water	0
Fat	–50 to –100
Air	–1,000

given a value of 0 and air is given a value of –1,000. Bone densities are very high, up to 1,000; soft tissue values falling in between (Table 1.2).

Recording Media

X-Ray Film

The most common type of recording medium used to be x-ray film. X-ray film is still used in many parts of the world. However, state-of-the-art radiology departments have replaced x-ray film with electronic recording media. X-ray film consists of a plastic sheet coated with a thin emulsion that contains silver bromide and a small amount of silver iodide. This emulsion is sensitive to light and radiation. A protective coating covers the emulsion. When the film is exposed to light or to ionizing radiation and then developed, chemical changes take place within the emulsion, resulting in the deposition of metallic silver, which is black. The amount of blackening on the film depends entirely on the amount of radiation reaching it and therefore on the amount attenuated or removed from the beam by the subject.

Other recording media include fluoroscopic screen and image intensification systems, photoelectric detector crystals, xenon detector systems, and computer-linked detectors that measure actual attenuation.

Fluoroscopic Screen

A fluoroscopic screen is coated with a substance (phosphor) that gives off visible light (or fluoresces) when it is irradiated. The brightness of the light is proportional to the intensity of the x-ray beam striking the plate and depends on the amount of radiation removed from the beam by the object being irradiated. Today, the fluoroscopic screen is combined with an electronic device that converts the visible light into an electron stream that amplifies the image (makes it brighter) by converting the electron pattern back into visible light. This system allows the radiologist to see the image clearly without requiring dark adaptation of the eyes, as was necessary in "conventional" (non–image-enhanced) fluoroscopy, described graphically earlier in the chapter. The technology of image intensification was originally developed around 1950 for military use at night. Intensifying screens, variants of fluoroscopic screens, were used in most film cassettes to reduce the amount of radiation needed to produce an acceptable exposure.

Photodetectors

Photons emitted by radioisotopes are detected with sodium iodide crystals. These crystals respond, when irradiated, by emitting light whose brightness is related to the energy of the photons striking them. Photodetectors, which are computer-linked, convert the light into an electronic signal, which is then amplified and converted into a variety of display images.

Computer-Linked Detectors

The twenty-first century is clearly the era of the computer and the age of the "information superhighway." Not surprisingly, computers are now essential components in radiology departments. CT and MR scanners and digital radiography units use electronic sensors that actually measure the attenuation coefficient of tissue through which the x-ray beam has passed and converts this mathematical value into a digitized shade of gray. The data are fed into a computer that plots the location of each of those measurements to produce the computer image. This is recorded on compact discs (CDs) or digital video discs (DVDs) and is displayed on a television monitor.

Picture Archiving and Communications System (PACS)

Computed radiography, a derivative of CT technology, has now replaced conventional film-screen radiography. It forms the basis for the *picture archiving and communications system* (PACS; Figs. 1.4 and 1.5) as well as for teleradiology. The typical PACS uses a photosensitive electronic plate that records the amount of radiation striking each location. This, as previously explained, depends on the density of the tissue through which the x-ray beam passes and the degree of attenuation of the beam. The radiation intensity at each site is recorded digitally to produce a digital image that can be transmitted directly to a high-resolution monitor. Storage is on CD or DVD.

Modern radiology departments no longer have conventional view boxes. Rather, the reading stations are a series of high-quality television monitors (see Fig. 1.5). Similarly, the clinical areas of the hospital and the physicians' offices have monitors. The problem of delay in transportation of x-ray films from the processing area to the file room and then to the reading areas is eliminated because the images are sent directly from the processing area to the reading areas electronically. Clinicians can view images by accessing them directly from the central archive to their work areas. Images that are too dark or too light can be electronically manipulated at the reading station (Fig. 1.6). Finally, having the diagnostic information in digital form enables the speedy electronic transfer of data for teleradiology.

Figure 1.4 Outline of a picture archiving and communications system (PACS). CT, computed tomography; DR, digital radiography; DSA, digital subtraction angiography; MRI, magnetic resonance imaging; QC, quality control.

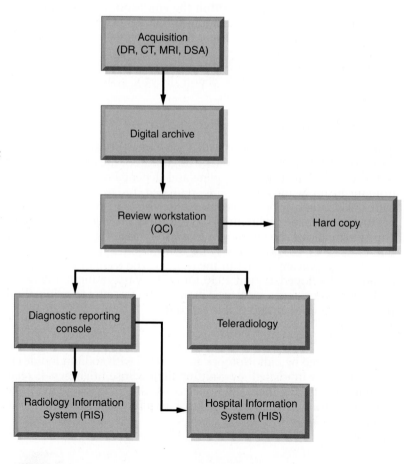

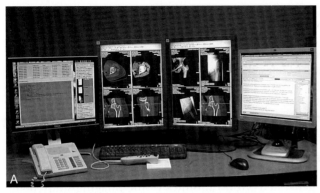
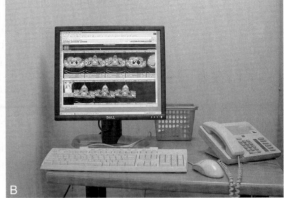

Figure 1.5 Picture archiving and communications system reading consoles. **A.** Diagnostic console in the radiology department. The far left screen holds the clinical information and the patient's imaging archive. The two center screens are high-resolution monitors for viewing the images and comparing studies. The far right screen shows the consultation report. **B.** Satellite console in an office. Only one screen is used for viewing.

State-of-the-art computerized imaging technology requires cooperation among members of the radiology department as well as those of the medical records department and hospital administration. In fully integrated systems, the *radiology information system* (RIS) communicates directly with the *hospital information system* (HIS). The RIS is used for scheduling examinations, communicating clinical data to the radiologists, archiving studies, and reporting the interpretations of those studies. The HIS provides all the medical information that a treating or consulting physician may need when seeing a patient. It is also an important resource for the radiologist, providing clinical information that may have been omitted from the request for the imaging study.

Teleradiology

Teleradiology is a natural offshoot of electronic imaging. Modern teleradiology systems are Web based. Among its many applications, teleradiology is probably most often used to provide after-hours ("night hawk") coverage when a department cannot have a radiologist on staff all night. Several enterprising companies have located in Sydney, Australia, or in Israel, where the time differences allow their radiologists to be working during the day while supplying information to U.S. doctors working at night.

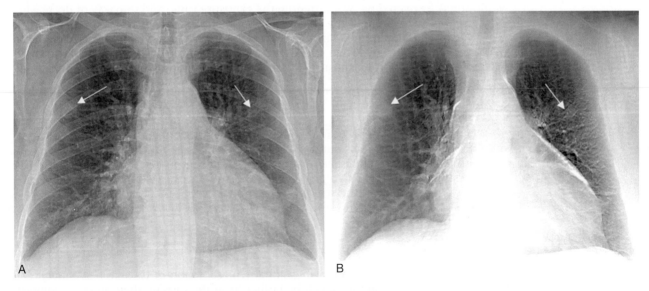

Figure 1.6 Electronic manipulations possible with picture archiving and communications system. **A.** Frontal radiograph of patient with known renal carcinoma shows suspected nodules in both upper lobes (*arrows*). **B.** Same image with bones electronically subtracted shows bilateral lung nodules (*arrows*). Other manipulations allow changes in density and contrast as well as reversal of densities.

As a rule, these companies provide "preliminary" interpretations for a set fee per study. The second application of teleradiology is providing coverage for facilities that do not have on-site radiologists. This may involve some night and weekend work as well. In this situation, images are sent to a central "command post," often at a university and typically staffed all night. The third use of teleradiology is for consultation. In this situation, images are sent from one facility to another to be reviewed by a more experienced radiologist. In our department, we use this mode for consultation between satellite facilities in our hospital system.

Voice recognition technology has further improved the turnaround time to produce a final report on imaging studies. Voice recognition programs produce quality reports with little need for editing by the radiologist, replacing the traditional method of dictation transcribed by a typist. When voice recognition is combined with PACS technology, final reports can be generated within minutes of the imaging study being performed.

Image Quality

Physical and geometric factors affect the radiographic image, regardless of the format. These factors include thickness of the part being studied, motion, scatter, magnification, and distortion.

FACTORS AFFECTING IMAGE QUALITY
- Motion
- Scatter
- Magnification

Thickness

The *thickness* of the part being imaged determines how much of the beam is removed or attenuated, as explained earlier. Thus, for adequate penetration, an obese patient requires more x-rays than does a thin patient, bone requires more x-rays than does the surrounding muscle, and a limb with a cast requires more x-rays, as does a wet plaster cast (because the water attenuates the x-ray beam).

Motion

Motion of the part being radiographed results in a blurred, nondiagnostic image. Motion may be overcome by shortening the exposure time, and one way of decreasing exposure time is to enhance the effectiveness of the recording medium. In the past this was done by using an intensifying screen—a device coated with a fluorescent material that gives off visible light when struck by x-rays. The visible light rather than the x-rays themselves produces the exposure. Modern digital imaging has replaced intensifying screens.

Scatter

Scatter is produced by deflection of some of the primary radiation beam; this can produce fog on the image and is undesirable. To eliminate as much scatter as possible, a grid with alternating angled slats of very thin radiolucent material combined with thin lead strips is used (Fig. 1.7). To prevent the lead strips from casting their own shadows as they absorb radiation, the whole grid is moved very quickly during the exposure, eliminating shadow lines. This system is known as the Bucky-Potter system, after the two men who invented it.

Magnification

The radiographic image is a two-dimensional representation of three-dimensional structures. Consequently, some parts will be farther from the cassette than others. Geometrically, x-rays behave similarly to light. Hence, *magnification* of objects will occur when they are at some distance from the cassette. The farther an object is from the cassette, the greater

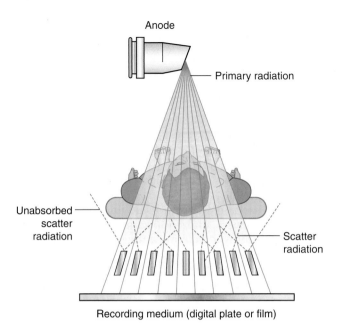

Figure 1.7 Grid function. A grid absorbs scattered radiation. Angling of the lead strips permits only the primary x-ray beam to pass through.

the magnification and the lesser the sharpness; the closer an object is to the cassette, the lesser the magnification and the greater the sharpness (Fig. 1.8). This has considerable importance in evaluating the heart on chest radiographs. On the standard chest radiograph, the x-ray enters the back of the patient and exits from the front; this is called a *posterior-to-anterior* (PA) radiograph. Because the heart is located anteriorly, relatively little magnification results. However, on an *anterior-to-posterior* (AP) radiograph of the chest, the beam enters the patient's front and exits from the back, and the heart appears somewhat larger because of its greater distance from the cassette. The best rule to follow to reduce the undesirable effect of magnification is to have the part of greatest interest closest to the cassette. This will produce the truest image of the region of interest.

Distortion

Distortion occurs when the object being radiographed is not perfectly perpendicular to the x-ray beam. The radiographic image of an object depends on the sum of the shadows

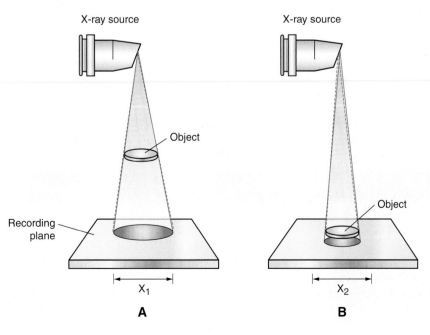

Figure 1.8 Magnification and image sharpness. **A.** The object is farther from the cassette, resulting in a larger image. However, its margin is not distinct. **B.** The object is closer to the cassette, resulting in a smaller and sharper image than in **A.**

produced by that object when x-rayed. Changes in the relationship of that object to the x-ray beam may distort its radiographic image (Fig. 1.9). For diagnostic clarity, therefore, it is best to have the part of major interest as close to and as perpendicular to the cassette as possible.

Radiographs ("Plain Film")

Radiography is the bread and butter of the diagnostic radiologist. The obsolete term *plain film* refers to radiographs in which no contrast material is used to enhance various body structures. In performing radiographic examinations, the natural contrast among the basic four radiodensities—air (gas), soft tissue (water), fat, and bone (metal)—is relied on to define abnormalities. Examples of radiographic studies with which you are familiar include chest, abdominal, and skeletal radiographs.

Fluoroscopy, a variant of radiography, is a useful modality for studying the diaphragm, heart motion, valve calcification within the heart, and localization of chest masses (Fig. 1.10). Despite being a fast and inexpensive way to determine the presence or absence of lung nodules, it is underutilized.

Figure 1.9 Distortion. The shape of an object on a radiograph depends on the angle at which the radiographic beam strikes it. A. Two objects of similar size cast distinct images when the x-ray beam is nearly perpendicular. The difference in size is the result of magnification. **B.** Angling the x-ray beam while the objects remain in the same relationship to one another results in an overlapping image that is not a true representation of the actual objects. **C.** Posterior-to-anterior (PA) radiograph of the chest in a patient with right middle lobe pneumonia. **D.** Lordotic view of the same patient made with the patient bending backward toward the film shows a dramatic change in the appearance of the heart, ribs, and infiltrate, which now appears as a mass adjacent to the heart border on the right (*arrow*).

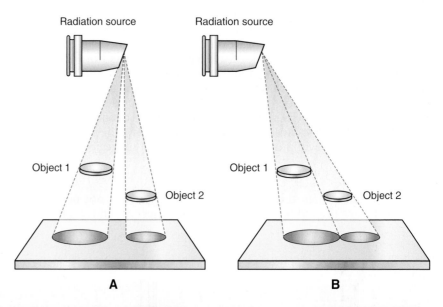

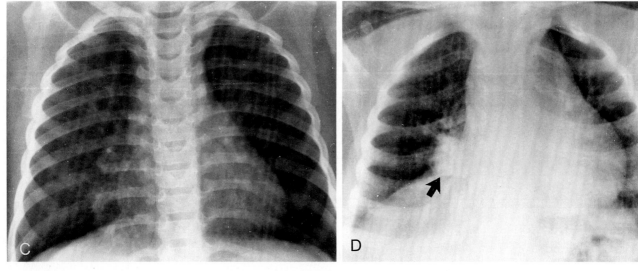

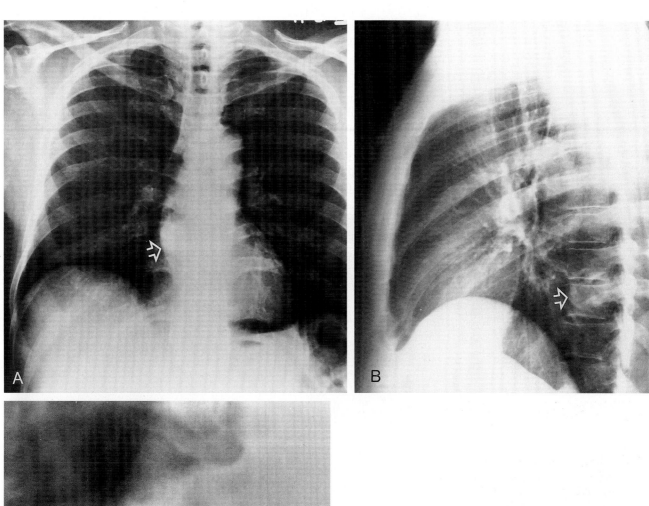

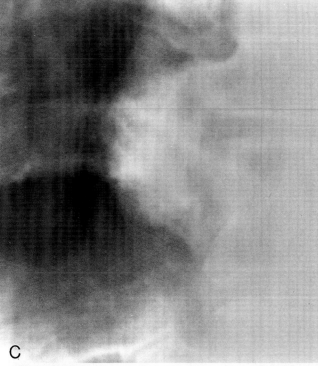

Figure 1.10   The value of chest fluoroscopy.   A. PA chest radiograph shows a "mass" through the cardiac shadow to the right of midline (*arrow*). **B.** Lateral view shows the mass to be posterior (*arrow*). **C.** Fluoroscopic spot film shows the density in question to be the result of bone spurs bridging the thoracic vertebral bodies. There was no tumor. Unfortunately, chest fluoroscopy has become a lost art, since CT is easier to obtain.

Contrast Examinations

Radiography is adequate for situations in which natural radiographic contrast exists between body structures, such as the heart and lungs, or between the bones and adjacent soft tissues. To examine structures that do not have inherent contrast differences from the surrounding tissues, it is necessary to use one of several contrast agents. Contrast examinations were used more extensively in the past to evaluate abdominal or intracranial masses.

CT and MR imaging have made most of these examinations obsolete. Three areas deserve specific mention: gastrointestinal tract, urinary tract, and blood vessels.

Gastrointestinal Tract

The most common contrast material used for gastrointestinal examinations is a preparation of barium sulfate mixed with other agents to produce a uniform suspension. They may be administered either by mouth (antegrade) or by rectum (retrograde) alone or, more commonly, in combination with air, water, and an effervescent mixture that produces carbon dioxide. Gas-enhanced studies are referred to as *air contrast* studies (Fig. 1.11).

In addition to barium preparations, water-soluble agents containing iodine are available for studying the gastrointestinal tract whenever there is the possibility of leakage

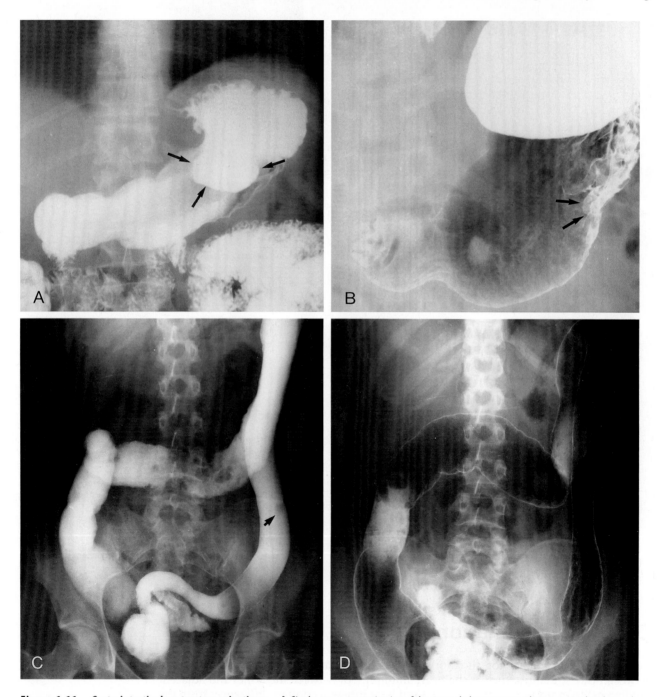

Figure 1.11   Gastrointestinal contrast examinations.   A. Single-contrast examination of the stomach demonstrates a large gastric ulcer (*arrows*). **B.** Double-contrast examination shows a tumor along the greater curvature (*arrows*). **C.** Single-contrast barium enema shows a polyp in the descending colon (*arrow*) in a patient with ulcerative colitis. Note the loss of haustral markings. **D.** An air contrast barium enema in the same patient.

of the contrast material beyond the bowel wall. Although barium is a chemically inert substance, it produces a severe desmoplastic reaction in tissues. Water-soluble agents, on the other hand, do not produce this type of reaction and are absorbed from the leakage site where they are excreted through the kidneys. Water-soluble agents, however, are not without hazard, because they can cause a severe chemical pneumonia if aspirated. They also cost more and thus are not used on a routine basis.

Urinary Tract

Urography is the radiographic study of the urinary tract. The contrast agents used for this study are primarily the ionic water-soluble salts of diatrizoic or iothalamic acids or the nonionic agents iopamidol or iohexol. These are administered intravenously (*intravenous urogram*) or retrograde to study the urethra, bladder, ureters, and renal pelvis. The physiology of these agents is discussed in Chapter 2. Intravenous urography largely has been replaced by CT.

Vascular System

Angiography is the study of the vascular system. Water-soluble agents similar to those used for urography are injected either intra-arterially or intravenously, and a rapid sequence exposure is made to follow the course of the contrast material through the blood vessels (Fig. 1.12). CT angiography using iodinated contrast and MR angiography (MRA) using gadolinium compounds are performed commonly. In these studies, the contrast is injected intravenously rather than through an arterial puncture, making the procedure safer and more tolerable for the patient.

A *sinogram (or fistulogram)* involves the injection of contrast material through an abnormal sinus tract into the body. Water-soluble agents are commonly used for these studies. In evaluating an empyema cavity in the chest, where there is a danger that a bronchopleural fistula may be present, an oil-soluble material such as propyliodone (Dionosil) is used because water-soluble contrast material entering the bronchial tree can produce a severe and often fatal chemical pneumonia.

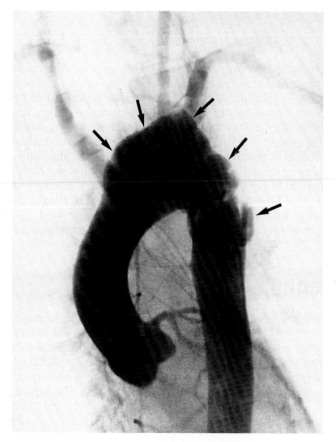

Figure 1.12   Arteriogram in a patient with posttraumatic rupture of the aorta.   This is a subtraction image in which black and white are reversed to improve contrast. Note the irregularity and ballooning of the aortic arch at the site of injury (*arrows*).

Figure 1.13   Herniated intervertebral disc.
Myelogram shows compression of the subarachnoid space by the herniated disc material (*arrows*). Today myelography is combined with computed tomography.

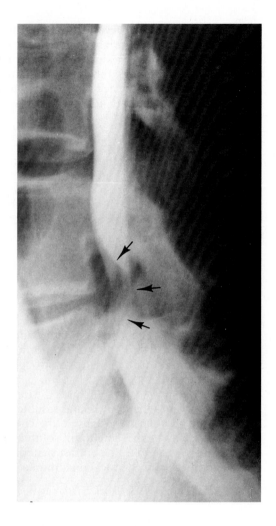

Diseases encroaching on the vertebral canal may be studied by *myelography*. The main indication is evidence of spinal cord or nerve root compression. The most common lesion is a herniated nucleus pulposus from a lumbar disc. Myelography is performed by inserting a needle between the spinous processes of lumbar vertebrae and entering the subarachnoid space. It may also be performed by puncture of the cisterna magna when there is a complete block within the vertebral canal and it is necessary to inject contrast medium above the lesion. Cerebrospinal fluid is also removed for study at this time. Nonionic, iodinated, water-soluble compounds are injected under fluoroscopic monitoring in varying amounts, and the patient is positioned for the study. Figure 1.13 shows a myelogram of a patient with a herniated lumbar disc. Note the compression of the thecal sac by the herniated material. Myelography is often performed in conjunction with CT. The development of MR imaging, however, has decreased the number of myelograms performed.

Computed Tomography

Under ordinary circumstances, the fleshy organs of the body, such as the heart, kidneys, liver, spleen, and pancreas, are considered uniform in radiographic density—like water, which produces a gray appearance on conventional radiographs. However, these tissues vary somewhat in their chemical properties, and it is possible, using computer-enhanced techniques, to measure those differences, magnify them, and display them in varying shades of gray or in color. This is the basis of CT. Godfrey Hounsfield was the first to develop the CT scanner in England. For his efforts, he was awarded the 1979 Nobel Prize in medicine.

Figure 1.14 **Principles of computed tomography (CT).** **A.** In the modern CT scanner, the x-ray tube rotates within the gantry. Detectors measure the amount of radiation removed from the x-ray beam. **B.** Modern CT scanners use arrays of detectors to shorten the time needed for the scan.

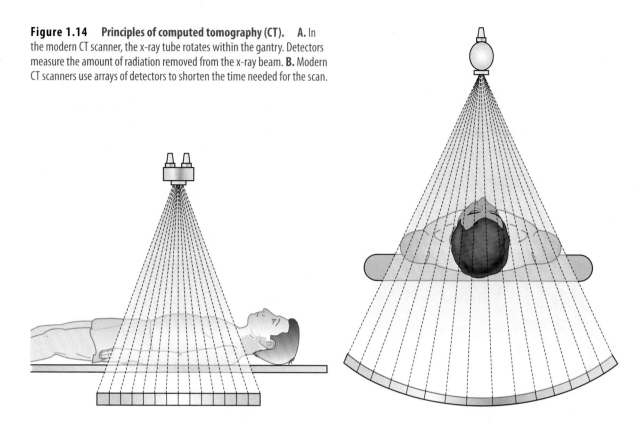

In CT (Fig. 1.14), an x-ray beam and a detector system move through an arc of 360°, irradiating the subject with a highly collimated (restricted) beam. This allows the detector system to measure the intensity of radiation passing through the subject. The data from these measurements are analyzed by a computer system that assigns different shades of gray (CT or Hounsfield numbers) to different structures based on their absorption or attenuation coefficients. The computer reconstructs a picture based on geometric plots of where these measurements were taken. Interestingly, although this system of diagnosis was developed in the early 1970s, the mathematical formula for the reconstruction of images based on measurements of their points in space was developed in 1917 by the mathematician Johann Radon.

Helical, or Spiral, Imaging

Modern CT is performed using helical or spiral technology. In earlier CT studies, multiple contiguous images were obtained to produce sections resembling the slices of a loaf of bread (Fig. 1.15A). In spiral CT, the data are acquired using technology that produces sections resembling an apple that has been peeled or sliced spirally (Fig. 1.15B). Furthermore, modern CT systems acquire data using banked rows of 64, 128, or 256 detectors at one time, thus the term *multislice* or *multidetector CT* (MDCT). The technology results in images that are obtained rapidly that, because of overlap of data, provide information on every square millimeter in the area of study. It is now possible to image an entire thorax or an entire abdomen in 20 seconds or less. This speed is important when breath holding is necessary to prevent motion artifacts. Rapid throughput of patients is made possible, as is rapid multiplanar and three-dimensional reconstruction of images (Fig. 1.16). Speed is particularly essential when trauma victims are imaged. In addition to the rapidity, another advantage of multislice technology is that additional studies may be derived from the data set obtained during the original acquisition. For example, a typical thorax–abdomen–pelvis (TAP) CT is usually reconstructed for interpretation using 5 mm slice thickness. It is possible to reconstruct a study of the thoracic and lumbar spine from the same data set at narrower (2 mm) slice thickness. The narrower sections allow greater detail to be shown of the bones, a feature critical for the diagnosis of spine fractures (Fig. 1.17).

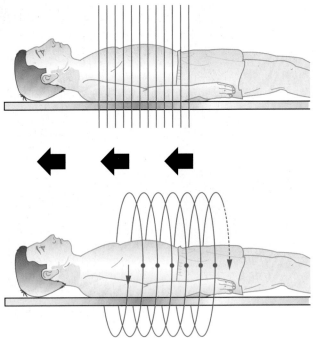

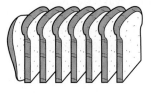

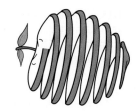

B

Figure 1.15　Conventional versus spiral computed tomography (CT).
A. Methods of acquisition of the data. In conventional CT (*top*), individual slices are obtained. In spiral CT (*bottom*), a continuous band of information is obtained. Horizontal arrows indicate the direction of patient travel through the gantry. **B.** Conventional CT obtains individual slices, much like the loaf of bread on the left. Spiral CT produces a continuous band of information, similar to the apple on the right. All state-of-the-art CT scanners use spiral and multidetector technology.

A

Digital Display and Picture Archiving and Communications System

The information obtained with CT systems is displayed digitally on a high-resolution monitor and stored on CD or DVD. Once the information has been recorded, it is possible to change the windows of the various densities to optimally demonstrate the lungs, soft tissues, or bone on the reading console (Fig. 1.18). The data from the study are linked to the PACS or teleradiology system. To enhance the appearance of certain viscera or vascular neoplasms, contrast material may be injected intravenously. The contrast agents used are identical to those used in angiography or urography.

Diagnostic Uses

Cranial scanning is performed to evaluate patients with various neurologic findings. This study is particularly useful in defining and localizing brain tumors (primary or metastatic) and in evaluating patients with neurologic emergencies such as intracerebral hemorrhage and subdural hematoma. Figure 1.19 shows the scan of a patient with a meningioma. Note how well the tumor is defined against the normal brain tissue. Figure 1.20 shows a patient with a subdural hematoma. Note the compression of normal brain tissue by the hematoma.

　　Scanning the rest of the body is particularly useful in evaluating visceral neoplasms (Fig. 1.21). Other uses include studies of patients with abdominal trauma (Fig. 1.22), investigation of patients with suspected pancreatic disease, mediastinal studies for defining the extent of tumors, evaluation of patients with Hodgkin disease or lymphoma for staging purposes, diagnosis of intra-abdominal abscess (Fig. 1.23), and scanning the musculoskeletal system for various bone and soft tissue disorders (Fig. 1.24).

Nuclear Imaging

Nuclear medicine traditionally has two divisions: nuclear imaging (radiology) and laboratory analysis. The diagnostic radiologist is concerned with the imaging aspect of the field. The use of isotopes for laboratory purposes and for evaluating physiologic functions is not discussed in this book. However, you should be aware that the laboratory aspect of nuclear medicine is equally as important as the imaging aspect.

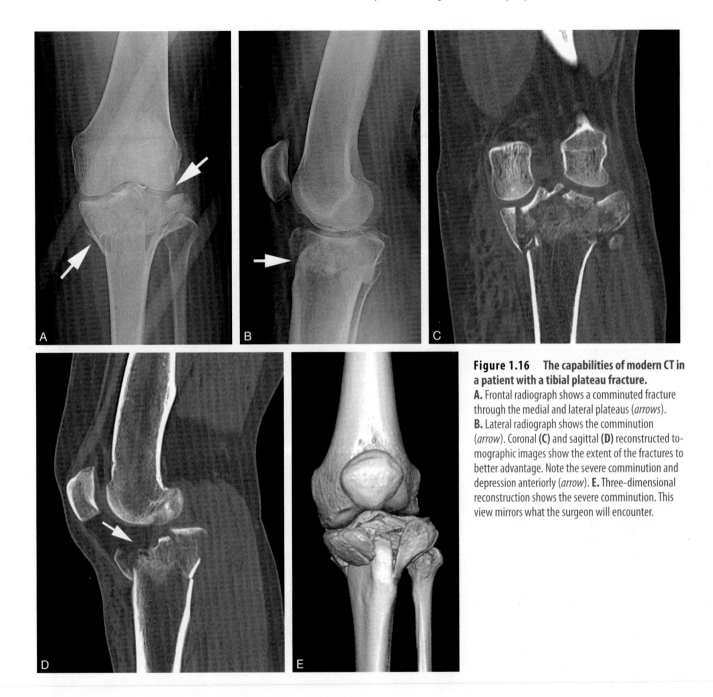

Figure 1.16   The capabilities of modern CT in a patient with a tibial plateau fracture.
A. Frontal radiograph shows a comminuted fracture through the medial and lateral plateaus (*arrows*).
B. Lateral radiograph shows the comminution (*arrow*). Coronal (**C**) and sagittal (**D**) reconstructed tomographic images show the extent of the fractures to better advantage. Note the severe comminution and depression anteriorly (*arrow*). **E.** Three-dimensional reconstruction shows the severe comminution. This view mirrors what the surgeon will encounter.

Radioactive Isotope Uptake

Nuclear imaging depends on the selective uptake of different compounds by different organs of the body. These compounds may be labeled with a radioactive substance of sufficient energy level to allow detection outside the body. The ideal isotope can be administered in low doses, is nontoxic, has a short half-life, is readily incorporated into "physiologic" compounds, and is relatively inexpensive. Technetium 99 m fulfills most of these requirements.

Half-Life

The *half-life* of an element is the time necessary for its degradation to one-half of its original activity. In medicine there are three types of half-lives: physical, biologic, and effective. The *physical half-life* is the period in which the element would decay on its own. This occurs naturally, whether the element is sitting on the laboratory shelf or has been

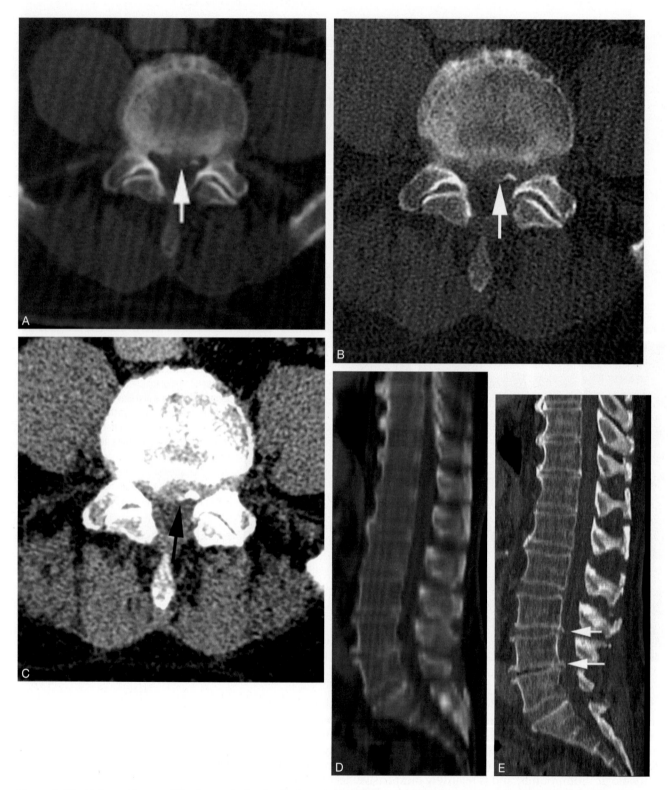

Figure 1.17   Reformatting capability in a study showing lumbar spinal stenosis.   An abdominal scan was performed at 5 mm slice intervals for suspected prostatitis. The patient also had leg paresthesias and a spine study was reconstructed from the same data set at 2 mm slice intervals. **A.** Detail view of axial CT abdominal image shows degenerative changes in the lower lumbar spine (*arrow*). **B** and **C.** Axial reconstructed images at bone and soft tissue windows, respectively, show the disc–osteophyte complex (*arrows*) much better than on the original study. **D.** Sagittal reconstructed image from original study shows poor detail. **E.** Sagittal reconstructed image using the narrow slice thickness shows multiple disc–osteophyte complexes (*arrows*) in much better detail. *Note the differences in the appearance in images made from the same data set.*

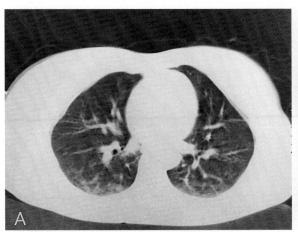 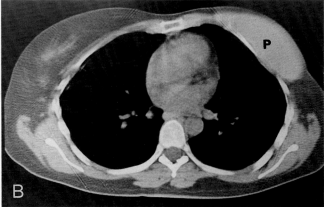

Figure 1.18   The effects of changes in window settings.   A. Image of a patient's thorax made at a window setting to enhance the lungs. **B.** The same section at soft tissue windows. Compare with part figure **A**. A breast prosthesis (*P*) is evident.

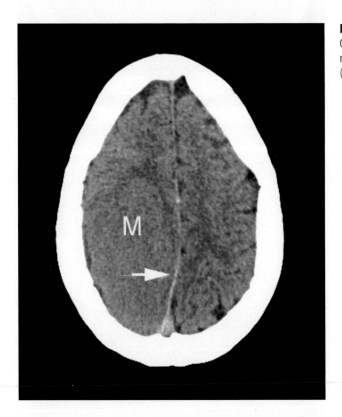

Figure 1.19   Meningioma. Cranial CT shows a mass (*M*) in the right occipital region. Note the bowing of the septum (*arrow*).

administered to a patient. *Biologic half-life* concerns the normal physiologic removal of the substance to which the isotope has been attached. For example, the sodium pertechnetate commonly injected for nuclear scanning is excreted into the urine and the gastrointestinal tract. Although the physical half-life of technetium 99m is approximately 6 hours, the biologic half-life is less. The *effective half-life* is a mathematical derivation based on a formula combining the biologic and physical half-lives. It measures the actual time the isotope remains effective within the body.

Static or Dynamic Imaging

Nuclear imaging is performed on either a static or dynamic basis. Static studies include the thyroid, liver, and conventional single photon emission computed tomography (SPECT) scans. Dynamic studies additionally include rapid sequence images to assess blood flow to organs such as the skeleton and the kidneys. Common types of scans are

Figure 1.20   Subdural hematoma on the right.   Note the compression of the right side of the brain by the low-density hematoma (*arrows*). There is loss of the sulci on the left as the result of compression. Compare with the left.

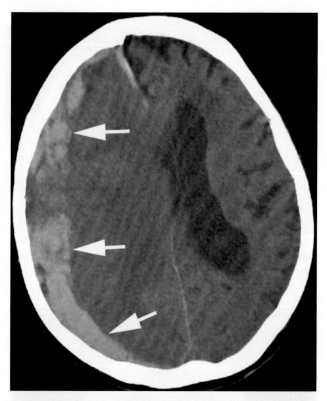

Figure 1.21   Abdominal CT showing a renal carcinoma on the right (*arrow*).   Note the difference in kidney contour and texture compared with the left.

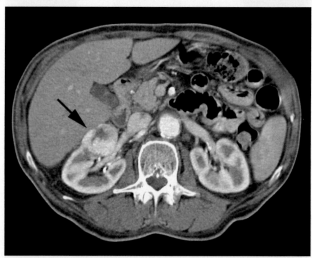

Figure 1.22   Abdominal trauma.   A. Axial CT image shows a large laceration (*asterisk*) in the middle of the liver. The dense areas in the laceration are hemorrhage. **B.** Left renal fracture showing a large retroperitoneal hematoma (*asterisk*) and active bleeding (*arrows*).

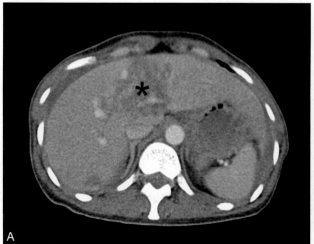

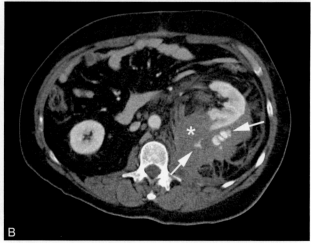

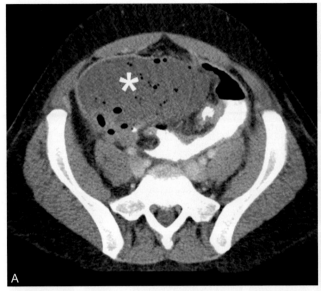

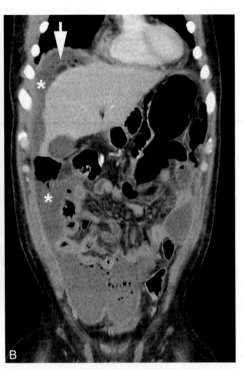

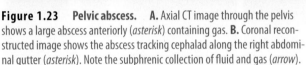

Figure 1.23   Pelvic abscess.   A. Axial CT image through the pelvis shows a large abscess anteriorly (*asterisk*) containing gas. **B.** Coronal reconstructed image shows the abscess tracking cephalad along the right abdominal gutter (*asterisk*). Note the subphrenic collection of fluid and gas (*arrow*).

listed in Table 1.3 and depicted in Figures 1.25 through 1.29. Equipment for detecting the uptake of isotopes and recording their images includes the γ-camera and the tomographic scanner.

There are basically five mechanisms of isotope concentration within the body:

1. Blood pool or compartmental localization (e.g., cardiac scan)
2. Physiologic incorporation (e.g., thyroid scan and bone scan)
3. Capillary blockage (e.g., lung scan)
4. Phagocytosis (e.g., liver scan)
5. Cell sequestration (e.g., spleen scan)

Positron Emission Tomography

Conventional nuclear scans use isotopes that produce γ- or x-rays. Positron emission tomography (PET) uses cyclotron- or generator-produced isotopes of relatively short half-life that emit positrons, which are significantly higher-energy particles. The initial application of PET scanning was primarily to evaluate brain metabolism by assessing blood flow to a specific part of the brain—for example, measuring focal decrease in epilepsy or differentiating between a tumor and radiation necrosis that might occur after treatment. Areas of increased brain activity show selective uptake of the injected isotope. It has been particularly useful in evaluating patients with senile dementia or Alzheimer disease (Fig. 1.30). PET scanning is more frequently used for oncologic imaging in diagnosis, staging, and restaging of malignancy after treatment. The reason for this is the ability of the PET scan to show increased use of glucose by the tumor (Fig. 1.31A). With newer technology, the PET image can be combined with a CT image (PET/CT) to allow more accurate localization for either surgery or biopsy of suspected metastases (Fig. 1.31B).

Magnetic Resonance Imaging

MR imaging is a noninvasive technique that does not use ionizing radiation. In the parameters used for medical imaging, it is without significant health hazard. MR imaging is based on the principles described by Felix Bloch and Edward Purcell in an experimental procedure they designed to evaluate the chemical characteristics of matter on a molecular level. For their work, Bloch and Purcell were awarded the Nobel Prize in physics in 1962.

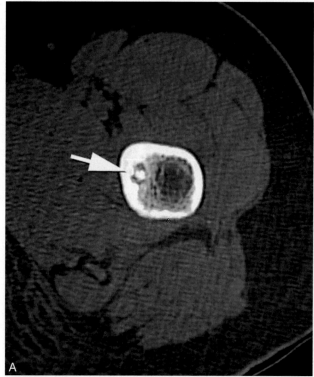

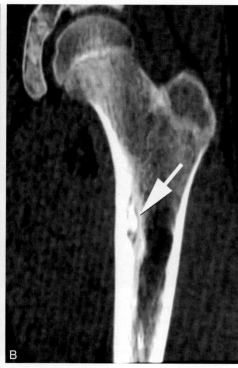

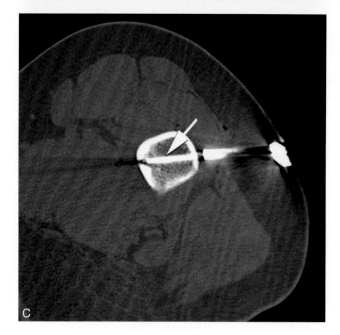

Figure 1.24   Osteoid osteoma.   Axial **(A)** and sagittal **(B)** reconstructed images show a lucent lesion in the medial proximal femur with a dense nidus (*arrows*). **C.** Axial image shows a probe (*arrow*) inserted into the tumor for percutaneous ablation.

Table 1.3 ISOTOPE SCANS AND COMMON USES

Type of Scan	Figure No.[a]	Common Indications
Lung	1.25	Pulmonary embolism, quantification of perfusion
Liver	1.26	Masses (hemangiomas), metastases, cholestasis
Bone	1.27	Metastases, pain, suspected child abuse
Thyroid	1.28	"Goiter" nodules, hyperthyroidism, cancer
Heart	1.29	Myocardial perfusion, function, and viability

[a]Scan illustrated in these figures.

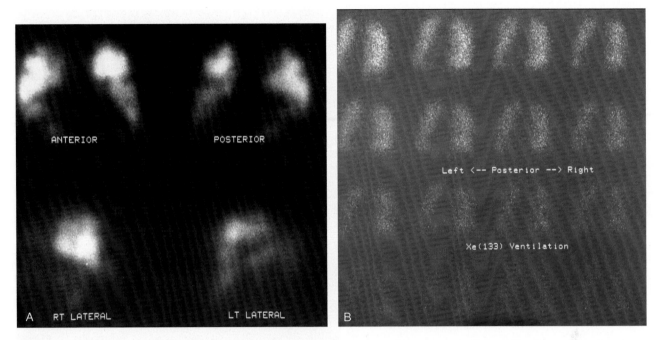

Figure 1.25   Ventilation-perfusion scan in a patient with pulmonary emboli.   A. Perfusion scan of the lungs shows many areas devoid of radioisotope (*photopenia*) bilaterally. **B.** The ventilation scan is normal. This combination of findings is diagnostic of pulmonary embolism.

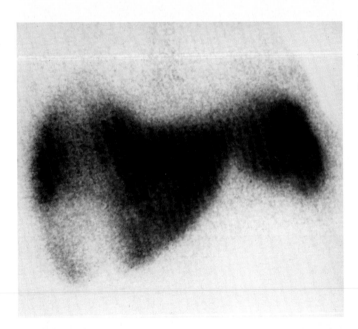

Figure 1.26   Liver scan in a patient with multiple metastases to the right lobe of the liver.   Note the large photopenic areas.

Raymond Damadian began investigating the possibilities of using MR for imaging in 1971. The development of computer imaging algorithms for CT accelerated the development of MR for medical diagnosis. Paul Lauterbur and Peter Mansfield were able to produce the first successful images using this technique, and for their efforts they received the 2003 Nobel Prize in medicine.

Magnetic Resonance Technology

MR imaging uses a pulsed radiofrequency (RF) beam in the presence of a high magnetic field to produce high-quality images of the body in any plane. The nuclei of any atoms with odd numbers of nucleons (protons and neutrons) behave like weak magnets in that they align themselves with a strong magnetic field. If a specific RF signal is used to perturb

Figure 1.27   Bone scan in a patient with metastatic disease.   Note the areas of the increased tracer concentration (*blackness*) throughout the skeleton.

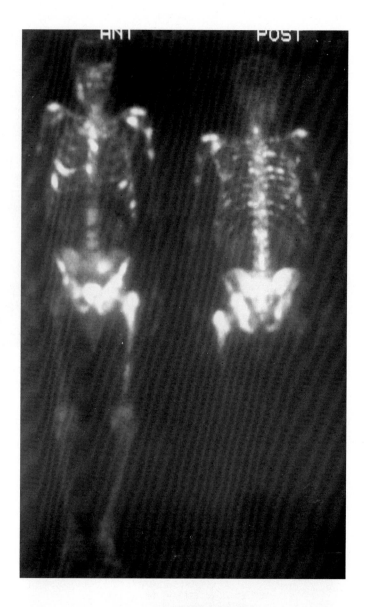

Figure 1.28   Thyroid scan showing a nodule as a photopenic area in the right lobe of the thyroid.

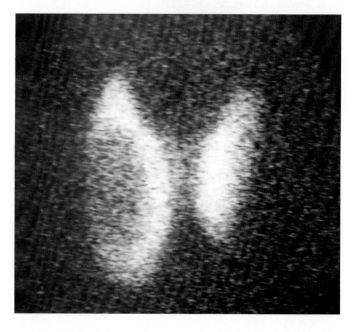

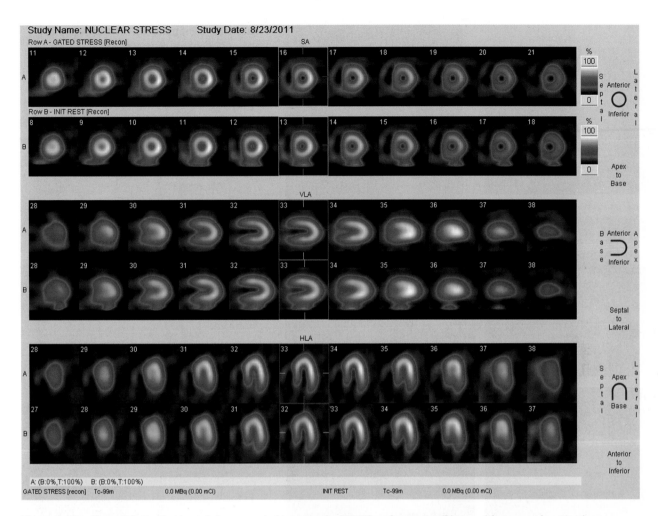

Figure 1.29 **Normal single photon emission computed tomography (SPECT) nuclear sestamibi scan with stress and rest testing.**
Distribution of blood flow is uniform over the left ventricle, as evidenced by the uniform distribution of the isotope between rest and stress. First row: short axis stress. Second row: short axis rest. Third row: vertical long axis stress. Fourth row: vertical long axis rest. Fifth row: horizontal long axis stress. Sixth row: horizontal long axis rest.

the nuclei under study, their relationship to the external magnetic field is altered and they will generate a radio signal of their own that has the same frequency as the signal that initially disrupted them (Fig. 1.32). This signal can then be amplified and recorded—the basis for MR imaging. Although many nuclei may be used for MR imaging, the most common is hydrogen because of its abundance in tissue and its sensitivity to the phenomenon of MR.

Multiple Planes and Contrast Manipulation

Like CT, MR imaging displays structures in a transverse or axial fashion. However, MR imaging can also produce images in any other planes. The common display parameters used are the sagittal, coronal, and axial planes. Furthermore, MR imaging has the advantage of being able to highlight the different pathologic changes in different tissues through contrast manipulation. This is accomplished by altering the pattern of RF pulses in a study. The MR image reflects the strength or intensity of the magnetic resonance RF signal received from the sample. Signal intensity depends on several factors, such as hydrogen density and two magnetic relaxation times: T1 and T2. The greater the hydrogen density, the more intense (bright) the MR signal will be. Tissues that contain very little hydrogen, such as cortical bone, flowing blood, and an air-filled lung, generate little or no MR signal and appear black on the images produced. Tissues high in hydrogen, such as fat or cartilage, have high signal intensity and appear white.

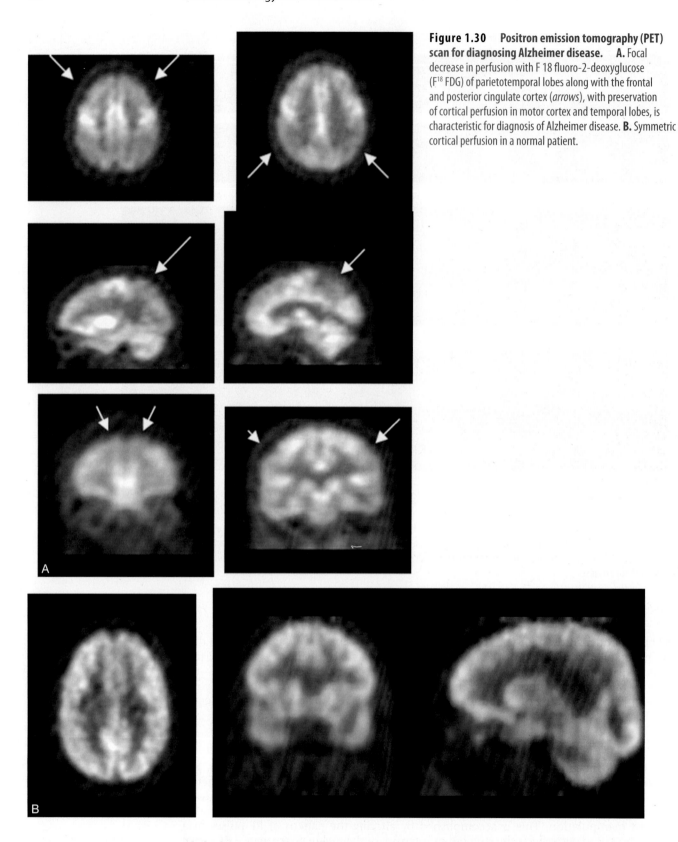

Figure 1.30   Positron emission tomography (PET) scan for diagnosing Alzheimer disease.   A. Focal decrease in perfusion with F 18 fluoro-2-deoxyglucose (F^{18} FDG) of parietotemporal lobes along with the frontal and posterior cingulate cortex (*arrows*), with preservation of cortical perfusion in motor cortex and temporal lobes, is characteristic for diagnosis of Alzheimer disease. **B.** Symmetric cortical perfusion in a normal patient.

Alphabet Soup: T1 and T2 and Other Magnetic Resonance Terms

Detailed explanation of the physics of MR and of T1 and T2 are beyond the scope of this text. An excellent reference is Bushong's *Magnetic Resonance Imaging*. However, in simple terms, these two measurements reflect quantitative alterations in MR signal strength owing to interactions of the nuclei being studied and their surrounding chemical and physical milieu. T1 is the rate at which nuclei align themselves with the external magnetic

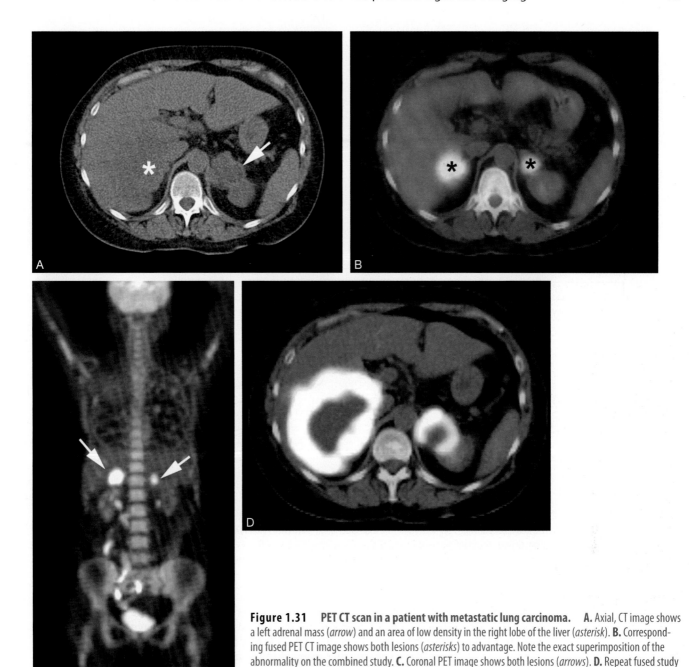

Figure 1.31   PET CT scan in a patient with metastatic lung carcinoma.   A. Axial, CT image shows a left adrenal mass (*arrow*) and an area of low density in the right lobe of the liver (*asterisk*). **B.** Corresponding fused PET CT image shows both lesions (*asterisks*) to advantage. Note the exact superimposition of the abnormality on the combined study. **C.** Coronal PET image shows both lesions (*arrows*). **D.** Repeat fused study 3 months later shows enlargement of both lesions.

field after RF stimulation. T2 is the rate at which the RF signal emitted by the nuclei decreases after RF perturbation. Other terms that you will encounter when discussing MR examinations with a radiologist or when reviewing the literature are:

- ○ *Tesla* (T): The unit of measure of magnetic flux density, or simply magnet strength; in the International System of Units (SI), 1 T equals 10,000 G.
- ○ *Echo time*: The time between the middle of the RF pulse and the middle of spin echo production.
- ○ *Repetition time*: The time between the beginning of one pulse sequence and the beginning of succeeding pulse sequences.
- ○ *Commonly used imaging parameters*: Spin echo, short T1 inversion recovery, and various acronymic gradient echo techniques (FISP, FLASH, etc.).

Again, for a detailed description, see Bushong's text.

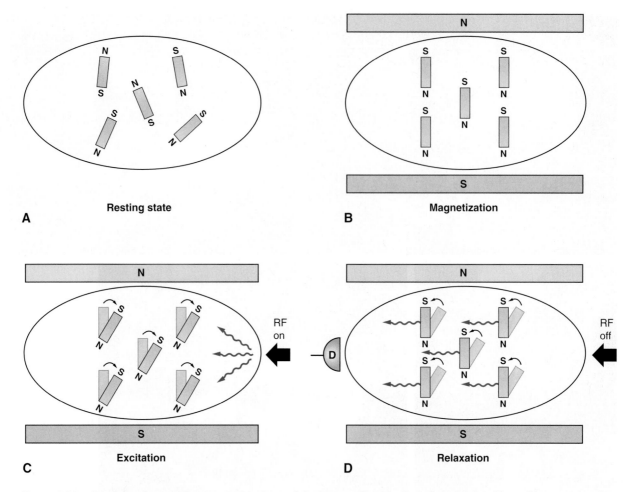

Figure 1.32   Principles of magnetic resonance imaging.   A. Resting state. The molecules in the body behave like small bar magnets and are arranged in a random fashion. **B.** Following magnetization. The molecules align themselves along the plane of magnetization. **C.** Excitation. A pulsed radiofrequency (*RF*) beam deflects the molecules as they absorb the energy from that beam. **D.** Relaxation. When the RF beam is switched off, the molecules return to their preexcitation position, giving off the energy they absorbed. This may be measured with a detector (*D*).

Magnet Strength

Typical high-field MR imaging units have a magnet strength of 1.5 to 3.0 T. Numerous smaller strength magnets are also on the market. Machines with magnet strength of 0.1 to 0.5 T have the advantage of being open and thus much less likely to produce claustrophobia in patients. However, studies done at lower magnetic strength take longer, raising the possibility of motion artifacts. Furthermore, images from lower strength magnets tend to be less detailed than those from the high-field units. A third type of magnet, designed primarily for office use, is the extremity magnet, which typically ranges between 0.1 and 1.5 T. This will accommodate knees, ankles, feet, hands, wrists, and elbows. Image quality varies with these units.

Diagnostic Uses

MR imaging is used primarily for studying intracranial (Fig. 1.33) and intraspinal (Figs. 1.34 and 1.35) pathology and for evaluating abnormalities of the musculoskeletal system (Figs. 1.36 and 1.37) and the heart. Additionally, it is used to evaluate abdominal visceral problems (Fig. 1.38). MRA is also commonly used for vascular abnormalities (Fig. 1.39).

Diagnostic Ultrasound

Diagnostic ultrasound is a noninvasive imaging technique that uses sonic energy in the frequency range of 1 to 10 MHz (1,000,000 to 10,000,000 cps). This is well above the normal human ear response of 20 to 20,000 Hz. Ultrasound is a nonionizing form of

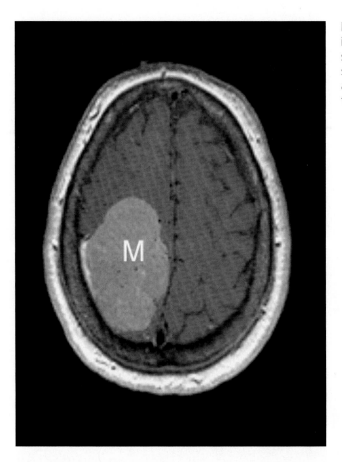

Figure 1.33 **Magnetic resonance imaging of meningioma.** (This is the same patient as in Fig. 1.19.) Axial image shows the tumor (*M*) to much better advantage. Note the internal structure of the tumor compared with Figure 1.19.

energy and, thus, is safe for use on pregnant patients and children. Echoes or reflections of the ultrasound beam from interfaces between tissues with various acoustic properties yield information on the size, shape, and internal structure of organs and masses. Ultrasound waves are greatly reflected by the interface between soft tissue and air or bone, thus limiting the use of this technique in the chest and musculoskeletal system. Figure 1.40 shows the components of an ultrasound machine. Most ultrasound machines are portable, allowing the examination to be brought to the patient's bedside.

STUDIES NO LONGER PERFORMED AND STUDIES THAT REPLACED THEM

❱ Conventional Tomography	CT
❱ Pneumoencephalography	CT, MRI
❱ Sweet's Eye Localization	CT
❱ Lymphangiography	CT
❱ Oral Cholecystectomy	CT
❱ Intravenous Cholangiography	CT, MRI
❱ Pelvimetry	Ultrasound
❱ Bronchography/Laryngography	CT, Endoscopy

"ENDANGERED" LIST AND STUDIES THAT WILL REPLACE THEM

❱ Upper GI Exam	Endoscopy
❱ Barium Enema	Endoscopy
❱ Intravenous Urogram	CT
❱ Ventilation/Perfusion Lung Scan	CT

Real-Time Imaging and Diagnostic Uses

Modern ultrasound equipment uses real-time imaging. A continuous stream of ultrasound waves are emitted from the transducer and reflected from the tissues being imaged. The transducer then acts as a receiver, receiving the returning waves and constructing a visual image. Real-time ultrasound allows dynamic scanning of moving objects such as a fetus

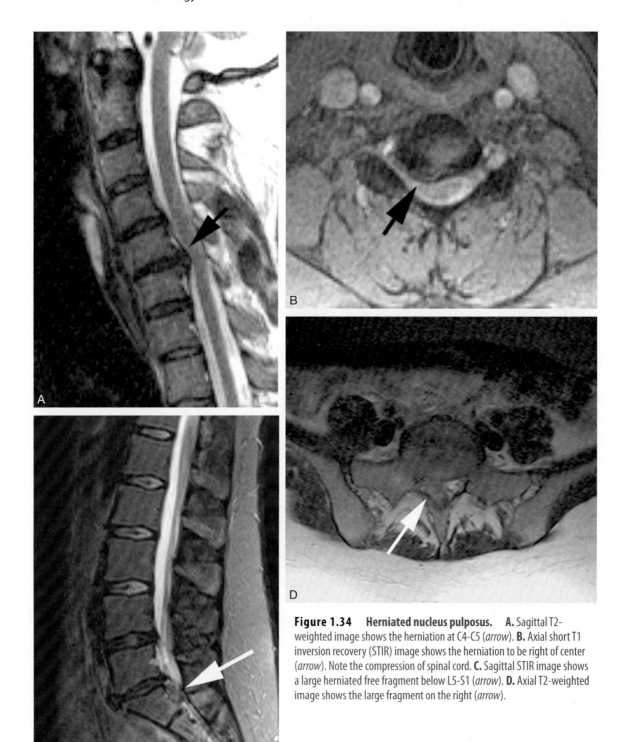

Figure 1.34   Herniated nucleus pulposus.   A. Sagittal T2-weighted image shows the herniation at C4-C5 (*arrow*). **B.** Axial short T1 inversion recovery (STIR) image shows the herniation to be right of center (*arrow*). Note the compression of spinal cord. **C.** Sagittal STIR image shows a large herniated free fragment below L5-S1 (*arrow*). **D.** Axial T2-weighted image shows the large fragment on the right (*arrow*).

in utero (Fig. 1.41) or a pulsating aorta. This technique also permits rapid and efficient screening of a body region (Fig. 1.42). In the past decade, ultrasound is being used more frequently for evaluating ligaments and tendons, or cystic lesions (Fig. 1.43). Ultrasound is an interactive modality. Observing moving body parts, such as the heart or an aorta, while performing the scan is often more useful than reviewing the static images afterward.

An additional feature of modern ultrasound is Doppler evaluation of blood vessels. With this technique, flow velocities within blood vessels can be measured, and screening for arterial stenosis can be performed. The technique is most commonly done in the

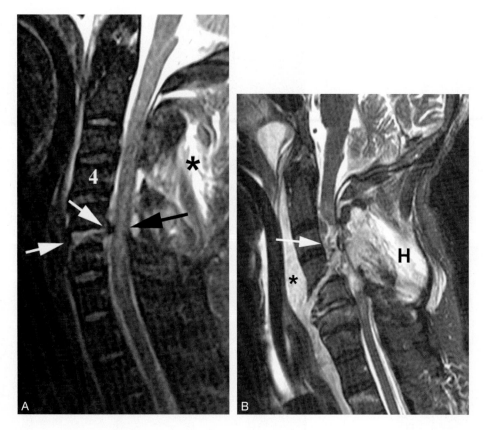

Figure 1.35 Spinal cord injuries (*arrows*). A. Cord edema (*black arrow*) in a patient with an extension injury at C5-C6. Note the ruptured anterior and posterior longitudinal ligaments (*white arrows*) and the posterior soft tissue hemorrhage (*asterisk*). **B.** Extension fracture dislocation at C4-C5. The spinal cord is transected posterior to C3 (*arrow*). Note the prevertebral (*asterisk*) hematoma and posterior hemorrhage (*H*).

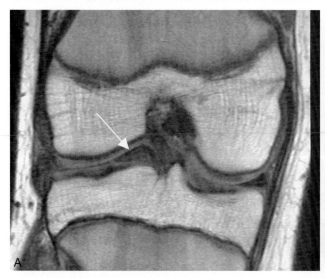

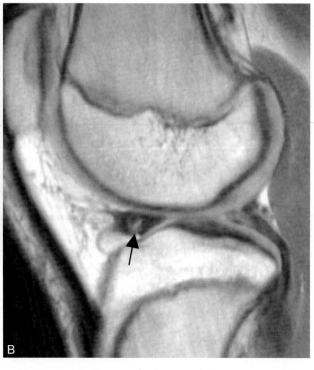

Figure 1.36 Bucket handle tear of medial meniscus. A. Coronal magnetic resonance image shows flipped fragment of medial meniscus (*arrow*) near the center of the joint. **B.** Sagittal image shows the torn anterior horn of the meniscus (*arrow*). Note the absence of a normal triangular meniscal image posteriorly.

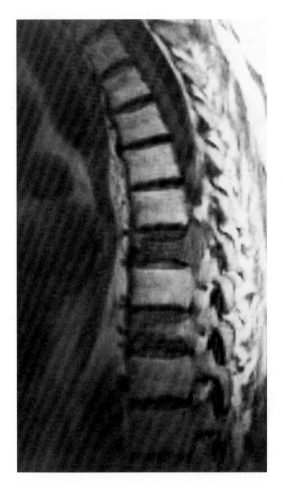

Figure 1.37   Metastatic disease of the spine.   Sagittal T1-weighted image shows areas of low signal (*dark*) as well as compression in two vertebrae. Other images showed the tumor to encroach on the subarachnoid space.

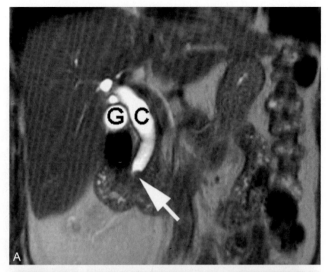

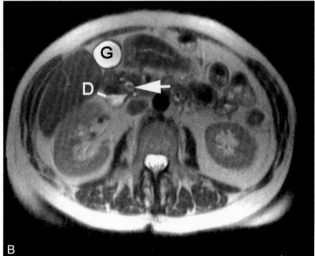

Figure 1.38   Magnetic resonance cholangiopancreatogram (MRCP).   A. Coronal T2-weighted (HASTE) image shows dilatation of the common bile duct (*C*) owing to a stone (*arrow*). Some contrast fills the gallbladder (*G*). **B.** Axial T2-weighted image shows the obstructing stone (*arrow*). The duodenum (*D*) and gallbladder (*G*) are also marked.

carotid arteries (Fig. 1.44). Additionally, Doppler evaluation of venous structures can be performed to rule out occlusion from deep venous thrombosis.

Ultrasound is also a useful tool in performing interventional procedures. Ultrasound-guided fluid aspirations, drainages, and biopsies are routinely performed quickly and safely in skilled hands.

Motion-mode (M-mode) ultrasound is used in echocardiography to study the dynamic changes of cardiac structures. The cardiac structures, including valves, form patterns in the M-mode ultrasound relating to their motion.

Drawbacks of Ultrasound

There are disadvantages to ultrasound. Ultrasound is unable to cross a tissue–gas or tissue–bone boundary, which renders it useless for evaluating the lung or bones. Furthermore, bony and gas-containing structures can obscure other tissues lying deeper to them. Finally, ultrasound, however, is an operator-dependent modality, and a high degree of technical skill is required to perform state-of-the-art examinations.

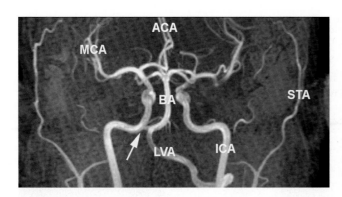

Figure 1.39   Cerebral magnetic resonance arteriogram in a patient with occlusion of the right vertebral artery (*arrow*).   Note the excellent demonstration of the normal vascular anatomy. The following arteries are demonstrated: anterior cerebral arteries (*ACA*); basilar artery (*BA*); internal carotid artery (*ICA*); left vertebral artery (*LVA*); middle cerebral artery (*MCA*); and superficial temporal artery (*STA*).

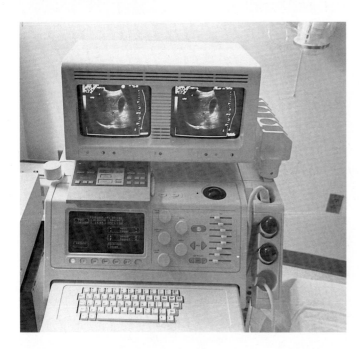

Figure 1.40   An ultrasound machine.

The "Radiologic Restaurant"

The impact that medical imaging has on the diagnosis and treatment of disease has changed dramatically in the past seven decades. It is also not surprising that the cost of the equipment to perform those imaging studies has also increased dramatically. In 1940, imaging (x-rays) influenced the management of 1 patient in 12. The cost of the most expensive piece of equipment (a fluoroscopic unit) was $9,500. In 1950, the ratio dropped to one patient in six, and the most expensive piece of equipment (usually an image-intensified fluoroscopic unit) was $25,000. By 1960, the ratio was one patient in three, and the cost of the most expensive piece of equipment (again fluoroscopy) was $85,000. In the 1970s, one patient in two needed imaging, and the cost of the most expensive piece of equipment (usually a CT scanner) topped $1,000,000. Since the 1980s, virtually all patients have been affected by imaging and the costs have risen to the $2,500,000-plus level, usually for MR imaging. However, digital radiography equipment frequently costs nearly $1,000,000. Table 1.4 summarizes these facts.

Three Approaches to Studies

This chapter has outlined the many studies available to solve various clinical problems. You have a large "menu" of studies that can be performed to evaluate your patient. The

Figure 1.41   Uterine ultrasound at 22 weeks of gestation. Note the placenta (*P*), fetal head (*H*), and torso (*T*). Ultrasound has become a primary diagnostic tool in obstetrics.

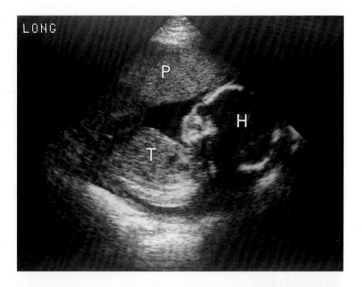

Figure 1.42   Cholelithiasis. Ultrasound examination in the longitudinal plane shows a gallstone measuring 0.97 × 1.20 cm (*arrow*) in the dependent portion of the gallbladder (*G*). The liver (*L*) lies immediately above the gallbladder.

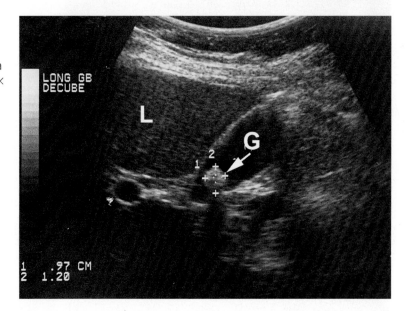

first choice you must make is the exact approach you wish to take toward this evaluation. Three approaches are currently in use: the "shotgun," the algorithmic, and the directed.

Shotgun Approach

The *shotgun approach* is one that is used too frequently. It takes little thought to order a battery of diagnostic laboratory and imaging studies for each patient in the hope that one or more of those tests will provide important diagnostic information. According to the "Law of Unintended Consequences," such an approach frequently results in findings that are either unexpected or are difficult to explain.

Algorithmic Approach

The *algorithmic approach* follows a more orderly selection of studies based on the patient's symptoms and the results of each study (Fig. 1.45). Although this approach requires some thought on the part of the clinician and study selectivity is possible, it is also probable that unnecessary studies will be performed just because they are in the protocol. For example, a patient with an acute, non-traumatic back strain usually needs no imaging and may be treated conservatively with rest, heat, and anti-inflammatory agents. Unfortunately, these patients often receive a complete radiographic evaluation of their lumbar spines and may even undergo MR imaging as well.

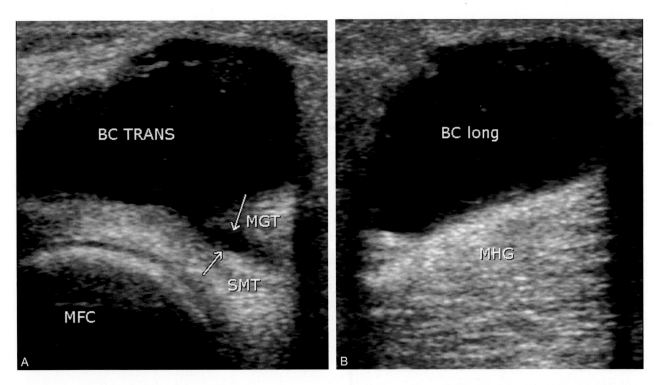

Figure 1.43   Baker cyst (*BC*) of popliteal area.   A. Transverse ultrasound image shows the cyst as a sonolucent area above the denser band of the semi-membranosus tendon (*SMT*). The arrows point to the neck of the cyst, which leads to the joint. **B.** Longitudinal image shows the cyst above the medial head of the gastrocnemius (*MHG*). MFC, medial femoral condyle; MGT, medial head of gastrocnemius. (Courtesy of Mihra Taljanovic, MD, University of Arizona, Tucson.)

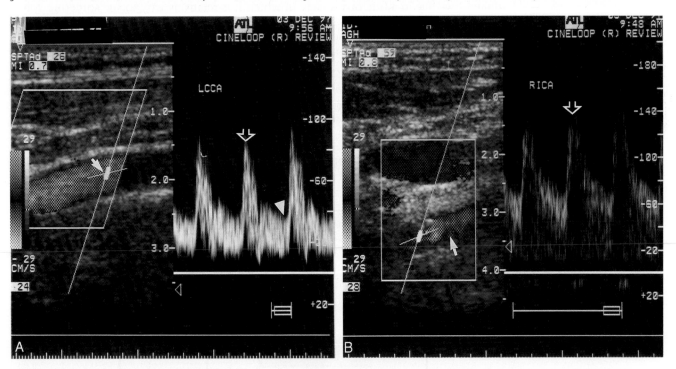

Figure 1.44   Carotid Doppler ultrasound examination.   A. Normal left common carotid artery (*LCCA*). The gray-scale image of a portion of the LCCA shows the vessel to be widely patent. The vessel walls are smooth without visible atheromatous plaques. The rectangle within the vessel lumen (*small arrow*) is the Doppler sample site from which the flow characteristics and velocities generate the Doppler waveform tracing shown to the right of the gray-scale image. There is a normal peak systolic flow velocity of approximately 90 cm/second (*open arrow*; normal ≤ 125 cm/second) as well as antegrade blood flow velocity of 40 cm/second at the end of diastole (*arrowhead*). The Doppler waveform also allows for evaluation of the degree of laminar flow disruption, or turbulence. This is reflected by the range of red blood cell velocities. The greater the velocity range, the greater the turbulence. In this instance, this normal vessel demonstrates a velocity range of 40 to 90 cm/second. **B.** Significant stenosis in a right internal carotid artery (*RICA*). The gray-scale image of a portion of an RICA shows gross vessel wall irregularity with significant stenosis near the Doppler sample site (*small arrow*). The Doppler waveform tracing shows an elevated peak systolic flow with velocities of 140 cm/second (*open arrow*). In addition, there is marked turbulence as a result of the increased red blood cell velocity. Compare these tracings and images with **A.**

Table 1.4 IMPACT OF MEDICAL IMAGING AND COSTS

Year	Ratio	Cost ($)	Equipment
1940	1:12	9,500	Fluoroscopy
1950	1:6	25,000	Fluoroscopy
1960	1:3	85,000	Fluoroscopy
1970	1:2	200,000	CT
1980	1:1	1,500,000	CT (MR)
1990–2013	1:1	2,500,000	MR

CT, computed tomography; MR, magnetic resonance.

Directed Approach

The *directed approach* is a carefully thought-out process in which the clinician has performed a thorough history and physical examination and *then* considers the diagnostic possibilities in that patient. The clinician chooses diagnostic studies based on *probability of diagnostic yield, safety* (invasive versus noninvasive study), *radiation dose, cost,* and *medicolegal concerns.* I prefer this approach and stress it daily to my consulting clinicians as well as to students and residents in all disciplines. Furthermore, in this age of cost containment, third-party payers demand that physicians follow this approach in an effort to reduce the soaring costs of medical care.

Medicolegal Concerns and Costs

I have raised two issues in the preceding paragraph: medicolegal concerns and costs. Unfortunately, we live in a litigious society in which it is relatively easy to sue someone. Many patients expect perfect results and, when they are not achieved, feel that somebody must be responsible and therefore somebody must pay. Moreover, the concept of contributory negligence on the part of the patient never enters into the equation. Feeding this is a tort

Figure 1.45 Algorithm for evaluation of low back pain. The clinical, laboratory, or imaging findings will determine the next step. Imaging studies are highlighted.

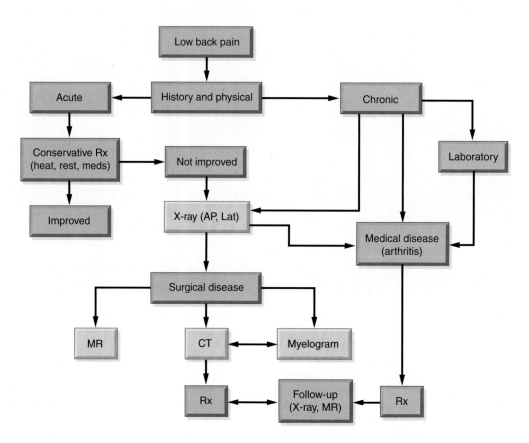

system that has too many lawyers as well as one that operates on the "contingency fee" system, in which plaintiffs owe nothing unless they win. As a result, the fear of being sued has prompted many physicians to practice "defensive medicine," which has been estimated to cost all U.S. citizens about $100 billion a year. Put another way, meaningful tort reform would reduce the cost of medical care by approximately 25%.

Not surprisingly, radiologists are being included in lawsuits more frequently, either as primary or, more commonly, as secondary defendants. In radiology, mammography generates the most lawsuits, followed by failure to diagnose other forms of cancer and failure to diagnose fractures. Issues that involve radiology in malpractice cases involve several areas: failure to diagnose, failure to recommend additional (appropriate) studies, failure to communicate, and improper or incomplete informed consent. As a clinician, you can protect yourself by taking the time to listen carefully to a patient, by performing thorough and complete examinations, and by documenting your actions in the patient's chart. When you order diagnostic imaging, you should clearly communicate to the radiologist the reasons for the examination and the diagnosis you suspect. I was an expert witness for the defense in a case involving delayed diagnosis of a fractured hip. The only clinical information given to the radiologist was "pain." Had the clinician added that the patient had fallen and was suspected of having a hip fracture, greater attention might have been paid to the femoral neck, where a subtle fracture was found.

Not only should you communicate with the radiologist, but also you should expect a complete interpretation of the study in a timely manner. The radiologist should immediately communicate any urgent findings back to you and should document the fact that such information was given, as well as the method (direct contact, telephone, etc.). You, the clinician, and your patients have the right to rapid consultation.

Cost-Effectiveness

When we mention the cost of a study we usually think of how much patients are billed for that service. Although it is helpful to consider costs in those terms, it is more useful to consider cost-effectiveness. Furthermore, the actual cost of a study is not what is charged for that examination but rather is based on a formula that takes into account the operating expenses for each machine, the technologist's time in performing the exam, any supplies used, and the efficacy of the diagnosis. For example, CT of the cervical spine has replaced radiography for screening patients suspected of having cervical injury. In addition to being much more sensitive at detecting fractures, CT takes less than half the time needed to do a complete radiographic examination. Numerous studies have validated the fact that CT is more cost-effective than radiography for patients with suspected spine injury. When considering performing a study, consult your radiologist for the most appropriate method of solving the patient's problem. Table 1.5 lists common imaging procedures, their costs, and their radiation doses.

American College of Radiology Task Force on Appropriateness Criteria

In 1993, the American College of Radiology (ACR) formed the ACR Task Force on Appropriateness Criteria. The task force consisted of 10 panels of expert radiologists and clinical consultants in each of the 10 subspecialties of diagnostic radiology. Each panel was charged with the task of developing a series of clinical conditions and variations that could serve as the basis for determining the appropriateness of imaging studies. For each clinical condition, the panel performed a literature search with a critical review of the data presented. The panel, after reviewing the data, then made recommendations on the appropriateness of each imaging study using the consensus method. The results were first published by the ACR in 1995. The recommendations, although not perfect, serve as guidelines for radiologists to help their clinical colleagues in making decisions regarding imaging. Additionally, each of the recommendations is subject to biannual review. Figure 1.46 shows a typical appropriateness chart. The full document may be viewed online and downloaded from the ACR web site at http://www.acr.org/ac.

Screening Examinations

One final issue to be discussed is that of so-called screening examinations. In recent years, a new industry has developed to provide "screening" whole-body CT or MR imaging on otherwise healthy persons. Entrepreneurs have flooded the airwaves, newspapers, and billboards with ads purveying their services. Of course, medical insurance does not cover these studies, but the imaging centers do take credit cards.

Table 1.5 COMMON IMAGING EXAMINATIONS, COSTS, AND DOSE

Examination	Cost ($)[a]	Dose (mR)
Chest (two-view)	290	108
Abdomen (two-view)	260	1,460
Femur	250	60
Pelvis	250	545
Wrist	24	04
Cervical (five-view)	410	194
Lumbar (five-view)	420	884
Mammogram (bilateral)	250	300
Upper gastrointestinal	460	1,700[b]
Barium enema	630	4,700[b]
Abdominal aortoiliac angiogram	3,300	151/image
Cranial CT	1,400	4,400
Chest CT	1,400	1,500
Abdominal CT	1,800	3,500
Lumbar CT	1,900	3,000
Abdominal ultrasound	900	0
Pelvic (obstetric) ultrasound	900	0
Cranial MR	2,000	0
Lumbar MR	2,400	0
Pelvic MR	2,200	0
Bone scan (isotope)	1,200	1,000 bone, 260 whole body
Lung scan (isotope)	1,000	900 lung, 61 whole body

CT, computed tomography; MR, magnetic resonance.

[a]2013 figures (includes technical and professional charges).

[b]Includes fluoroscopy time.

Is there a value in such screening? The generic answer is no. Three areas have demonstrated their ability to diagnose malignancies in early stages: mammography, colonoscopy or barium enema, and chest radiography. Screening mammography is effective in identifying small cancers, including ductal carcinoma in situ. Colonoscopy or barium enema is also effective in finding polyps, which have the potential to become malignant. *"Remove a polyp, cure a potential cancer,"* goes the popular saying. Finally, chest radiography, particularly in patients with certain risk factors such as smoking or occupational exposure to certain substances, has been effective in identifying lung cancers while they are small and potentially curable. There is no credible evidence that whole-body CT or MR screening of the general population is effective at identifying early malignancies or other abnormalities.

The Radiologist as a Consultant

The complexity of today's diagnostic imaging studies makes it imperative that the radiologist be more than an interpreter of those studies. As the practice of radiology has become more organ–system oriented in larger hospitals, radiologists have gravitated to subspecialty

American College of Radiology
ACR Appropriateness Criteria®

Clinical Condition: Chronic Neck Pain

Variant 1:   Patient without or with a history of previous trauma, first study.

Radiologic Procedure	Rating	Comments	RRL*
X-ray, cervical spine	9	AP, lateral, open mouth, both obliques.	☢☢
MRI cervical spine without contrast	2		O
Facet injection/arthrography cervical spine selective nerve root block	2		☢☢
X-ray myelography cervical spine	2		☢☢☢
CT cervical spine without contrast	2		☢☢☢
Tc-99m bone scan neck	2		☢☢☢
Myelography and post myelography CT cervical spine	2		☢☢☢☢
MRI cervical spine without and with contrast	1		O
CT cervical spine with contrast	1		☢☢☢
CT cervical spine without and with contrast	1		☢☢☢
Rating Scale: 1, 2, 3 usually not appropriate; 4, 5, 6 may be appropriate; 7, 8, 9 usually appropriate			*Relative radiation level

Figure 1.46   Representative American College of Radiology Appropriateness Criteria table for suspected spine trauma. (From the American College of Radiology Task Force on Appropriateness Criteria. Appropriateness Criteria for Imaging and Treatment Decisions. Reston, VA: American College of Radiology, 2012. Reprinted with permission.)

areas through additional training after residency. Large radiology groups have members who are specialists in neuroimaging, angiography and other invasive procedures, body imaging, musculoskeletal imaging, pulmonary imaging, trauma, gastrointestinal imaging, uroradiology, pediatric radiology, and nuclear imaging. These radiologists work closely with specific groups of clinicians to solve their special diagnostic problems. The clinicians, for their part, consult with their radiologic colleagues on a daily basis, either for interpretation of studies or to determine the best method of working up a particular diagnostic problem. Radiologic subspecialists are often on call to perform studies after normal working hours. They make themselves available to consult on request with the clinician. They often participate in multidisciplinary conferences, such as a surgery–radiology–pathology conference, and give lectures to clinicians on topics of mutual interest.

Radiologists have been extensively trained in each of the imaging modalities. They also adhere to the ACR Practice Guidelines and Technical Standards®. These documents specify indications for studies, qualifications for personnel performing and interpreting them, and the technical specifications for equipment. Like the ACR Appropriateness Criteria®, the Practice Guidelines and Technical Standards are subject to periodic review and revision. They, too, may be accessed online at the ACR web site.

You should learn to make use of this most valuable resource, the radiologist. Keep in mind, however, that he or she can best help you when informed of clinical or laboratory data on a patient. This means that requests for diagnostic studies should contain pertinent clinical information. The radiologist may be better able to tailor an examination to the exact needs of the patient. This will result in time saved in both the studies obtained and the hospital stay. A secondary benefit will be cost containment—a topic of continuing importance. Many studies provide similar information. There is little benefit in ordering expensive studies that will duplicate the diagnostic information. Finally, one of the greatest benefits of using your radiologist is that he or she views the patient and the clinical problem without the "tunnel vision" that medical or surgical specialists often exhibit by focusing solely on the structures within their particular area of expertise. A good example is the patient with back pain. The orthopaedist focuses on the skeletal causes; the urologist concentrates on the kidneys and ureters. However, the radiologist looks at the entire area under study and does not have any ego investment in the diagnosis. Remember, your prime consideration should be the welfare of your patient. Consultation with the radiologist is as important for helping that patient as consulting with any other specialist.

Summary and Key Points

▶ Diagnostic radiology has emerged over the past 100 years to become a vital link in the patient care chain. Diagnostic imaging is performed on nearly all patients seen in medical practice.

▶ Cross-sectional imaging can demonstrate organs and their diseases that previously could be seen only surgically or at the time of necropsy.

▶ The radiologist has a large variety of studies available to use and is in the best position to recommend the appropriate study based on consultation with the clinician.

▶ This chapter described the various imaging studies offered, reviewed their principles, and made recommendations regarding their appropriate use.

▶ Blind or protocol-driven ordering of any diagnostic test is to be discouraged. It is best to tailor each examination to the needs of patients.

Suggested Additional Reading

American College of Radiology Task Force on Appropriateness Criteria. Appropriateness Criteria for Imaging and Treatment Decisions. Reston, VA: American College of Radiology, 2012. Available at: http://www.acr.org/ac.

Bushburg JT, Seibert JA, Leidholdt EM Jr, Boone JM. Essential Physics of Medical Imaging. 3rd Ed. Philadelphia, PA: Lippincott Williams & Wilkins, 2011.

Bushong SC. Magnetic Resonance Imaging. 3rd Ed. St. Louis, MO: Mosby, 2003.

Edelman RR, Hesselink JR, Zlatkin MB, Crues JV. Clinical Magnetic Resonance Imaging. 3rd Ed. Philadelphia, PA: WB Saunders, 2006.

Eisenberg RL. Radiology: An Illustrated History. St. Louis, MO: Mosby-Year Book, 1991.

Fishman EK, Jeffrey RB Jr. Multidetector CT: Principles, Techniques, and Clinical Applications. Philadelphia, PA: Lippincott Williams & Wilkins, 2003.

Gagliardi RA, McClennan BL. A History of the Radiological Sciences: Diagnosis. Reston, VA: Radiology Centennial, 1996.

Mettler FA Jr, Guiberteau MJ. Essentials of Nuclear Medicine Imaging. 6th Ed. Philadelphia, PA: Saunders Elsevier, 2012.

Rumack CM, Wilson SR, Charboneau JW, Levine D. Diagnostic Ultrasound. 4th Ed. St. Louis, MO: Mosby, 2011.

Ziessman HA, O'Malley JP, Thrall JH. Nuclear Medicine: The Requisites. 4th Ed. St. Louis, MO: Mosby Elsevier, 2013.

chapter 2

Radiographic Contrast Agents

Matthew S. Hartman   Richard H. Daffner

Various structures within the body are recognizable on imaging studies either because of their inherent densities (e.g., bone distinguished from muscle) or because they contain one of the basic natural materials (e.g., air). However, because most of the internal viscera are of the radiographic density of water or close to it, it is necessary to introduce into these structures a material that will outline walls, define anatomy, and demonstrate any pathologic conditions. Chapter 1 briefly mentioned these agents and some of the studies for which they are used. This chapter and our online supplement describe their physiology and pharmacology, define indications and contraindications for their use, and discuss the treatment of reactions to them.

Barium Preparations

Barium sulfate (USP), in one of its many forms, provides the mainstay for radiographic examinations of the gastrointestinal (GI) tract. Barium is of high atomic weight, which results in considerable absorption of the x-ray beam, thus providing excellent radiographic contrast. In the usual preparation, finely pulverized barium mixed with dispersing agents is suspended in water.

When administered orally or rectally, it provides excellent coating and distention of the GI tract. When compared with water-soluble contrast agents, barium provides better mucosal detail, is more resistant to dilution, and is less expensive.

Alternatives

Although barium itself is chemically inert, when it is extravasated outside the GI tract, a severe desmoplastic reaction may theoretically develop. This is most likely to occur in a patient with a perforation of the GI tract. As a result, water-soluble contrast material, which will be absorbed rapidly from the interstitial spaces and peritoneal cavities should be used as the first-line agent to rule out a leakage (Fig. 2.1).

Contraindications

Barium is contraindicated in patients in whom you suspect a large bowel obstruction. As opposed to water-soluble contrast, barium will not be absorbed or be diluted by water, a big advantage. However, if barium is allowed to remain within the colon for a long time proximal to an obstruction, it may inspissate and compound the patient's problem. In addition, retained barium in the GI tract will make any subsequent computed tomography (CT) scan nondiagnostic because of the backscatter.

 ▶ Barium should never be used in patients in whom you suspect a large bowel obstruction.

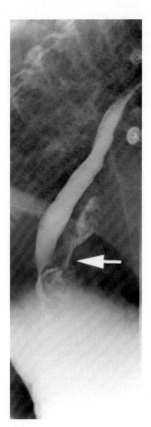

Figure 2.1   Extravasation of oral contrast (arrow) from the gastroesophageal junction into the mediastinum. A water soluble contrast agent was used.

Water-Soluble Contrast Media

The common chemical structure of all water-soluble contrast media is an iodinated benzene ring (Fig. 2.2). Like barium, iodine has a high atomic number, will absorb the x-ray beam, and be white on the x-ray images. Water-soluble contrast agents can be categorized based on their osmolality: *high-osmolality* contrast media (HOCM), *iso-osmolality* contrast media (IOCM), and *low-osmolality* contrast media (LOCM), which have different biochemical profiles and prices. As a non-radiologist you will not need to know the finer details about these different contrast agents, which are usually determined by the radiology department's protocol or by the radiologist performing the study.

Water-soluble contrast agents can be injected directly or indirectly into the body to provide contrast enhancement. With respect to CT examinations, contrast is injected intravenously. After the contrast has had time to pass through the body (30 to 60 seconds), contrast-enhanced CT images can be taken with excellent resolution of soft tissue organ and vascular detail (Fig. 2.3). Water-soluble contrast can also be injected into various body parts with subsequent diagnostic imaging, including the blood vessels (*angiography*), the spinal canal (*myelography*), and joints (*arthrography*). Water-soluble contrast can also be injected into the GI tract (enemas, fistulograms, postoperative leak studies, etc.) and into the genitourinary tract (cystogram, nephrostogram, hysterosalpingogram, etc.) for detailed fluoroscopic evaluation which will be discussed in Chapters 8 to 10.

Adverse Reactions

Extravasation

Contrast does not always end up in the intended location. For example, when a patient is injected with intravenous contrast for a CT examination, it is possible for that agent to extravasate into the subcutaneous tissues of the arm. This can be a painful condition, which can lead to morbidity with skin necrosis if not treated correctly (Fig. 2.4). Treatment for such incidents should be performed by the radiology personnel who have been fully trained to manage such emergencies. Please note that treatment for such events may vary from hospital to hospital but there are several general principles. The first line of treatment involves assessing the situation with respect to the volume of contrast extravasated, a physical examination with respect to skin breakdown, and a neurovascular assessment of the involved extremity. The IV needle/catheter should be removed. Then measures should be taken to decrease the swelling by elevating the extremity and also applying a warm or cold compress. Surgical consultation is only required for large-volume (>100 mL) extravasations, where there is high risk of skin breakdown. We will expand on the treatment of extravasation in our online module.

With respect to the GI tract, water-soluble contrast is commonly used when there is a suspected perforation (see Fig. 2.1). These agents do not cause any of the undesirable side effects that barium is known to produce when outside the GI tract. However, water-soluble contrast media result in less distention and poorer coating of the GI tract when compared with barium. Barium is often administered to obtain additional diagnostic images after the radiologist has initially ruled out a leak with water-soluble contrast. Water-soluble contrast has one important contraindication: suspected communication between the GI tract and the tracheobronchial tree (esophago-airway fistula or aspiration risk). As mentioned in Chapter 1, water-soluble materials can be irritating to the tracheobronchial mucosa and produce a severe chemical pneumonia that may result in death. In these rare instances,

Figure 2.2   Prototypical iodinated contrast molecule (diatrizoate sodium).   All have at least three iodine atoms (I). Differences in various types of contrast will depend on the makeup of the remaining radicals.

COONa

I

I

CH₃CONH

NHCOCH₃

I

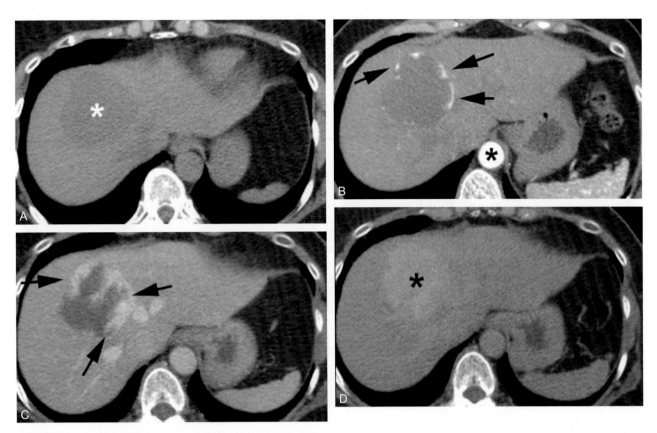

Figure 2.3   The value of contrast.   A. The first image is taken without intravenous contrast and demonstrates a hypodense central liver lesion (*asterisk*). Intravenous contrast was administered. At 30 seconds **(B)** the arterial phase imaging shows intense enhancement of the aorta (*asterisk*) and some peripheral enhancement of the lesion (*arrows*). At 60 seconds **(C)** there is peripheral nodular enhancement of the lesion (*arrows*). At 2 minutes **(D)** the lesion (*asterisk*) has filled in completely. This is diagnostic of a hemangioma.

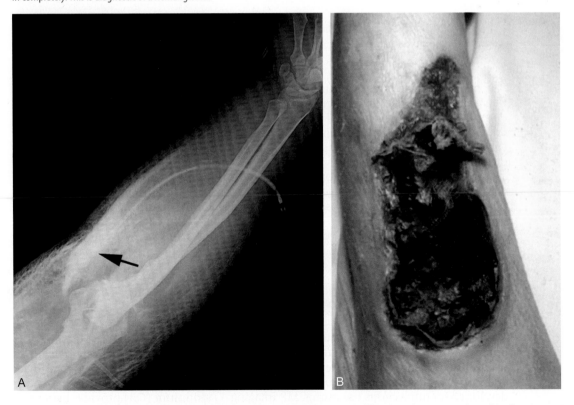

Figure 2.4   Contrast extravasation.   A. Approximately 20 mL of intravenous contrast (*arrow*) extravasated into the subcutaneous tissues of the right arm. Note the IV tubing. **B.** Tissue necrosis at the site of extravasation.

an oil-based contrast may be used. Older formulations of water-soluble contrast had high osmolality (HOCM) and could also cause a sudden pulmonary edema which can result in death, especially in newborns and the elderly if aspirated into the lungs. This risk of death is lower with the new formulations using the lower osmolar agents (LOCM).

▶ Water-soluble contrast is contraindicated in patients with suspected esophago-airway fistula or with an aspiration risk.

Allergic Reaction

Although normal persons may not suffer any severe, long-lasting effects from the administration of contrast, one must remember that contrast, like any drug or medication, can result in an allergic reaction which can potentially result in death. Depending on the severity of the allergy, which should be documented, the patient can be premedicated with a combination of steroids and diphenhydramine before receiving the intravenous contrast. As with a bee sting or any other allergen, subsequent exposures to the same allergen can have increasing severity and precautions should be taken or an alternative study should be considered. Specific premedication protocols and treatment algorithms will be discussed in our online module.

Contrast-Induced Nephropathy

Excretion of these intravenous agents is largely performed by glomerular filtration within the kidney. In the kidneys, especially in a dehydrated patient and patients with borderline renal function (including diabetics), glomerular and tubular damage may result in temporary impairment of renal function and oliguria, which has been labeled *contrast-induced nephropathy* (CIN). We check glomerular filtration rate and creatinine clearance in all patients prior to intravenous contrast administration. In patients with poor renal function (excluding those already on dialysis) contrast is contraindicated and the radiologist needs to discuss the case with the referring physician and the patient.

▶ Contrast is contraindicated in patients with poor renal function (unless already on dialysis).

Patients with borderline renal function are often hydrated prior to and after administration of intravenous contrast. Alternatively, the radiologist and the ordering physician may deem the risk of long-term renal impairment to be too high. Diagnostic options include doing the study without intravenous contrast, performing dialysis immediately after the contrast-enhanced study or using a different modality such as ultrasound to answer the diagnostic question.

Another related concern is found in patients with known borderline renal function who are taking the antihyperglycemic agent, metformin. Metformin is cleared from the body by tubular secretion and has the potential to result in life-threatening lactic acidosis if it accumulates in the bloodstream, as would happen with CIN. To decrease this risk, most radiology departments have specific metformin protocols whereby a patient is asked to withhold his/her metformin after a contrast-enhanced study until the patient's renal function has normalized.

Paramagnetic Agents

Despite the variety of pulse sequences available for magnetic resonance (MR) imaging, difficulties still exist for differentiating between neoplasms and chronic cerebral infarctions, tumors and perifocal cerebral edema, or recurrent herniated intervertebral discs and surgical scars. For these reasons, a number of paramagnetic contrast agents have been developed for intravenous use during MR imaging. Gadolinium (Gd) provides better soft tissue and vascular detail for MR images in much the same way that water-soluble contrast does for CT (Fig. 2.5).

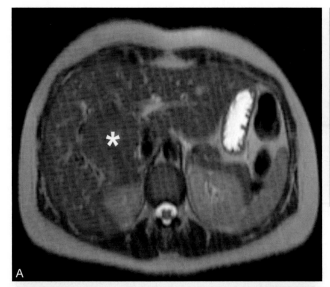

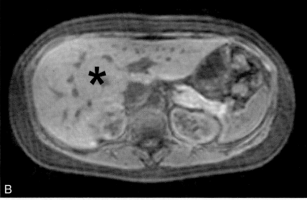

Figure 2.5   Nodular hyperplasia of the liver.   The lesion (*asterisks*) is barely perceptible on (**A**) T2- and (**B**) T1-weighted imaging without contrast. The lesion (*asterisk*) brightens intensely on the contrast-enhanced image (**C**). Note how much brighter the aorta (*arrow*) is because of the contrast.

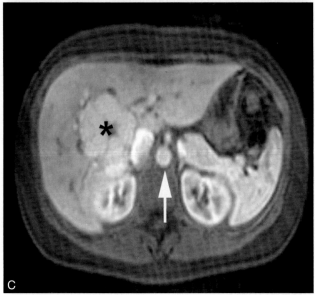

Gadolinium-diethylenetriamine pentaacetic acid (Gd-DTPA) is most commonly used. Gadolinium was chosen because of its strong effect on the relaxation time in the scanning sequence. Chelation with DTPA prevents the inherent toxicity of the free Gd ion. In diagnostic doses, Gd-DTPA increases the signal in vascular structures, similar to the effect of conventional water-soluble contrast media. For MR arthrography, a very dilute mixture of Gd (0.4%) is used because of its intense paramagnetic effect. Gadolinium solution may be safely mixed with iodinated contrast materials for needle localization.

Adverse Reactions

Gadolinium compounds also carry a different risk of adverse reactions. Like any medication that is administered, there is a risk of anaphylaxis/true allergy; however, the risk is lower compared with iodinated compounds. It was originally thought that Gd compounds had no nephrotoxicity and could be used in azotemic patients and dialysis patients. Unfortunately, a small number of renal patients who received Gd under this supposition developed a debilitating condition called *nephrogenic systemic fibrosis* (NSF). NSF is a rare and progressive fibrosing syndrome, involving the skin, joints, eyes, and internal organs. Its pathophysiology is not fully understood; however, there is a strong association with Gd use in patients with renal impairment. Gadolinium has been identified at the microscopic level in these areas of fibrosis.

We do not administer Gd to patients with poor renal function or on dialysis without discussing the risks and benefits of the procedure with the patient and referring physician.

This chapter touched on some of the highlights of contrast media with respect to how it works and some pitfalls related to administration of certain types of contrast. We have developed an online interactive module which goes into more depth, with respect to allergies, contrast reactions, extravasations, and treatment of reactions.

Summary and Key Points

▶ Commonly used contrast agents may be categorized as particulate (barium), water soluble, and paramagnetic.

▶ Barium remains the mainstay for radiographic evaluation of the hollow organs of the GI tract. However, barium may be toxic outside the lumen of the bowel.

▶ Water-soluble contrast agents can be injected intravenously, resulting in enhancement of vessels and organs for CT examinations.

▶ Water-soluble contrast agents can be injected directly into various body parts for multiple examinations: angiography, myelography, arthrography, fistulograms, leakage studies, loopograms, cystograms, nephrostograms, and hysterosalpingograms.

▶ Contrast agents may cause life-threatening allergic reactions.

▶ The radiologist and ordering physician should work together to decide the risk and benefit of administering contrast with respect to renal function and allergy/need for premedication.

▶ Paramagnetic agents such as Gd are used for many of the same indications as iodinated agents for MR studies.

▶ Avoid using Gd in patients with renal failure and on dialysis because of the risk of NSF.

▶ The types of reactions to contrast media, how to recognize them, and how to treat them were briefly discussed.

▶ Thorough familiarity with the technique of cardiopulmonary resuscitation is advised.

Suggested Additional Reading

ACR Manual on Contrast Media, Version 8.0. Reston, VA: American College of Radiology, 2012.

ACR-SPR Practice Guideline for the Use of Intravascular Contrast Media. Reston, VA: American College of Radiology, 2012 rev.

Bettman MA, Heeren T, Greenfield A, et al. Adverse events with radiographic contrast agents: results of SCVIR contrast agent registry. Radiology 1997;203:611–620.

Bush WH, Swanson DP. Acute reactions to intravascular contrast media: types, risk factors, recognition, and specific treatment. AJR 1991;157:1153–1161.

Cochran ST, Bomyea K, Sayre JW. Trends in adverse events after IV administration of contrast media. AJR 2001;176:1385–1388.

Cohan RH, Dunnick NR, Bashore TM. Treatment of reactions to radiographic contrast material. AJR 1988;151:263–270.

Dunnick NR, Sandler CM, Newhouse JH. Textbook of Uroradiology. 5th Ed. Philadelphia, PA: Lippincott Williams & Wilkins, 2012:57–74.

Katayama H, Yamaguchi K, Kozuka T, et al. Adverse reactions to ionic and nonionic contrast media. Radiology 1990;175:621–628.

Lasser EC, Lyon SG, Berry CC. Reports on contrast media reactions: analysis of data from reports to the U.S. Food and Drug Administration. Radiology 1997;203:605–610.

Martin, DR, Semelka RC, Chapman A, et al. Nephrogenic systemic fibrosis versus contrast-induced nephropathy: risks and benefits of contrast-enhanced MR and CT in renally impaired patients. J Magn Reson Imaging 2009;30:1350–1356.

McClennan BL. Ionic and nonionic iodinated contrast media: evolution and strategies for use. AJR 1990;155:225–233.

Runge VM. Safety of approved MR contrast media for intravenous injection. J Magn Reson Imaging 2000;12:205–213.

chapter 3

Interventional Radiology

Elmer Nahum   Richard H. Daffner

Introduction

Interventional radiology (IR) is a specialty that uses image guidance to assist in the performance of minimally invasive procedures. The diagnostic and therapeutic procedures offered by interventional radiologists cover a wide variety of organ systems requiring knowledge and interaction with many different subspecialties. Angiography was first described by Moniz in 1927 after he injected contrast directly through a needle into a blood vessel. Diagnostic angiography advanced in 1953, when Seldinger described accessing the femoral artery with a needle and guidewire to allow passage of catheters for angiography. The first interventional radiological procedures were pioneered by Dotter and Judkins in 1964 by using sequential dilators over a guidewire to restore patency to arteries. Other early important refinements included the development of catheter balloon angioplasty, the addition of CT and ultrasound for guidance, the use of coaxial microcatheters (small diameter catheters placed through a larger base catheter), and improvement in guidewire technology. IR applications further broadened with the development of embolization coils, catheter-directed thrombolytic medications, stents, and vena cava filters. The image quality and efficiency improved with dedicated angiography equipment that used digital imaging and digital subtraction replacing cumbersome film-based imaging. With innovation as its cornerstone, IR continues to broaden its scope of treatment. Table 3.1 lists the many vascular and nonvascular IR procedures.

Tools of the Trade

There are numerous devices that an interventional radiologist can employ during a particular procedure. Each of these is often modified for the particular application.

Table 3.1 INTERVENTIONAL RADIOLOGY PROCEDURES

Vascular	Nonvascular
Angiography	Biopsy
Stenting	Abscess drainage
Embolization	Biliary drainage
Chemotherapy infusion	Gastrostomy tube placement
Thrombolysis	Nephrostomy
Transjugular intrahepatic portosystemic shunts	Stone extraction
Venous access	Foreign body retrieval
Vena cava filter placement	Screw placement

Catheters

Catheters allow the interventional radiologist to access a specific area in the body from another entry point in the body. Angiographic catheters are usually composed of poly-ethylene or polyurethane and can be divided into flush catheters and selective catheters (Fig. 3.1). *Flush catheters* are typically used for aortic injections and have multiple side holes near the tip to allow for a rapid high-volume injection to opacify the large diameter vessel. The catheter typically contains a curve that prevents its tip from inadvertently lodging into a small vessel. *Selective catheters* contain only a single end hole and have no side holes. Selective catheters can have a single bend or curve, and multiple bends or a reverse curve. The diameter of the catheter is measured in French (Fr) size: 3 Fr is equivalent to 1 mm. Most diagnostic catheters are 4 or 5 Fr. One of the limitations of these catheters is their inability to track within multiple curved segments. Thus, microcatheters, which are 3 Fr or less, and more supple, can be placed through the 4 or 5 Fr base catheter in a telescoping manner to reach distant vascular beds, such as the hepatic artery, distal splenic artery, and branches of the internal iliac artery (Fig. 3.2).

Guidewires

Guidewires are metallic or plastic wires that serve two general roles: exchange and guidance within a vessel or lumen. Not only can the guidewire be used during the exchange of the access needle to a catheter, but it can be used to exchange different catheters. In order to negotiate the various curves in a vessel and not damage the intima, a guidewire is placed ahead of the catheter tip.

Angioplasty Catheters

Angioplasty catheters are specialized catheters with a balloon placed near its leading end to allow for dilation of stenoses (Fig. 3.3). The balloon is inflated through a side port and typically connected to a pressure gauge. The manufacturer will note on the packaging the balloon diameter, length, nominal pressure, and burst pressure. The nominal pressure is the pressure needed to achieve the stated diameter. The burst pressure is a recommendation by the manufacturer of the maximal inflation pressure before balloon rupture might occur. Various factors are involved when selecting the appropriate angioplasty catheter, including trackability, compliance (ability of balloon to stretch more than its nominal diameter), strength of balloon material, and cost.

Stents

Stents are metallic cylindrical devices that are placed within a vessel or other lumen to provide a scaffolding to decrease the likelihood of recurrent stenosis (Fig. 3.4).

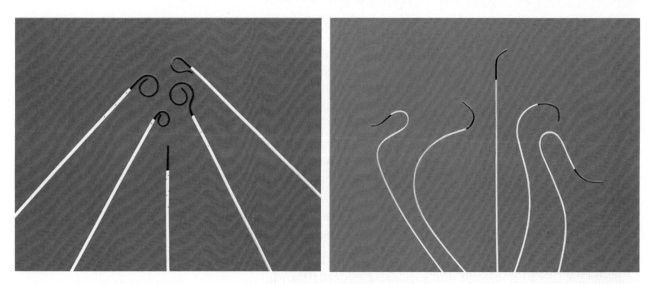

Figure 3.1   Angiographic catheters.   A. Flush catheters have multiple side holes with the tip pointing inward to allow for rapid contrast injection without allowing the catheter to enter into small vessels. **B.** Selective catheters of various configurations facilitate access into branch vessels. The standard diameter of these catheters is 4 to 5 Fr.

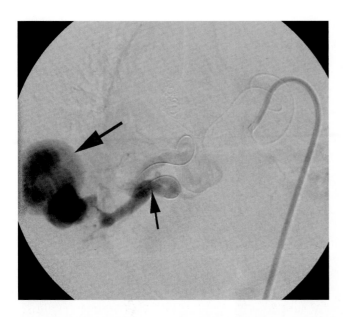

Figure 3.2 Microcatheter. A 2.4 Fr microcatheter (*small arrow*) has been advanced through the 5 Fr base catheter into a very tortuous bronchial artery in preparation for embolization of an unusual bronchial artery to pulmonary vein fistula (*large arrow*).

Stents can be made of bare metal or can be covered with a fabric (covered stent or stent graft). A *balloon-expandable* stent is mounted on an angioplasty catheter. When that stent is positioned in the proper location, the balloon is inflated, expanding the stent. Alternatively, *self-expandable* stents can be used. This stent is housed between two layers of thin catheters. The stent is deployed by unsheathing the outer layer. The metal in a

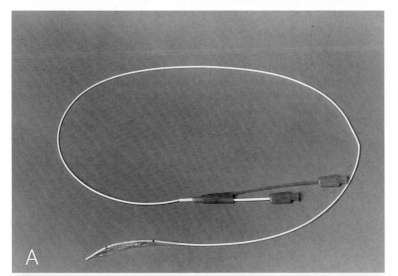

Figure 3.3 Angio-plasty catheters.
A. The catheter contains one port through which a guidewire is placed and another port for balloon inflation. **B.** Close-up of inflated balloon.

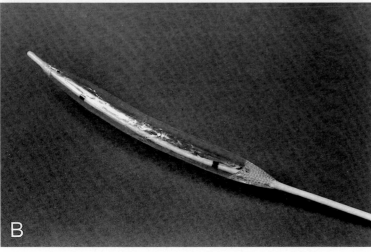

Figure 3.4
Stents. **A.** Left to right: two types of graft covered self-expandable stents (*stent grafts*); a bare metal self-expandable stent in the center; and a pair of balloon stents. **B.** Endovascular stent grafts for abdominal aortic aneurysm repair.

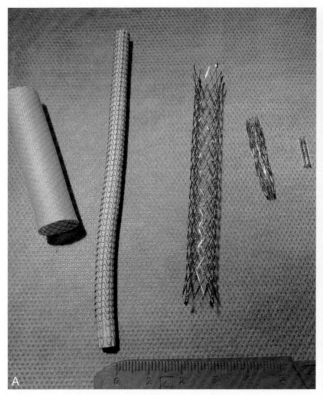
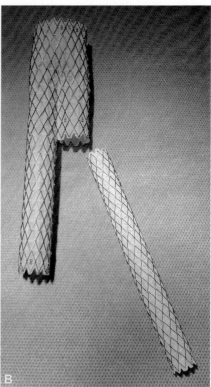

self-expandable stent has a memory to prevent it from collapsing. Balloon-expandable stents are used when precise positioning is needed, such as at the origin of a renal artery. However, balloon-expandable stents have no memory to stay expanded and they are not used in parts of the body where extrinsic compression could occur (i.e., neck and extremities).

Embolic Materials

Various materials can be delivered through a catheter to purposely occlude a specific vessel or deliver a specific therapeutic agent (Fig. 3.5). Curled metallic wires with or without embedded fibers called embolization coils are delivered by pushing the coil through a catheter with a guidewire. Polyvinyl alcohol (PVA) beads, ranging in size from 50 to 1,000 μm, are often used for tumor embolization. Cyanoacrylate glue and other adhesives can be injected for vascular malformations and other indications. Yttrium 90 radioactive beads and chemotherapeutic agents combined with PVA particles can treat liver neoplasms.

Percutaneous Ablation Devices

These are specialized instruments for ablating tumors in the liver, kidney, lung, and bone percutaneously (Fig. 3.6). These devices are used to freeze (cryoablation) or burn (radiofrequency ablation and microwave ablation) tumors.

Other devices, including biopsy needles (Fig. 3.7), vena cava filters, drainage catheters, and venous access devices, will be discussed later in this chapter.

Diagnostic Angiography

Angiography is the visualization of the blood vessel lumen using fluoroscopy and x-ray imaging (conventional angiography), computed tomography (CT) (CT angiography or CTA) or magnetic resonance imaging (MRI) (MR angiography or MRA). Angiography can be divided into arteriography and venography. Over the last decade, CTA and MRA have improved enough that the role of conventional angiography solely for

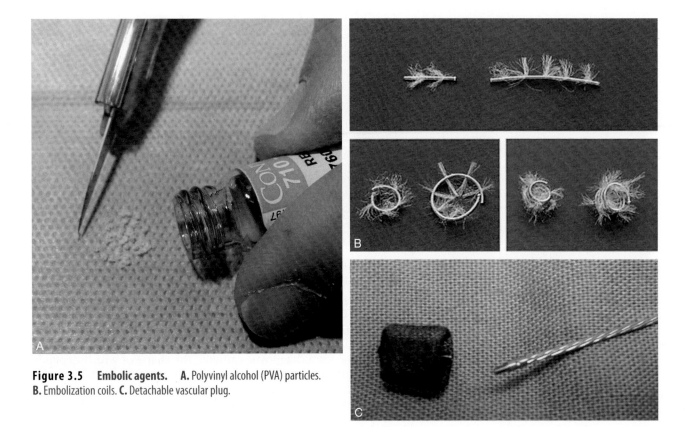

Figure 3.5 Embolic agents. A. Polyvinyl alcohol (PVA) particles. **B.** Embolization coils. **C.** Detachable vascular plug.

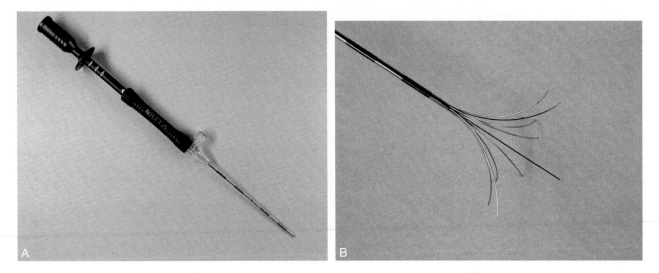

Figure 3.6 Radiofrequency ablation probe. A. Probe with electrodes retracted. **B.** Tip of probe with electrodes deployed. These are placed directly into the lesion.

diagnosis is now fairly limited. However, conventional angiography remains vital for guiding vascular interventions.

General applications of angiography include:

- Delineating anatomy prior to intervention or surgery
- Detecting vascular stenoses or occlusions
- Detecting a specific site of bleeding
- Detecting abnormal arteriovenous communications
- Identifying neoplasms

Figure 3.7   Biopsy devices.

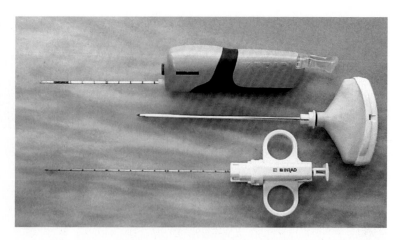

Arteriography Technique

The vast majority of conventional arteriograms are performed by accessing the common femoral artery with an 18G to 21G needle (Fig. 3.8), using either manual palpation of the vessel or ultrasound. Alternative sites of access include the brachial artery or through surgical incisions. Once pulsatile blood is encountered, a guidewire is placed through the needle. The needle is then exchanged for a diagnostic catheter, the shape of which depends on the artery being studied. In some instances, an arterial sheath is placed to facilitate the exchange of multiple different catheters and improves maneuverability of the catheter. A thorough knowledge of normal and variant angiographic anatomy is important to help select the vessel and choose the correct catheter shape and size.

 ▶ A thorough knowledge of normal and variant angiographic anatomy is important to help select the vessel and choose the correct catheter shape and size.

Digital technology allows superimposition of a previously obtained angiogram over the live fluoroscopy to facilitate guidance of the catheter (*roadmapping*). Once the

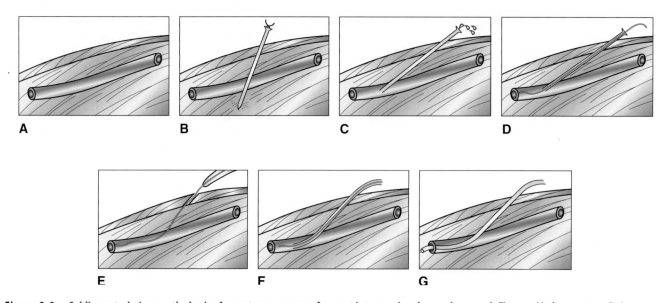

Figure 3.8   Seldinger technique—the basis of percutaneous access for most interventional procedures.   A. The vessel before puncture. **B.** A two-part needle consisting of a central stylet and an outer sheath punctures the vessel through both walls. **C.** The stylet is removed, and the sheath is withdrawn until blood is obtained. **D.** A guidewire is threaded through the sheath into the vessel. **E.** The sheath is removed, and a catheter is advanced over the guidewire. **F.** The guidewire and catheter are advanced in the vessel. **G.** The guidewire is removed, leaving the catheter in the vessel ready for injection or infusion of medication.

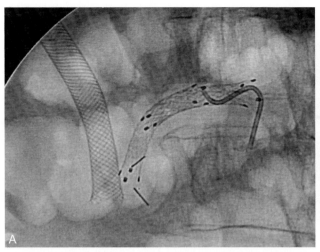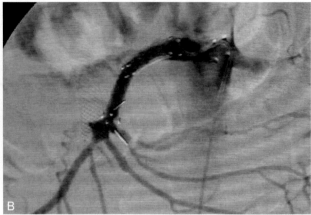

Figure 3.9   Digital subtraction angiography.   A. Mask before contrast injection. **B.** Digitally subtracted image during contrast injection into the superior mesenteric artery. The mask is "subtracted" from the image obtained with contrast, leaving an image which accentuates the contrast from the background.

catheter is positioned properly, contrast is injected to opacify the vessels downstream from the catheter tip. The amount of contrast injected will vary depending on the size of the vessel and number of vessels to be visualized. Digital subtraction angiography (DSA) is typically used to improve contrast resolution. It is common practice to use *subtraction technique* when performing angiography. Historically, in this process, a "mask" was made of a preliminary radiograph of the area in question by using a special film that reversed the densities (i.e., white becomes black and vice versa). This mask was placed over a radiograph taken after injection of contrast. The whites and blacks canceled each other when additional subtraction was performed, leaving the extra densities—the injected contrast in the vessels. This process is now performed digitally instead of with film, using a technique known as DSA. On the traditional subtraction angiogram, the vessels are better visualized and little or none of the background structures are visible (Fig. 3.9).

Once the angiogram is completed, and the catheter is removed, either manual compression is applied to the artery or one of a variety of closure devices is used. Closure devices typically use plugs or sutures to provide hemostasis (Fig. 3.10). Patients usually require 2 to 6 hours of bed rest after catheter removal. The risks of angiography include bleeding or pseudoaneurysm at the access site, vascular injury, allergic reaction, and contrast-induced nephropathy.

Trauma

Various arterial and venous injuries can occur from trauma and they can be detected by CTA or conventional angiography. CTA is performed for most cases of suspected vascular injury. Conventional angiography can be helpful when bullet fragments or surgical hardware is present that often degrades a CT image. Additionally, if there is an intent to treat based on clinical findings, the patient might go directly to the angiography suite. The following vascular injuries may be encountered:

- Extravasation
  - Vessel transection or tear (Fig. 3.11A and B)
  - Pseudoaneurysm (Fig. 3.11C and D)
- Stenosis
  - Intramural hematoma (Fig. 3.11E)
  - External compression (Fig. 3.11F)
  - Dissection (Fig. 3.11G)
- Arteriovenous fistula (Fig. 3.11H and I)

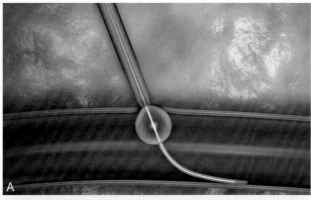

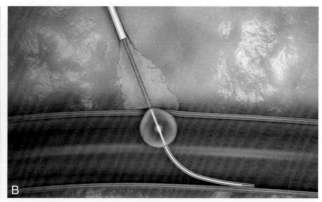

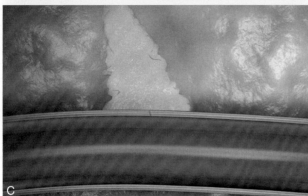

Figure 3.10   Arterial closure device.   A variety of devices are available. Some are suture mediated, while others use a material such as collagen or ethylene glycol delivered through a tube and placed on the external surface of the artery. The device shown here uses an anchoring balloon within the artery to prevent placement of closure material within the arterial lumen. **A.** Device in place. **B.** Catheter withdrawn and occlusive material is injected. **C.** Device withdrawn. (*Courtesy of Access Closure.*)

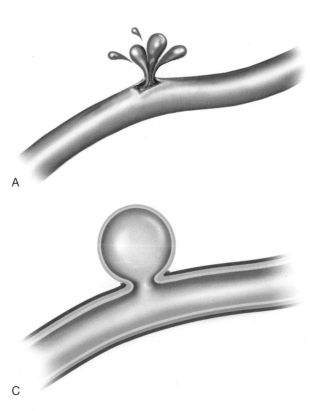

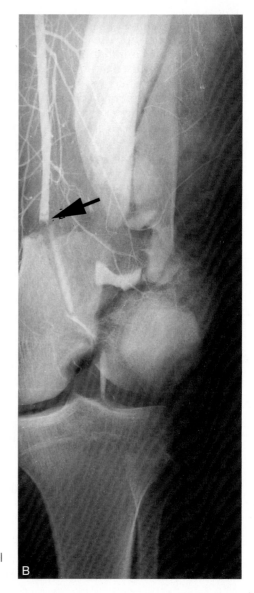

Figure 3.11   Vascular injuries.   A. Rupture. **B.** Transection of the distal femoral artery (*arrow*) due to a fracture. **C.** Pseudoaneurysm.

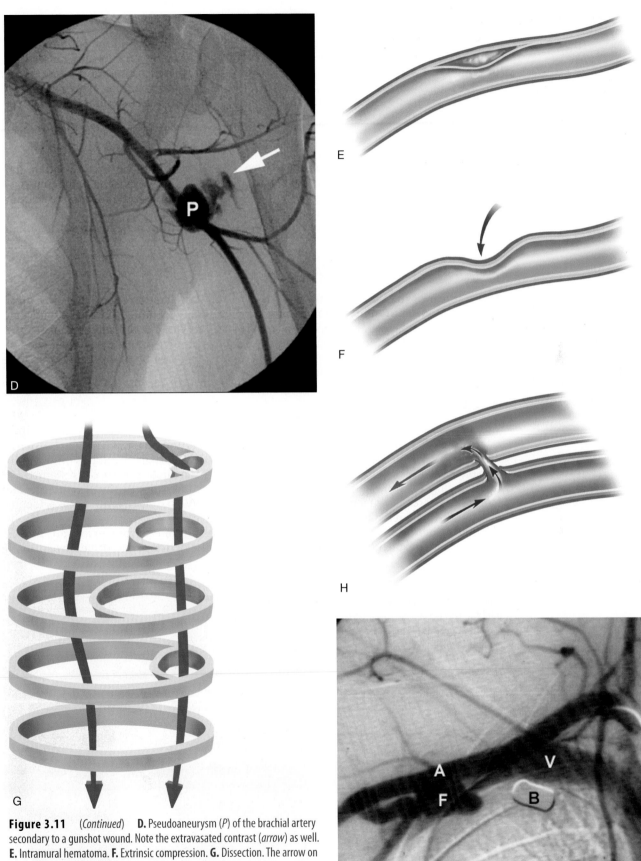

Figure 3.11 (*Continued*)   **D.** Pseudoaneurysm (*P*) of the brachial artery secondary to a gunshot wound. Note the extravasated contrast (*arrow*) as well. **E.** Intramural hematoma. **F.** Extrinsic compression. **G.** Dissection. The arrow on the right shows blood dissecting into the wall of the vessel and then reentering the true lumen. **H.** Arteriovenous (AV) fistula. **I.** AV fistula due to gunshot wound. Note the bullet (*B*) and contrast passing freely through the fistula (*F*) from the subclavian artery (*A*) into the subclavian vein (*V*).

Extravasation

Contrast *extravasation* is encountered when contrast is found beyond the confines of the expected location of the vessel. Extravasation may be caused by a frank tear (transection) or a pseudoaneurysm. A *pseudoaneurysm* is a confined leak occurring from a tear in the arterial wall. The leak can be contained by adventitia or surrounding tissues. Contrast flows into the pseudoaneurysm sac and back into the blood vessel. Besides trauma, pseudoaneurysms can also occur with infection.

Stenosis

A stenotic vessel in the trauma setting can be a manifestation of vasospasm, intramural hematoma, extrinsic compression, stretch injury, or dissection. It must be noted that classic arterial dissections, which involve a longitudinal tear through the media, are seldom encountered in trauma of the chest, abdomen, or extremities.

Arteriovenous fistulae can occur when there is a breach from penetrating trauma of an adjacent artery and vein.

Acute Traumatic Aortic Injury

This is a tear of the thoracic aorta caused by a rapid deceleration (Fig. 3.12). The most common location of injury in survivors is the proximal descending thoracic aorta. Fatality rates are high before arrival to the hospital. Of those victims who survive to reach the hospital, 40% die within 24 hours. The lesions are typically complete or partial tears of the aorta. Repair can be performed by open surgical repair or by inserting endovascular stent graft via a femoral approach (Fig. 3.13).

Splenic Trauma

The spleen can fracture with blunt or penetrating trauma. If the patient is hemodynamically stable and no extravasation or pseudoaneurysm is found on CT, the patient is usually managed conservatively. If the injury produces a pseudoaneurysm or extravasation within the spleen, or the patient is hemodynamically unstable, an angiogram is often warranted. If the angiogram shows a focal pseudoaneurysm or extravasation within the spleen, the lesion can be treated via a microcatheter using coils or PVA particles. If no lesion is identified, but the patient remains hemodynamically unstable or has continued blood loss from the injury, the bleeding rate may be below the detection rate of the angiogram. In this instance, a main splenic artery coil embolization can be performed to decrease perfusion

Figure 3.12   Acute traumatic aortic injury. Chest CT shows a small collection of contrast medial to the proximal descending aorta (*arrow*).

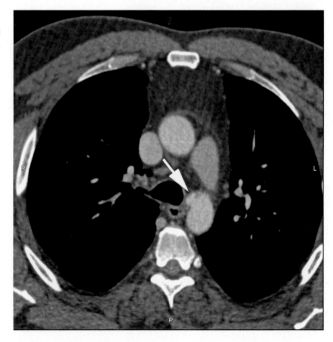

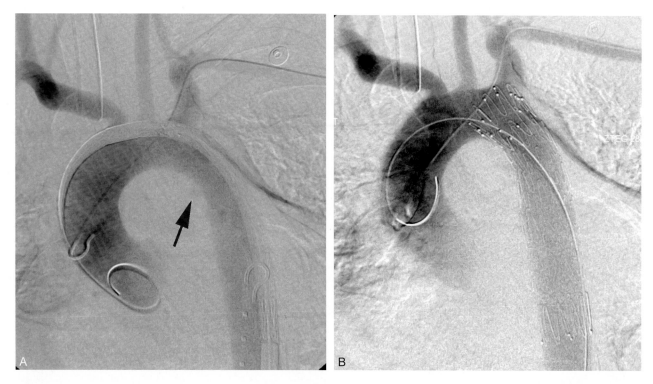

Figure 3.13   Acute traumatic aortic injury.   Same patient as in Figure 3.12. **A.** Aortogram prior to endovascular stenting shows the extravasation (*arrow*). **B.** Aortogram following stenting shows the leak is no longer present.

pressure to the spleen. Flow will be redirected (via the gastroepiploic artery arcade) at a lower pressure and splenic function will remain (Fig. 3.14). Complications of splenic embolization include splenic abscess and delayed rupture.

Hepatic, Renal, Pelvic, and Extremity Trauma

Main vessel injury may need to be treated surgically or can be treated with a covered stent. Branch vessel injuries may be treated with embolization (Fig. 3.15).

Oncology

Liver Tumors and Catheter-Directed Therapies

Malignant liver lesions can be managed in some instances with various IR liver-directed therapies, including chemoembolization, radioembolization, and percutaneous ablation.

Transarterial Chemoembolization

Transarterial chemoembolization (TACE) may be an option for non-surgical candidates, with hepatocellular carcinoma (HCC), neuroendocrine liver metastases, and other hypervascular tumors. Prospective randomized controlled studies have shown survival benefits with TACE for HCC. For TACE, a microcatheter is advanced into the right or left hepatic artery with a combination of chemotherapeutic agents administered along with embolic agents. Lipiodol, which is iodinated poppyseed oil, is often added to the mixture. Lipiodol serves both as a selective carrier of the chemotherapeutic agents and as a selective embolic agent. The oil will be metabolized by the areas of normal liver that contain Kupffer cells. Tumors, which lack Kupffer cells, will remain embolized by the oil and will receive a higher relative dose of the chemotherapy (Fig. 3.16).

Radioembolization

Radioembolization is now approved by the Food and Drug Administration for treating colorectal metastases and HCC. Millions of minute particles of β-emitting yttrium 90

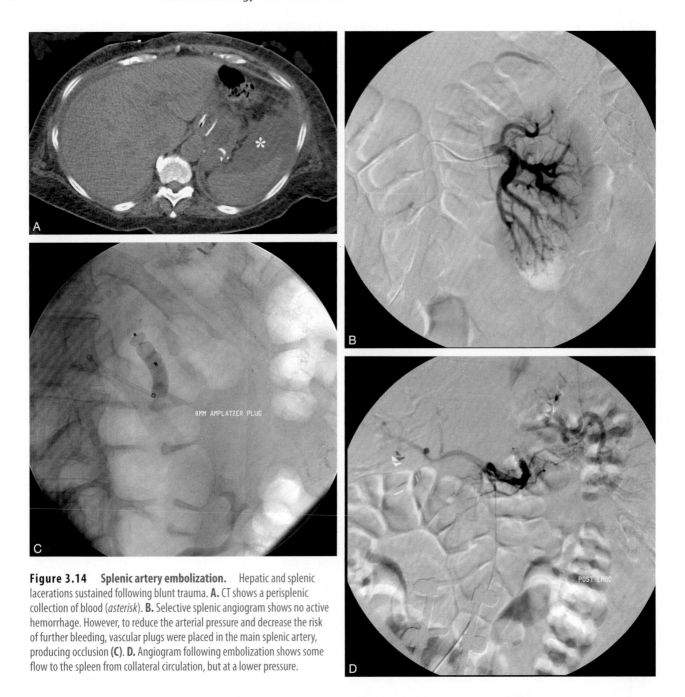

Figure 3.14   Splenic artery embolization.   Hepatic and splenic lacerations sustained following blunt trauma. **A.** CT shows a perisplenic collection of blood (*asterisk*). **B.** Selective splenic angiogram shows no active hemorrhage. However, to reduce the arterial pressure and decrease the risk of further bleeding, vascular plugs were placed in the main splenic artery, producing occlusion **(C). D.** Angiogram following embolization shows some flow to the spleen from collateral circulation, but at a lower pressure.

are injected into one or both lobes. Both TACE and radioembolization require careful attention to anatomy to ensure that these agents are not delivered outside of the liver. Anomalous branches or extrahepatic branches close to the injection point (such as the gastroduodenal and right gastric arteries) are often present, which require coil embolization to prevent damage by the delivered agent. Severe ulcerations of the stomach or bowel may occur with non-target (outside of the liver) embolization. The post-embolization syndrome (nausea, vomiting, pain, and low-grade fever) that often occurs following TACE is managed medically.

Tumor Ablation

Small liver lesions (typically less than 5 cm) can also be treated with various CT or ultrasound-guided ablative techniques using specialized probes to perform radiofrequency and cryo- or microwave ablations. These percutaneous devices are also used for the lung, kidney, and bone tumors.

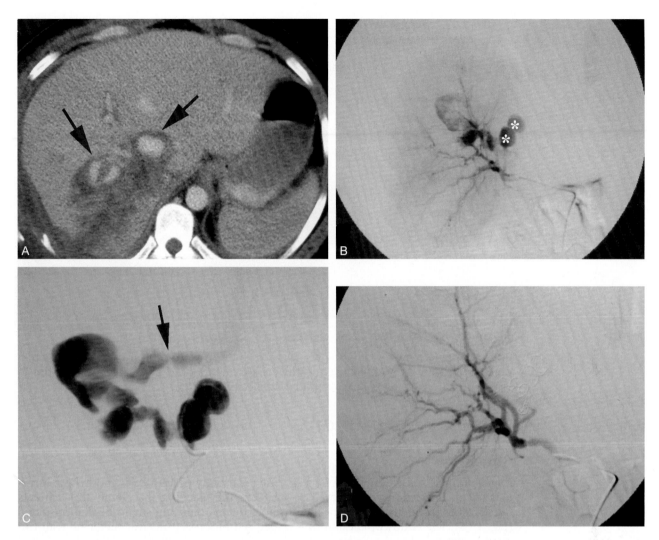

Figure 3.15   Hepatic vascular injury.   A. CT image shows abnormal contrast pooling in the central liver (*arrows*). **B** and **C.** Selective angiography shows a combination of aneurysms (*asterisks*) and rapid filling into a hepatic vein (*arrow*) from an arteriovascular fistula. **D.** Following coil embolization the fistula is closed. Blood flow to the embolized segment of liver will be through collateral vessels.

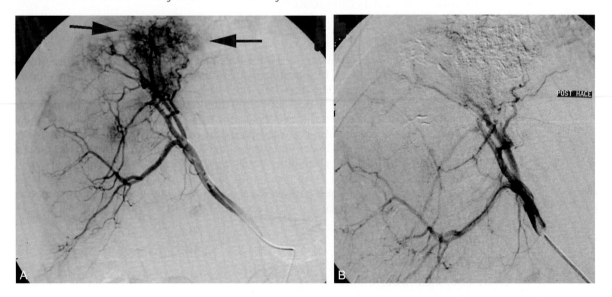

Figure 3.16   Hepatocellular carcinoma in the right lobe of the liver.   A. Right hepatic angiogram shows neovascularity in the upper portion of the right lobe (*arrows*). **B.** Angiogram following chemoembolization shows there is little flow to the area. The white areas within the tumor represent subtraction artifacts from the lipiodol. The flow will improve over a few weeks, which will allow hepatic recovery and retreatment, if necessary.

Figure 3.17 Subcutaneous chest ports for long-term venous access.

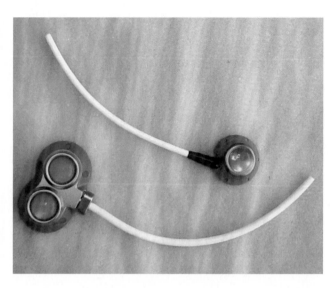

Venous Access for Oncology

Because chemotherapy can be highly toxic to the vein wall, central vein access is often needed. Chest ports or central vein catheters are often placed by interventional radiologists using fluoroscopic and ultrasound guidance (Fig. 3.17).

Arterial Interventions

Bleeding

Angiography for gastrointestinal tract bleeding is usually performed if endoscopic measures fail or if bleeding is too severe to visualize the bleeding site (Table 3.2). Patients usually need to be hemodynamically unstable for the bleeding site to be demonstrated (Fig. 3.18). The endoscopic exam or a tagged red blood cell nuclear medicine scan can assist in determining the location of the bleeding so that branch vessels can be selected with a microcatheter to increase the chances of success. Embolic agents for gastrointestinal bleeding include coils, PVA particles, gelfoam sponge, and glue. Infarction of bowel is a very rare complication after embolization.

Mesenteric Ischemia

Acute mesenteric ischemia is characterized by abdominal pain out of proportion to physical findings in combination with bloody diarrhea. Etiologies include embolus, thrombotic occlusion in a patient with existing atherosclerotic disease, dissection, and non-occlusive mesenteric ischemia (Fig. 3.19). Most cases are treated surgically, although in high-risk selected patients, catheter-directed thrombolysis may be an option. In non-occlusive mesenteric ischemia, there is generalized vasoconstriction of the superior mesenteric artery (SMA), typically in a setting of shock. Patients are treated by volume resuscitation and a continuous catheter infusion of a vasodilator such as papaverine.

Chronic mesenteric ischemia is almost always due to an atherosclerotic stenosis or occlusion at or near the origin of the SMA. These lesions are amenable to treatment with a stent (Fig. 3.20). If the lesion cannot be crossed with a guidewire, a surgical bypass may be needed.

Peripheral Vascular Disease

Embolic or Thrombotic Occlusions

Acute embolic or thrombotic occlusion of the iliac or lower extremity arteries can lead to motor and sensation loss resulting in eventual amputation if untreated. Emboli most often arise from a cardiac source, such as in a patient with atrial fibrillation. Thrombotic

Table 3.2 CAUSES OF ANGIOGRAPHICALLY DETECTABLE GASTROINTESTINAL HEMORRHAGE

Upper GI Bleeding

- Esophagus
- Mallory-Weiss tear
- Varices
- Stomach
- Ulcer
- Varices and portal hypertensive antral gastropathy
- Gastritis
- Dieulafoy lesion
- Duodenum
- Ulcer
- Pancreatitis—GDA, PDA
- Hemobilia
- Aortoenteric fistula
- Tumor
- Arteriovenous malformation
- Post-surgical/post-biopsy

Lower GI Bleeding

- Diverticula
- Angiodysplasia
- Meckel diverticulum
- Aortoenteric fistula
- Tumor
- Post-surgical/post-biopsy

GI, gastrointestinal; GDA, gastroduodenal artery; PDA, pancreaticoduodenal artery.

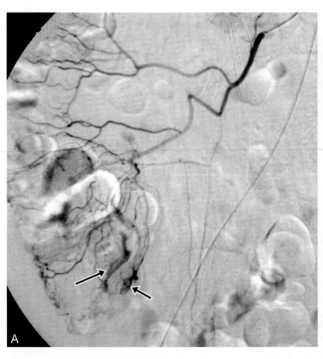
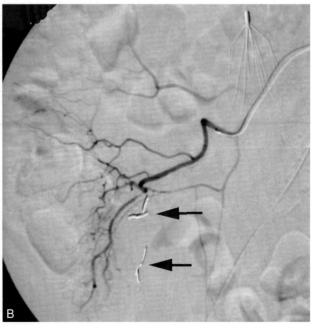

Figure 3.18   Embolization for GI bleeding.   A. Selective injection of the right colic artery shows contrast extravasation into the cecum (*arrows*). **B.** Selective injection following embolization of bleeding vessels with microcoils (*arrows*) shows no further extravasation.

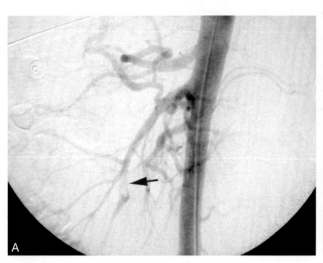
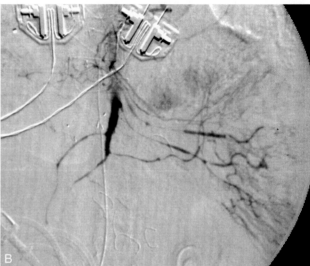

Figure 3.19   Acute mesenteric ischemia.   A. Superior mesenteric artery (SMA) embolus. Lateral aortogram shows a filling defect in the distal main trunk of the SMA (*arrow*). **B.** Non-occlusive mesenteric ischemia (NCOMI). There is a pruned appearance of the SMA branches. NOMI is usually a complication of shock and can be treated with a continuous infusion of a vasodilator through a catheter.

occlusions may occur after a stenosis from atherosclerotic disease becomes so severe that flow has stopped. Alternatively, a thrombus may occur as a result of a plaque that has an irregular surface promoting in situ thrombosis.

A different type of embolus can arise from atherosclerotic plaque fracture in the aorta that travels distally. These emboli typically are small and lodge in distal pedal artery branches resulting in blue or black multifocal lesions on the tips of the toes, known as the blue toe syndrome. These patients are usually managed with anticoagulation or antiplatelet medications with possible stenting of the culprit plaque (Fig. 3.21).

Angiographic findings that suggest an acute arterial thrombosis include a lack of collateral vessels, an intraluminal filling defect, and a stagnant column of contrast within the vessel. Catheter-directed therapies include thrombolysis with *tissue plasminogen activator* (TPA) through a multi-side hole infusion catheter or mechanical thrombectomy with specialized devices that aspirate thrombus. The advantages compared with a surgical approach include a more complete thrombus removal (especially in the tibial arteries below the knee) and quicker time to recovery. TPA can lead to serious bleeding complications or embolization of distal arteries. Thrombolysis infusions require many hours for the occlusion to resolve. Patients are sent to an intensive care unit with a continuous infusion of TPA through the catheter. The patient is then brought back to the angiography suite, typically the following day, for follow-up angiography (Fig. 3.22). Once complete thrombolysis has occurred, persistent stenosis that would require angioplasty or stenting may be demonstrated. Patients who have significant sensory or motor loss should be considered for emergent surgical thromboembolectomy and possible bypass.

Stenoses

Atherosclerosis is the most common etiology of stenoses or occlusions leading to claudication. These lesions may be amenable to angioplasty or stenting. Stenting is favored over angioplasty for stenoses longer than 2 cm, eccentric or irregular plaque or occlusions. Stenting across joint spaces is generally avoided due to potential injury of the stent from repetitive movement. Table 3.3 lists the causes of lower extremity arterial insufficiency.

Surgical bypass grafts are prone to developing intimal hyperplasia at the anastomotic sites. TPA, stenting, or thrombolysis may be needed to restore patency.

Abdominal Aortic Aneurysm

Abdominal aortic aneurysms (AAA) occur as a result of atherosclerotic degeneration of the elastic lamina, resulting in dilation of the lumen. By definition, an aneurysm is present when the diameter of the vessel is greater than 1.5 times its normal diameter.

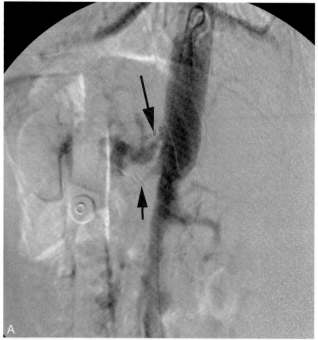

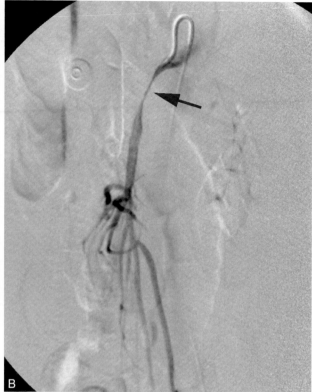

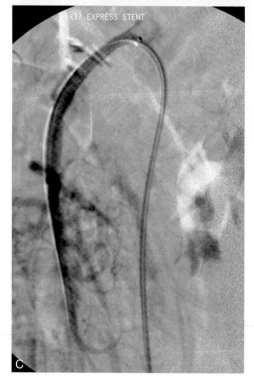

Figure 3.20 Chronic mesenteric ischemia. Typical signs of this condition include anorexia and postprandial abdominal pain. **A.** Lateral aortogram shows a high-grade stenosis at the origin of the celiac artery (long arrow) and a significant stenosis of the superior mesenteric artery (SMA) (*short arrow*). **B.** Selective injection of the SMA shows the stenosis (*arrow*). **C.** Lateral selective injection following stent placement shows no residual stenosis. The patient's symptoms improved post stenting.

Most AAA are repaired when they reach a diameter of 5.0 cm. Open surgical repair and endovascular repair are the two treatment options. Open surgical repair of AAA is generally performed on patients whose AAA extends above the level of the renal arteries because the visceral arteries arising from the aneurysm need to be surgically reimplanted onto the aneurysm graft. If the aneurysm is located infrarenally (with 1–2 cm of normal diameter aorta below the renal arteries and the start of the sac and no severe angulation), an endograft can be placed. Endovascular repair is performed after surgical exposure of both common femoral arteries. A typical endograft contains a main body with a single iliac limb (similar to a pair of pants with one of the legs removed) which is first deployed so that the main body of the graft is immediately below the renal arteries and the iliac

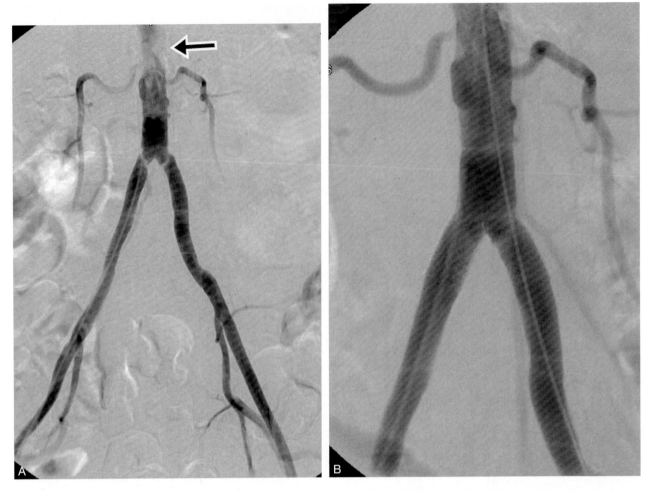

Figure 3.21   Atheroemboli.   A. An eccentric stenosis from an atherosclerotic plaque (*arrow*) created a nidus for thromboemboli resulting in bilateral ischemic toes. **B.** Aortogram showing improvement following aorto-iliac stenting.

Table 3.3 CAUSES OF LOWER EXTREMITY ARTERIAL STENOSES OR OCCLUSIONS

- Atherosclerosis
- Embolus
- Trauma
- Vasculitis (Buerger's disease, drug-induced)
- Thrombosed popliteal artery aneurysm
- Popliteal artery entrapment
- Adventitial cystic disease
- Persistent sciatic artery

limb terminates in the iliac artery. The second iliac limb is then deployed from the contralateral access so that a portion of it is placed within the shortened limb while its distal end is in the iliac artery (Fig. 3.23).

Endoleaks

Following placement of the graft, patients will need to undergo serial CT or MRI to ensure that the excluded aneurysm sac is not enlarging. Most enlarging aneurysms post endovascular stent grafting are due to endoleaks. Endoleaks are identified by finding contrast in

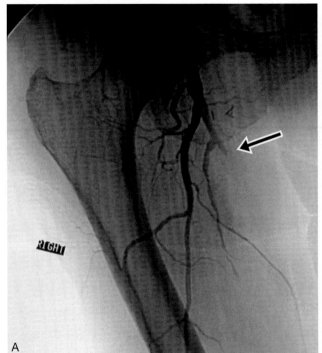

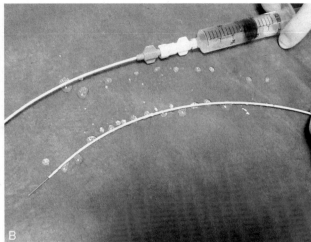

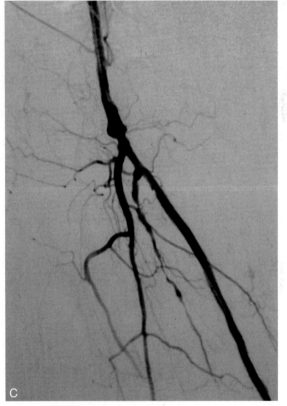

Figure 3.22 Thrombolysis. **A.** Acute occlusion of femoral artery bypass graft (*arrow*). **B.** Multi-side hole infusion catheter used for tissue plasminogen activator (TPA). **C.** Post TPA infusion angiogram shows blood flow restored.

the aneurysm sac that was supposed to be excluded (Table 3.4). Repairing an endoleak can be quite challenging since the excluded aneurysm sac needs to be accessed via collaterals or direct percutaneous puncture (Fig. 3.24).

Renal Artery Stenosis

Atherosclerotic disease can result in stenoses near the origin of the renal arteries. This may result in decreased systolic pressure to that kidney with subsequent increase in renin and angiotensin causing hypertension. These stenoses are typically repaired by placement of a balloon-expandable stent (Fig. 3.25). Stenting has also been performed to attempt to improve renal function in those patients with renal insufficiency and hemodynamically significant stenoses. There has been much debate about the benefits of renal artery stenting for both hypertension and renal insufficiency.

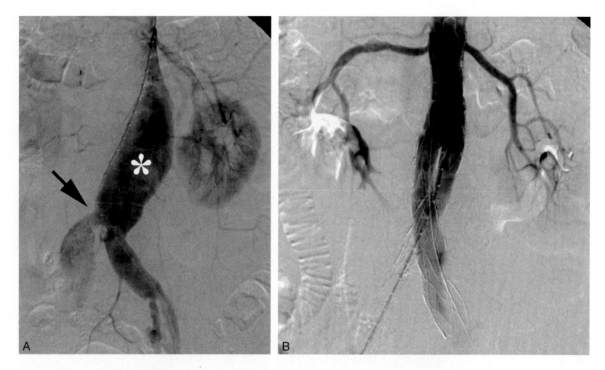

Figure 3.23   Repair of an infrarenal abdominal aortic aneurysm with an endovascular stent graft.   A. Presenting aortogram shows the aneurysm (*asterisk*) and stenosis of the right common iliac artery (*arrow*). **B.** Aortogram following stenting shows normal lumens in the aorta and the iliac arteries. The upper portion of the stent is positioned immediately below the renal arteries. The iliac limbs can terminate either in the common or external arteries, depending on the presence or absence of a common iliac artery aneurysm.

Table 3.4 TYPES OF ENDOLEAKS

1. Contrast emanating from the proximal or distal landing zone of the graft
2. Contrast arising from a collateral artery (inferior mesenteric or lumbar artery), which feeds into the sac
3. Tear or discontinuity of graft
4. Graft porosity (seen with some types of grafts during initial placement as blood flows through the interstices of the graft fabric)

Venous Disease

Vena Cava Filters

An inferior vena cava (IVC) filter may be placed in patients who have lower extremity deep venous thromboses (DVT) or pulmonary embolism (PE) with a contraindication for anticoagulation, or in patients who have developed a worsening PE or DVT despite anticoagulation. Sometimes a filter is placed prophylactically in high-risk patients with expected long-term immobility.

First, access is gained into the femoral, jugular, or antecubital veins. A venacavagram is performed to determine caval diameter, caval anomalies, renal vein location, and the presence of caval thrombus. A self-expanding filter is deployed through a 6 to 12 Fr catheter and placed just below the level of the renal veins (Fig. 3.26).

Various permanent and optional filters are available (Fig. 3.27). Permanent filters have been available for decades, while retrievable (optional) filters have only been available over the last several years. Some early models of optional filters showed significant migration issues. Newer models seem to show more stability. Besides migration, other complications include strut penetration through the IVC wall, strut fracture, thrombosis, and intimal hyperplasia with resultant IVC stenosis. Serious complications, however, are rare.

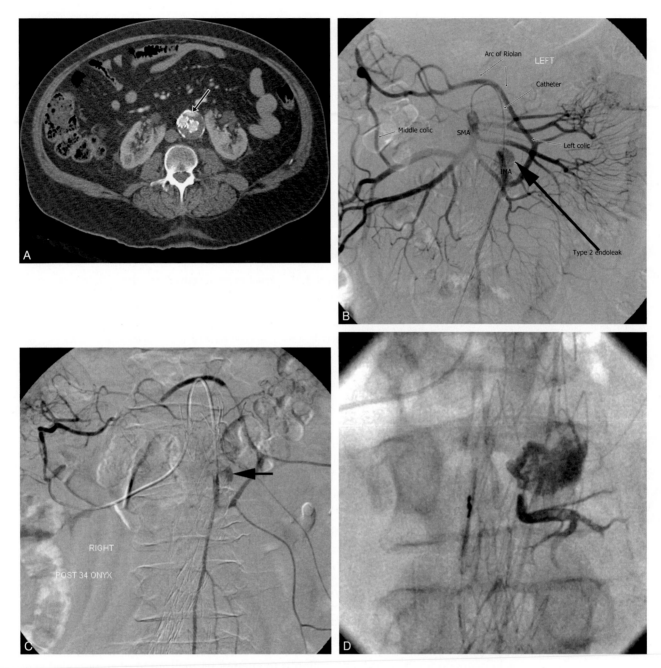

Figure 3.24   Type 2 endoleak repair in same patient as in Figure 3.23.   A. CT image shows an enlarging aneurysm with a type 2 endoleak (*arrow*) in the anterior portion of the aneurysm sac. The two limbs of the endograft are immediately posterior to the leak. **B.** After injecting the superior mesenteric artery (SMA), contrast fills the middle colic and left colic arteries. The left colic and inferior mesenteric artery (IMA) fills retrograde and the endoleak is noted from the IMA (*long arrow*). **C.** Glue was injected through a microcatheter that was placed within the leak (*arrow*). **D.** Fluoroscopic image of the injected embolic agent.

Vascular Access

Interventional radiologists are frequently asked to establish venous access routes in patients needing long-term intravenous medications, hemodialysis, or chemotherapy or in patients with difficult venous access (Fig. 3.28). The use of ultrasound and fluoroscopic guidance and knowledge of vascular anatomy greatly improves success with fewer complications. Commonly placed devices include peripherally inserted central catheters, subcutaneous ports, dialysis catheters, and nontunneled triple- or quad-lumen catheters. These devices may result in thrombosis at the access site or intimal hyperplasia. This can result in a more challenging access when a future venous catheter is needed. For central vein access, ultrasound-guided right internal jugular vein access is preferred because it provides the

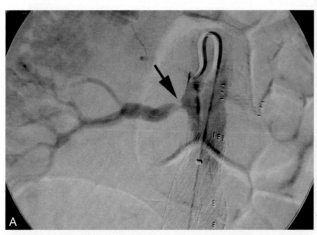

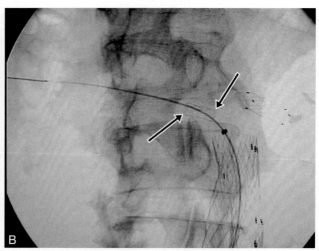

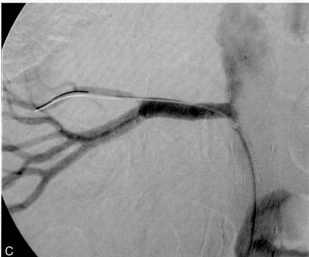

Figure 3.25   Renal artery stenosis and stenting.   This patient underwent prior abdominal aortic aneurysm endovascular repair and left renal artery stenting. **A.** Selective right renal artery injection shows a high-grade stenosis at the ostium (*arrow*). **B.** Following guidewire placement across the stenosis, a balloon-mounted stent is introduced. Arrows show the stent position. **C.** After the balloon is inflated and removed the stent is deployed showing full patency of the artery.

straightest catheter course to the superior vena cava—right atrial junction and minimizes the risk of pneumothorax. The order of access following right internal jugular occlusion might be left internal jugular, external jugular, subclavian, femoral or saphenous, translumbar (direct access under fluoroscopy, ultrasound, or CT into the IVC), and transhepatic veins (direct percutaneous access into the right lobe of the liver's right hepatic vein). To help maintain future access, one option is to attempt recanalization of an occluded vein with angioplasty to allow passage of a catheter.

Interventional radiologists are, on occasion, consulted to remove fragmented or displaced catheters and guidewires, using specialized snares.

Transjugular Intrahepatic Portosystemic Shunt

Patients with portal hypertension who present with variceal hemorrhage or intractable ascites may benefit from creation of a *transjugular intrahepatic portosystemic shunt* (TIPS). Variceal hemorrhage is treated first pharmacologically and endoscopically. If these measures fail, a TIPS procedure is often needed. Following right internal jugular vein access and sheath placement, a long, curved needle is advanced from the right hepatic vein to the right portal vein (Fig. 3.29), allowing placement of a self-expandable bare or covered stent between the two vessels and decompressing the portal venous system. Before this procedure was developed, these high-risk patients had to undergo surgery for which the morbidity and mortality were high. The procedure is not without risk. Besides bleeding, encephalopathy and liver failure can occur in high-risk patients since more blood flow is

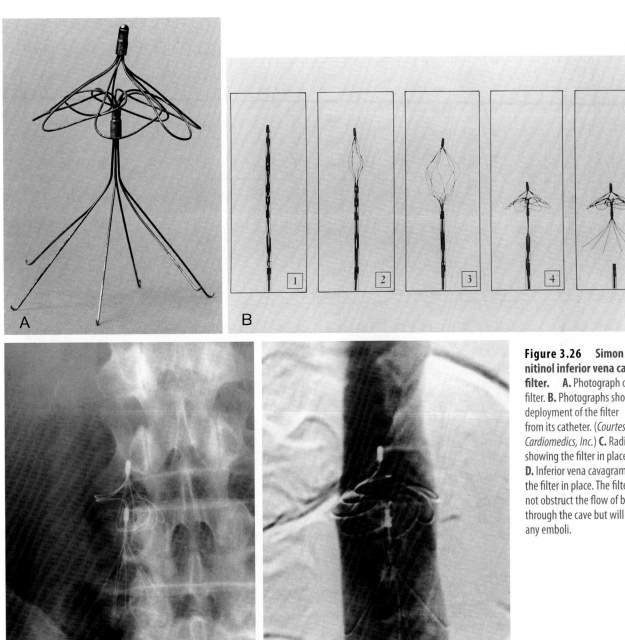

Figure 3.26 Simon nitinol inferior vena cava filter. A. Photograph of the filter. **B.** Photographs showing deployment of the filter from its catheter. (*Courtesy of Cardiomedics, Inc.*) **C.** Radiograph showing the filter in place. **D.** Inferior vena cavagram shows the filter in place. The filter does not obstruct the flow of blood through the cave but will trap any emboli.

directed away from the liver parenchyma. At our institution, patients usually require general anesthesia for the procedure.

Uterine Artery Embolization

Uterine artery embolization is a treatment option for management of leiomyomas that have resulted in menorrhagia, pelvic pain, or mass effect symptoms such as urinary incontinence. Other options include hormonal therapy, myomectomy, and hysterectomy. Embolization of both uterine arteries using particles (PVA and variations)

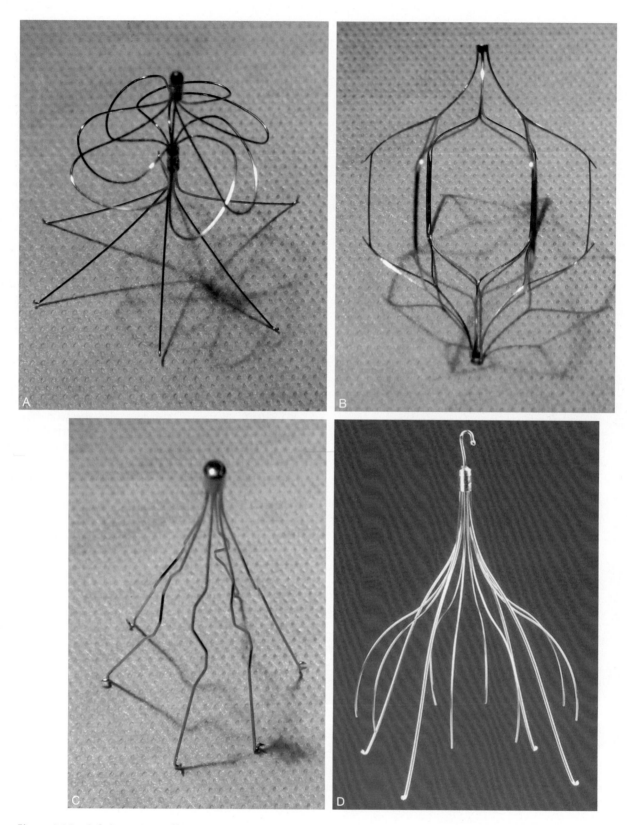

Figure 3.27   Inferior vena cava filters.   A–C. Permanent filters. **D.** Optional filter with a hook that allows removal with a snare from a jugular approach.

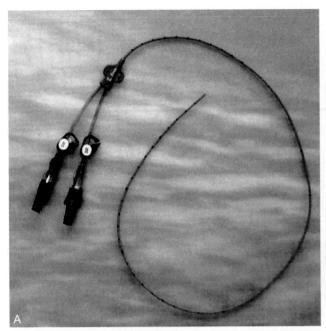 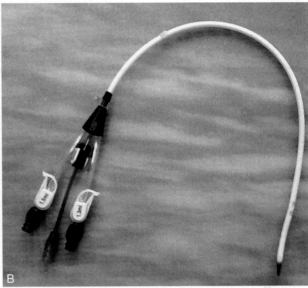

Figure 3.28 Central venous catheters. A. Peripherally inserted central catheter (PICC). **B.** Tunneled catheter used for plasmapheresis.

is performed until there is stasis in the artery (Fig. 3.30). A post-embolization syndrome (nausea, vomiting, pain, and low-grade fever) often occurs following these treatments and are managed medically. Patients are typically discharged within 24 hours after the procedure. Rare complications include passage of sloughed off fibroids and endometritis.

Percutaneous Biopsy

Biopsy procedures are performed using various needles throughout the body. Percutaneous biopsy has prevented countless surgeries for which the sole purpose was to obtain tissue. Biopsies can be performed using whatever imaging modality shows the lesion to best advantage. Fluoroscopy can be used for some bone lesions. Ultrasound guidance provides real-time visualization of the biopsy needle, but is limited to organs or areas that can be shown well with this modality. The liver, thyroid gland, breast, and kidney are some of the areas suitable for access with ultrasound. CT guidance is helpful for deeper lesions or for very precise positioning, especially when trying to avoid other nearby structures such as bowel.

In our department, we have a dedicated CT scanner that is used solely for interventional procedures. In addition, we have provided space for our cytopathologist to have a small "wet lab" to provide immediate assessment of the tissues removed during biopsies.

Decompression and Drainage

Decompression and drainage is performed as a variation of the Seldinger technique. A needle is placed into the fluid collection using imaging (usually ultrasound or CT) guidance (Fig. 3.31). A guidewire is then advanced through the needle, the needle is removed, and a drainage catheter is introduced into the fluid-filled space. The catheter is either taped or sutured in place and then attached to a drainage bag or vacuum bottle. Variations of this technique may be used to drain obstructed renal collecting systems (*nephrostomy*) (Fig. 3.32), obstructed biliary ducts (Fig. 3.33), and gastric outlet obstruction or as feeding tubes (*percutaneous gastrostomy*). For obstructing biliary or ureteral lesions, IR procedures may be used to correct the obstruction by placing temporary catheters or permanent metallic stents or by performing angioplasty. Benign strictures can be dilated, and malignant obstructions can be stented open.

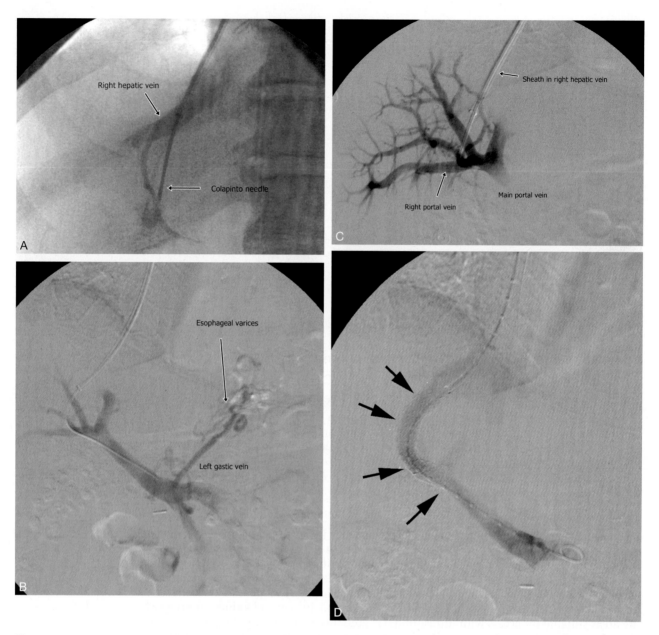

Figure 3.29   TIPS procedure.   A. A sheath is introduced via the right internal jugular vein and is advanced to the right hepatic vein. There, a Colapinto needle is advanced fluoroscopically toward the right portal vein. **B and C.** After opacifying the right portal vein, a guidewire and a catheter are placed into the main portal vein. Note the filling of the left gastric vein in **B. D.** A self-expandable stent (*arrows*) is then deployed between the right hepatic and right portal veins. The left gastric vein is now decompressed and no longer fills with contrast.

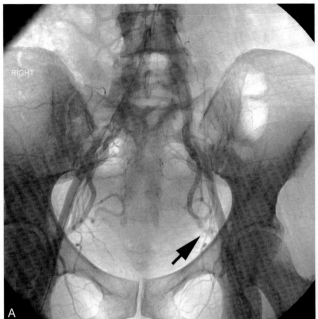

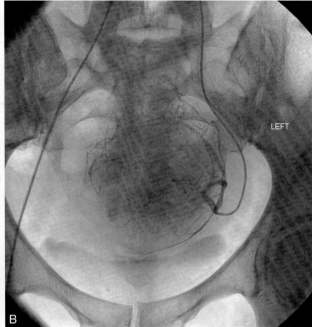

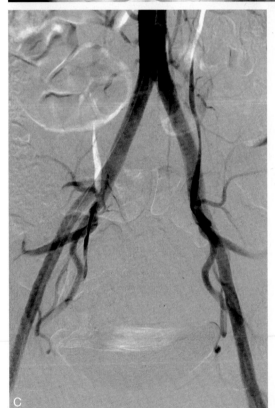

Figure 3.30   Uterine artery embolization.   A. Pelvic angiogram shows bleeding from a uterine vessel on the left (*arrow*). **B.** Embolic particles are selectively injected into the uterine arteries. **C.** Post-embolization angiogram shows the bleeding to have been stopped. Compare with **A.**

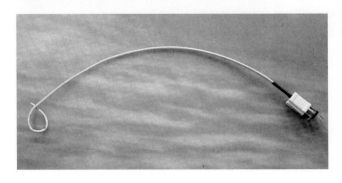

Figure 3.31   Drainage catheter with a locking pigtail loop controlled by pulling a string near the catheter hub.

Figure 3.32   Percutaneous nephrostomy set. **A,** guidewire; **B,** dilator; **C,** pigtail drainage catheter; **D,** needle and stylet; **E,** thin-walled needle.

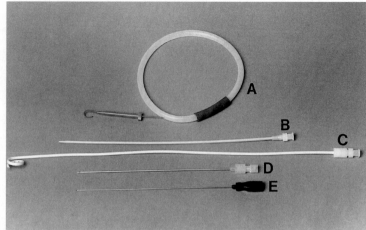

Figure 3.33   Percutaneous transhepatic cholangiogram and biliary drainage in a patient with pancreatic carcinoma.   An endoscopic retrograde cholangiogram was attempted but the distal common bile duct stricture could not be crossed by the endoscopist. **A.** A long small diameter needle (*arrow*) is advanced from the right lateral abdomen between the ribs toward the central liver under fluoroscopic guidance. This needle was used to opacify the biliary ducts, which are dilated. A second needle (*arrowhead*) was then placed in a more peripheral duct to decrease the chance of bleeding from a large central blood vessel. **B.** A wire is then negotiated into the duodenum (*arrow*) followed by a stiffening dilator. **C.** Multi-side hole drainage catheter, which is introduced over the dilator. **D.** Cholangiogram following catheter placement shows decompression of the biliary tree.

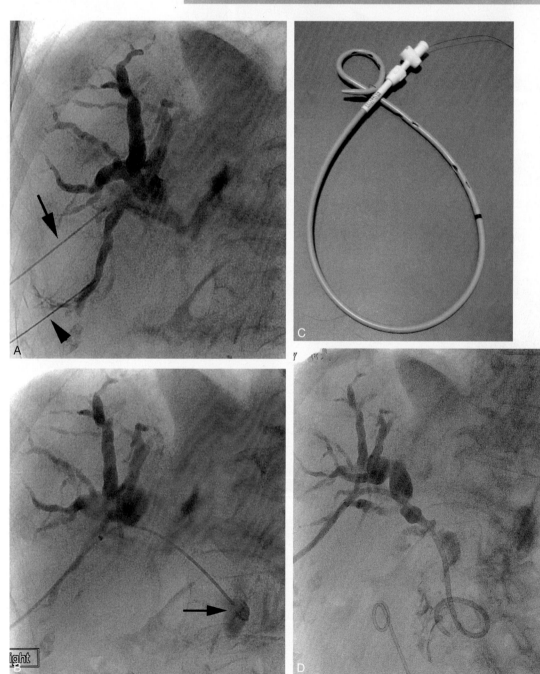

Extraction procedures for biliary and renal stones can also be performed percutaneously. The procedure is a variant of that used for decompression, with the exception being the use of an extraction instrument through the catheter within the lumen of the occluded duct.

Percutaneous Screw Placement

Musculoskeletal radiologists have been called upon to assist orthopaedic surgeons in the placement of screws across unstable sacroiliac joints or across acetabular fractures. Traditionally, these procedures have been performed under fluoroscopic guidance by the orthopaedists in the operating room. Radiologists have been asked to perform these procedures using CT guidance on obese patients who were unsuitable candidates for fluoroscopic-guided placement. CT has the advantages of permitting precise localization, accurate determination of angles, and exact depth measurements for screw placement (Fig. 3.34).

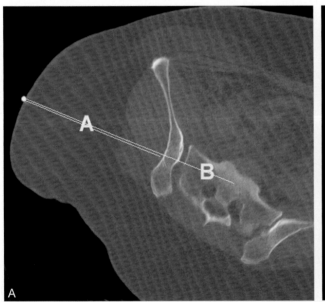

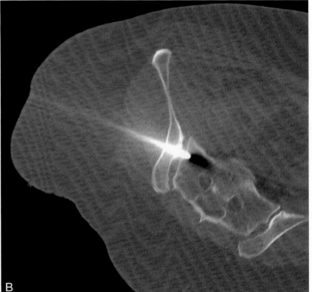

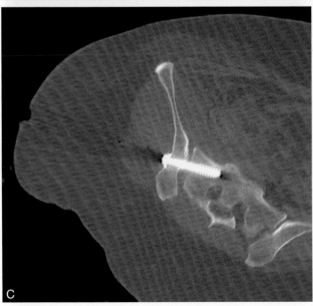

Figure 3.34   CT-guided screw placement across an unstable sacroiliac joint.   A. CT image shows a wide right sacroiliac joint. Lines are for measurement of depth from the skin to the iliac bone (*A*) and for screw length (*B*). **B.** CT image shows the screw being placed. **C.** CT image showing final position of the screw. Note that the sacroiliac joint is now narrower.

Suggested Additional Reading

Fenton DS. Image-Guided Spine Intervention. Philadelphia, PA: WB Saunders, 2003.
Kandarpa K. Handbook of Interventional Radiologic Procedures. 4th Ed. Philadelphia, PA: Lippincott Williams & Wilkins, 2010.
Kaufman JA, Lee MJ. Vascular and Interventional Radiology. The Requisites. St. Louis, MO: Mosby/Elsevier, 2004.
Uflacker R. Atlas of Vascular Anatomy: An Angiographic Approach. 2nd Ed. Philadelphia, PA: Lippincott Williams & Wilkins, 2006.
Valji K. The Practice of Interventional Radiology with Online Cases and Videos. Philadelphia, PA: Elsevier, 2012.

Chest Imaging

Jeffrey S. Mueller   Richard H. Daffner

The chest radiograph is the examination you will be requesting and observing with the greatest frequency. In addition, it is the examination that you will most likely be reviewing alone. Chest radiographs account for slightly less than half of all the examinations performed in any radiology practice. One of the reasons for this is that the chest is considered the "mirror of health or disease." Besides giving information about the patient's heart and lungs, the chest radiograph provides valuable information about adjacent structures such as the gastrointestinal tract, the thyroid gland, and the bony structures of the thorax. Furthermore, metastatic disease from the abdominal viscera, head and neck, or skeleton frequently manifests itself in the lungs. Thus, the "routine" chest radiograph should not be considered quite so "routine." Figures 4.1 through 4.4 illustrate some of these entities.

Technical Considerations

The Patient

The first technical consideration for any imaging study is to be certain that the examination is of the *correct* patient (Fig. 4.5). In the past, it was important to check the patient's name, gender, age, and medical identification number on the study with that given on the requisition slip. However, most radiology departments now use digital imaging and every exam is available for immediate review on a computer or workstation through the PACS or picture archiving and communication system. These have minimized the common problem of accidentally assigning a radiograph to the wrong patient. Nevertheless, mismatches still occur. Furthermore, because many critically ill patients have multiple studies performed the same day, it is important to check the time of each examination (Fig. 4.6). Actual patient identification is checked by looking for congruent bony structures, soft tissue characteristics such as breast shadows (or their absence), and the presence of life-support equipment (i.e., lines and/or tubes) or surgical hardware (see Fig. 4.5). *Always use old studies (films) for comparison, whenever they are available.* Old studies are your best friends in radiology!

 ▶ Old imaging studies are your best friends in radiology.

Analysis

All radiographic images should be analyzed for *density*, *motion*, and *rotation*. A determination should be made as to whether the entire thorax is displayed. Be sure that the technologist has not cut the costophrenic angles off the image. On a properly exposed radiograph, the thoracic vertebrae should be barely discernible through the image of the heart. The medial ends of the clavicles should be equidistant from the patient's midline, indicating no rotation.

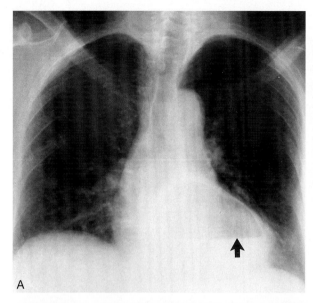

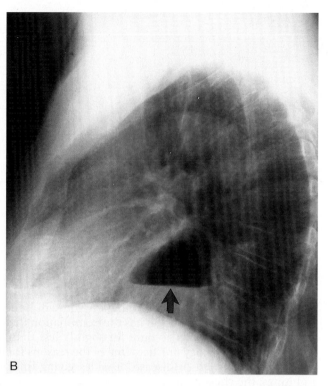

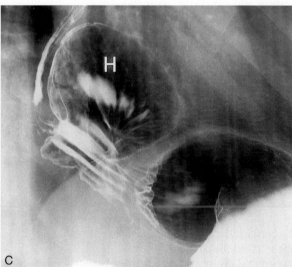

Figure 4.1   Large paraesophageal hiatal hernia detected on a "routine" chest examination.   Frontal **(A)** and lateral **(B)** radiographs demonstrate a mass behind the heart with a large air–fluid level (*arrows*). **C.** Detail image from upper gastrointestinal exam shows barium and air within the hernia sac (*H*).

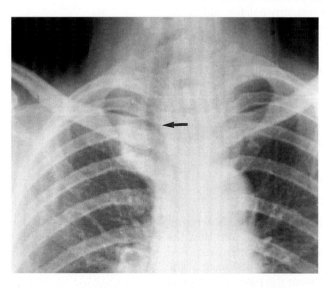

Figure 4.2   "Routine" chest radiograph showing a thyroid mass (goiter) on the left displacing the trachea to the right (*arrow*).

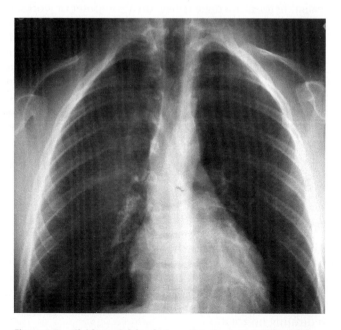

Figure 4.3   Cleidocranial dysplasia.   Note the absence of the clavicles.

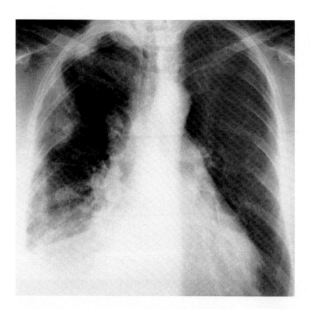

Figure 4.4   Multiple pulmonary and mediastinal metastases in the right hemithorax detected on a "routine" chest radiograph.

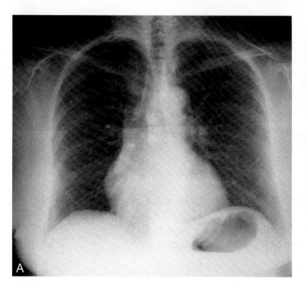

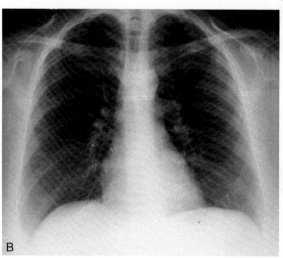

Figure 4.5   Mislabeled chest radiographs.   A and **B.** Consecutive radiographs from the outpatient imaging center were both labeled with the same patient identification. Note the differences between each patient with regard to heart and aortic configuration, clavicle shape, and breast size. Although this error has become less common with picture archiving and communication system, it can still occur.

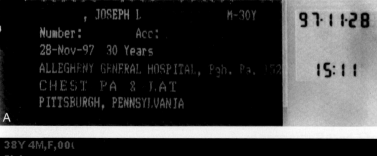

Figure 4.6   Identification labels.   A. Film screen technique. The information on the dark part of the label is printed on the film at the time it is processed. The top line contains the patient's name and to the right, gender and age. The next line has the patient's hospital identification number and immediately adjacent the film accession number (*Acc*) that refers only to the current examination. The next line contains the date of the examination, and the patient's age, once again. The fourth and sixth lines give the identification of the hospital. The fifth line tells what type of examination was performed. The numbers in the light portion of the label include the date on top and the time of the examination on the bottom. This is important if a patient has multiple examinations in 1 day. **B.** Digital technique. Same information displayed digitally (name and other patient ID data intentionally blacked out for Health Insurance Portability and Accountability Act compliance).

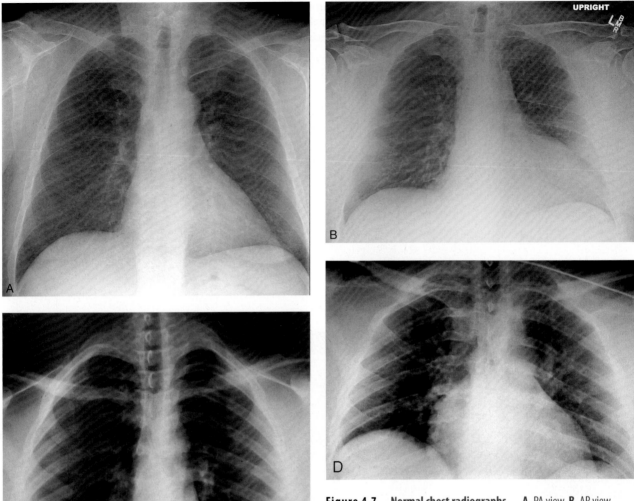

Figure 4.7   Normal chest radiographs.   A. PA view. **B.** AP view.
(See text for description.) Upright PA **(C)** and supine AP **(D)** views on another patient. Note the differences in the appearance of the heart and skeletal structures caused by the changes in position.

The next step is to decide what *type of examination* has been performed. The ordinary chest radiograph is made with the patient in the erect position with the anterior portion of the chest against the film cassette. The x-ray tube is positioned 6 feet behind the patient, and the horizontal beam enters from the back (posterior) and exits through the front (anterior): the *PA radiograph*. If the patient turns completely around and the beam enters from the front, the resulting image is termed an *AP radiograph*. Figure 4.7**A** is a PA erect radiograph of a young patient; Figure 4.7**B** is an AP erect image of the same patient. Figure 4.7**C** and **D** illustrates the differences between erect and supine radiographs.

Common Features of Chest Radiographs

In general, the following are features that commonly identify PA chest radiographs: the lung markings are more distinct, the heart is smaller, the clavicles are superimposed over the upper lungs, and the cervical and thoracic vertebrae are more clearly visible. These findings suggest an AP radiograph: the heart appears larger than usual, the lung volumes are shallow, and the clavicles are usually higher.

Full Inspiration

One of the most important technical considerations in evaluating the chest radiograph is determining whether or not the study demonstrates optimal *inspiration*. Figure 4.8, a frontal image of a healthy man, was deliberately made in forced expiration. Failure to observe that the image was obtained with shallow lung volumes could easily lead to a mistaken diagnosis of congestive heart failure (CHF). After all, the heart appears large, the pulmonary vessels are more prominent, and there is blunting of both lung bases, suggesting pleural effusions. Figure 4.9 is a maximal inspiratory radiograph of the same individual; it is perfectly normal.

There are many reasons why a study may not be obtained in full inspiration. Obesity is a common mechanical cause; acute abdomen or recent surgery results in voluntary restriction; the cardiac patient with CHF is unable to displace the edema fluid in the "waterlogged" lungs; and the patient with chronic restrictive lung disease cannot expand his/her chest to expected maximum because of scarring and loss of compliance in the lung tissues. For all these reasons, the terms *"shallow lung volumes"* and *"poor inspiratory result"* are used rather than *"poor inspiratory effort."* In most instances, these patients will have made a good inspiratory *effort*, but the lung volumes (the *result*) are low.

A chest radiograph is considered to have adequate lung volumes when the diaphragm crosses the tenth rib or interspace posteriorly or the eighth rib anteriorly. The reader is cautioned not to fall into the pitfall of diagnosing "nondisease" in a patient without full inspiration.

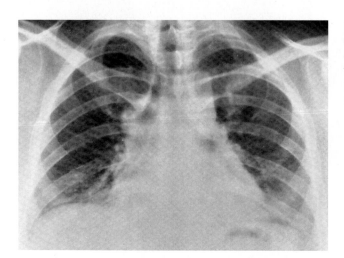

Figure 4.8   Expiratory chest radiograph.   This image was made in deliberate expiration. There is elevation of the diaphragm, crowding of the lower lung markings, and apparent heart enlargement. (Compare with Fig. 4.9.)

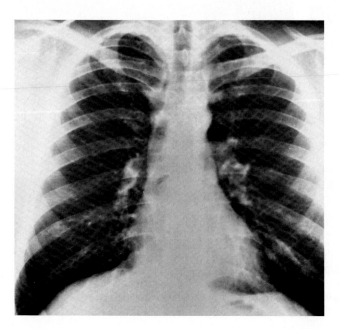

Figure 4.9   Normal inspiratory chest radiograph.   (Same patient as in Fig. 4.8.) Note the differences in full inspiration.

Expiration

Interestingly enough, there are certain circumstances in which it is desirable to deliberately perform a study in *expiration*. These include evaluation of the patient with a suspected foreign body in a bronchus, a "ball-valve" type of bronchial obstruction, or a suspected pneumothorax. In the first instance (Fig. 4.10), the PA inspiratory image is normal; the expiratory radiograph demonstrates no change in the volume of the lung on the obstructed side. The normal lung decreases in volume, and the mediastinum swings toward the normal side. In the second instance, the pneumothorax is enhanced by the decrease in lung volume (Fig. 4.11). If the patient such as a toddler or a sedated patient cannot cooperate, decubitus views are useful (see below).

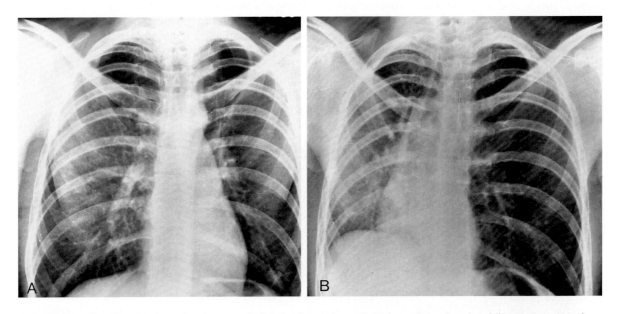

Figure 4.10   Use of inspiratory and expiratory technique in obstruction.   A. PA chest radiograph made in full inspiration is normal. **B.** Radiograph made in expiration shows the mediastinum and heart to shift to the right. There is no volume change on the left. These findings indicate an obstructing lesion in the mainstem bronchus on the left, found to be a bronchial adenoma on subsequent bronchoscopy.

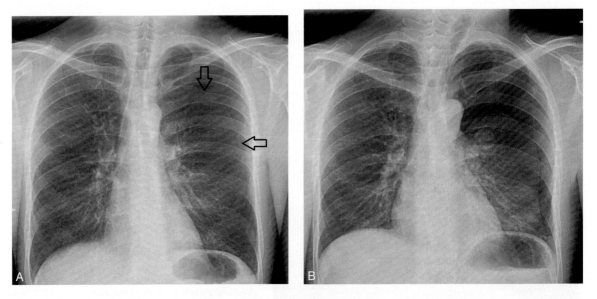

Figure 4.11   Use of inspiratory and expiratory technique in pneumothorax.   A. Inspiratory radiograph shows a pneumothorax on the left (*arrows*). **B.** Expiratory radiograph shows enlargement of the pneumothorax.

Rotation

Rotation of the patient or angulation may result in distortion of normal anatomic images. As mentioned previously, you should be able to detect rotation by observing the position of the medial ends of the clavicles.

Lordotic views have been advocated as a means of examining abnormalities in the lung apices. The examination is made by having the patient lean backward toward the cassette while a horizontal beam is used to make the exposure (Fig. 4.12). Use of a position marker at the edge of the cassette indicates the angulation of the patient (Fig. 4.13). We do not use this view frequently because CT is more definitive and is more easily available.

Portable Technique

Another technical consideration is the analysis of radiographs made by *portable technique.* Studies of this kind are performed on severely debilitated or critically ill patients who cannot be safely transported to the radiology department. In reviewing these studies, it is important to recognize these studies are limited. There may be motion (the patient cannot

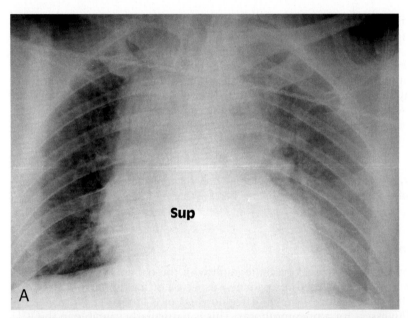

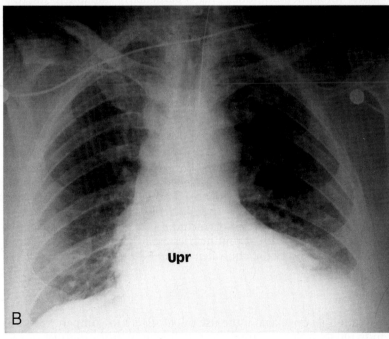

Figure 4.12   Lordotic positioning.   A. Supine lordotic image shows the clavicles to be positioned high. The mediastinum appears widened, and the heart is egg shaped. **B.** Upright radiograph on the same patient shows striking differences.

Figure 4.13   Position markers. Radiographic appearance of a vial of dilute radiographic contrast in the erect (left), 45° recumbent (center), and supine (right) positions.

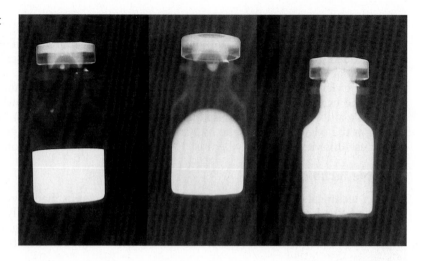

hold his/her breath) or the patient may be rotated. In fact, these exams were originally designed to validate appropriate positioning of the life-support equipment, not to diagnose lung or cardiac disease. There are countless examples of missed lung cancers and pneumonia not seen on portable chest x-rays that are clearly demonstrated on a two-view chest x-ray. Remember that a portable chest x-ray should be obtained immediately following insertion of any central line, endotracheal tube, and other life-support equipment in the intensive care setting. If the patient needs a chest x-ray for anything other than tube and line position, a two-view chest x-ray should be performed in the radiology department if possible.

▶ A portable chest radiograph should be obtained immediately following insertion of any life-support device in the intensive care setting.

Decubitus Position

Occasionally it may be useful to make a radiograph with the patient lying on one side (*decubitus position*). This study is used for patients suspected of having pleural effusions to determine whether the effusion layers out (free flowing) or is loculated. However, it is even more helpful to assess for a pneumothorax. This is particularly valuable in the ICU (intensive care unit) setting where portable exams will miss most small pneumothoraces. Lastly, decubitus views are extremely valuable in the pediatric setting of a suspected aspirated foreign body. Toddlers rarely cooperate with inspiratory and expiratory views to show air trapping distal to a foreign body. This problem is easily circumvented with bilateral decubitus views. The lung with the aspirated foreign body will trap air and will not compress or deflate on the ipsilateral decubitus view.

Dual-Energy Subtraction

Some chest radiographs use dual-energy subtraction, which allows one to selectively subtract the bones to display only the lungs and heart, or conversely, to subtract the heart and lungs to display the bones. This exam has four views: PA, lateral, PA subtracted (lungs), and PA bone (Fig. 4.14). This technique increases the sensitivity for detecting lung nodules and pneumonia that would be obscured by the ribs. It can also differentiate between a calcified and noncalcified nodule; the former is usually benign and the latter is potentially malignant. There are disadvantages, however, including longer examination times and slightly higher radiation dose. Of course, a routine chest x-ray has the lowest radiation dose of any ionizing medical imaging exam, equivalent to an 8-hour plane ride or 1 day of natural background radiation.

Old Studies as Comparison

A final technical consideration is, once again, the use of *old studies* to compare with the current study. Many individuals have abnormal chest radiographs from inactive or old

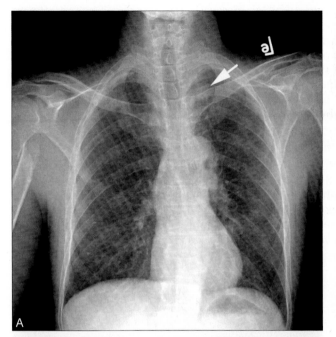

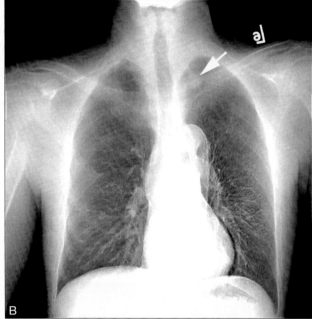

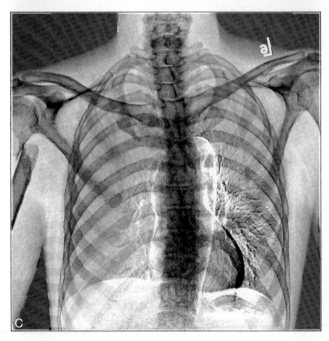

Figure 4.14   Dual-energy chest x-ray views showing left upper nodule (*arrows*, A and B).   A. Normal frontal. **B.** Frontal lung window, bones subtracted. Note how much better the nodule can be seen. **C.** Frontal bone window, lungs subtracted. The nodule cannot be seen.

diseases. The most common conditions encountered are old granulomatous disease, scarring, and chronic obstructive pulmonary disease. Without the old radiographs for comparison, the patient may have to undergo extensive (and expensive) evaluation that may include a biopsy. Every effort should be made to obtain old studies. *Every* current study should be compared with a previous one if it is available. If old studies are not available, you should place a note to that effect in the medical record.

Other Imaging Modalities

Although chest radiography is the mainstay for diagnosing thoracic disease, other imaging modalities are also used. Chest fluoroscopy is a valuable technique for assessing diaphragmatic paralysis. Otherwise known as the "sniff" test, a radiologist can quickly differentiate between a paralyzed diaphragm versus an elevated diaphragm. Normally, the diaphragm contracts and moves downward with inspiration or "sniffing." If the diaphragm rises, the diaphragm is paralyzed.

Computed Tomography

Computed tomography (CT) with multidetector technology is an extremely valuable technique for assessing a wide array of pulmonary, mediastinal, cardiovascular, and chest wall pathology (Fig. 4.15). Chest CT should be performed with iodinated intravenous contrast in the setting of suspected or known neoplasm, adenopathy, pleural disease, pulmonary arterial, cardiovascular disease, or trauma (Fig. 4.16). Intravenous contrast can be safely withheld for lung disease or pulmonary nodule follow-up.

Magnetic Resonance Imaging

Magnetic resonance imaging (MRI) has only a few indications for assessing chest disease but should always be performed with contrast if possible. The best indications for chest MRI include aortic disease, diaphragmatic injury, and staging certain lung cancers such as Pancoast tumor in the lung apex or mesothelioma (Fig. 4.17). Chest MRI can detect pulmonary emboli but CT is more sensitive and the new gold standard. MRI can also be gated to the heart cycle to assess for a variety of cardiac diseases (see next chapter).

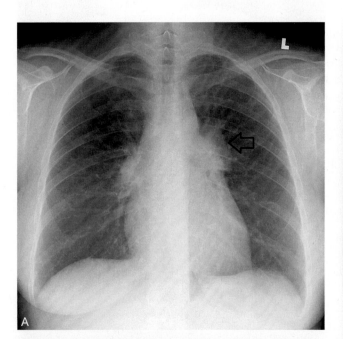

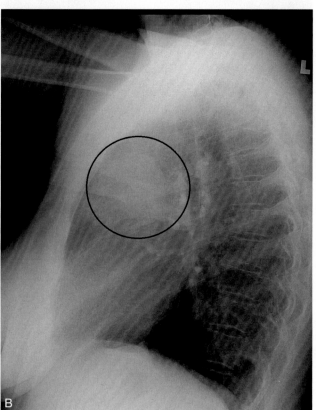

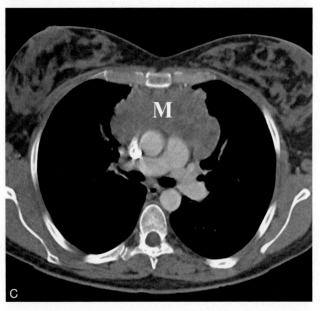

Figure 4.15   Mediastinal mass.   A. Frontal radiograph shows a left-sided mediastinal mass (*arrow*). This is a case of "too many bumps." **B.** Lateral radiograph shows the mass to be in the anterior mediastinum (*circle*). **C.** Axial CT image confirms the anterior mediastinal mass (*M*).

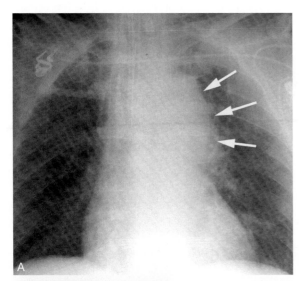

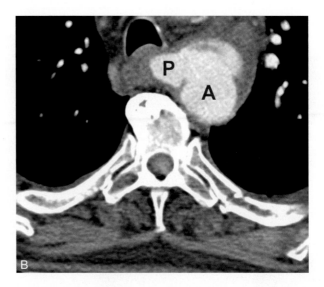

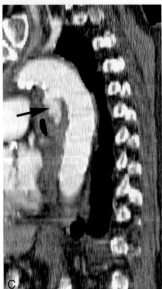

Figure 4.16   Posttraumatic aortic tear.   A. Frontal chest radiograph shows widening of the superior mediastinum and straightening and irregularity of the aortic knob (*arrows*). **B.** Axial contrast-enhanced CT image just below the aortic arch (*A*) shows extravasation of contrast anteriorly, and a pseudoaneurysm (*P*) medially. **C.** Sagittal reconstructed CT image shows the hemorrhage and pseudoaneurysm (*arrow*).

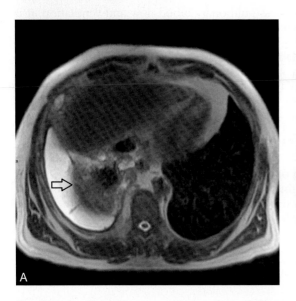

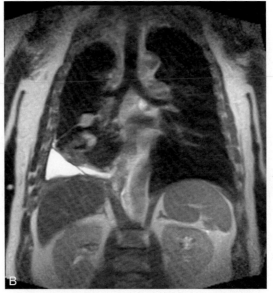

Figure 4.17   Magnetic resonance image of mesothelioma.   A. Axial T2-weighted MR image shows a bright pleural effusion and adjacent pleural mass (*arrow*). **B.** Coronal T2-weighted MR image shows disease is confined to the right chest with no extension below the diaphragm. MR is valuable for staging mesothelioma with its superior contrast resolution.

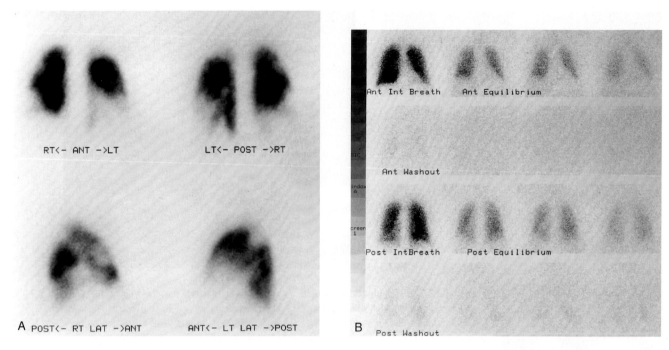

Figure 4.18   Perfusion–ventilation (V/Q) scan in a patient with pulmonary emboli.   A. Perfusion scan of the lungs demonstrates many areas devoid of radioisotope (photopenia) bilaterally. **B.** Ventilation scan is normal. This combination of findings is diagnostic of pulmonary emboli, particularly when the chest radiograph is normal or near normal.

Ultrasound

Ultrasound is used to diagnose suspected pleural fluid collections, particularly on the right side, where imaging is performed in the transhepatic plane. Ultrasound is not useful for lung lesions because the sound waves cannot cross tissue–air borders. Nevertheless, ultrasound is commonly used to guide thoracentesis or placement of pigtail catheters to drain pleural effusions. Some radiologists occasionally use ultrasound to biopsy chest wall and peripheral lung masses. Ultrasound is also very useful for the biopsy of axillary and supraclavicular adenopathy.

Nuclear Imaging

Finally, *nuclear imaging* is performed to assess pulmonary blood flow and ventilation. It is most commonly used to diagnose suspected pulmonary emboli. The typical ventilation–perfusion (V/Q) scan uses inhaled xenon133– or technetium 99m–labeled DTPA for ventilation imaging followed by technetium 99m–labeled macroaggregated albumin particles injected intravenously for perfusion imaging (Fig. 4.18). However, V/Q scans do not perform well in the setting of obstructive lung disease or if the patient has an abnormal chest x-ray. Therefore, it is always recommended to obtain a two-view chest x-ray before ordering a V/Q study.

Anatomic Considerations

A logical approach to the interpretation of chest radiographs is predicated on the observer developing an orderly system for scanning each image. It matters not whether the review begins from the outside and proceeds inward or vice versa. What is important is to be consistent and thorough evaluating the following structures every time:

- Trachea and mediastinum
- Heart and great vessels
- Lungs and pulmonary arteries
- Pleura and costophrenic angles
- Diaphragm and abdomen
- Bones and soft tissues

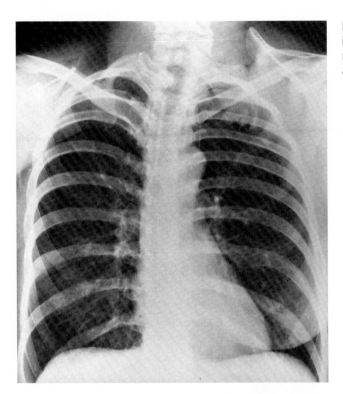

Figure 4.19 Order of visual scan in a patient with a right radical mastectomy and a left shoulder anomaly. (See text for description.)

The order of visual scan is illustrated in Figure 4.19, which shows a patient who has had a right radical mastectomy and has a congenital anomaly of the left shoulder. The analysis of this study and its reporting is as follows: "The heart and mediastinal structures are normal. The pulmonary vessels and aorta are normal. The lungs, costophrenic angles, pleura, and diaphragm are normal. The patient has had a right radical mastectomy as indicated by the absence of the right breast shadow and increased lucency from the missing pectoralis muscle. A bony anomaly is present in the left shoulder: elevation of the scapula, the presence of an omovertebral bone, and a cleft vertebra at C6. This particular type of anomaly is called Sprengel deformity."

The lateral chest radiograph should receive the same attention as the PA film and is analyzed similarly. Consider the report on the lateral chest radiograph in a patient with known esophageal carcinoma (Fig. 4.20): "...on the lateral chest view, the trachea is deviated anteriorly by a soft tissue mass that contains an air-fluid level. This is most consistent with the diagnosis of an obstructing esophageal mass. The cardiac silhouette is normal. The lungs, costophrenic angle, posterior recesses, and diaphragm are normal. There are no significant vertebral abnormalities."

Structures

Let us now review the normal anatomic structures found on the chest radiograph in the same order as the image analysis.

Trachea

The *trachea* is a midline structure whose air-filled image stands out in bold contrast to the surrounding soft tissues of the neck and mediastinum. On a well-penetrated frontal radiograph, the *carina* (tracheal bifurcation) may be found at the level of the T4–T5 interspace. In young children, it is not uncommon for the tracheal air column to bow to the right. A trachea deviated to the left should be considered abnormal and CT of the chest should be performed to determine the cause. On the lateral view, the tracheal air column may be seen slowly angling down from the thoracic inlet. The soft tissue line (*retrotracheal line*) along its posterior wall should not be bowed and should not exceed 3 mm in thickness (Fig. 4.21).

Figure 4.20   Carcinoma of the esophagus.   A. lateral chest radiograph shows an air–fluid level (*arrow*) immediately behind the trachea. There is thickening of the retrotracheal line. Compare with Figure 4.21. **B.** Esophagogram shows nearly complete obstruction to the passage of barium (*arrow*).

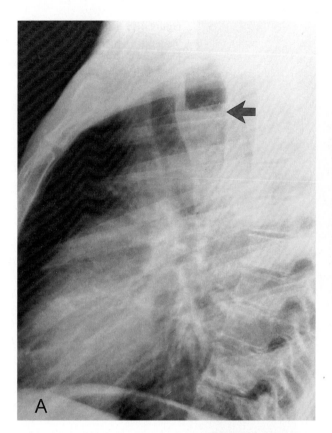

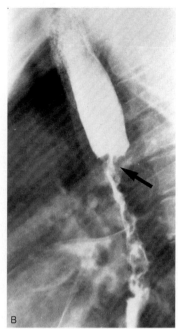

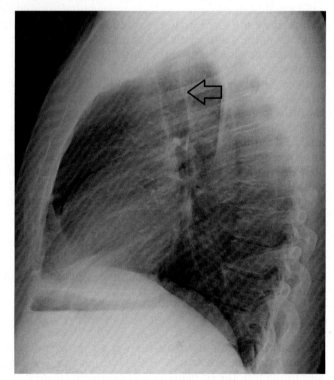

Figure 4.21   Normal lateral chest radiograph.   Arrow points to the posterior tracheal line which should be less than 3 mm in thickness.

Mediastinum

The *mediastinum* is the central thorax between lungs, including the heart. To help classify abnormalities and narrow the differential diagnosis, the mediastinum has been divided into three regions: anterior, middle, and posterior (Fig. 4.22). The anterior mediastinum is found immediately behind the sternum and anterior to the great vessels and heart. The posterior mediastinum is located behind the heart and trachea including the vertebral

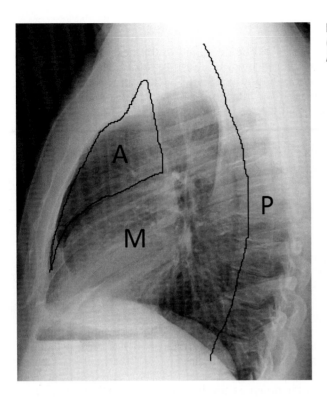

Figure 4.22 Mediastinal compartments.
(See text for description.) *A,* anterior mediastinum; *M,* mediastinum; *P,* posterior mediastinum.

bodies. The middle mediastinum is located between the anterior and posterior pericardium and contains the critical structures of the chest, including the pericardium, heart, aortic arch and proximal brachiocephalic vessels, pulmonary arteries and veins, trachea and main bronchi, and lymph nodes. Be aware, other mediastinal classifications exist using different landmarks (Fig. 4.23). Pathologic aspects of these compartments will be discussed in the following section.

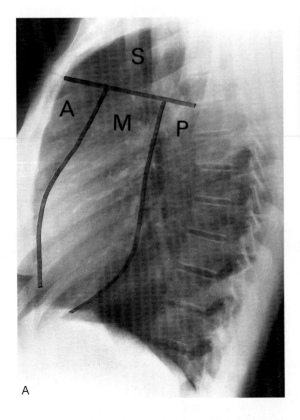

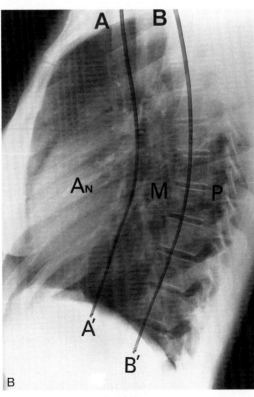

Figure 4.23 Other mediastinal classifications.
A. The anatomic mediastinum: anterior (*A*), middle (*M*), posterior (*P*), and superior (*S*) segments. **B.** Different radiological mediastinal classification: *A*N, anterior mediastinum; *M,* middle mediastinum; *P,* posterior mediastinum.

Heart and Great Vessels

The anatomy of the *heart and great vessels* will be described in the next chapter. It is sufficient to say at this point, however, that all lung markings found on the normal chest radiograph are made by pulmonary arteries and veins and not by bronchi. After all, the blood-filled vessels are of water density; air-filled bronchi, which normally have thin walls, provide no significant contrast to the aerated lungs.

 ❯ All lung markings found on the normal chest radiograph are made by pulmonary arteries and veins and not by bronchi.

Lungs and Pulmonary Arteries

There are three lobes in the right *lung* and two in the left. Each lobe is divided into anatomic segments supplied by its own bronchus and blood vessels (Fig. 4.24). In the right upper lobe are the apical, anterior, and posterior segments; the middle lobe has medial and lateral segments. The right lower lobe contains a superior segment and, in clockwise fashion, posterior, medial, anterior, and lateral basal segments.

The left upper lobe consists of a fused apical-posterior segment, an anterior segment, and superior and inferior lingular segments. The left lower lobe is similar to the right lower lobe except that the anterior and medial basal segments are fused. A knowledge of the location of these segments is important in localizing disease. The reader is advised to note that there is a significant portion of lung contained in the costophrenic recesses posteriorly. These recesses extend as far down as the level of L2. Occasionally, tumors occur within the lung in this location. These abnormalities often will not be seen on chest radiographs but may be detected on an abdominal radiograph (Fig. 4.25) or on CT.

Figure 4.24   Segmental bronchial anatomy.
Right upper lobe: *A*, apical; *P*, posterior; *An*, anterior. Right middle lobe: *L*, lateral; *M*, medial. Right lower lobe: *S*, superior; *Ab*, anterior basal; *Lb*, lateral basal; *Pb*, posterior basal; *Mb*, medial basal. Left upper lobe: *AP*, apical–posterior; *A*, apical; *P*, posterior; *An*, anterior; *Sl*, superior lingular; *I*, inferior lingular. Left lower lobe: *S*, superior; *AMb*, anterior-medial basal; *Lb*, lateral basal; *Pb*, posterior basal.

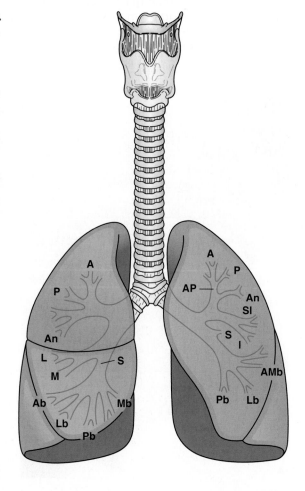

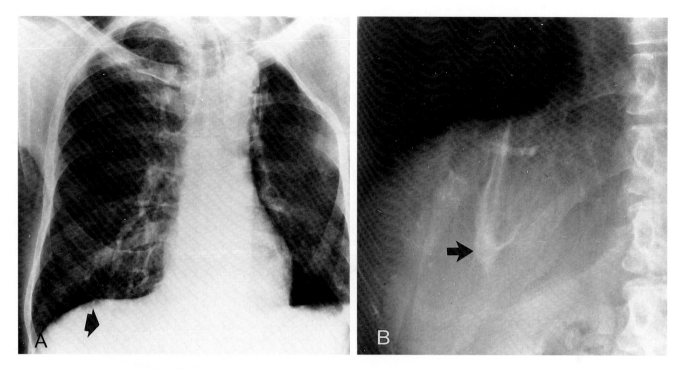

Figure 4.25 Carcinoma of the right lower lobe in an extreme basal segment. **A.** PA chest radiograph barely shows a lesion beneath the diaphragm on the right (*arrow*). **B.** Detail view from an abdominal radiograph shows an irregular mass (*arrow*) in an extreme basal segment of the right lower lobe.

 ▶ There is a significant portion of lung contained in the costophrenic recesses posteriorly.

The basic anatomic and functional pulmonary unit is the *acinus*, the portion of lung distal to the terminal bronchiole where gas exchange takes place. It contains respiratory bronchioles, alveolar ducts, alveolar sacs, and alveoli. Anatomically and radiographically, a consistently recognizable structure results from the grouping of three to five acini together to form the *secondary pulmonary lobule*. The typical lobule is approximately 1 cm in diameter in adults. Each of these lobules is surrounded by its own interlobular septa and interstitial structures (Fig. 4.26). Diseases that affect the air spaces are referred to as having an *acinar- or alveolar-type* pattern; diseases that affect the interstitial tissues are referred to as having an *interstitial* pattern.

The interlobular septa are not seen normally. However, when they become edematous or thickened, they become visible as faint linear lines known as septal or *Kerley* lines (Fig. 4.27).

There are microscopic communications between the distal portions of the bronchiolar tree and surrounding alveoli known as the *canals of Lambert*. They provide an accessory route for air passage from the bronchioles to the alveoli. Another connection is the *pores of Kohn*, which are small openings in the alveolar wall about 10 to 15 μm in diameter. These permit the lung distal to an obstructed bronchus or bronchiole to be ventilated by a process known as *collateral air drift*. They also allow infection to spread.

Pleura

The *pleura* consists of two layers, the visceral pleura and the parietal pleura. The visceral pleura encases the lungs. Under normal circumstances, the pleura is not visualized with the exception of the normal *interlobar fissures* (Fig. 4.28). On the right, there are two fissures, the oblique (major) and the horizontal (minor). The left lung contains an oblique fissure only. The oblique fissure begins at the level of the fourth thoracic vertebra, extending obliquely downward and forward and ending approximately at the level of the sixth rib anteriorly. The horizontal or minor fissure begins roughly at the level of the sixth rib

Figure 4.26   The pulmonary lobule.   This consists of a terminal bronchiole (*TB*), several levels of respiratory bronchioles (*RB*), alveolar ducts (*AD*), and alveolar sacs (*AS*). Each acinus is surrounded by its own interstitial structures and interlobular septum.

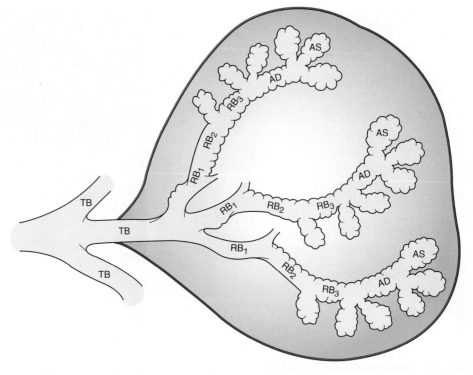

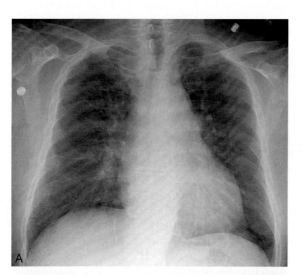

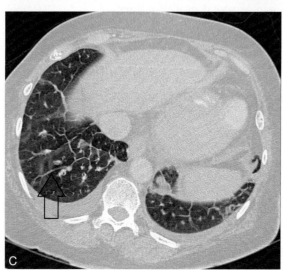

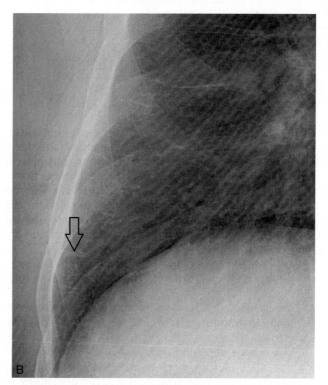

Figure 4.27   Kerley lines in patients with congestive heart failure.
A. AP radiograph shows subtle Kerley B lines in the peripheral lung.
B. Detail view shows the linear horizontal Kerley B lines in the periphery (*arrow*). **C.** CT shows interlobular septal thickening.

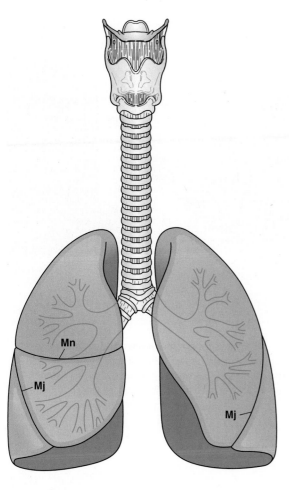

Figure 4.28   Division of the lungs by fissures. *Mn*, minor fissure; *Mj*, major fissure.

laterally and extends anteriorly and slightly downward to end near the medial portion of the fourth rib. Occasionally, an accessory fissure may be found bordering a segment of lung that has become partially or completely separated from its adjacent segments. The best known of these is the *azygous fissure*, which is created by the downward migration of the azygous vein through the apical pleura of the right upper lobe. In doing so, the vein invaginates a portion of pleura and results in a comma-shaped structure seen in the vicinity of the right upper lobe (Fig. 4.29). It is a normal variant.

The pleura is frequently involved in inflammatory, neoplastic, and traumatic insults to the chest. These may result in areas of thickening or distortion along the pleural surface or in the *costophrenic or cardiophrenic angles.* Pleural calcification may also occur (Fig. 4.30).

Diaphragm

The *diaphragm*, which separates the thoracic from the abdominal cavities, appears most often as a smooth, dome-shaped structure on either side. There may be scalloping or irregularities along the diaphragmatic surface, a frequent finding considered to be of little significance. The right hemidiaphragm is slightly higher than the left. Occasionally, gaseous distension of the stomach or colon produces elevation of the left hemidiaphragm above the right. The reason for the lower left hemidiaphragm is the contiguity of the left ventricle of the heart with it and not the bulk of the liver elevating the right hemidiaphragm.

Soft Tissues

Soft tissue images commonly visible on the routine chest radiograph are the axillary fold produced by the pectoral muscles, supraclavicular and neck soft tissues, and breast tissue. In addition, nipple shadows are frequently seen over the lower thorax. They may be mistaken for a lung nodule, but are distinguished by their characteristic location and frequently a second nipple shadow overlying the opposite lung. When this poses a problem, a repeat radiograph with markers on the nipples is indicated (Fig. 4.31).

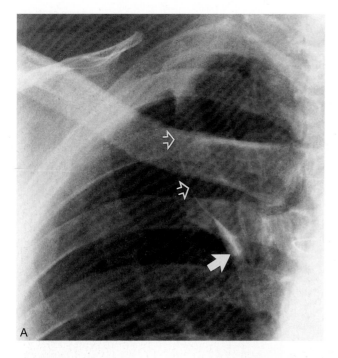

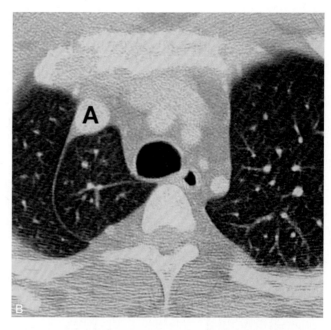

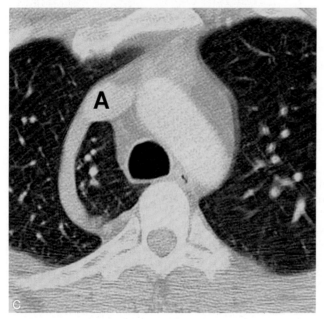

Figure 4.29   A. Azygous fissure (*open arrows*) and azygous vein (*solid arrow*).   This is a normal variant. **B** and **C.** CT images show the azygous vein (*A*) traversing the thorax. The azygous fissure, which represents pleural invagination around the vein as it descends, is seen just posterior to the vein in **B**.

Bony Structures

Bony structures visible on the chest radiograph include the ribs, thoracic vertebrae, lower cervical vertebrae, clavicles, scapulae, and occasionally the heads of the humeri. In addition, the sternum is clearly visible on the lateral chest film. Occasionally, the manubrium projects as a prominence just to the right of the midline. It should not be mistaken for a pulmonary mass. Not uncommonly, cervical ribs are encountered. An abnormal-appearing rib in the cervicothoracic region can be considered a cervical rib if the transverse process to which it is articulating points inferiorly. *Cervical transverse processes point down; thoracic transverse processes point up* (Fig. 4.32).

 ❫ Cervical transverse processes point down; thoracic transverse processes point up.

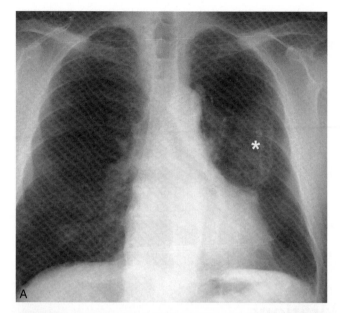

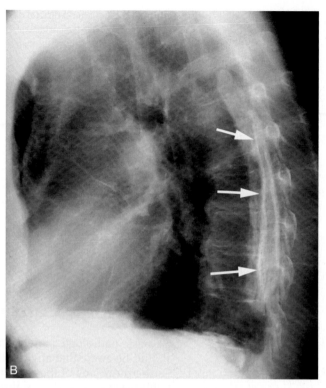

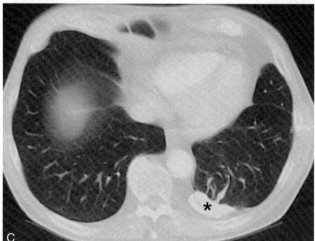

Figure 4.30   Pleural calcification.   A. Frontal radiograph shows a "mass" in the left midlung field (*asterisk*). **B.** Lateral radiograph shows the "mass" to be an area of thick pleural calcification posteriorly (*arrows*). **C.** CT image shows the dense pleural calcification posteriorly (*asterisk*).

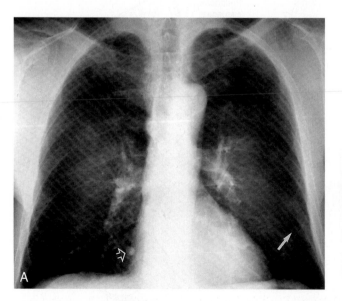

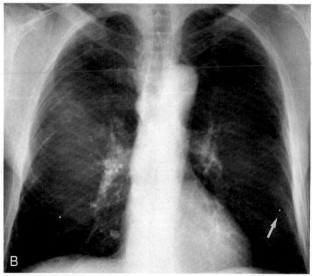

Figure 4.31   Use of nipple markers.   A. Frontal radiograph shows a rounded density in the left midlung field (*solid arrow*). There is a granuloma in the right lower lobe (*open arrow*). **B.** Repeat radiograph made with markers on both nipples. Note how the rounded density on the left corresponds to the nipple shadow (*arrow*).

Figure 4.32   Bilateral cervical ribs (*open arrows*). The cervical transverse processes (*C*) point downward; the thoracic (*T*) point upward.

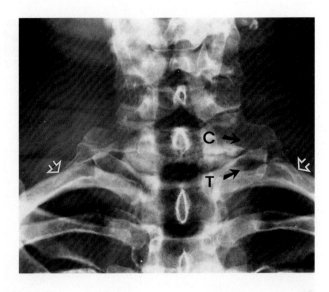

Pathologic Considerations

Six basic pathologic patterns may alter the normal appearance of the lungs. The reader should be aware that any or all of these may be present at one time in the same patient. Furthermore, any of these entities may be combined with abnormalities of the heart and pulmonary vessels. The six abnormalities are as follows:

- Air space disease—consolidation
- Atelectasis—collapse
- Pleural fluid accumulation—effusion
- Masses—tumors and tumor-like abnormalities
- Emphysema—overinflation
- Interstitial changes—fibrosis and/or edema

Figure 4.33 illustrates the effect of these abnormalities on the pulmonary lobule.

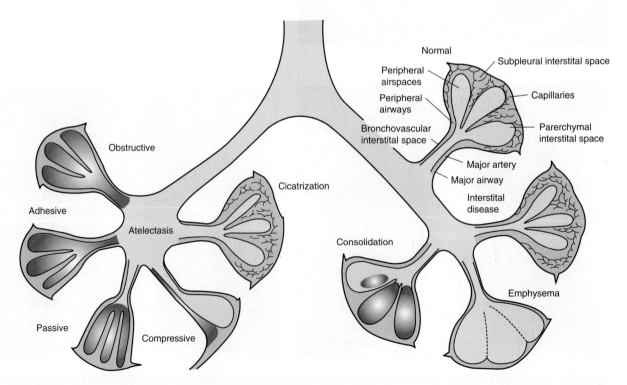

Figure 4.33   Schematic drawing of the four basic pathologic patterns affecting the lungs, atelectasis (five variations), consolidation, emphysema, and interstitial disease, compared with a normal pulmonary lobule.

Air Space Disease—Consolidation

When the air spaces become filled with fluid (inflammatory exudate, blood, edema, or aspirated fluid), they lose their normal lucency and become opaque, fluffy, or cloudlike appearance. By knowing the location of the lung segments and their relationship to the mediastinum and diaphragm, it is possible to accurately localize an area of consolidation by noting the loss of these normal anatomic landmarks.

The basis for visualization of the border of a structure depends on its contiguity with another structure of *different radiographic density.* Hence, we normally see the *silhouette* of the mediastinal structures and the diaphragm because they are of soft tissue density and are outlined by the adjacent air density in the lung. Consolidations adjacent to these borders result in the loss of the normal-appearing borders or silhouettes. This concept was first described by Fleischner and popularized by Felson as the *silhouette sign.*

Silhouette Sign

Fleischner's famous experiment demonstrating the silhouette sign is illustrated in Figure 4.34: An empty x-ray film box was tilted on end; liquid paraffin was poured into it and allowed to congeal into a triangular density. A second empty film box was taped behind the first box, and both were radiographed (see Fig. 4.34A). The gray image of the solid paraffin represents a "cardiac border," and the blackness of the air within both boxes represents "aerated lung," creating a model for demonstrating the effects of consolidation on the silhouette of the "heart." The boxes were again radiographed in the upright position after mineral oil (of approximately the same radiographic density as solid paraffin) was poured into the empty box behind the one containing the paraffin (see Fig. 4.34B). Note

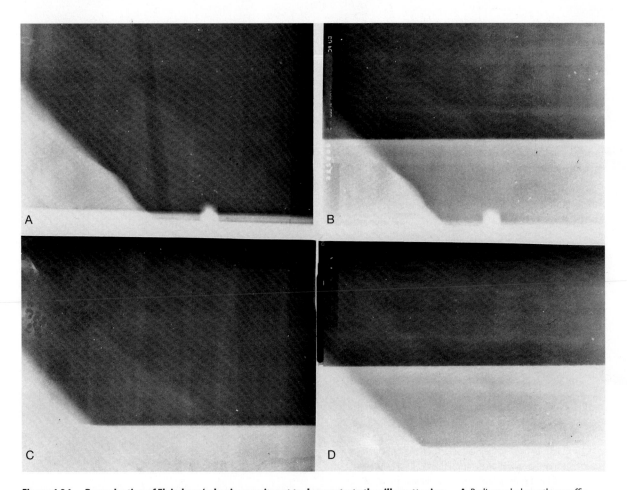

Figure 4.34   Reproduction of Fleischner's classic experiment to demonstrate the silhouette sign.   A. Radiograph shows the paraffin in one box with air in the second. **B.** Radiograph shows paraffin in one box with mineral oil in the second box. The border of the paraffin is still visible. **C.** Radiograph shows mineral oil added to the box with paraffin. The silhouette of the lower portion of the paraffin now disappears. **D.** Radiograph shows mineral oil in both boxes. The only portion of the paraffin obscured is that covered by mineral oil sitting immediately adjacent to it (lower air–fluid level).

the air–fluid level at the border between the mineral oil and the air in the second box. More importantly, the image of the "heart" is still clearly visible because of the air adjacent to its border. Thus, an area of consolidation behind the heart does not obliterate its border.

The mineral oil was then poured out of the back box and into the box containing the paraffin. A radiograph of this (see Fig. 4.34C) shows obliteration of a portion of the border of the "heart" image because of the contiguity of the two structures of similar radiographic density. This is analogous to pneumonia in the right middle lobe or in the lingula obliterating the cardiac border (Fig. 4.35).

Finally, mineral oil was poured into the second box, with the resultant radiograph (shown in Fig. 4.34D). Note the obliteration of the lower "cardiac" border by the "consoli-

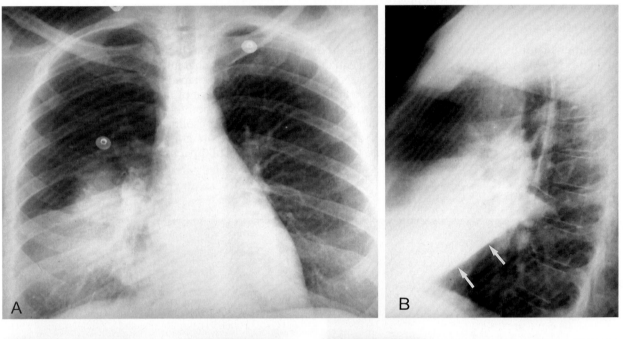

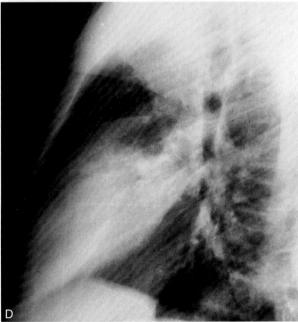

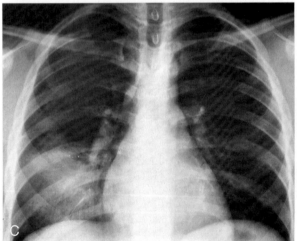

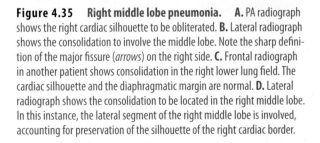

Figure 4.35   Right middle lobe pneumonia.   A. PA radiograph shows the right cardiac silhouette to be obliterated. **B.** Lateral radiograph shows the consolidation to involve the middle lobe. Note the sharp definition of the major fissure (*arrows*) on the right side. **C.** Frontal radiograph in another patient shows consolidation in the right lower lung field. The cardiac silhouette and the diaphragmatic margin are normal. **D.** Lateral radiograph shows the consolidation to be located in the right middle lobe. In this instance, the lateral segment of the right middle lobe is involved, accounting for preservation of the silhouette of the right cardiac border.

dated" area adjacent to it. However, the upper "cardiac" border is clearly visible along with an air–fluid level behind it because this upper border is still surrounded by air.

In summary, an intrapulmonary abnormality that is contiguous with the border of the heart, aorta, or diaphragm will result in the loss of that border on the radiograph. This border will not be obliterated unless the lesion is anatomically contiguous with it. These principles apply not only to the PA or AP chest radiograph but also to the lateral view and, in addition, to certain abdominal radiographs that show loss of the psoas margin with retroperitoneal inflammation or hemorrhage.

> ▶ An intrapulmonary abnormality that is contiguous with the border of the heart, aorta, or diaphragm will result in the loss of that border on the radiograph.

The following consolidations are illustrated: right middle lobe (see Fig. 4.35), right upper lobe (Fig. 4.36), right lower and middle lobe (Fig. 4.37), left upper lobe and lingual (Fig. 4.38), lingula (Fig. 4.39), and left lower lobe (Fig. 4.40).

On the lateral radiograph, we can identify each hemidiaphragm because of a normal-appearing silhouette sign. The anterior portion of the cardiac border lies in contiguity with the left hemidiaphragm. Therefore, the anterior one-third of the left diaphragmatic image is obliterated by the cardiac border. This is one reliable way to identify each hemidiaphragm (Fig. 4.41). Since the x-ray beam penetrates the chest from right to left, the right posterior costophrenic angle is always larger due to the magnification effect. The gastric air bubble usually resides underneath the left hemidiaphragm. A summary of localization using the silhouette sign is in Table 4.1. Although the localizing signs are extremely useful, the reader is cautioned that they are not always infallible. For example, an area of consolidation in the lateral segment of the right middle lobe will not always obliterate the right cardiac border (see Fig. 4.35**C** and **D**). It is therefore important to use two views at all times when evaluating patients with lung disease.

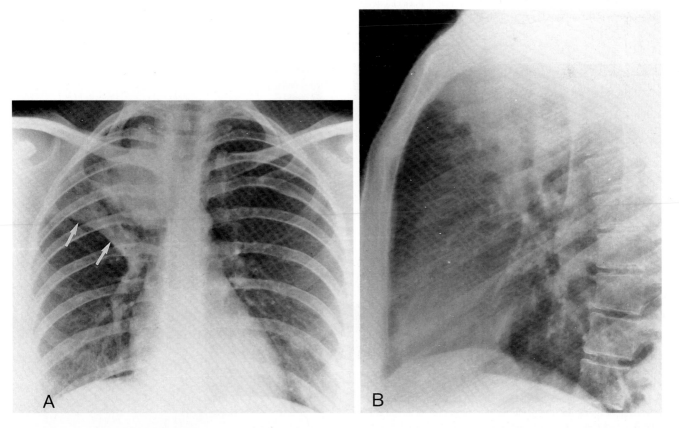

Figure 4.36   Right upper lobe consolidation and atelectasis.   A. Frontal radiograph shows obliteration of the superior mediastinal silhouette on the right. Volume loss is present as evidenced by elevation of the minor fissure, which is well demarcated (*arrows*). **B.** Lateral radiograph shows the upper lobe consolidation.

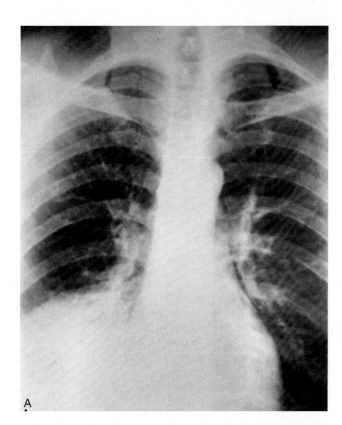

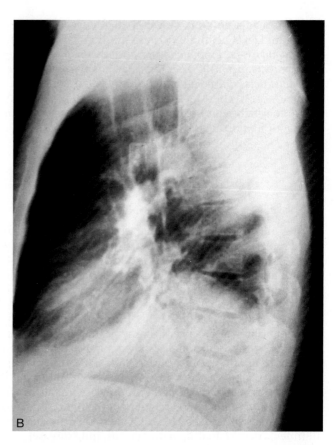

Figure 4.37   Right lower and middle lobe infiltration.   A. Frontal radiograph shows increased density in the right lower lung field that obscures the right hemidiaphragm and also a portion of the right heart border. **B.** Lateral view shows the right hemidiaphragm to be obscured by the right lower lobe infiltrate. The lower portion of the cardiac silhouette shows increased density as a result of the involvement of a portion of the right middle lobe as well.

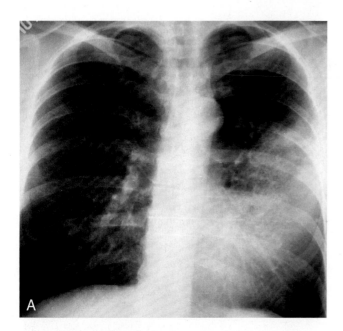

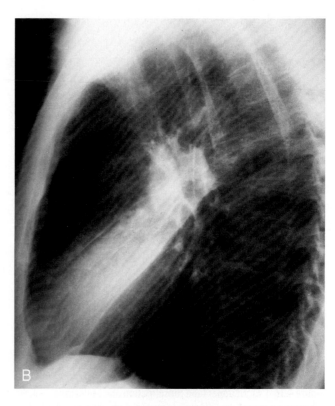

Figure 4.38   Combined left upper lobe and lingular consolidation.
A. Frontal radiograph shows the left cardiac border obscured. Consolidation extends above the cardiac shadow into the anterior segment of the left upper lobe. **B.** Lateral radiograph shows consolidation to mostly overlap the heart.

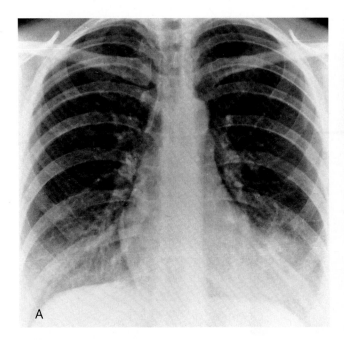

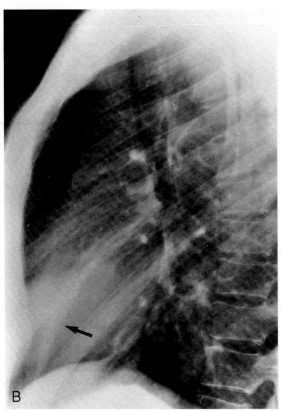

Figure 4.39   Consolidation in the lingula.   A. Frontal radiograph shows the silhouette of the apex of the heart to be obscured by the overlying consolidation. **B.** Lateral radiograph shows the consolidation anteriorly (*arrow*).

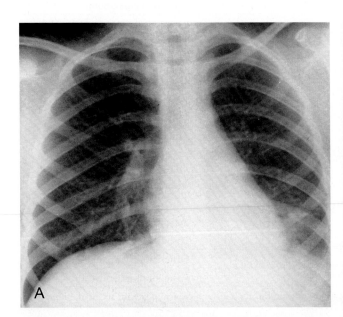

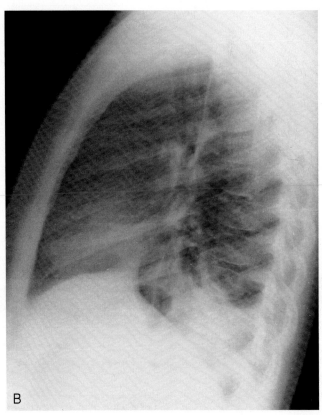

Figure 4.40   Left lower lobe pneumonia.   A. Frontal radiograph shows the silhouette of the diaphragm on the left to be obliterated. **B.** Lateral radiograph shows the posterior consolidation.

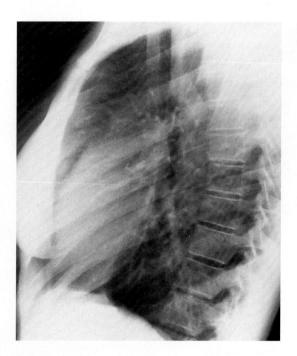

Figure 4.41   Normal lateral radiograph showing the diaphragm.   (See text for description.)

Table 4.1 LOCALIZATION USING THE SILHOUETTE SIGN

Structure	Obliteration/ Overlap	General Location	Anatomic Location of Border
Heart	Obliteration	Anterior	Middle lobe
			Lingula
			Anterior mediastinum
			Anterior segment of an upper lobe
			Lower end of oblique fissure
			Anterior portion of pleural cavity
	Overlap	Posterior	Lower lobe
			Posterior mediastinum
			Posterior portion of pleural cavity
Ascending aorta (right border)	Obliteration	Anterior	Anterior segment, right upper lobe
			Right middle lobe
			Right anterior mediastinum
			Anterior portion, right pleural cavity
	Overlap	Posterior	Superior segment, right lower lobe
			Posterior segment, right upper lobe
			Posterior mediastinum
			Posterior pleural cavity
Aortic knob (left border)	Obliteration	Posterior	Apical-posterior segment, left upper lobe
			Posterior mediastinum
			Posterior pleural cavity
	Overlap	Anterior	Anterior segment, left upper lobe
			Far posterior portion mediastinum or pleural cavity
Descending	Obliteration	Posterior	Superior and posterior basal segments, aorta left lower lobe

Cervicothoracic Sign

The *cervicothoracic sign*, a variant of the silhouette sign, is useful in determining whether a mass that is seen above the level of the clavicles is intrapulmonary or mediastinal. If this mass is seen in its entirety, it must lie *posteriorly* because it is surrounded by air and therefore must be entirely within the thorax. If it is located *anteriorly*, its border will be obliterated by the images of the neck structures and will seem to disappear into the neck. Therefore, it is cervicothoracic, lying partially in the anterior part of the mediastinum and partially in the neck. Figure 4.42 illustrates this in a patient with a prominent brachiocephalic artery, the most common cause of this finding.

Air Bronchogram

Another useful sign that indicates consolidation in the lung is the *air bronchogram*. As previously mentioned, normal bronchi are not visible on the chest radiograph. This is because they have thin walls, contain air, and are surrounded by air in the lung parenchyma. However, parenchymal consolidation that results in a water density in the alveolar spaces in the lung may demonstrate adjacent bronchi because the air within their lumens will stand out in stark contrast to the dense lung (Fig. 4.43). The formation of the air bronchogram sign is illustrated in Figure 4.44. Plastic tubing sealed at each end was placed in an empty plastic container and radiographed (Fig. 4.44**A**). The walls are barely discernible, because the tubing contains air and there is air surrounding it. Water was then added to the container to cover the tubing (Fig. 4.44**B**). The wall is now barely visible.

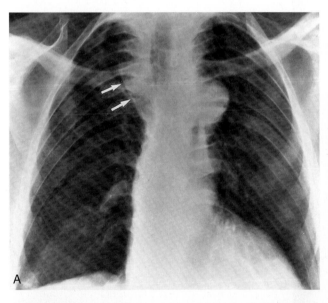

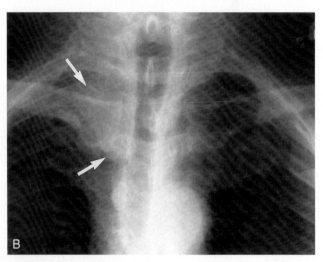

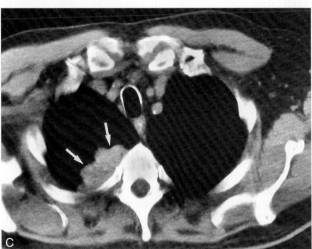

Figure 4.42 Cervicothoracic sign. A. Frontal radiograph shows a right paratracheal density (*arrows*). Note that the image of this density disappears as it crosses the clavicle. This indicates that the structure in question is located anteriorly and has entered the neck. This density is, in fact, the tortuous right brachiocephalic artery. If this structure were located posteriorly, it would be seen in its entirety above as well as below the clavicle, as in **B**. **B.** A right paratracheal density (*arrows*) extends above as well as below the clavicle. **C.** CT scan shows the density to be located in the posterior aspect of the apical segment of the right upper lobe (*arrows*).

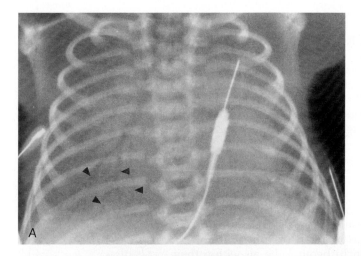

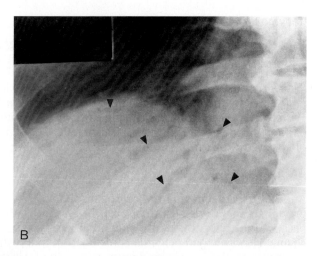

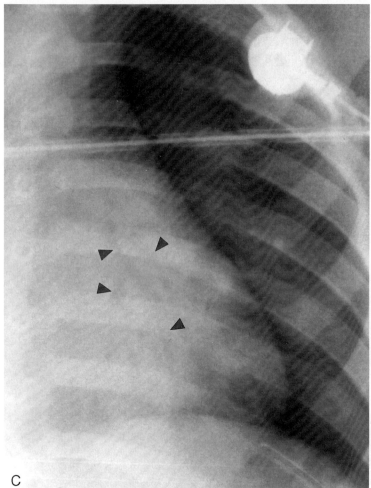

Figure 4.43   Air bronchograms.   A. Air bronchograms in the right lung (*arrowheads*) in an infant with hyaline membrane disease. **B** and **C.** Detail views of the lower lobes in two other patients with pneumonia show multiple air bronchograms (*arrowheads*).

However, the air within the tubing defines its lumen (air bronchogram). Water was then poured into the tubing with the resultant radiographic appearance (shown in Fig. 4.44**C**). As illustrated here, there is no difference between the water inside the tube and the outside (no air bronchogram).

The air bronchogram is a valuable sign that, when present, is virtually diagnostic of air space (acinar) disease. A pleural or mediastinal mass may be excluded because there are no bronchi traversing these lesions. Similarly, a mass in the lung should engulf, occlude, or displace bronchi, and therefore the air bronchogram would not occur. If an air bronchogram is seen within a round pulmonary density, the lesion is most likely an

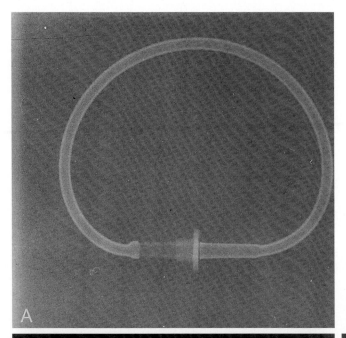

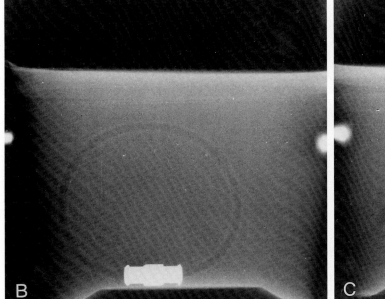

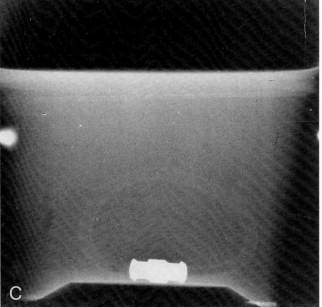

Figure 4.44   Air bronchogram formation.   A. Radiograph of a plastic tube shows its walls. **B.** When the tube is submerged in water, the lumen and walls are still visible as would be seen in an air bronchogram. **C.** When water fills the tubing, the lumen is obscured.

inflammatory process, an infarct, a contusion, or, more rarely, an alveolar cell carcinoma or lymphoma. All of these are acinar lesions. Rare exceptions to this rule are bronchiectasis and chronic bronchitis, in which thickening of the bronchial walls may result in tubular air profiles (Fig. 4.45).

Atelectasis—Collapse

Atelectasis is a condition of volume loss of some portion of the lung. It may be massive, with complete collapse of an entire lung or, more commonly, less extensive and involve a lobe, segment, or subsegment. Atelectasis results from a number of causes, which are illustrated in Figure 4.33.

- ○ *Obstructive* atelectasis, the most common type, results when a bronchus is obstructed by a neoplasm, foreign body, or mucous plug (Fig. 4.46). Quite often, there is associated pneumonia distal to the site of obstruction.
- ○ *Compressive* atelectasis is a purely physical phenomenon in which the normal lung is compressed by a tumor, emphysematous bulla, or an enlarged heart (Fig. 4.47).

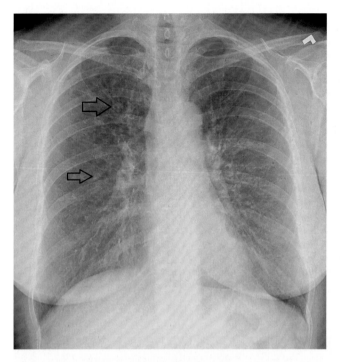

Figure 4.45   Bronchiectasis.   Thickened bronchial walls produce a tubular pattern in a patient with bronchiectasis (*arrows*).

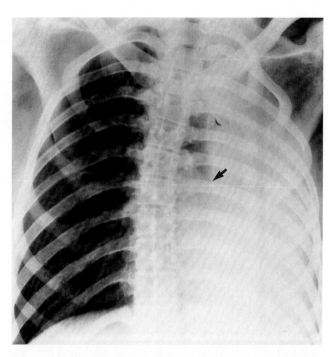

Figure 4.46   Obstructive atelectasis on the left.   There is complete collapse of the left lung caused by a central obstructing lesion in the left mainstem bronchus (*arrow*). The heart and mediastinum have shifted to the left.

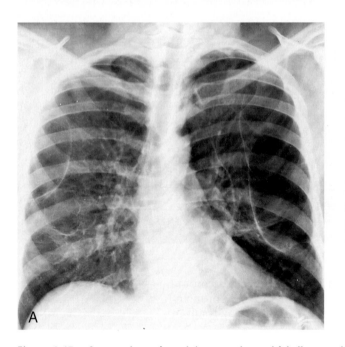

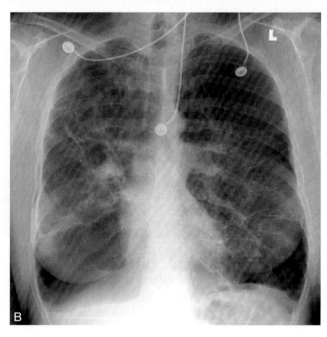

Figure 4.47   Compressive atelectasis in two patients with bullous emphysema.   The large bullae in each lung compress and displace the remaining lung markings.

○ *Cicatrization* atelectasis is produced by organizing scar tissue (Fig. 4.48). This occurs most often in healing tuberculosis (TB) and other granulomatous diseases, as well as in entities such as pulmonary infarct and pulmonary trauma.

○ *Adhesive* atelectasis is a unique type of volume loss that occurs in the presence of patent airways. The mechanism involved is believed to be the inactivation of surfactant. A common example of this is hyaline membrane disease (HMD) (Fig. 4.49).

○ *Passive* atelectasis results from the normal compliance of the lung in the presence of either pneumothorax or pleural effusion. The airways remain patent (Fig. 4.50).

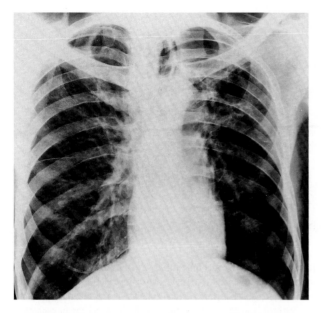

Figure 4.48   Cicatrization atelectasis.   Scarring in the left lung has produced atelectatic changes in the left upper lobe. Note the left lower lung lucency indicating left lower lobe hyperinflation compensating for the collapsed left upper lobe.

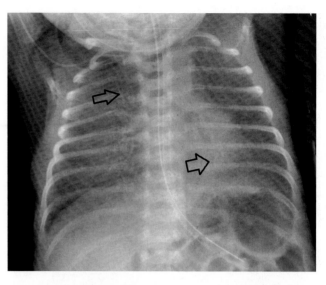

Figure 4.49   Adhesive atelectasis in a premature newborn with hyaline membrane disease.   There is a "ground glass" opacification to both lungs with air bronchograms (*arrows*).

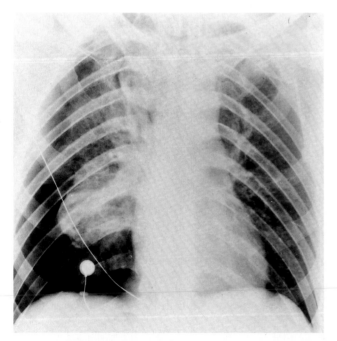

Figure 4.50   Passive atelectasis.
There is partial collapse of the right lung in a patient with large right pneumothorax.

Direct and Indirect Signs

The radiographic signs of lobar collapse are of two types: *direct* and *indirect*. The only direct sign is displacement or deviation of an interlobar fissure. There are several indirect signs, including increased density of the collapsed lobe, compensatory hyperinflation of an adjacent lobe, hilar deviation toward the collapsed lobe (superior with upper lobe collapse, inferior with lower lobe collapse), diaphragmatic elevation, contralateral hyper-inflation, ipsilateral mediastinal or tracheal shift, ipsilateral rib approximation, shift of a granuloma in an adjacent lobe, and sometimes absence of an air bronchogram in the involved lobe. In any patient, one or all of these signs are usually present (Figs. 4.51 and 4.52). Of the indirect signs, the most reliable is displacement of the hilar vessels, which shift in the direction of the collapse.

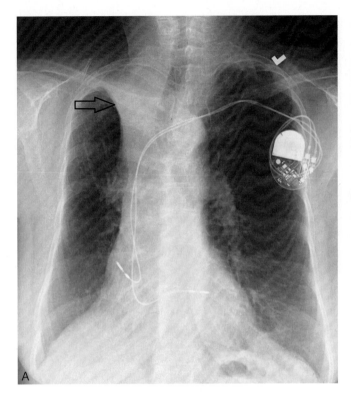

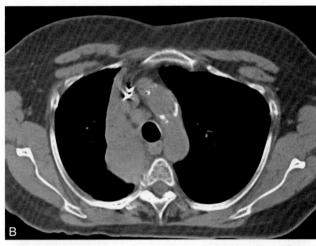

Figure 4.51   Right upper lobe collapse in a patient with a central lung carcinoma.   A. There is consolidation in the atelectatic right upper lobe. The minor fissure is elevated (*arrow*) and there is a mass in the right hilar region. The mediastinum is shifted to the right. **B.** These findings are confirmed on the CT.

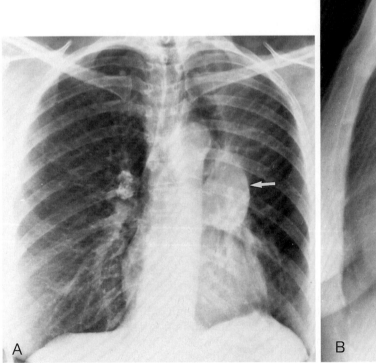

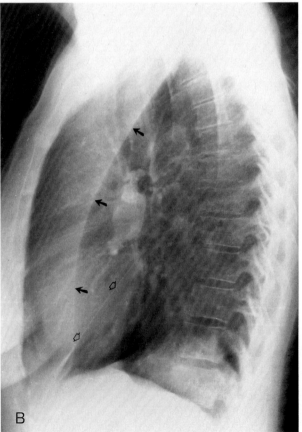

Figure 4.52   Left upper lobe collapse in a patient with a central carcinoma.   A. Frontal radiograph shows a mass in the left hilar region (*arrow*). Note the shift of the left-sided pulmonary vessels upward. **B.** Lateral radiograph shows anterior bowing of the major fissure on the left (*solid arrows*). The normal right-sided major fissure is also shown (*open arrows*).

In general, the upper lobes collapse medially, upward, and anteriorly. On the right side, the most reliable signs are an increase in density with obliteration of the right mediastinal border and shift of the minor fissure superiorly (see Fig. 4.51). On the left, a characteristic sign is a vague increased density in the left lung with preservation of the aortic knob. In both instances, the ipsilateral diaphragm is usually elevated. On the lateral view, the major fissure is displaced anteriorly and superiorly (see Fig. 4.52).

The right middle lobe and lingula collapse downward and medially obscuring the cardiac border on the frontal film. On the lateral view, a triangular-shaped density is seen overlying the cardiac silhouette (Fig. 4.53).

The lower lobes collapse posteriorly, medially, and downward. On a frontal radiograph, the classic lower lobe collapse is a triangular-shaped density behind the cardiac shadow. The ipsilateral hemidiaphragm is also obscured. On the lateral view, a fissure shift may also be appreciated. In total collapse, a wedge-shaped density occurs posteriorly and inferiorly, extending down to the diaphragm (Fig. 4.54). In some instances, lower lobe collapse is difficult to detect on the frontal radiograph. Regardless, atelectasis may signify a centrally obstructing tumor and CT may be necessary. In the inpatient or critical care setting, a patient with acute dyspnea who also has atelectasis will frequently have an obstructing mucous plug that needs to be cleared with pulmonary toilet or bronchoscopy.

> A patient with acute dyspnea who also has atelectasis will frequently have an obstructing mucous plug that needs to be cleared.

Linear Atelectasis

Linear or *"plate-like"* atelectasis, a less severe form of partial collapse, may occur throughout the lungs and appears as a dense line in one or more lobes (Fig. 4.55). Dependent atelectasis involving a portion of the lower lobe frequently silhouettes or obscures the adjacent hemidiaphragm (Fig. 4.56). This can be a cause of low-grade fever, but it is frequently difficult to distinguish this from pneumonia without a lateral projection.

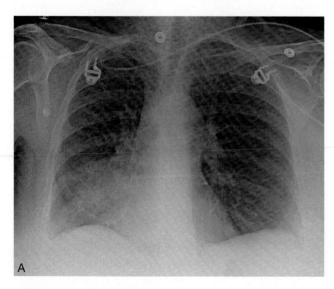

A

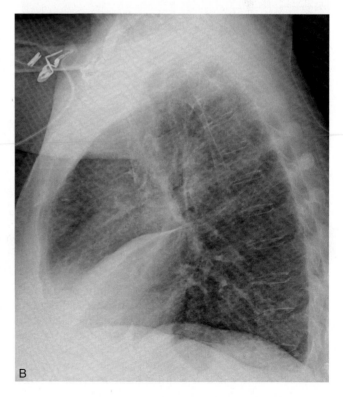

B

Figure 4.53   Right middle lobe collapse.   A. Frontal radiograph shows obliteration of the right heart border. **B.** lateral view shows an anterior linear stripe which represents the collapsed right middle lobe.

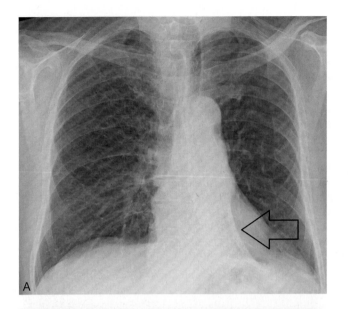

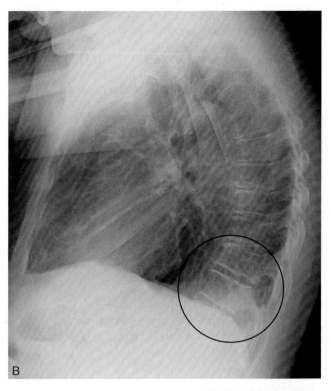

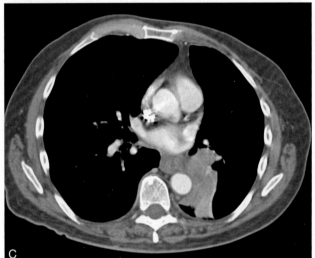

Figure 4.54   Left lower lobe atelectasis.   A. PA radiograph shows retrocardiac consolidation (*arrow*) with an obscured left medial hemidiaphragm and a left hilar mass ("too many bumps"). **B.** Lateral view shows subtle consolidation overlying the lower spine (*circle*). **C.** Left lower lobe atelectasis and left hilar mass are confirmed on the CT.

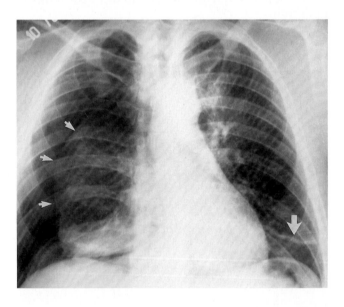

Figure 4.55   Linear atelectasis in the left lower lobe (*large arrow*) in a patient with a tension pneumothorax on the right (*small arrows*).

Pleural Fluid Accumulation—Effusion

Pleural effusions occur in a variety of pathologic conditions, including infection, embolism, neoplasm, CHF, and trauma. Pleural fluid may be either free or loculated within the pleural space. Free pleural fluid occupies the most dependent portion of the pleural cavity and can appear as a meniscus or apparent "elevation of the diaphragm" on an upright radiograph (Fig. 4.57**A**) or as an increase in the overall opacity of one hemithorax on a recumbent film. A decubitus view can quantify the amount of pleural fluid and determine if it is loculated (Fig. 4.57**B**).

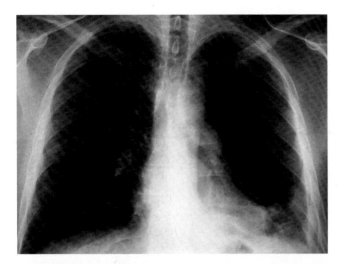

Figure 4.56 Left basilar atelectasis. Left basilar consolidation silhouettes out the adjacent diaphragm. Distinguishing atelectasis from pneumonia on a frontal view only is difficult.

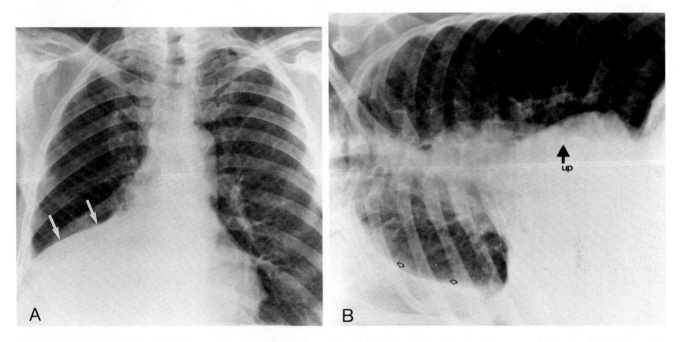

A

B

Figure 4.57 Large right pleural effusion. **A.** Frontal radiograph shows right middle and lower lobe atelectasis with a suspected right pleural effusion (*arrows*). **B.** Right lateral decubitus view shows most of the fluid layers out (*open arrows*).

Loculated Pleural Fluid

Loculated pleural fluid occurs when fibrous adhesions form. Occasionally, the fluid will collect in a fissure to form a *"pseudotumor"* or "phantom tumor" (Figs. 4.58 and 4.59). This usually occurs in patients with CHF and clears when that condition resolves. A pseudotumor may be recognized by its tapered margins at a fissure as well as the fact that it changes shape with positioning.

▶ A pseudotumor may be recognized by its tapered margins at a fissure as well as the fact that it changes shape with positioning.

Other Signs

Other signs of pleural effusion include widening of the pleural space, blunting of the costophrenic angle, and mediastinal shift in massive effusion. It is estimated that up to

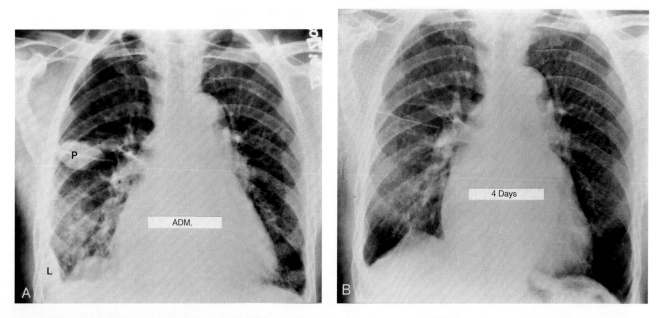

Figure 4.58   Pseudotumor caused by pleural effusion.   A. Radiograph taken on admission (*ADM*) shows a mass-like collection of fluid along the minor fissure (*P*). There is loculated fluid (*L*) in the right costophrenic angle in this patient with congestive heart failure. **B.** Radiograph made 4 days later shows a decrease in the cardiac size. The pleural effusion is also diminished. The pseudotumor is no longer present.

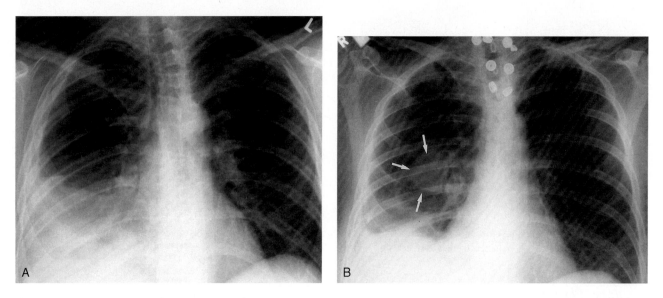

Figure 4.59   Pulmonary pseudotumor.   A. Initial radiograph shows a large right pleural effusion. **B.** One day later, the overall effusion is less. However, loculated pleural fluid in the major fissure produces a pseudotumor (*arrows*).

300 mL of pleural fluid may accumulate in the costophrenic sulcus posteriorly before an effusion is apparent on the frontal radiograph! Therefore, lateral and decubitus views are more sensitive for the detection of small pleural effusions.

 ▶ Up to 300 mL of pleural fluid may accumulate in the costophrenic sulcus posteriorly before an effusion is apparent on the frontal radiograph!

Patients with unexplained pleural effusions should be carefully studied for neoplasm or empyema (infection of the pleural space). In addition to cytologic and microbiology

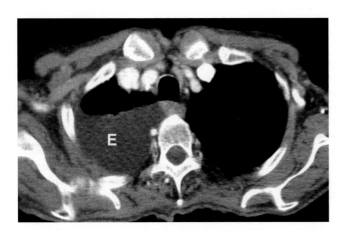

Figure 4.60 Right-sided pleural effusion (*E*) as demonstrated on a CT scan.

studies of the fluid itself, it is important to look for associated lung masses, adenopathy, pleural enhancement, or pleural nodularity on CT. Simple pleural fluid on CT is commonly associated with atelectasis of the adjacent lung (Fig. 4.60).

Masses—Tumors and Tumor-Like Abnormalities

Lung and mediastinal masses are a very important and unfortunately a common group of diseases. In general, a variety of clinical, historic, and radiologic findings are used to predict the nature of the mass. Ultimately, the diagnosis rests in the hands of the pathologist. The most common etiologies of the solitary pulmonary nodule are either tumors or granulomas. Table 4.2 lists the differential diagnoses of common and uncommon pulmonary nodules.

Table 4.2 DIFFERENTIAL DIAGNOSES OF PULMONARY NODULES

Diagnosis	Solitary	Multiple	Growth[a]
Common			
Bronchial adenoma	X		0/I
Carcinoma, primary	X	X	I
Granuloma—tuberculosis, fungus	X	X	0
Hamartoma	X	X	0/I
Metastases	X	X	I
Simulated nodule (nipple, bone lesion, skin tumor, foreign body, artifact)	X	X	0
Uncommon			
Abscess	X	X	D
Hematoma	X	X	D
Infarct	X	X	D
Loculated pleural fluid	X	X	D
Cryptogenic organizing pneumonia	X	X	0/D
Pneumoconiosis, conglomerate mass	X	X	0
Sarcoidosis		X	0/D
Sequestration	X		0
Vascular lesion	X	X	0/I

[a]I, increase in time; D, decrease in time; 0, no growth.

Cavitary Masses

Some nodules may cavitate (Fig. 4.61). The most common masses that cavitate are lung carcinoma (Fig. 4.61**A** and **B**), necrotizing infections (abscess), and metastatic lesions (usually squamous cell). TB or fungal pneumonia (Fig. 4.61**C**), hematomas, and pneumatoceles are other cavitary masses that may be encountered. Much has been made of the thickness of the wall of a cavitary mass regarding its pathogenesis. A cavitary mass with a wall thickness greater than 15 mm is more likely to be malignant. A cavitary mass with a wall thickness less than 4 mm is likely benign. However, this criterion is not specific enough to reliably differentiate between a benign and malignant process. Percutaneous CT-guided needle biopsy or bronchoscopy is usually necessary for histologic confirmation. In some instances, such as trauma or infection, it may be possible to observe cavitation develop as in a pneumatocele (Fig. 4.62). In most instances, the cavity will be detected on the initial chest radiograph. An air–fluid level in a mass is pathognomonic of cavitation.

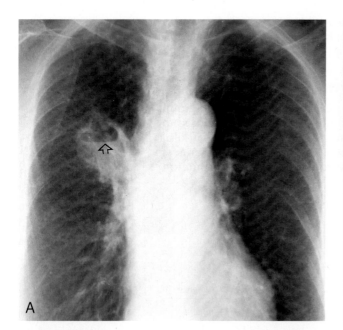

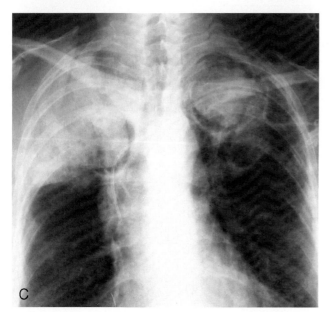

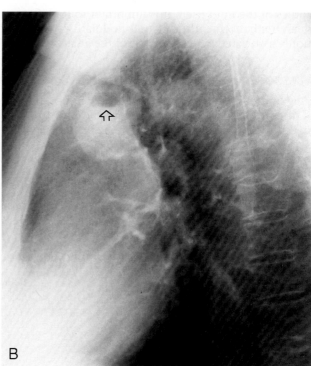

Figure 4.61   Cavitating lung lesions.   Frontal (**A**) and lateral (**B**) views show cavitation in a right upper lobe carcinoma. Note the air–fluid level within the cavity (*arrows*). **C.** Aspergillosis with bilateral upper lobe cavities containing large mycetomas ("fungus balls").

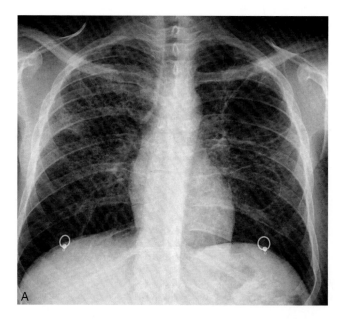

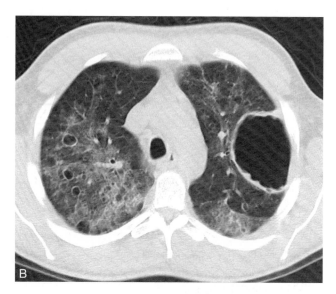

Figure 4.62 **Left upper lobe pneumatocele in an area of pulmonary hematoma secondary to trauma.** **A.** Frontal radiograph shows a thin-walled cavity (pneumatocele) in the left lung. **B.** CT shows bilateral pneumatoceles and associated ground glass opacities. The combination is suspicious for *Pneumocystis carinii* pneumonia.

 ▶ An air–fluid level in a mass is pathognomonic of cavitation.

Evaluating Pulmonary Nodules

The first step in evaluating a pulmonary mass (nodule) is to locate its epicenter. Doing so will allow one to determine whether the mass began in the lung, the mediastinum, the pleura, or the chest wall. A similar analysis is made when confronted with masses anywhere else in the body.

 ▶ The first step in evaluating a pulmonary mass (nodule) is to locate its epicenter.

When evaluating solitary pulmonary nodules, the following studies are useful: an old chest radiograph, CT, MR, and PET imaging. As mentioned previously, the most valuable study a radiologist can have for evaluating a solitary nodule is the patient's old chest x-ray. The reader should be cautioned, however, that in reviewing serial chest images, it is necessary to examine not only the most recent old chest study but also one that dates back a considerable period of time. A very slowly growing nodule may not appear to have grown from one exam to the next. However, when comparing studies *out of sequence*, the difference may be quite dramatic. Figure 4.63 shows a series of circles, each differing in diameter by 1 mm. It is difficult to tell the difference between consecutive circles. However, by comparing drawings out of sequence a significant difference is apparent. A change in size also represents a change in volume, which increases by the cube power of its radius. Thus, a lesion that doubles in its diameter has actually increased eightfold in volume!

 ▶ A lesion that doubles in its diameter has actually increased eightfold in volume.

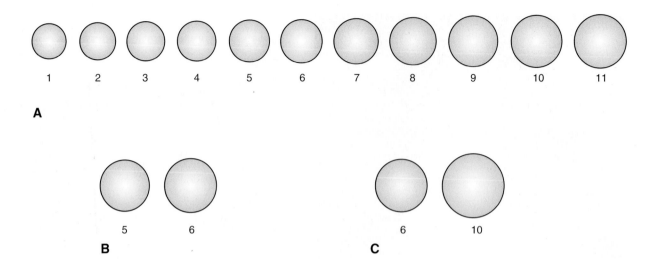

A

Figure 4.63   Importance of viewing serial radiographs out of sequence.   A. Each of these circles varies in diameter by 1 mm. **B.** Comparing circles 5 and 6 shows the difference to be minimal, if any. **C.** Comparing circles 6 and 10 shows a significant change. Often the human eye cannot detect the small changes in the size of nodules.

Spiculated Margins

A spiculated margin in any mass is a sign of malignancy (Figs. 4.64 and 4.65). It indicates that the mass is invading the surrounding tissue. This finding is similar to that seen at the border of a breast carcinoma (Fig. 4.66). Calcification in a lesion is suggestive of a benign entity, especially when it is centrally located or "popcorn shaped" (Fig. 4.67). The reader is cautioned, however, in using calcification as the sole criterion of the nature of the lesion, because a scar carcinoma may engulf a calcified granuloma. In these instances, the calcification may be eccentric or stippled.

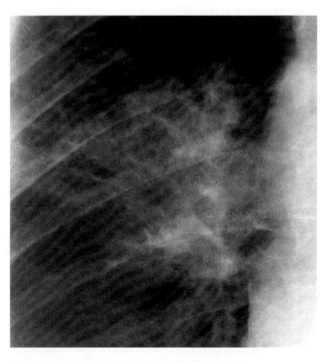

**Figure 4.64   Spiculation in a lung carcinoma.   Detail view of a perihilar carcinoma shows the speculated irregular margin.

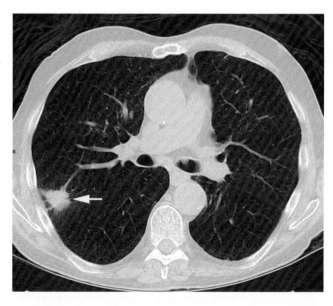

**Figure 4.65   Spiculation in a lung carcinoma.   CT image shows a right upper lobe mass (*arrow*) with a spiculated margin.

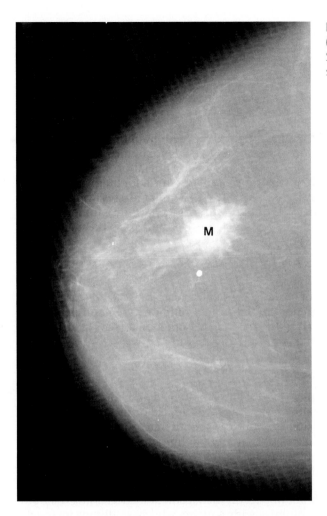

Figure 4.66   Carcinoma of the breast (*M*) showing irregular spiculated margins.
Spiculation indicates invasion. Note the similarity to Figure 4.64.

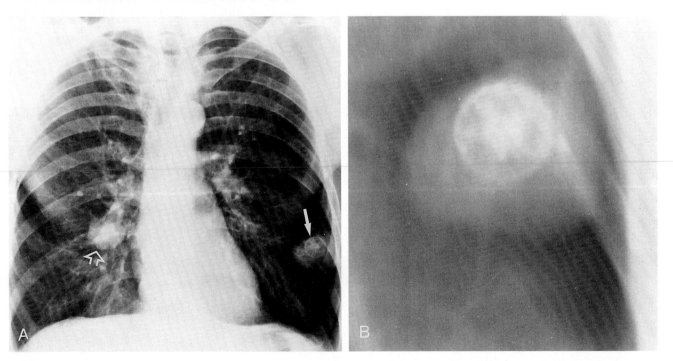

Figure 4.67   Calcification in a lung lesion.   A. Frontal radiograph shows bilateral lung masses. The mass on the right (*open arrow*) contains no calcification. There is calcification on the left (*solid arrow*). **B.** Tomogram of the left-sided mass shows the calcification. This lesion was a granuloma that was later engulfed by a carcinoma.

▶ Spiculated margins of any mass suggest malignancy and indicate that the mass is invading the surrounding tissue.
▶ Calcification in a pulmonary mass suggests a benign process.

Computed Tomography

CT is the most useful imaging tool for evaluating patients with pulmonary and mediastinal masses (Fig. 4.68). The information gained includes evidence of mediastinal invasion (Fig. 4.69), chest wall invasion (Fig. 4.70), presence of peripheral or multiple nodules (Fig. 4.71), and calcification (Fig. 4.72). This information is critical for lung cancer staging purposes. Contrast-enhanced CT may be used to differentiate hilar masses from dilated or enlarged pulmonary vessels. The latter will opacify with contrast, while a tumor will not. CT is also useful for detecting multiple metastases (Fig. 4.73) and is also the mainstay for guided percutaneous biopsy (Fig. 4.74).

Magnetic Resonance Imaging

As previously mentioned, chest MRI of the chest is useful for cardiovascular disease, including aortic aneurysms, dissection, intramural hematoma, pulmonary embolism, helping stage patients with a Pancoast (apical) lung cancer or mesothelioma (see Fig. 4.17), and assessing for diaphragmatic tears with trauma.

Positron Emission Tomography Scan

Finally, positron emission tomography (PET) scan has emerged as a critical modality in oncological diagnosis. PET measures the level of glucose uptake or metabolic activity of tissues. Due to their rapid cell division and nuclear mitotic rate, cancer cells generally have higher activity or standard uptake value than normal human cells. PET scans can be performed to facilitate the workup of a suspicious pulmonary nodule. Second, the fact that a "whole-body" PET scan is performed allows simultaneous initial staging evaluation of a wide array of thoracic cancers, including lung, esophageal, and breast cancer as well as lymphoma. This has had a significant impact on management by decreasing the number of unnecessary or "futile" thoracotomies with patients who have distant metastatic disease. PET exams are commonly combined with a simultaneous CT that help localize abnormalities and decrease scan time.

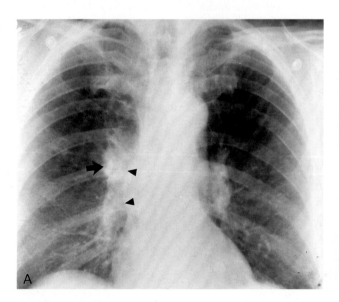
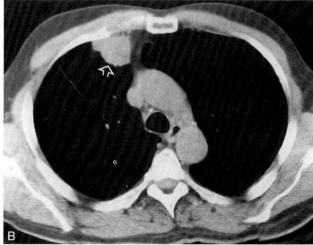

Figure 4.68   Lung carcinoma, right upper lobe.   A. Frontal radiograph shows a mass (*arrow*) just above the right hilum. The mass does not obscure the image of the ascending aorta (*arrowheads*), indicating a location either anterior or posterior to that structure. **B.** CT image shows the mass to be located in the anterior segment of the right upper lobe (*arrow*) adjacent to the pleura.

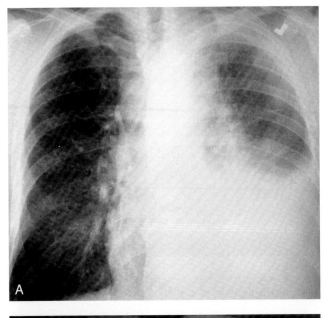

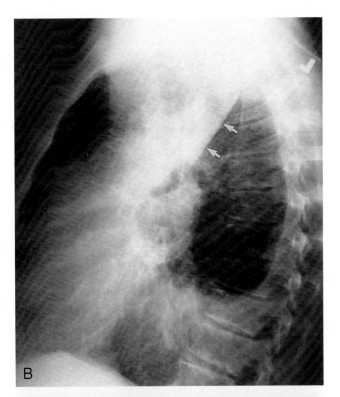

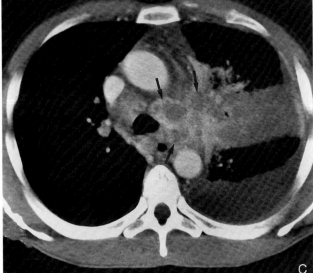

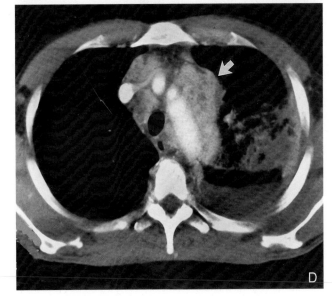

Figure 4.69   Mediastinal invasion from metastatic carcinoma.
A. Frontal radiograph shows consolidation in the lingula and left lower lobe. There is a large left pleural effusion. The upper mediastinum is widened, particularly on the left, where the aortic arch is indistinct. **B.** Lateral radiograph shows increased density along the upper major fissure on the left (*arrows*) as well as over the area of the aortic arch. **C.** CT image shows a broad area of consolidation in the left upper lobe as well as necrotic (*gray*) foci of tumor in mediastinal lymph nodes (*arrows*). **D.** CT section adjacent to the aortic arch shows the mediastinal invasion (*arrow*). Note the pleural effusions in **C** and **D**.

Biopsy

Patients with pulmonary nodules are often submitted to a battery of diagnostic studies, including chest and abdominal CT, bone scans, and PET. These are performed before histologic confirmation of the lesion in the hope that a primary lesion will be found, thus indicating that the pulmonary lesion is metastatic. The final diagnosis, however, is predicated on tissue examination. It is now routine to perform a biopsy of a pulmonary nodule percutaneously or transbronchially under fluoroscopic or CT guidance (see Fig. 4.74). We have a cytology "minilab" in our department where a cytopathologist examines aspirated

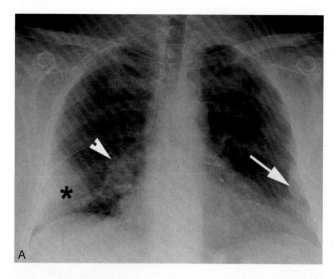
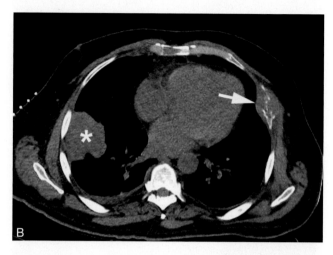

Figure 4.70   Lung carcinoma with chest wall invasion.   A. Frontal radiograph shows a large peripheral mass in the right lower lung (*asterisk*), a smaller adjacent mass (*arrowhead*), and another mass along the left chest wall (*arrow*). **B.** CT image shows the large right peripheral mass (*asterisk*). The left-sided mass is invading the chest wall (*arrow*).

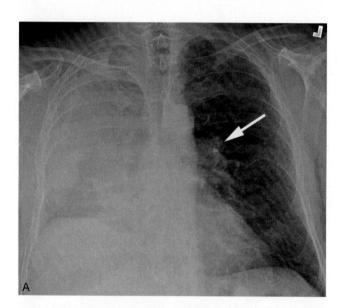
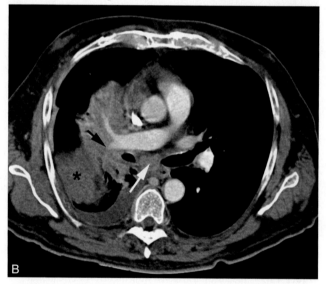

Figure 4.71   Lung carcinoma with multiple pulmonary nodules.   A. Chest radiograph shows opacification of the right hemithorax from a central obstructing carcinoma of the right mainstem bronchus. There is a metastatic nodule (*arrow*) on the left. **B.** CT image shows the mass on the right pinching the bronchus closed (*black arrow*). Note the collapsed right lower lobe (*asterisk*) and metastatic deposit in a subcarinal lymph node (*white arrow*).

material and "touch" preparations to determine whether (1) the biopsy or aspiration is adequate; (2) the sample is neoplastic or inflammatory; and (3) malignant cells are present. If any of these aforementioned studies fail to provide an adequate answer, thoracotomy with excision of the lesion is usually the next step.

Mediastinal Masses

Mediastinal masses are sometimes difficult to separate from pulmonary parenchymal masses. However, most show extrapulmonary signs such as obtuse margins with the pleura and centered outside the lung. The majority of all primary mediastinal masses occur in the anterior compartment, one-third occur in the middle compartment, and the remainder occur in the posterior compartment. Most patients with mediastinal

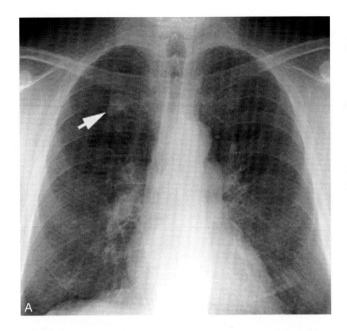

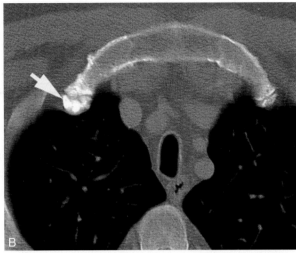

Figure 4.72 **Calcified granuloma.** **A.** Chest radiograph shows a "nodule" in the right upper lobe (*arrow*). **B.** CT image shows the "nodule" to be a hypertrophied and calcified granuloma (*arrow*) immediately beneath the first costochondral junction.

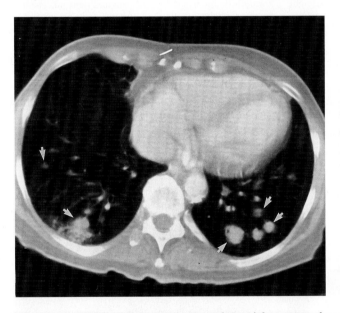

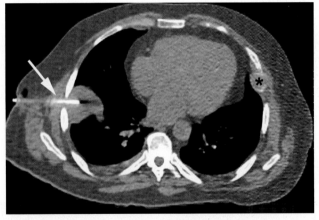

Figure 4.73 **Multiple pulmonary metastases (*arrows*) demonstrated by CT.** These nodules are too large in that location to be considered vessels.

Figure 4.74 **Use of CT guidance for biopsy of a lung mass.** (Same patient as in Fig. 4.70.) A needle (*arrow*) has been placed into the right-sided mass. Note the left-sided mass invading the chest wall (*asterisk*).

masses are asymptomatic. Table 4.3 lists abnormalities found in each compartment of the radiologic mediastinum.

The most common neoplasms in the anterior mediastinum are lymphoma (Fig. 4.75), thymomas (Fig. 4.76), and teratomas. Other anterior abnormalities that may occur include foramen of Morgagni hernias (Fig. 4.77) and pericardial cysts (Fig. 4.78).

The majority of masses arising in the middle mediastinum are lymph nodes, representing lymphoma, metastatic disease, sarcoidosis (Fig. 4.79), or response to infection or chronic inflammatory lung disease. Hiatal or paraesophageal hernias are the most common masses located immediately behind the heart. If they contain an air–fluid level, the diagnosis is confirmed (Fig. 4.80). In some instances, it may be necessary to administer oral barium or perform CT to establish the diagnosis.

The most likely cause of a posterior mediastinal mass is a neurogenic tumor (Fig. 4.81). These generally appear as a paraspinous mass and are often associated with changes in the

Table 4.3 CONDITIONS FOUND IN EACH MEDIASTINAL COMPARTMENT

Category of Disease	Compartments		
	Anterior	Middle	Posterior
Neoplasm	Lymphoma	Metastasis (lung and esophagus)	Neurogenic tumor (nerve sheath tumor and paragangliomas)
	Metastasis	Lymphoma	Lymphoma
	Thyroid neoplasm	Metastasis (distant)	Pheochromocytoma
	Thymic neoplasm		Myeloma
	Teratoma		Metastasis (lung and esophagus)
	Parathyroid adenoma		
Cystic Lesions	Thymic cyst	Bronchogenic cyst	Neurenteric cyst
	Pericardial cyst	Esophageal duplication cyst	Thoracic duct cyst
			Lateral meningocele
Vascular Abnormalities	Aortic aneurysm (ascending)	Aortic aneurysm (root, ascending arch)	Aortic aneurysm (descending)
	Cardiac aneurysm (right ventricle and left apex)	Tortuous or aneurysm brachiocephalic vessels	Aberrant right subclavian artery
		Cardiac aneurysm	
		Vascular ring (double aortic arch)	
		Sinus of Valsalva aneurysm	
Other	Anterior diaphragmatic hernia (Morgagni)	Hiatal hernia (sliding and paraesophageal)	Posterior diaphragmatic hernia (Bochdalek)
	Postoperative hematoma	Lymphadenopathy (inflammatory)	Extramedullary hematopoiesis
	Mediastinitis	Mediastinitis	Distended esophagus
	Abscess	Abscess	Mediastinitis
		Hematoma	Abscess

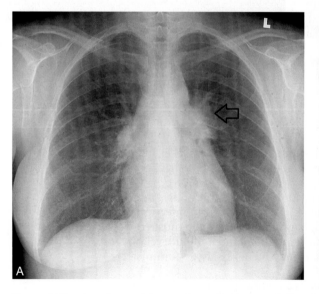

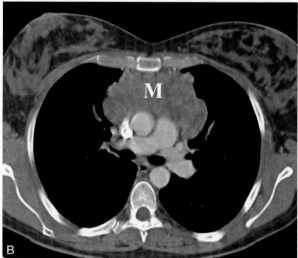

Figure 4.75   Lymphoma of the anterior mediastinum.   A. Frontal radiograph shows a lobular mass in the mediastinum (*arrow*). **B.** CT image shows the mass (*M*) to be anteriorly.

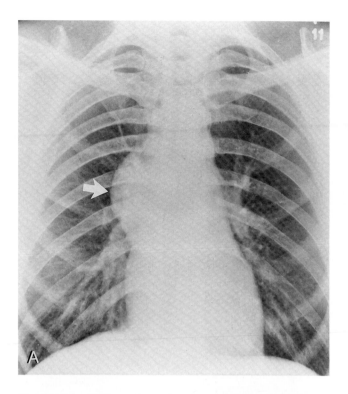

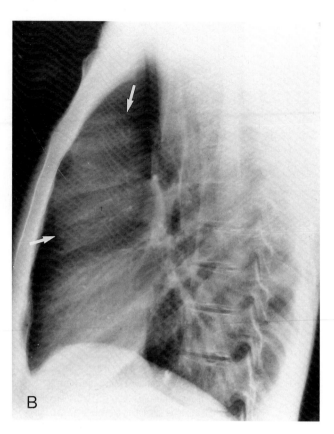

Figure 4.76   Thymoma (*arrows*).   A. Frontal radiograph. **B.** Lateral radiograph.

vertebrae or of the posterior ribs. Neurofibromas and schwannomas frequently enlarge the neural foramina. Calcification may occur in neuroblastomas in children.

Bronchogenic carcinoma may occur as a mediastinal mass in *any* compartment. This diagnosis should always be considered in any adult with a mediastinal mass.

Multiple pulmonary nodules may be granulomas or metastases. If the lesions contain calcium and are widely disseminated (Fig. 4.82), the diagnosis is old granulomatous disease. Multiple large nodules, particularly of varying sizes and randomly distributed (Fig. 4.83), are usually metastases. Metastases may also occur in a "lymphangitic" form as a result of lymph node infiltration and lymphedema producing a prominent interstitial pattern (Fig. 4.84).

Emphysema—Overinflation

One does not need a chest radiograph to make a diagnosis of emphysema. There are adequate physical findings for that. However, there are certain radiographic findings that corroborate those of the physical examination. A better use of the chest x-ray in the emphysematous patient is to detect localized bullae, peribronchial infiltrates, and pneumothorax or pneumomediastinum.

The radiographic findings of classic emphysema reflect the overinflation, loss of compliance, and parenchymal destruction that denote the pathophysiology of the disease. The most reliable radiographic sign of emphysema is decreased ("pruned") vascularity. Other signs are hyperlucency; increased retrosternal clear space; increased lung volume; depression, flattening, or reversal of the curvature of the diaphragm; decreased diaphragmatic excursion; presence of prominent central pulmonary arteries with rapid tapering ("marker") vessels; bowing of the sharply defined trachea ("saber trachea"); and vertical cardiac configuration. Bullae may be present to a greater or lesser extent (Figs. 4.85 and 4.86). CT is particularly useful for showing some of the more subtle findings of emphysema, particularly the centrilobular form.

▶ The most reliable radiographic sign of emphysema is decreased ("pruned") vascularity.

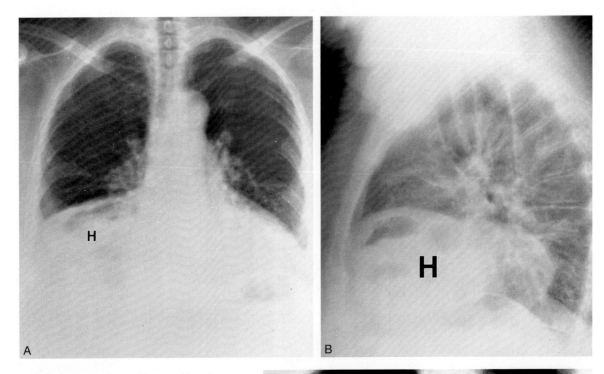

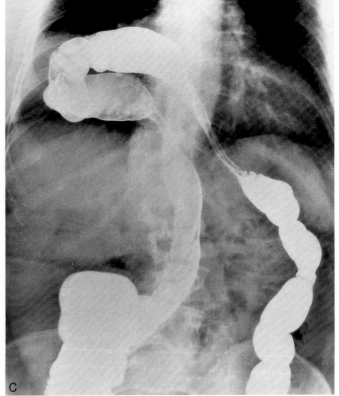

Figure 4.77   Foramen of Morgagni hernia.
A. Frontal radiograph shows apparent consolidation in the right lower lobe containing gaseous shadows. This is the hernia sac (*H*). **B.** Lateral radiograph shows the gas-containing hernia (*H*). **C.** Barium enema shows the herniated colon in the right hemithorax.

Chronic Pulmonary Disease

Patients with chronic pulmonary disease may not have all the classic findings of emphysema. Some may have prominent interstitial markings, the so-called dirty lung seen particularly in smokers. In some younger individuals, the only finding may be hyperlucency, representing early overinflation (Fig. 4.87). Emphysematous changes are often combined with other abnormalities.

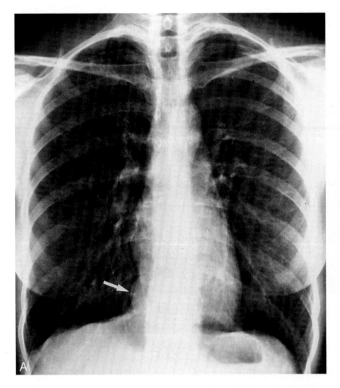

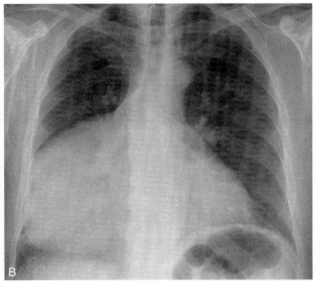

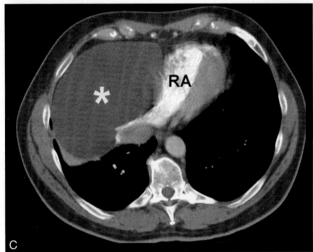

Figure 4.78   Pericardial cysts.   A. Frontal radiograph shows a small bump along the right cardiophrenic angle (*arrow*). **B.** Frontal radiograph shows a large mass adjacent to the heart on the right. **C.** CT image shows the mass (*asterisk*) compressing the contrast-filled right atrium (*RA*). (**B** and **C**, courtesy of Carl Fuhrman, M.D.)

Interstitial versus Acinar Disease

Diseases that primarily involve the interlobular connective tissue with or without secondary involvement of the air spaces are called interstitial diseases. They constitute a group of disorders that have recognizable radiographic patterns:

- Reticular
- Nodular
- Combined reticulonodular
- Cystic or honeycombing

The etiologies vary and include pulmonary edema, fibrosis, metastatic neoplastic (lymphangitic), and primary inflammatory conditions (early viral pneumonia and interstitial pneumonia). Many of these diseases produce some degree of air space or acinar pattern as they progress.

Acinar Lesions

Pure acinar or alveolar lesions produce a pattern characterized by fluffy or "cloudlike" margins, coalescence, a segmental or lobar distribution, a "butterfly" appearance (radiating out from the hila), and air bronchograms. Conditions that produce acinar patterns include acute alveolar edema (pneumonia, CHF with pulmonary edema, toxic or chemical reaction), bleeding (idiopathic pulmonary hemorrhage), aspiration of any fluid, and alveolar cell carcinoma. A rare condition that produces this pattern is alveolar proteinosis.

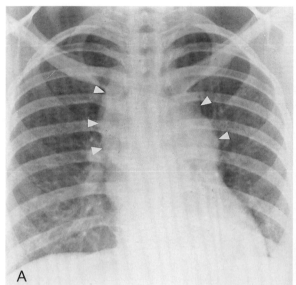

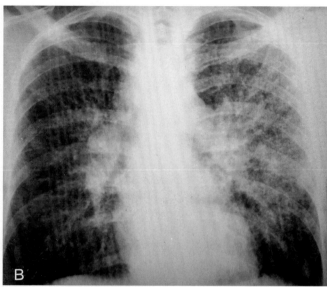

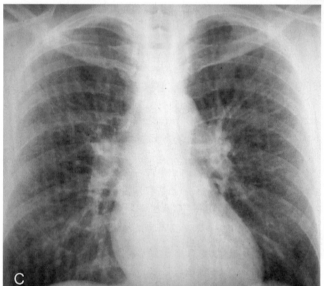

Figure 4.79   Sarcoidosis.   A. Nodal pattern. There are too many "bumps" (*arrowheads*). **B.** Mixed parenchymal and nodal pattern in another patient. Note the enlargement of mediastinal and hilar lymph nodes as well as diffuse interstitial disease, particularly on the left. **C.** The same patient 2 months after treatment. The nodes are smaller and the peripheral lungs are normal.

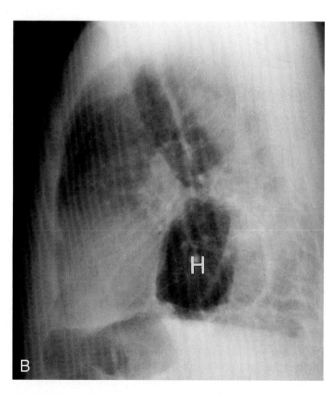

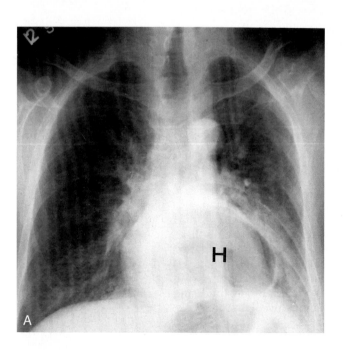

Figure 4.80   Hiatal hernia.   Frontal (A) and lateral **(B)** radiographs show the large hernia sac (*H*) behind the heart.

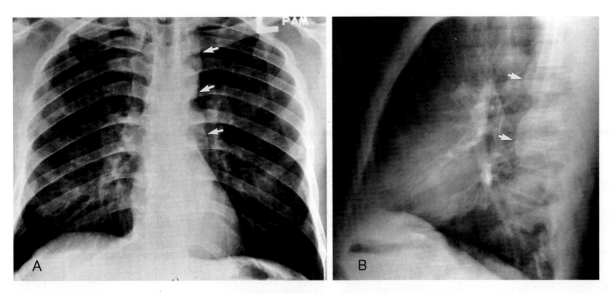

Figure 4.81   Posterior mediastinal widening in a patient with neurofibromatosis.   A. Frontal radiograph shows lobulation in the left paraspinal region (*arrows*). **B.** Lateral radiograph confirms the posterior location of the masses (*arrows*).

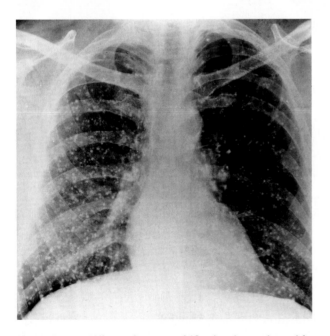

Figure 4.82   Diffuse pulmonary calcifications in a patient with histoplasmosis.

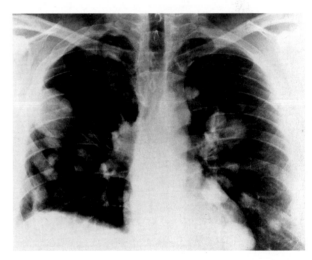

Figure 4.83   Multiple metastases.

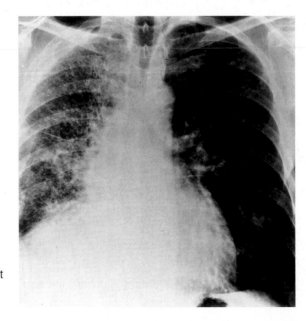

Figure 4.84   Lymphangitic spread of carcinoma.   There is enlargement of the right hilum and a prominent interstitial pattern on the right that indicates lymphedema and lymphangitic spread of tumor.

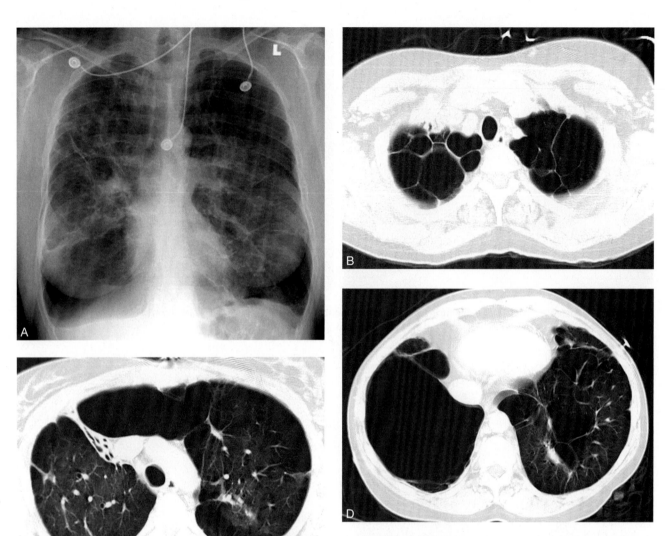

Figure 4.85   Bullous emphysema.   Note the large bilateral blebs.
A. Radiograph. **B to D.** CT images. Note the large areas devoid of lung markings.

Pulmonary Edema

It is possible to differentiate many of the more common acinar diseases on the basis of pattern, distribution, and time course. Pulmonary edema is one of the most common acinar diseases encountered. The causes include CHF, fluid overload (iatrogenic), central nervous system depression or stroke, and inhalation of noxious gases. Pulmonary edema in the presence of cardiac enlargement is usually of cardiac origin (Fig. 4.88). Edema in the presence of a normal sized heart is generally from some other cause. Upper lobe distribution occurs more with neurologic abnormalities. The pattern changes rapidly, often on a daily basis. In more severe cases, usually of cardiac origin, interstitial edema may also be present.

 Pulmonary edema in the presence of cardiac enlargement is usually of cardiac origin; edema in the presence of a normal sized heart is generally from some other cause.

Pneumonia

Pneumonia, on the other hand, may involve any lobe, an entire lung, or be unilateral or bilateral. There are few distinguishing features of the acute bacterial pneumonias.

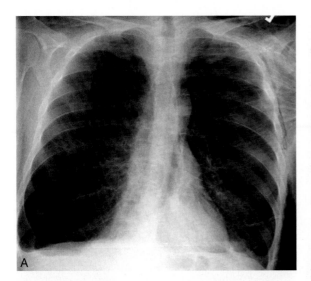

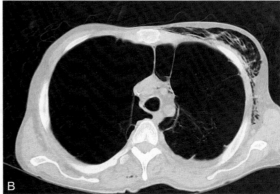

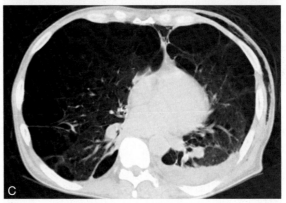

Figure 4.86   Bullous emphysema.   A. Frontal radiograph shows large bullae in both upper lobes in the periphery of the lower lobes. Note the absence of lung markings in these areas. **B** and **C.** CT images show the large cystic bullae. Note the crowding of the normal lung by the bullae, otherwise known as vanishing lung disease.

However, those caused by an unusual organism tend to produce a more widespread acinar pattern. *Klebsiella* pneumonia often produces bulging of a fissure away from the consolidated lobe; *Staphylococcus aureus* may produce multiple cavities and pneumatoceles. Pneumonic consolidations, as a rule, clear by slowly fading. The acinar consolidation often remains visible on the chest radiograph after the patient has become clinically better. *You should be careful to treat your patient and not the radiograph.* Nevertheless, in middle aged and elderly patients, a follow-up two-view chest x-ray should be obtained 6 weeks after the initial diagnosis to exclude an underlying neoplasm. Pneumonia is a common presentation for lung cancer, which can be difficult to diagnose even with CT given the adjacent pulmonary infection and consolidation. Failure to arrange proper follow-up may lead to a delay in cancer diagnosis and put the clinician at risk for legal indemnification.

Other Acinar Disease

Other acinar processes have the same appearances as pneumonia or pulmonary edema. The pattern and timing of the clearing often may provide clues to their cause. Consolidation from a lung infarct is peripheral and wedge shaped. Lung contusions from trauma (Fig. 4.89) generally clear within 24 to 48 hours. Any trauma patient who develops consolidation more than 24 hours after trauma should be suspected of having pneumonia or aspiration. Widespread and persistent consolidation in an intubated patient may mean the onset of adult respiratory distress syndrome (ARDS, see below).

Distinguishing Pure Acinar Disease from Pure Interstitial Disease

Pure acinar disease may frequently be distinguished from pure interstitial disease by pattern recognition. For demonstration purposes, consider the lung to be analogous to a piece of chicken wire, where the wire hexagons represent the interstitial tissues and the spaces represent the air spaces. Under normal circumstances, there is a uniform black background with thin interlacing strands of gray (Fig. 4.90A). In acinar disease, the air spaces are filled in. Unless there is total consolidation of a lobe or a lung, an acinar process will appear as *white dots* (representing the so-called acinar shadows) *on a black background* of aerated lung (Fig. 4.90B). If, however, the disease is primarily interstitial,

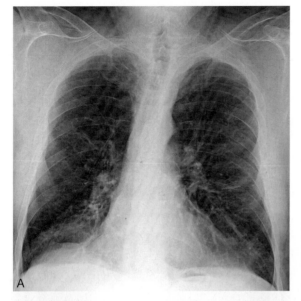

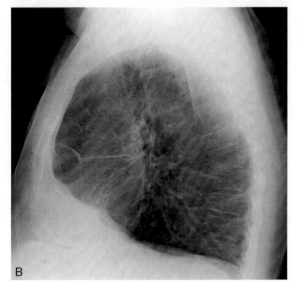

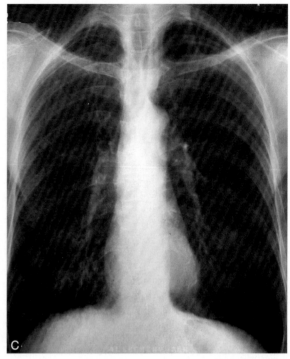

Figure 4.87   Chronic obstructive pulmonary disease (COPD).   Frontal **(A)** and lateral **(B)** radiographs show hyperinflation with flattening of the diaphragms on the lateral projection. **C.** Frontal radiograph in another patient shows the heart appearing small, a finding not uncommon in many COPD patients.

Figure 4.88   Pulmonary edema. There are fluffy alveolar densities throughout both lungs. The cardiac silhouette is obscured in this patient with congestive heart failure.

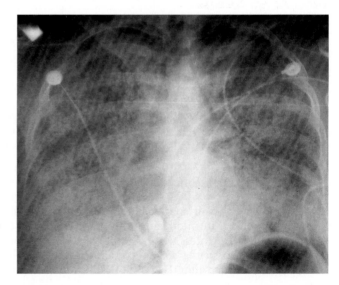

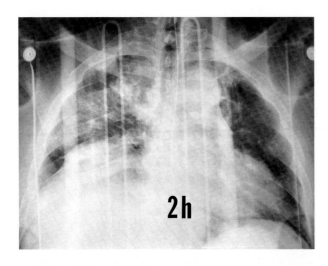

2h

Figure 4.89   Pulmonary contusions in a trauma victim.   Radiograph made 2 hours after the accident shows multiple areas of consolidation throughout the right lung. A right pleural effusion is present.

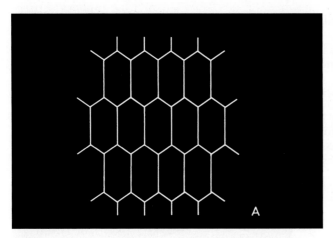

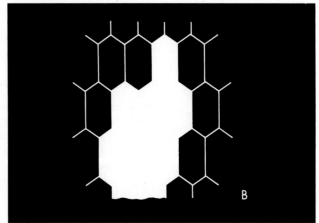

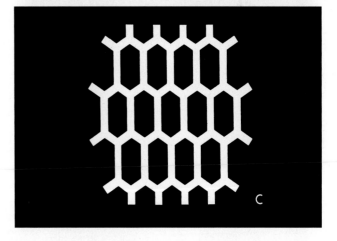

Figure 4.90   Acinar pattern versus interstitial pattern.   A. The normal parenchymal pattern is a uniform black background ("air spaces"), with thin interlacing white strands ("interstitial tissues"). **B.** In acinar disease, the air spaces are filled in, producing a pattern of white dots on a black background. **C.** In interstitial disease, there is thickening of the interstitial tissues resulting in a pattern of black dots on a white background.

there is thickening of the borders around the acini and the resulting pattern is that of *black dots* (representing aerated acini) *surrounded by a white background* of the thickened interstitial tissue (Fig. 4.90**C**). Concomitant airway and interstitial disease produce a combined pattern. The following outline lists some of the more common interstitial diseases:

Primary Pulmonary Interstitial Diseases

　○ Infections ·
　　• TB
　　• Histoplasmosis
　　• Coccidioidomycosis

○ Inhalation disorders
- Inorganic dust
  - Silicosis
  - Asbestosis
  - Pneumoconiosis (mixed dust)
  - Siderosis
  - Other inorganic dust diseases
- Organic dust
  - Farmer's lung
  - Mushroom worker's disease
  - Bagassosis
  - Other organic dust diseases

○ Miscellaneous
- Sarcoidosis
- Drug-induced disease
- Rheumatoid arthritis
- Scleroderma
- Hemosiderosis
- Chronic thromboembolism
- Histiocytosis
- Desquamative interstitial pneumonia
- Idiopathic interstitial pneumonia (form of ARDS)

Combining Clinical, Radiologic, and Histologic Findings

A chest CT is indicated to narrow the diagnostic possibilities. The morphology, distribution, and time course of the CT abnormalities can often narrow the diagnosis to less than three or four entities. However, sometimes an open lung biopsy is required for histologic diagnosis. Nevertheless, interstitial lung disease can often be confusing with overlapping appearances not only at CT but histologically as well. A good clinical history is also essential, especially if one is

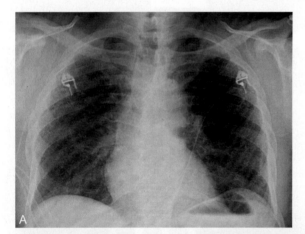

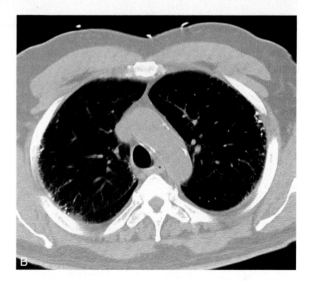

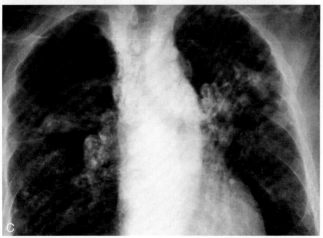

Figure 4.91   Silicosis.   A. Thickening and calcification of the interstitial markings in the periphery of both upper lobes. **B.** The peripheral interstitial thickening and calcification is better demonstrated on the CT. **C.** In a different patient, confluent parenchymal densities and "egg shell" calcifications of hilar and paratracheal lymph nodes are present.

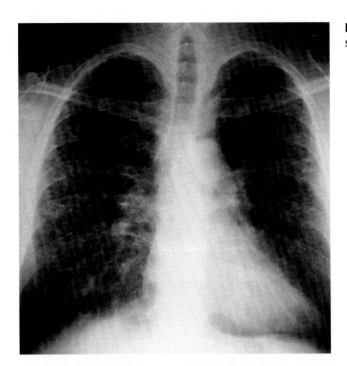

Figure 4.92 Increased interstitial lung markings in both midlungs suspicious for fibrosis.

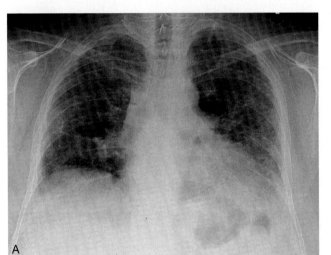

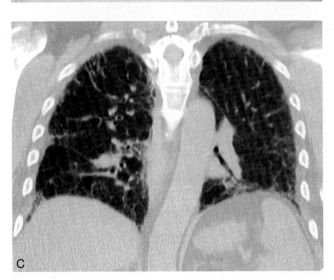

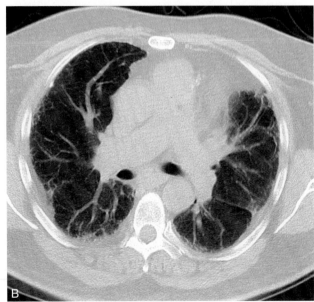

Figure 4.93 **Pulmonary fibrosis and "honeycombing."** **A.** Frontal radiograph shows extensive interstitial disease and shallow lung volumes. **B.** Axial CT shows the peripheral nature of the interstitial thickening and honeycombing typical for the most severe and devastating of the interstitial pneumonias; usual interstitial pneumonia. **C.** Coronal CT shows the same findings.

entertaining a diagnosis of pneumoconiosis or other industrial exposure. Therefore, the clinical, radiologic, and histologic findings should be combined in a multispecialty forum to make a unifying diagnosis. In past years, a "high-resolution chest CT" or more detailed examination of the lung would be necessary to complete the workup. However, with newer generation CT scanners, the resolution of routine chest CT provides comparable detail of a high-resolution chest CT. Therefore, a specialized high-resolution exam is now frequently unnecessary. Figures 4.91 through 4.93 show representative examples of pure interstitial disease.

Pneumothorax

Pneumothorax may result from a variety of causes, including trauma (laceration by fractured rib, stab, or bullet wound) and iatrogenic factors (following thoracentesis, lung biopsy, or placement of subclavian catheter), or may occur spontaneously. The most common radiographic findings are absence of pulmonary vessels extending to the chest wall, a visible pleural line displaced from the chest wall, and increased lucency of one

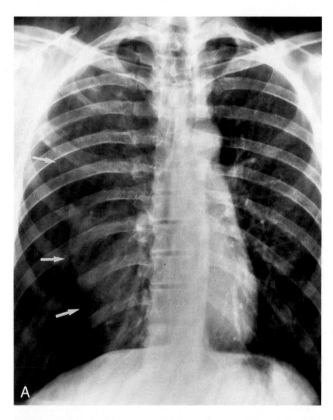

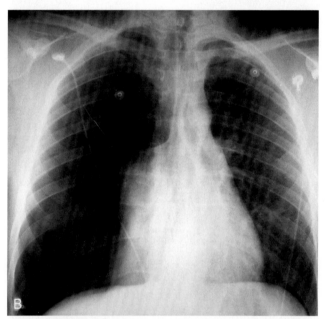

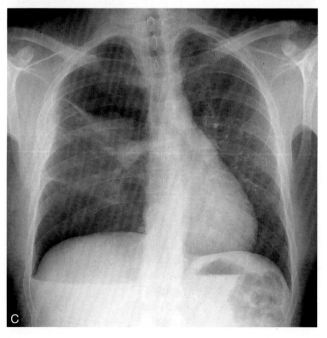

Figure 4.94   Tension pneumothorax in three patients.   There is displacement of the mediastinum (*arrows*) toward the left in **A**. The density on the right in **B** is the collapsed lung. In **C**, there is incomplete collapse of the right lung due to pleural scarring. The mediastinum is shifted to the left, however.

CHAPTER 4 Chest Imaging

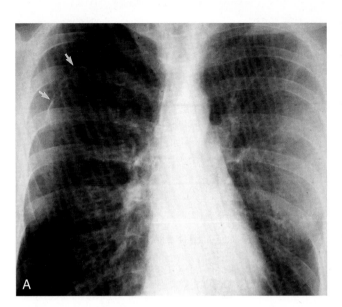
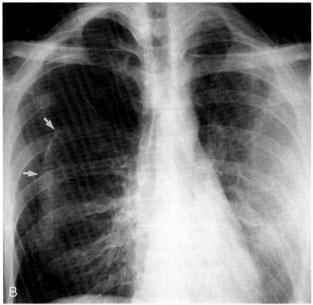

Figure 4.95 **Right-sided pneumothorax (*arrows*) demonstrating the use of inspiratory (A) and expiratory (B) radiographs.** Note how the pneumothorax is "enlarged" on the expiratory film **(B)**.

hemithorax. If the patient has a tension-type pneumothorax, air continuously enters the pleural space and builds up pressure, which compresses the mediastinum toward the opposite lung. This may result in severe respiratory distress unless immediately recognized. The most common sign of tension pneumothorax is a shift of the mediastinum away from the abnormal side (Fig. 4.94). This is a true emergency and requires immediate tube decompression. An ancillary sign in tension pneumothorax is depression of the affected hemidiaphragm. A pneumothorax may be made more visible by an expiratory radiograph (Fig. 4.95). Decubitus views are also valuable in the critical care setting.

Some pneumothoraces are not as obvious. Pleural air will be found over the apex of a lung on erect radiographs (Fig. 4.96). CT is very sensitive for identifying pneumothorax. In supine patients, free air collects anteriorly and superiorly (Fig. 4.97).

Pulmonary Embolus

It is estimated that pulmonary embolus is the most common abnormality found on autopsies of hospitalized patients who die. Fortunately, in most cases, embolism occurs without infarction because of the double blood supply to the lung from the pulmonary arteries and bronchial arteries. Pulmonary emboli are most likely to occur in severely ill patients who are bedridden and cancer patients who are hypercoagulable.

 ▶ Pulmonary embolism is the most common abnormality found at autopsies of hospitalized patients.

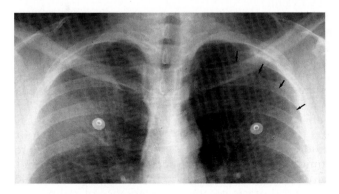

Figure 4.96 Left apical pneumothorax (*arrows*).

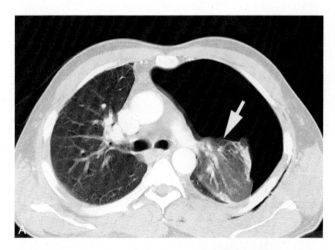
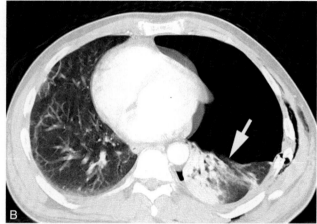

Figure 4.97   Tension pneumothorax as demonstrated on CT.   A and **B.** Two CT images show the large collection of free air on the left. The mediastinum is shifted to the right. Note the collapsed lung posteriorly (*arrows*).

Radiographic Findings

Interestingly, there may be few radiographic findings of pulmonary embolus in any particular patient. Clinicians and radiologists should have a high index of suspicion to make this diagnosis because a common radiographic finding is a "normal" chest, which is incompatible with a patient in acute cardiopulmonary distress. Radiographic signs that may be seen, however, include pleural effusion, peripheral or bibasilar infiltrates, focal atelectasis, elevation of the diaphragm, and hypovascular peripheral lung segments. Infiltration and formation of a "mass" may occur with infarction. With healing, these areas of peripheral consolidation shrink in the same pattern as a melting ice cube, retaining its original outline, only becoming smaller.

Ventilation–Perfusion Lung Scintigraphy

V/Q lung scintigraphy, although used infrequently, is still a useful diagnostic procedure in patients suspected of having pulmonary emboli. Injected particles are trapped in the capillary bed, and thus give an index of pulmonary arterial perfusion. Inhaled particles demonstrate the ventilation pattern of the lungs. Patients with emphysema, pneumonia, pulmonary fibrosis, or pleural effusions may demonstrate displacement of vessels, physiologic shunting of blood flow, or poorly ventilated areas. However, a "mismatched" decrease in perfusion of a lung zone that is receiving ventilation is a very reliable sign of an intrinsic vascular defect, i.e., a pulmonary embolus obstructing blood flow (Fig. 4.98). It is critical to assess the V/Q scan with contemporaneous chest radiographs to reduce the likelihood of false-positive outcomes. The utility of V/Q scan decreases with consolidation, pleural effusion, or obstructive lung disease (chronic obstructive pulmonary disease or asthma). Nevertheless, it may still be used as a first-line imaging modality in patients with a normal chest radiograph and no obstructive lung disease who are suspected of having pulmonary emboli. V/Q scans are also valuable for those patients with impaired renal function who are at high risk for developing acute renal failure from iodinated contrast injection that is administered for a CT exam.

Chest CT has largely replaced the V/Q scan for diagnosing pulmonary emboli and now is considered the gold standard for diagnosis. The main reasons for this are the "indeterminate" outcome of V/Q scans in patients with known lung diseases and the ready availability of CT, particularly at night and on weekends when nuclear medicine facilities are not immediately available. In most instances, the CT can be obtained in a significantly shorter period of time than that required to call in a nuclear medicine technologist and have the technologist prepare the isotope for injection. Modern CT is fast and more importantly, more effective in demonstrating small peripheral emboli, as well as the larger more central ones (Figs. 4.99 and 4.100). With modern multidetector CT scanners, the thorax may be studied in as little as 5 to 8 seconds. Most patients are able to breath hold in that short time period. Thus, the advantages of CT lie in its availability, high sensitivity for clinically significant emboli, as well as its ability to provide more information about the lungs and thoracic organs in the absence of pulmonary

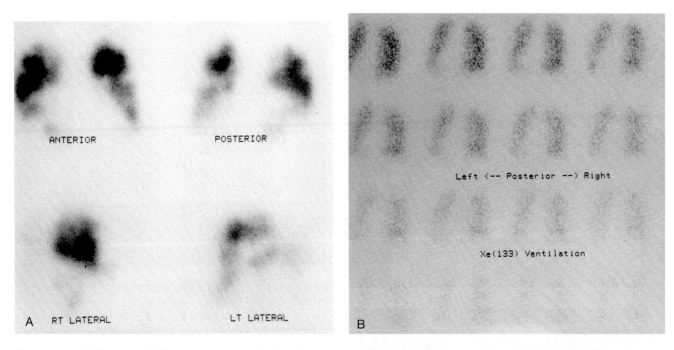

Figure 4.98 Pulmonary embolism. **A.** Perfusion scan shows photopenic areas throughout both lungs, representing regions of lack of perfusion. **B.** Ventilation scan shows that these areas are normally ventilated.

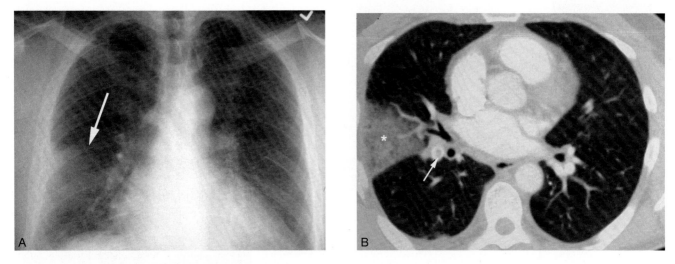

Figure 4.99 CT of small pulmonary embolism. **A.** Radiograph shows a wedge-shaped area of increased density in the right middle lobe (*arrow*). **B.** CT image shows the wedge-shaped area in the right middle lobe (*asterisk*) representing an infarct. Note the small filling defect in the adjacent pulmonary artery (*arrow*).

emboli. There are, however, some limitations in the use of CT. In approximately 2% to 5% of patients, the study is suboptimal. This may be the result of patient obesity, poor contrast opacification of the pulmonary arteries, or respiratory motion. According to the PIOPED II trial which used 4- and 16-slice multislice detectors for the examination, the sensitivity of CT for pulmonary embolism is 86% with a specificity of 96%. However, the sensitivity and specificity has likely increased as a result of better spatial resolution and shorter breath holds with more advanced 64 or higher slice technology.

Pulmonary Arteriography

Pulmonary arteriography was used as the old "gold standard" for diagnosing pulmonary emboli (Fig. 4.101) prior to the emergence of CT. However, given the rapid improvement in CT technology and low mortality rates following a negative chest CT, pulmonary angiography has been relegated to a therapeutic modality with catheter-directed thrombolysis or mechanical thrombectomy for large or saddle pulmonary emboli.

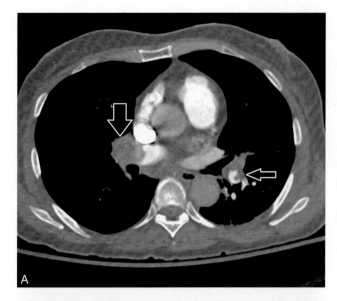

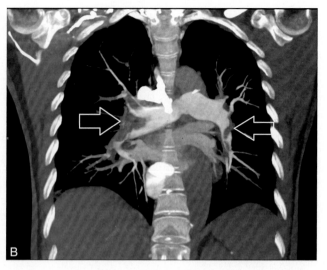

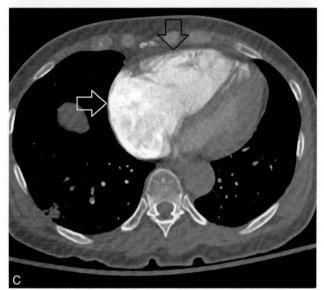

Figure 4.100   CT of large pulmonary embolism with right heart strain.   A. Axial CT image shows large filling defects in both pulmonary arteries (*arrows*). **B.** Coronal maximum projection CT image shows bilateral thrombi (*arrows*). **C.** Axial CT image shows enlargement of the right ventricle (*black arrow*) and right atrium (*white arrow*). If the patient's vital signs are unstable, right ventricular strain in the setting of pulmonary embolism is an indication for thrombolytic therapy.

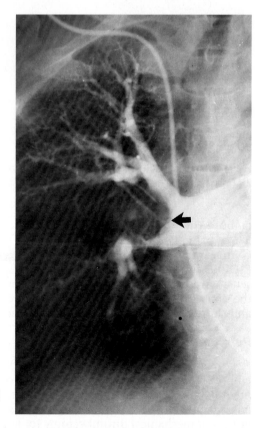

Figure 4.101   Pulmonary embolism.   Pulmonary arteriogram shows a large saddle embolus (*arrow*). Note the poor perfusion of the right middle and lower lobes as opposed to the upper lobe.

Appearance of the Chest after Surgery

Monumental advances have been made in thoracic surgery in the past 50 years: development of new techniques for cardiopulmonary bypass, lung surgery, and coronary revascularization procedures; stents; development of new prosthetic heart valves; advancements in heart transplantation; and perfection of new techniques for esophageal bypass surgery. These changes have reduced the morbidity and mortality in patients who undergo cardiothoracic surgery.

You should familiarize yourself with the various appearances of the chest postoperatively. Remember, once the patient has recovered and is free of symptoms of the previous disease, we can consider this chest "normal" for that individual. In addition, it is crucial to compare any postoperative chest radiographs with old studies to facilitate the detection of complications or new disease. In some cases, it may necessitate obtaining those studies from another institution.

The appearance of the chest radiograph in a patient who has undergone cardiac, thoracic, or esophageal surgery is characteristic of the procedure following recovery from surgery. In the immediate postoperative period, there are many generic findings common to all procedures. Operative manipulation of the lung may result in areas of patchy consolidation. Pleural effusion is a common finding following both cardiac and pulmonary surgery. Patients who have undergone cardiac surgery often show enlargement of the cardiac silhouette. CHF, pneumonia, atelectasis (particularly the left lower lobe), and pneumothorax are frequent findings in the immediate postoperative period (Fig 4.102).

Foreign Objects

Following heart or lung surgery, a variety of foreign objects may be seen in the thorax. These include chest tubes placed anteriorly in the supine patient for drainage of air and posteriorly for drainage of fluid, staple lines representing areas of resected lung, surgical clips, sternotomy wires, mediastinal drains, a variety of intravascular catheters, and prosthetic heart valves. Furthermore, pacemaker leads may be either endocardial or epicardial in attachment. Electrocardiographic leads may also be seen on the chest wall. Some of these "foreign bodies" are illustrated in Figure 4.102.

We can divide the discussion of the chest during the postoperative period into four categories:

- Primary lung surgery
- Primary cardiac surgery
- Primary esophageal surgery
- Mastectomy

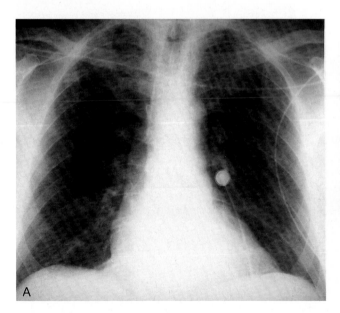 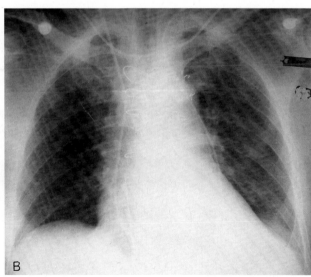

Figure 4.102   Changes of cardiac surgery.   A. Preoperative portable frontal radiograph is normal. **B.** Following cardiac surgery, there are multiple sternal wires present. There are surgical clips adjacent to the aorta. An endotracheal tube, Swan-Ganz catheter, and mediastinal drains are also present.

Primary Lung Surgery

Patients undergo *lung surgery* in basically three types of procedures: wedge or segmental resection, lobectomy, and pneumonectomy.

The most common radiographic manifestation of excisional wedge or segmental resection of a pulmonary abnormality is a line of wire staples across the lung (Fig. 4.103A). These procedures are commonly performed with video-assisted thoracoscopic surgery (VATS), which utilizes a small incision and insertion of a fiberoptic thoracoscope. In general, VATS is less traumatic to the chest wall than a traditional thoracotomy without muscle incision and rib removal allowing patients faster operative recovery with fewer complications.

Lobectomies can be performed with VATS or traditional thoracotomy depending on the stage of disease and complexity of the abnormality and depending on whether neoadjuvant chemotherapy (chemotherapy before resection) was administered. On chest films, metal clips and/or a staple line representing the line of resection across the bronchus is seen. There is a shift of fissures as with atelectasis, the directions being the same as in atelectasis of the affected lobe. Hyperinflation of the remaining lobes on the side of a lobectomy is also seen. These findings are illustrated in Figure 4.103B.

Following pneumonectomy, the affected hemithorax fills with fluid (Fig. 4.104A and B). Air within the affected side gradually resorbs, leaving an opaque hemithorax. As healing ensues, the heart and mediastinum are drawn toward the side of surgery. Often the cardiac silhouette is not well seen. The remaining lung hyperinflates to fill the space vacated by the shifted heart and mediastinum, as illustrated in Figure 4.104C. Any patient with persistent air, no mediastinal shift, or multiple air–fluid levels should be suspected for an empyema and dehiscence of the bronchial resection margin (Fig. 4.105).

Thoracoplasty and plombage are procedures that were once performed to eliminate dead space within the chest. These procedures were commonly performed to treat TB before the advent of antimicrobial therapy. A patient who has undergone thoracoplasty exhibits deformity of the upper chest wall on the affected side (Fig. 4.106A). Patients who have undergone plombage will exhibit foreign material, as in Figure 4.106B.

Primary Cardiac Surgery

Cardiac surgery is performed most often to replace damaged heart valves, bypass stenotic coronary arteries, palliate congenital heart disease, and for cardiac transplantation. The majority of the patients following cardiac surgery will have wire sutures in the sternum. If the sternotomy wires are small, the surgery was likely performed for congenital heart disease when the patient was a child.

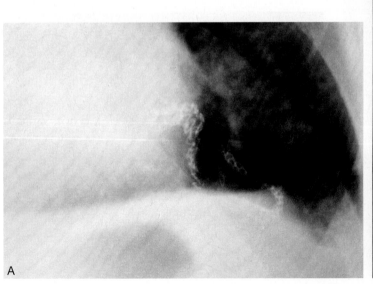

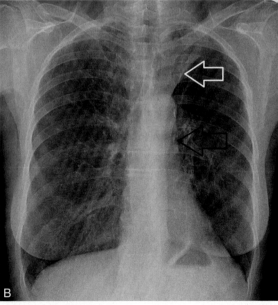

Figure 4.103   Changes following left lung resection.   A. Surgical staple lines in the left lower lobe from a wedge resection. **B.** Frontal radiograph shows a left upper lung opacity (*white arrow*), left lung volume loss, and left hilar surgical clips (*black arrow*) from a left upper lobectomy.

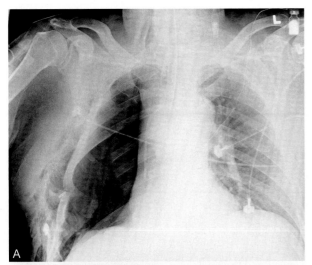

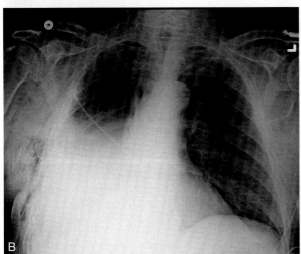

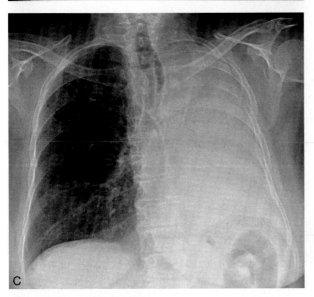

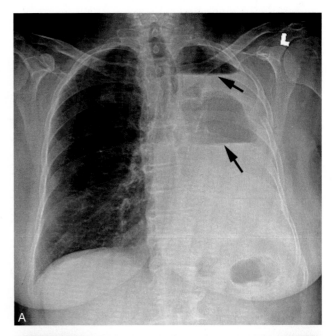

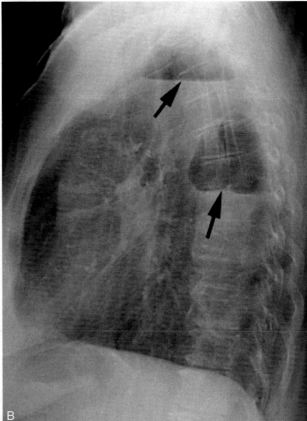

Figure 4.105 Complication from left pneumonectomy. Frontal (A) and lateral (B) films show two air–fluid levels (*arrows*) in the pneumonectomy cavity. This indicates fluid loculation which is suspicious for an empyema.

Figure 4.104 Changes following pneumonectomy. **A.** Frontal radiograph demonstrates lucency completely replacing the right lung and multiple right rib deformities from a recent right thoracotomy and pneumonectomy. **B.** Follow-up study a few days later shows development of a right pleural effusion. **C.** Different patient several months after left pneumonectomy. Note complete resorption of the air. The hemithorax has filled with fluid and the mediastinum is shifted.

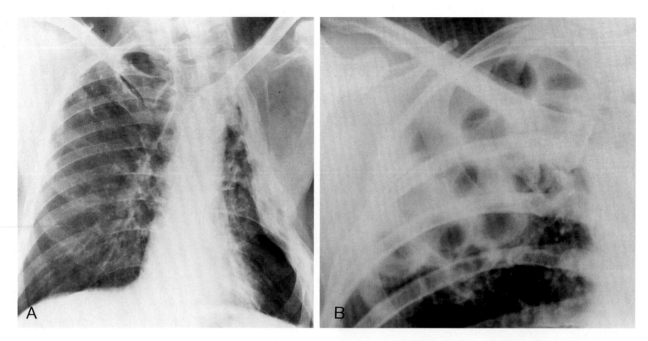

Figure 4.106   Unusual postoperative appearances.   A. Thoracoplasty. **B.** Changes after plombage in which plastic balls were placed in the right hemithorax.

Prosthetic valves are either mechanical or bioprosthetic and come in several varieties. When observing these valves on radiographs, one can easily appreciate the location of the mitral and aortic rings (Figs. 4.107 and 4.108).

Patients who undergo bypass surgery of the coronary arteries often show multiple metal clips along the left lateral margin of the cardiomediastinal silhouette indicating a left internal mammary dissection and anastomosis usually to the left anterior descending

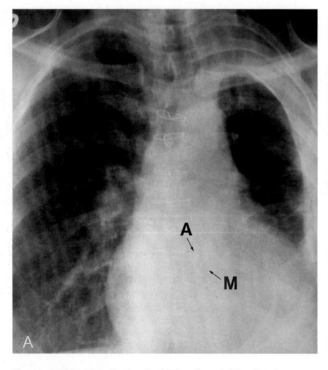

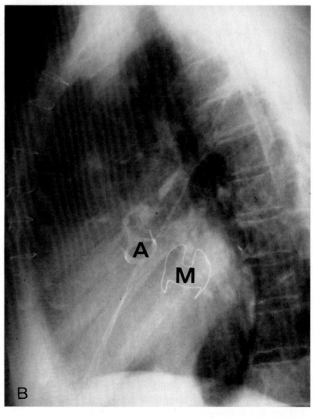

Figure 4.107   Prosthetic mitral (*M*) and aortic (*A*) valves.
A.   Frontal view. **B.** Lateral view shows the valves to better advantage.

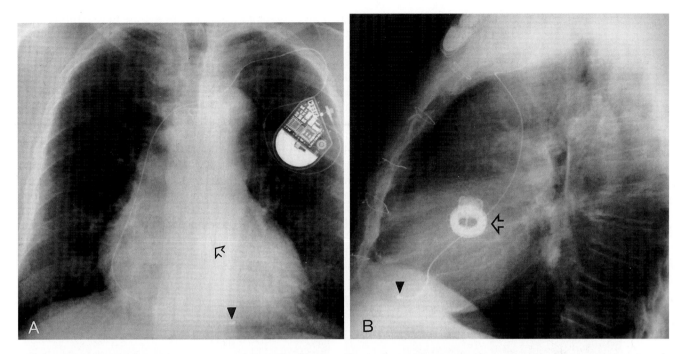

Figure 4.108 Prosthetic aortic valve (*arrows*) and transvenous pacemaker. The tip of the pacing lead (*arrowheads*) is in the right ventricle. **A.** Frontal view. **B.** Lateral view.

coronary artery. On occasion, small metal rings indicate the position of each saphenous vein grafts originating off the aorta. In some patients, the chest x-ray indicates the number of coronary bypass grafts. These findings are illustrated in Figure 4.109. Coronary artery stents may also be seen on a well-penetrated radiograph.

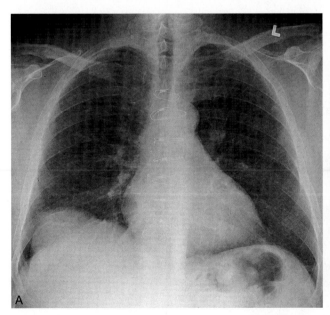

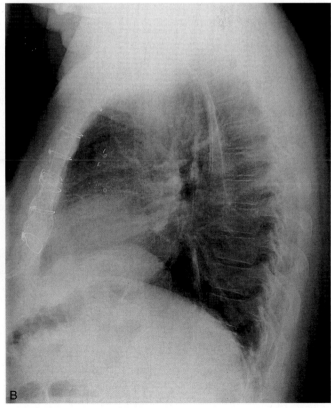

Figure 4.109 Changes following cardiac surgery. Note the presence of sternal wires, mediastinal vascular clips, and circular markers indicating the proximal anastomosis of each saphenous vein coronary bypass graft. **A.** Frontal view. **B.** Lateral view.

Patients who have had palliative surgery for congenital heart disease may exhibit a variety of changes, depending on the surgical procedure. In some instances, as with palliation of a septal defect or ligation of a patent ductus arteriosus, the appearance may be perfectly normal if the surgery has been successful.

Pacemaker technology has dramatically evolved with both pacing and defibrillator functions now available. Pacemakers have two components: the pacemaker generator which is the oval metal box usually in the upper chest wall and the pacemaker leads. Pacemaker leads are either endocardial and epicardial. The endocardial leads are generally placed into the right atrium and right ventricle. When seen on the routine PA and lateral chest radiographs, there should be a gentle curve to the catheter (see Fig. 4.110). Any kinking or odd course of the lead should suggest that the catheter is not in the right position. The pacemaker generator is usually in the anterior chest wall. Pacemaker lead fracture usually occurs near the clavicle where the lead enters the subclavian vein. Biventricular pacemakers are indicated for patients with severe CHF and have three leads: right atrial, right ventricular, and coronary sinus. Epicardial leads are placed along the outside of the heart usually to treat heart block or dysrrhythmias that develop during cardiac surgery. Generally, these wires go through the diaphragm to the battery pack, which is in the abdominal wall (Fig. 4.111).

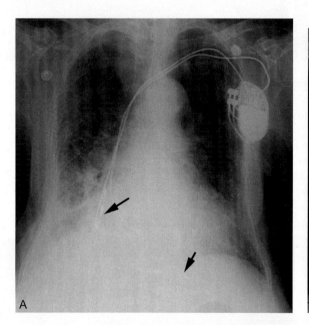
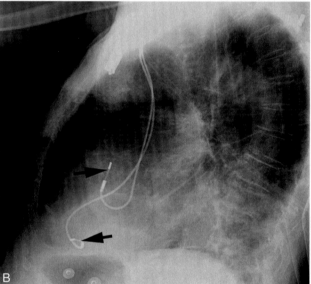

Figure 4.110   Intracardiac pacemaker showing the leads (*arrows*) in the right atrium and right ventricle.   **A.** Frontal view. **B.** Lateral view.

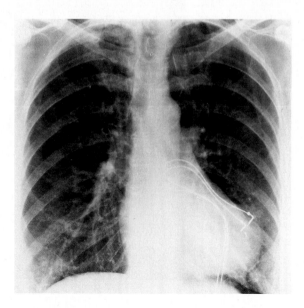

Figure 4.111   **Epicardial pacemaker leads on the left side.**

An automatic implantable cardiac defibrillator is often combined with a pacemaker or may be implanted alone. When ventricular tachycardia or fibrillation occurs, the device automatically discharges a cardioverting shock. The intracardiac defibrillator may be recognized by the coiled spring appearance of the defibrillating leads (Fig. 4.112).

Primary Esophageal Surgery

Numerous procedures have been devised for palliation of esophageal disease. There are basically two types, esophagectomy and hiatal hernia repair. In an esophagectomy, the esophagus is removed and the stomach is pulled up from the abdomen, otherwise known as a gastric pull through (Fig. 4.113). In some cases, a segment of colon is used to replace the esophagus, otherwise known as a colonic interposition. *Hiatal hernia repair* may on occasion show a mass in the immediate postcardiac region. This represents the fundus of the stomach, which has been plicated around the distal esophagus to create a competent esophageal sphincter. Metal clips may also be seen in this region. Various types of stents may also be used to bypass the obstructed esophageal segment.

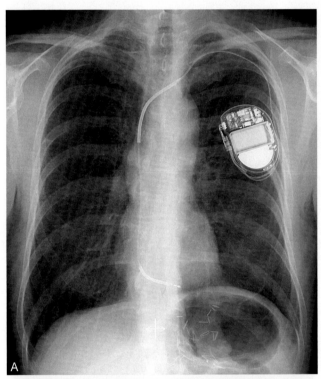

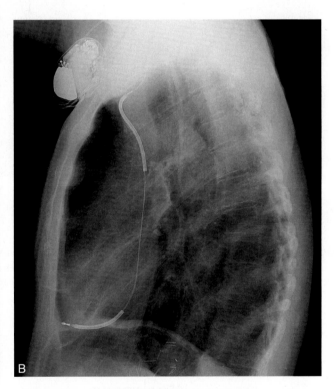

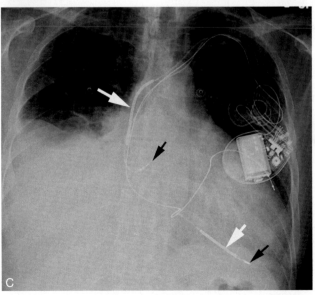

Figure 4.112   Automated internal cardiac defibrillator.   PA **(A)** and lateral **(B)** views show the generator box overlying the left chest wall. The defibrillating leads are in the superior vena cava and the right ventricle. **C.** Another patient with a combined pacemaker and defibrillator. The coiled defibrillating leads are in the superior vena cava and the right ventricle (*large white arrows*). The pacing leads are in the right atrium and right ventricle (*small black arrows*) as well as a third lead in the coronary sinus making this a biventricular pacemaker.

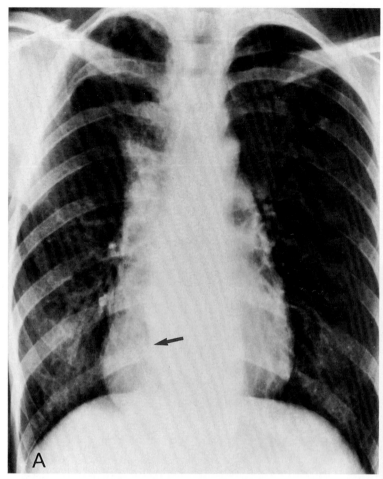

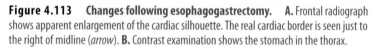

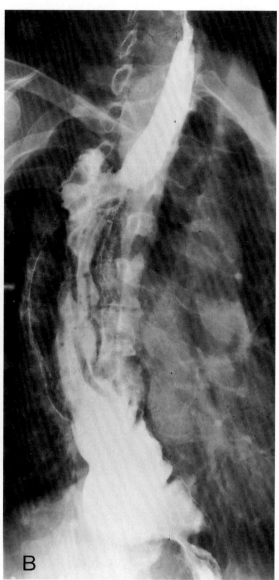

Figure 4.113   Changes following esophagogastrectomy.   A. Frontal radiograph shows apparent enlargement of the cardiac silhouette. The real cardiac border is seen just to the right of midline (*arrow*). **B.** Contrast examination shows the stomach in the thorax.

Mastectomy

You should also be familiar with postoperative appearance of the patient following radical mastectomy for breast carcinoma. After mastectomy, the operative side is more lucent on frontal chest x-ray. This is because of the absence of the breast shadow and pectoralis major muscle. If we follow the soft tissue lines of the axilla on the normal side, we can see that the axillary fold merges imperceptibly with that of the breast shadow. However, on the affected side, the axillary fold extends up to and crosses over onto the thorax (Fig. 4.114). Occasionally, a lymph node dissection has also been performed and surgical clips are present in the axilla. These changes are now less common since the introduction of breast conservation therapy (lumpectomy combined with radiation and chemotherapy).

Other Considerations

Postoperative patients or any other patient in an ICU usually have numerous tubes and lines for life support. Many times endotracheal tubes are inadvertently inserted into the right mainstem bronchus or the esophagus. A nasogastric or feeding tube may be inadvertently placed into the airway (Fig. 4.115) or lung. Similarly, intravenous or arterial catheters occasionally end up in an unintended position. Chest tubes may be kinked or have

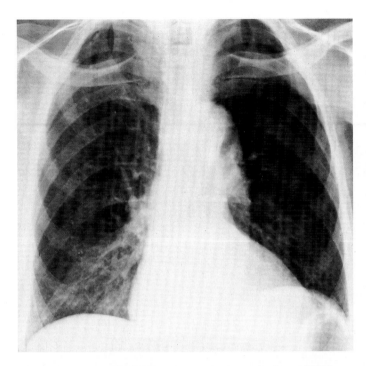

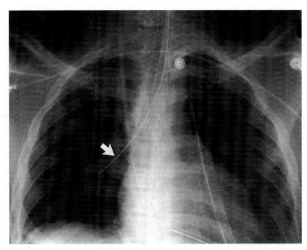

Figure 4.115 Nasogastric tube in right mainstem bronchus (*arrow*).

Figure 4.114 **Changes following left radical mastectomy.** The left hemithorax is hyperlucent due to an absent pectoral muscle and breast. Note the differences in soft tissues between right and left.

their tips of side holes in the axilla. Wayward support devices may have disastrous results. A malpositioned tube or line that is not quickly rectified commonly results in litigation. A portable chest x-ray should be performed to validate the position of any newly placed endotracheal tube, feeding tube, or central line to verify proper positioning.

> A portable chest radiograph should be performed to validate the position of any newly placed endotracheal tube, feeding tube, or central line to verify its position.

Radiation Pneumonitis

Radiation pneumonitis is a form of inflammatory lung disease that is usually found 1 to 6 months after radiation therapy for lung or breast cancer as well as lymphoma. The likelihood of radiation pneumonitis increases if chemotherapy is delivered at the same time. In the acute stage, there are nonspecific areas of consolidation, air bronchograms, and sometimes pleural effusions. In the late stages, fibrosis occurs. A radiographic clue to the diagnosis is that the distribution of the abnormalities is usually nonanatomic following the borders of the radiation therapy port that was used. These borders are usually well defined (Fig. 4.116). Radiation usually produces hilar and/or fissure displacement, depending on the ports. Obtaining a history of previous radiation therapy is key to making the diagnosis. On occasion, there may be skeletal changes from radiation therapy as well.

Acquired Immunodeficiency Syndrome–Related Abnormalities

Acquired immunodeficiency syndrome (AIDS) is the result of infection with the human immunodeficiency virus (HIV). Patients with this disease suffer a variety of pulmonary infections and neoplasms, although the frequency of these diseases has diminished with the successful use of antiretroviral therapy. *Pneumocystis carinii* pneumonia (PCP) is one of the more common infections. Chest radiographs show nonspecific bilateral ground glass opacities (Fig 4.117**A**), but can be normal in early infection. CT is actually very specific and should be ordered if PCP infection is suspected. CT shows a combination of ground glass opacities and pneumatoceles (Fig. 4.117**B**).

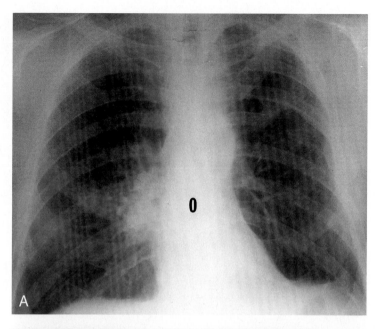

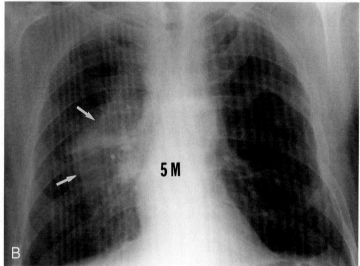

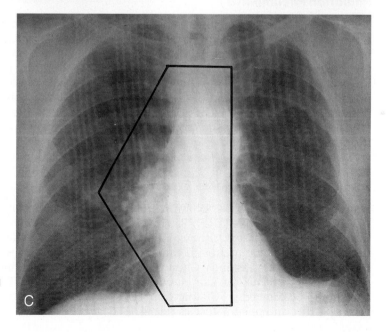

Figure 4.116   Radiation pneumonitis.   A. Pretreatment radiograph shows a large mass in the right hilum. **B.** Five months after radiation therapy, there is a sail-like sharply outlined density in the right lung (*arrows*). **C.** Pretreatment radiograph with radiation port superimposed. Note the similarity of the density in **B** to the treatment port.

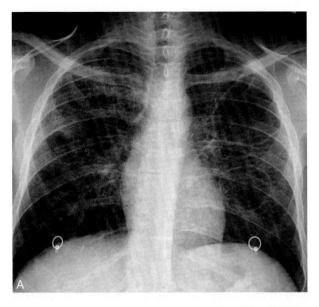
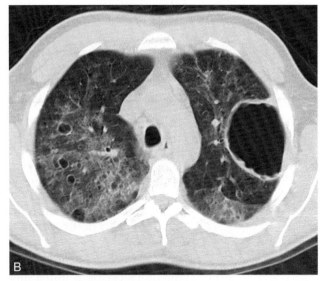

Figure 4.117   *Pneumocystis carinii* **pneumonia (PCP) edema pattern in an acquired immunodeficiency syndrome patient.**   **A.** Radiograph shows bilateral ground glass opacities and pneumatoceles. **B.** CT shows the same findings in greater detail.

Pneumocystis infection is not the only pathogen to infect HIV patients. Pyogenic organisms, most commonly *Haemophilus influenzae* and *Streptococcus pneumoniae*, also cause pneumonia. In addition, fungal, nocardial, and mycobacterial infections (*Mycobacterium tuberculosis* and *Mycobacterium avium-intracellulare*) are not uncommon. The pulmonary patterns produced by these organisms are similar to those seen in other immunocompromised patients, such as those who have hematologic malignancies (leukemia and lymphoma), patients on chemotherapy for malignancies, organ and bone marrow transplant patients, and those receiving high-maintenance doses of steroids for chronic systemic diseases such as rheumatoid arthritis or systemic lupus erythematosus.

Kaposi sarcoma and lymphoma are common in AIDS patients. Radiographically, this usually presents as pulmonary nodules, consolidation, mediastinal or hilar adenopathy, and pleural effusion. Figure 4.118 illustrates some of these findings.

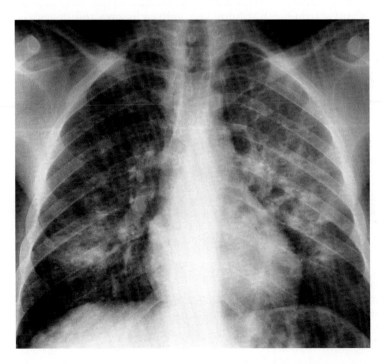

Figure 4.118   Pulmonary Kaposi sarcoma in a patient with acquired immunodeficiency syndrome.   Note the bilateral parenchymal and interstitial pulmonary densities. (Courtesy David Epstein, M.D., from Radiology 1982;183:7−10. Reproduced with permission.)

Tuberculosis

TB has been one of the scourges of humankind. This disease, which had been in decline in the United States, began to make a dramatic comeback in the early 1980s. The reasons for this included a number of medical and social factors, such as an increasing incidence of drug abuse, increasing numbers of homeless people, and the rise in the number of patients infected with HIV. TB has always been known as "the great imitator" because of its propensity to mimic other diseases.

 ▶ TB is known as "the great imitator" because of its propensity to mimic other diseases.

The evaluation of a patient with suspected TB should begin with a Mantoux skin test (purified protein derivative [PPD]) and a chest x-ray. Pulmonary TB has primary or secondary forms with a variety of radiographic appearances depending in the stage of disease and the integrity of the patient's immune system.

Primary Tuberculosis

Primary TB begins as initial inoculation in the lungs. Most healthy patients will contain the infection with no radiographic abnormality. Therefore, most PPD-positive patients will have a normal chest radiograph. Some primary infections will create enough of an inflammatory response to produce calcified nodule(s) and thoracic lymph node(s). When this occurs, it leaves a characteristic radiographic pattern known as the "*primary inflammatory complex*" or *Ranke complex* (Fig. 4.119). However, this complex is not specific for TB. It is also commonly seen with fungal or histoplasmosis infection, particularly in the central and eastern regions of the United States. Nevertheless, it does indicate inactive disease.

Immunocompromised or chronically ill patients with primary TB usually have radiographic abnormalities. This includes nonspecific consolidation, cavitary nodules and masses (Fig. 4.120), small miliary nodules (Fig. 4.121), necrotizing adenopathy, and pleural effusions. In fact, in a patient with known TB, a cavitary nodule or mass with an air–fluid level is considered diagnostic for transmissible disease and the patient should be immediately isolated in a negative pressure environment.

Secondary Tuberculosis

The secondary form of TB involves reactivation of dormant foci of infection. The infection thrives in areas of high oxygen concentration, particularly the upper lobes. Fibronodular consolidation may occur with or without cavitation and adenopathy. In end stage of reactivation TB, there is fibrosis and scarring with volume loss, shift of fissures and/or vessels,

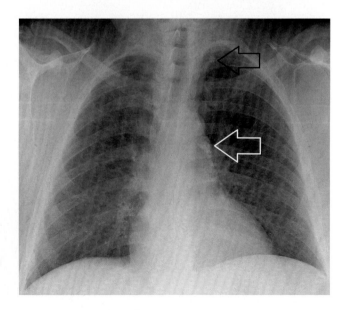

Figure 4.119   Ranke complex.
Frontal view shows a calcified left upper lobe pulmonary nodule (*black arrow*) from the initial infection and spread of disease to a left hilar lymph node (*white arrow*).

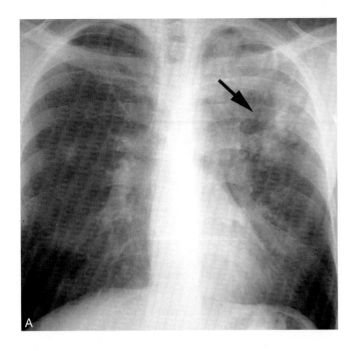

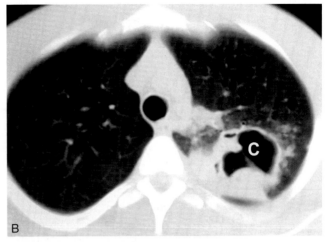

Figure 4.120   Tuberculosis left upper lobe.   A. Frontal radiograph shows consolidation and cavitary disease (*black arrow*). **B.** Axial CT better characterizes the cavitary abscess.

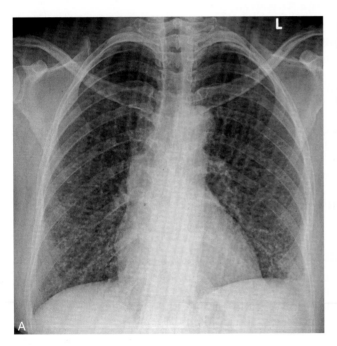

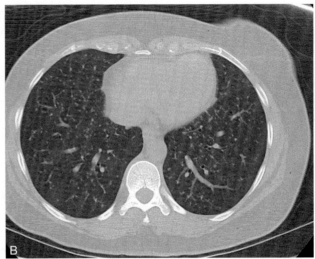

Figure 4.121   Miliary tuberculosis in a patient with acquired immunodeficiency syndrome.   **Note the fine diffuse nodular pattern throughout both lungs. **A. Frontal radiograph. **B.** Axial CT.

and calcification (Fig. 4.122). Once again, old chest radiographs are crucial in these cases to assess for interval change. Any patient with a radiograph suggestive of TB should have a study at least 6 months prior made available for review. Any new changes may indicate reactivation disease.

TB in pediatric patients commonly presents with thoracic and neck adenopathy.

Lastly, TB can disseminate anywhere in the body. If a patient is suspected of having TB, complete systemic evaluation is recommended.

▶ TB in children commonly presents with thoracic and neck adenopathy.

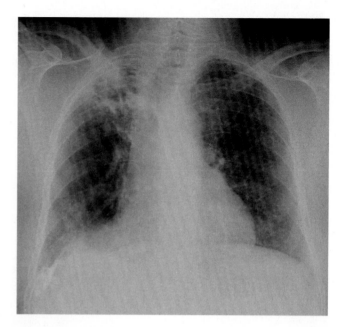

Figure 4.122   Old tuberculous infection.   Right upper lobe consolidation, fibronodular scarring, and ipsilateral mediastinal shift characteristic for granulomatous infection. This could represent active or inactive disease. Old studies would be helpful to assess for new disease.

Adult Respiratory Distress Syndrome

Critically ill patients frequently develop a serious pulmonary complication known as *ARDS*. These patients suffer prolonged anoxia, receive extended ventilatory assistance, and develop an evanescent pulmonary pattern that combines features of pneumonia, pulmonary edema, and mild fibrosis. The pattern changes little on a daily basis. Any intubated patient with persistent multilobar consolidation on chest x-ray should be suspected of having ARDS. CT will show bilateral consolidation with traction bronchiectasis elucidating the fibrotic and stiffness of the diseased lungs (Fig. 4.123). Since these patients require high positive pressure respiratory support, a small airway can rupture producing a pneumothorax or pneumomediastinum. Otherwise known as barotrauma, this can be a deadly. Since the patient is receiving high-pressure ventilation, the pneumothorax can quickly enlarge producing a tension pneumothorax and cardiopulmonary collapse. Therefore, any intubated patient who develops a new pneumothorax should be strongly considered for new chest tube insertion regardless of the size of the pneumothorax to avoid this devastating complication.

Special Pediatric Considerations

Chest radiographs make up at least one-third of all radiologic examinations performed at most children's hospitals. Although many of the diseases, such as pneumonia and atelectasis, produce changes that are identical in children and adults, there are a number of entities that are unique to newborns, infants, and children.

Upper Airway Obstruction

Choanal atresia is an obstruction to the posterior wall of the nasopharynx. It is a threat to newborns who are obligate nasal breathers, particularly during feeding. In approximately 90% of patients the obstruction is bony. Thirty-three percent are bilateral. CT is the best modality for making the diagnosis.

Tonsillar and adenoidal enlargement may be found in asymptomatic healthy children. A neck radiograph showing such enlargement and airway narrowing (Fig. 4.124) usually does not provide any more information than a good clinical examination.

Epiglottitis and *croup* are upper airway diseases that produce respiratory stridor, cough, fever, and irritability. True epiglottitis is less common but more dangerous than croup. The peak incidence is around age 3½. It is usually caused by infection with *H. influenzae*. A lateral radiograph of the neck typically shows increase in the size of the epiglottis and thickening of the aryepiglottic folds (Fig. 4.125). It is this thickening of these folds that obstructs the airway.

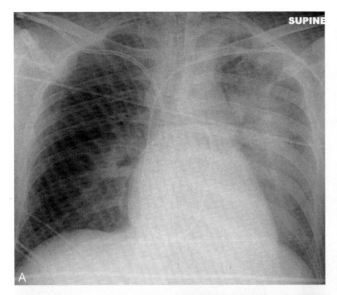

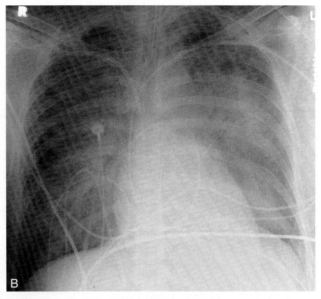

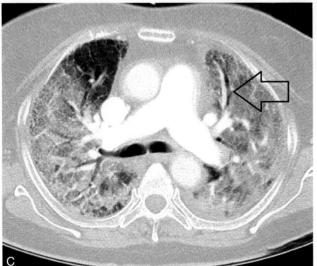

Figure 4.123   Adult respiratory distress syndrome (ARDS).
A. Portable chest radiograph on a trauma victim shows multilobar consolidation in both lungs. Note the presence of an endotracheal tube and Swan-Ganz central venous catheter. **B.** Twelve hours later the portable radiograph shows a dramatic increase in consolidation throughout both lungs. The cardiac size remains normal. **C.** CT image in a different patient shows bilateral consolidation and dilated bronchi (*arrow*). Both signs together in an intubated patient are characteristic for ARDS.

Most cases of croup are caused by viral pathogens. Frontal radiographs of the neck show loss of the lateral contours of the subglottic trachea. On the frontal view, there is narrowing of the airway to produce an inverted "V" that has been called the "steeple sign" (Fig. 4.126).

Disorders of the Newborn

There are a number of conditions that affect newborn infants, especially those who are premature or of extremely low birth weight. These entities are respiratory distress syndrome (RDS), bronchopulmonary dysplasia (BPD), transient tachypnea of the newborn (TTN), neonatal pneumonia, and meconium aspiration.

Respiratory Distress Syndrome

RDS, also known as *HMD*, is a disorder of hypoventilation and pulmonary immaturity with inadequate surfactant production. It occurs predominantly in newborns under 32 weeks of gestation and incidence decreases with advanced gestational age. It is the leading cause of death in newborns. Radiologically, the disease produces a diffuse coarse granular alveolar pattern with shallow lung volumes and air bronchograms (Fig. 4.127). Complications of RDS include pneumothorax, pneumomediastinum, and interstitial emphysema. In many instances, the patient develops BPD.

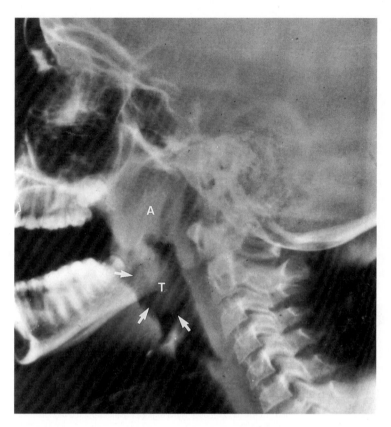

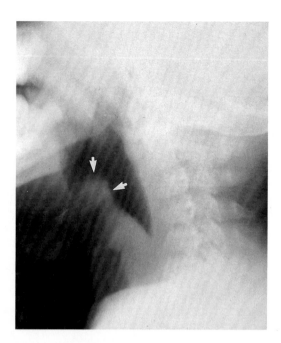

Figure 4.125   Epiglottitis.   There is blunting and thickening of the epiglottis (*arrows*). This has severely narrowed the airway immediately below. Note the dilated hypopharynx.

Figure 4.124   Enlarged tonsils (*T*) (*arrows*) and adenoids (*A*) in an 8-year-old.
The adenoidal enlargement has virtually occluded the nasopharynx.

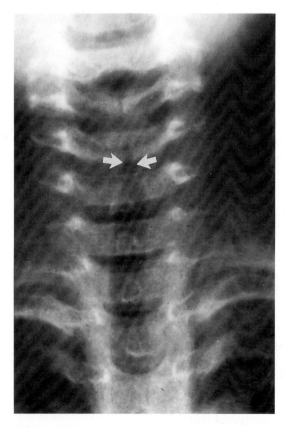

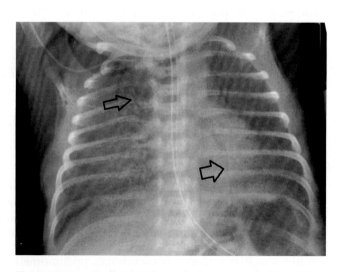

Figure 4.126   Croup.   Frontal radiograph of the neck shows a "steeple sign" of the subglottic region (*arrows*).

Figure 4.127   Hyaline membrane disease.   There is a "ground glass" appearance to both lungs with air bronchograms (*arrows*).

Bronchopulmonary Dysplasia

BPD, also known as chronic lung disease of premature infants, is a complication of prolonged ventilator therapy and RDS. This disease is assigned to infants older than 30 days who required extensive ventilator support, have ongoing pulmonary dysfunction, and characteristic chest x-ray findings. Classically, radiographs show coarse pulmonary opacities with cystic changes and hyperinflation (Fig. 4.128).

Transient Tachypnea of the Newborn

TTN ("wet lung") is caused by delayed resorption and clearing of fetal lung fluid. It is a common cause of respiratory distress in the newborn with babies delivered by cesarean section. Radiographically, there is a pattern of fluid in the lungs with bilateral perihilar infiltrate effusions that can mimic RDS (Fig. 4.129). However, the two diseases are quickly distinguished by their radiographic course. At 10 to 12 hours, TTN begins to clear, whereas RDS usually shows persistent or worsening consolidation. The chest radiograph is usually normal by 48 hours of age in TTN. In addition, TTN usually has increased lung volumes and sometimes a pleural effusion. RDS generally has shallow lung volumes with no pleural effusion. *One important clinical clue to the diagnosis is that the findings occur in a newborn of normal size and birth weight.*

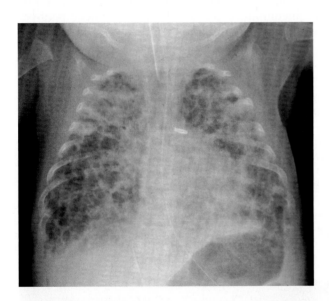

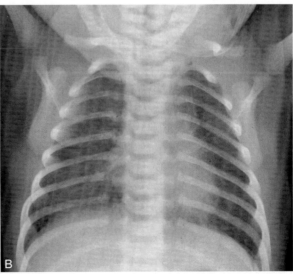

Figure 4.128 Bronchopulmonary dysplasia. Coarse pulmonary lung markings and cystic lung disease commonly develop after 30 days in premature neonates requiring prolonged ventilator assistance. Note the endotracheal and orogastric tubes as well as the ductus arteriosus clip.

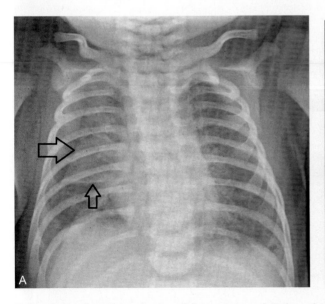

Figure 4.129 Transient tachypnea of the newborn. A. Radiograph immediately after delivery shows ill-defined vascularity consistent with pulmonary edema. Note a normal thymus overlying the right lung otherwise known as the sail sign (*arrow*). **B.** Follow-up radiograph the next day is normal.

Meconium Aspiration Syndrome

Meconium aspiration syndrome occurs as the result of meconium aspiration at the time of birth producing a chemical bronchiolitis with obstruction. This produces patchy areas of atelectasis and segmental hyperinflation. Over time, the opacities will migrate and typically the lungs are overinflated. Pneumothorax or pneumomediastinum may occur in as many as 25% of patients. Because of the chemical nature of the inflammation, radiologic clearing is slower than other pneumonias. The diagnosis is usually assured when the clinical picture includes a history of meconium staining at birth.

Pneumonia

Neonatal pneumonia can be a difficult radiographic diagnosis. Any neonate with persistent and asymmetric consolidation that fails to regress should raise the possibility of a neonatal pneumonia (Fig. 4.130). Nevertheless, RDS and meconium aspiration can have a similar appearance.

Pneumonia in toddlers can have a radiographic pattern similar to those seen in older children and adults. The reader is cautioned not to "overcall" a pneumonia on a crying child, in whom the radiograph is obtained in *expiration*. In these instances, crowding of markings, particularly in the right lower lobe, may be misinterpreted as an infiltrate. Always assess the lung volumes in any child to avoid overcalling a bacterial pneumonia. With a sufficiently aerated film, viral pneumonia produces ill-defined bilateral perihilar infiltrates (Fig. 4.131). Community-acquired pneumonia shows consolidation usually confined to one lobe.

Bronchiolitis and Asthma

Bronchiolitis is a clinical condition in patients over 1 year of age caused by a virus (usually respiratory syncytial virus). Patients typically have a syndrome of wheezing, tachypnea, and low-grade fever. Radiographically, the condition is characterized by hyperinflation, peribronchial cuffing, with or without perihilar linear opacities. The chest radiograph becomes normal once the disease resolves.

Asthma typically occurs in older patients, but can be seen in toddlers as well. The radiographic findings are typically hyperinflation and peribronchial cuffing (Fig. 4.132). With acute asthmatic exacerbations, lobar or segmental atelectasis can occur secondary to mucoid impaction. Pneumonia is an unusual complication unless the patient has a fever or other clinical findings suspicious for infection.

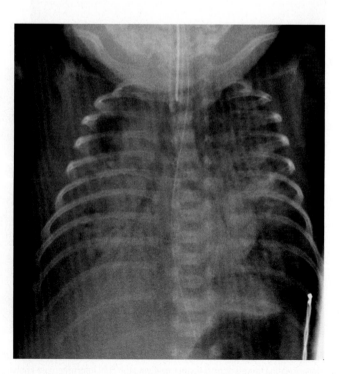

Figure 4.130   Neonatal pneumonia.
Frontal view demonstrates asymmetric bilateral consolidation in a neonate with streptococcal pneumonia.

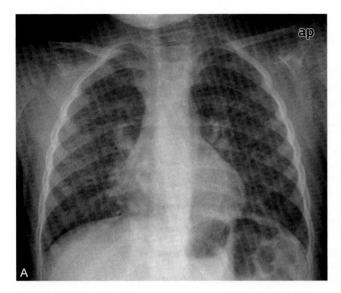

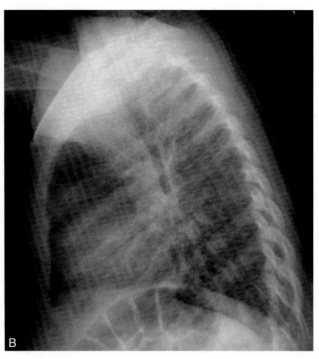

Figure 4.131   Viral pneumonia.   Frontal **(A)** and lateral **(B)** views show interstitial perihilar infiltrates in a patient with a fever characteristic for a viral pneumonia.

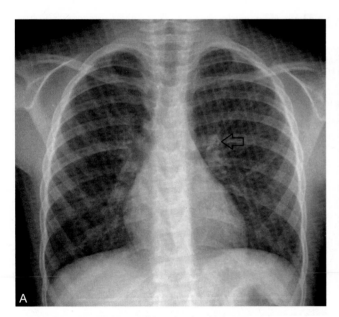

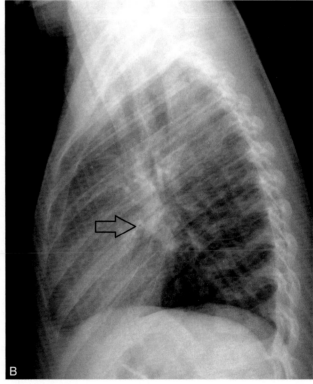

Figure 4.132   Asthma in a child.   Frontal **(A)** and lateral **(B)** views show hyperinflation with peribronchial cuffing (*arrows*).

Summary and Key Points

▶ Chest radiography is the most common imaging examination performed today.

▶ Chest CT is an integral technique in characterizing lung abnormalities and delineating the extent of their involvement. It is particularly important in the diagnosis of pulmonary emboli, aortic dissection, trauma, and neoplasm.

▶ The unit of structure and function in the lung is the pulmonary lobule. This serves on a macroscopic and microscopic level to explain lung pathology.

▶ Pathologic alterations seen in the lung include consolidation, atelectasis, pleural fluid, masses, emphysema, fibrosis, pneumothorax, and pulmonary embolus. Each of these abnormalities produces clearly recognizable patterns.

▶ The concepts of the silhouette sign and the air bronchogram were described as was their importance in localizing pulmonary consolidations.

▶ Acinar (air space) disease produces "fluffy" or "cloudlike" opacities as opposed to reticular or linear abnormalities characteristic for interstitial disease.

▶ Specific entities discussed include postoperative appearances, effects of radiation, diseases that occur in AIDS patients, and pulmonary TB.

▶ Conditions specific to newborns and older children include HMD, BPD, TTN, meconium aspiration, and bronchiolitis.

▶ Community-acquired pneumonias and asthma appear similar in the pediatric age group as well as in adults.

Suggested Additional Reading

Fraser RS, Colman N, Muller N, Paré PD. Synopsis of Diseases of the Chest. 3rd Ed. Philadelphia, PA: WB Saunders, 2005.

Goodman LR. Felson's Principles of Chest Roentgenology Text with CD ROM. 3rd Ed. Philadelphia, PA: Saunders/Elsevier, 2007.

Hansell D, Armstrong P, Lynch D, McAdams HP, Bankier AA. Imaging of Diseases of the Chest. 5th Ed. St. Louis, MO: Mosby/Elsevier, 2009.

Ketai L, Meholic A, Lofgren R. Fundamentals of Chest Radiology. 2nd Ed. Philadelphia, PA: W.B. Saunders, 2006.

Kirks DR, Griscom NT, eds. Practical Pediatric Imaging. Diagnostic Radiology of Infants and Children. 3rd Ed. Philadelphia, PA: Lippincott-Raven, 1998.

McLoud T, Boiselle PM. Thoracic Radiology. The Requisites. 2nd ed. St. Louis, MO: Mosby/Elsevier, 2010.

Reed JC. Chest Radiography: Plain Film Patterns and Differential Diagnoses. 6th Ed. St. Louis, MO: Mosby/Elsevier, 2010.

chapter 5

Cardiac Imaging

Jeffrey S. Mueller   Richard H. Daffner

Cardiac imaging technology has greatly advanced in the last 40 years allowing rapid assessment of coronary artery disease, congenital heart disease, and structural heart disease. The new technology not only accurately quantifies the severity of cardiac disease but assesses responses to treatment and provides important prognostic information.

Cardiac imaging is a subspecialty shared by radiologists and cardiologists. Cardiologists typically perform echocardiography and cardiac catheterization. Radiologists interpret most chest radiographs. Nuclear imaging (single photon emission computed tomography [SPECT] and positron emission tomography [PET]), MRI, and CT are interpreted by either specialty depending on local expertise and referral patterns. As discussed in the following sections, developments in imaging technology have made it possible to make accurate diagnoses using noninvasive techniques.

This chapter discusses the criteria for certain *categories* of diseases rather than describing specific entities. For a complete discussion of those entities, you should consult a comprehensive text on cardiology.

Technical Considerations

The advances in diagnostic imaging techniques in the past four decades have revolutionized cardiac imaging. Radiography, cardiac series, cardiac fluoroscopy, and cardiac catheterization were the mainstays of cardiac imaging before 1975. However, echocardiography, radionuclide cardiac perfusion studies (SPECT and PET), computed tomography (CT), and magnetic resonance imaging (MRI) have become standard evaluation tools in the hands of the cardiovascular radiologist and the cardiologist. Precise cardiac CT images allow the demonstration of coronary arteries with a high degree of accuracy, approaching that for coronary angiography. MRI is extremely valuable for the assessment of myocardial viability following myocardial infarction, valvular heart disease, and myocardial function. CT and MRI are also important tools for the assessment of congenital heart disease. Consequently, clinicians now have a number of options available to evaluate patients. As with any other organ system, your choice of diagnostic studies will depend on getting the most information in the safest way at the lowest cost. Therefore, consulting with your local radiologist or cardiologist is mandatory.

 ▶ Your choice of diagnostic studies will depend on getting the most information in the safest way at the lowest cost.

The same technical considerations for chest radiography that were discussed in Chapter 4 for pulmonary disease apply when evaluating the heart radiographically. You should first decide if the radiograph is a posterior–anterior (PA) or anterior–posterior (AP) view, if the patient is lordotic, and if rotation is present. The degree of penetration (darkness or lightness), the presence of motion, and the degree of inspiration are also important factors to consider. A radiograph made with the patient in a slightly lordotic position will falsely distort and magnify the cardiac size. One that is too light will accentuate the pulmonary vessels. A study with the patient not in maximum inspiration may result in further accentuation of pulmonary vessels and cause an appearance of cardiac enlargement and/or an erroneous diagnosis of congestive heart failure (Fig. 5.1).

It is also necessary to pay close attention to the patient's body habitus. A narrow AP diameter of the chest or a pectus excavatum deformity may result in anterior compression of the heart and a spurious appearance of cardiac enlargement (Fig. 5.2).

The next important step is to assess for the presence of the complications of heart disease. This includes the development of pulmonary edema, pleural effusions, pulmonary hypertension, aortic disease, and, in rare cases, rib notching from collateral vessel formation.

Figure 5.1   Expiratory view.   PA radiograph made in forced expiration. The diaphragm is flat and the heart appears enlarged. The pulmonary vessels appear prominent.

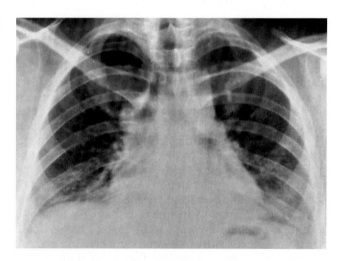

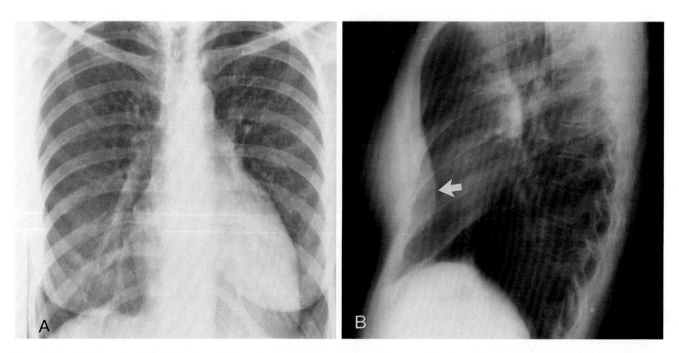

Figure 5.2   Pectus excavatum deformity.   A. Frontal radiograph shows apparent enlargement of the heart. The ribs are slightly more horizontal posteriorly and steeper anteriorly. **B.** Lateral radiograph shows a prominent pectus excavatum deformity (*arrow*). The sternal deformity compressed the heart and gave the spurious appearance of enlargement.

The basic imaging techniques used for evaluating the heart are:

- chest radiography;
- cardiac catheterization and coronary arteriography;
- echocardiography;
- radioisotope studies (SPECT and PET);
- CT; and
- MRI.

Each modality will be described in detail.

Chest Radiography

Chest radiography is the most frequently ordered imaging examination in patients with suspected cardiac disease. By knowing the normal anatomy portrayed on the PA and lateral images and by analyzing the sizes of pulmonary arteries and veins, you can frequently tell if the patient has heart disease.

Cardiothoracic Ratio

A popular method used to determine cardiac size is the *cardiothoracic ratio*: the maximum width of the cardiac shadow on the PA chest radiograph divided by the maximum width of the thorax. This method has received criticism because a true determination of cardiac enlargement requires evaluating the cardiac silhouette on *both* the PA and lateral views. Generally, however, the cardiac width should never exceed half the width of the thorax on the PA image. Keep in my mind that assessing heart size on an AP or portable chest radiograph is inaccurate and often misleading.

 ▶ The cardiac width should never exceed half the width of the thorax on the PA radiograph.

Cardiac Catheterization and Coronary Arteriography

Left heart catheterization and coronary arteriography are invasive procedures performed by interventional cardiologists. These procedures allow accurate evaluation of the size and configuration of the cardiac chambers, the great vessels, and the coronary arteries. The most common use is in patients with known or suspected coronary artery disease. Real-time echocardiography has decreased the number of catheterizations used to determine cardiac chamber size and configuration. Cardiac CT may further decrease the number of catheterizations performed for patients with chest pain. Right heart catheterization is performed to evaluate patients with pulmonary hypertension in order to measure right heart and pulmonary arterial pressures and resistance. A pulmonary arterial wedge pressure can also be obtained to estimate left atrial pressure.

Echocardiography

Echocardiography is an ultrasound examination of the heart and great vessels, primarily using one of three techniques: motion mode (M mode), cross-sectional (two-dimensional) imaging, or Doppler technique. It can be obtained with a probe on the chest wall (*transthoracic*) or with an esophageal probe (*transesophageal*). The echocardiogram is the principal diagnostic tool for investigating valvular disease, assessing heart function and wall motion abnormalities, calculating ejection fraction, and characterizing pericardial effusions.

Conventional ultrasound of the solid viscera relies on the principle of the velocity of sound traveling through a medium, reflecting off a tissue interface, and returning to the transducer. An internal computer calculates the distance of that interface from the transducer and displays the image on a monitor. Moving interfaces, such as would be encountered in the beating heart, produce echographs that change as a result of variations in the distance to the transducer. For this reason, cardiac and vascular (Doppler) ultrasound studies are significantly different from those of static organs.

Motion-Mode Echocardiography

All forms of cardiac ultrasound evolved from M-mode echocardiography. M-mode ultrasound displays cardiac motion as a one-dimensional recording over a time period that can be displayed on a paper strip tracing (Fig. 5.3). This allows for measuring the depth of each structure as well as displaying its motion (Fig. 5.4). Two-dimensional cross-sectional echocardiography provides real-time images of the moving heart chambers. By shifting the transducer and altering the depth of penetration of the ultrasound beam, a tomographic image of the heart and its chambers can be obtained.

Doppler Echocardiography

Doppler echocardiography allows the study of interruptions or obstruction of flowing blood and thus is used primarily to assess the direction and velocity of blood flow in the heart, great vessels, and peripheral arteries and veins. It is particularly useful in evaluating the integrity and motion of the cardiac valves. Color Doppler superimposes a color-coded, real-time depiction of the direction of blood flow on a two-dimensional image. The added color helps in the interpretation of the study. Spectral Doppler estimates velocity and direction. Information can be plotted on a graph showing changes in velocity of moving blood versus time. Abnormally elevated velocities are the key components to estimating the severity of valvular or vascular stenosis (Fig. 5.5).

Transthoracic Echocardiography

Transthoracic echocardiography is performed by placing the transducer on the neck, chest, and abdomen to obtain parasternal long-axis and short-axis, apical, subcostal, and suprasternal images (Figs. 5.6 and 5.7). Figure 5.8 illustrates some of the normal anatomic structures demonstrated by this technique. Transesophageal echocardiography obtains images by inserting a probe down the esophagus while the patient is sedated. The advantage is a better acoustical window providing more detailed and accurate imaging. Either technique can also be enhanced by intravenous contrast or gas-filled microbubbles. This improves the contrast resolution of the exam and also allows for better detection of right to left intracardiac shunts. For greater detail, consult the excellent texts by Armstrong or Bonow listed at the end of this chapter.

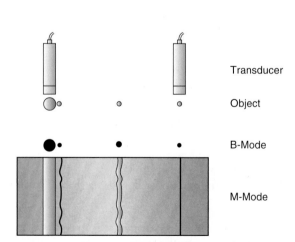

Figure 5.3   Ultrasound display modes.   The transducer passing over objects of varying size portrays those objects in a different fashion depending on the display mode. In brightness mode (B mode), the objects appear as dots; in motion (M mode), they appear as a series of wavy lines.

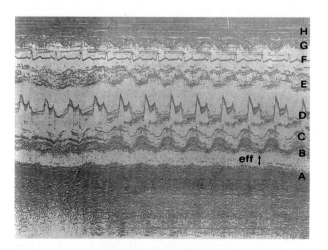

Figure 5.4   M-mode echocardiogram showing a pericardial effusion (*eff*).   Anatomic structures and motion are displayed on a tracing. The vertical column is distance from the transducer which is at the top. The ultrasound sound waves propagate from the top of the tracing to the bottom displaying the acoustical impedance of different anatomical structures. The horizontal axis is time. The waveforms indicate motion of the different cardiac valves. **A.** Pericardium. **B.** Left ventricular wall. **C.** Chorda tendinea. **D.** Mitral valve. **E.** Septal wall. **F.** Electrocardiogram. **G.** Right ventricular wall. **H.** Chest wall.

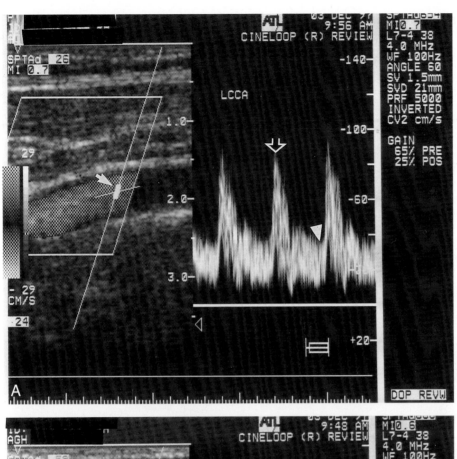

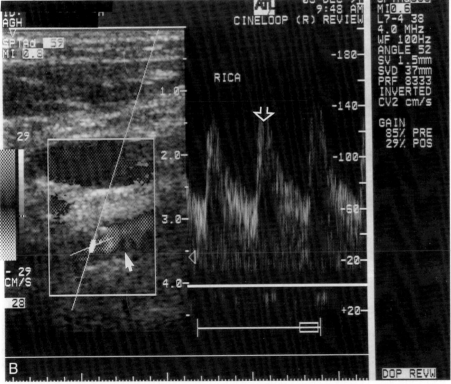

Figure 5.5 Carotid Doppler ultrasound examination. **A.** Normal left common carotid artery (LCCA). The gray-scale image of a portion of the LCCA shows the vessel to be widely patent. The vessel walls are smooth, without visible atheromatous plaques. The rectangle within the vessel lumen (*small arrow on left*) is the Doppler sample site from which the flow characteristics and velocities generate the Doppler waveform tracing shown to the right of the gray-scale image. There is a normal peak systolic flow velocity of 90 cm/second (*open arrow;* normal ≤125 cm/second) as well as antegrade blood flow velocity of 40 cm/second at the end of diastole (*arrowhead*). The Doppler waveform also allows for evaluation of the degree of laminar flow turbulence, otherwise known as spectral broadening. This is reflected by the range of red blood cell velocities. The greater the velocity range, the greater the turbulence. This normal vessel demonstrates a velocity range of 40 to 90 cm/second. **B.** Significant stenosis in a right internal carotid artery (RICA). The gray-scale image of a portion of the RICA shows gross vessel wall irregularity with significant stenosis near the Doppler sample site (*small arrow on left*). The Doppler waveform tracing shows an elevated peak systolic flow with velocities of 140 cm/second (*open arrow*). In addition, there is marked spectral broadening which are bright pixels between the top of the waveform and the horizontal axis. Compare these tracings and images with **(A)**.

Stress Test Assessment

The cardiologist can also assess for ischemic heart disease. Typically, the patient exercises on a treadmill to stress the heart. If the patient cannot exercise, dobutamine can be infused, which elevates the patient's heart rate and cardiac output. The exercise or pharmacologic "stress" raises the metabolic requirements of the heart and under normal

Figure 5.6   Normal planes of echocardiographic scans.
LA, left atrium; *LV,* left ventricle; *RA,* right atrium; *RV,* right ventricle.

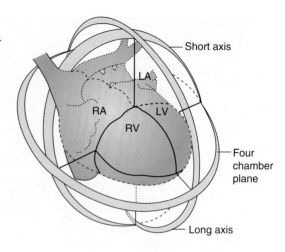

Parasternal Long Axis View

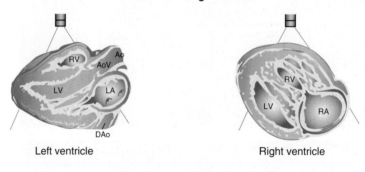

Left ventricle   Right ventricle

Parasternal Short Axis View

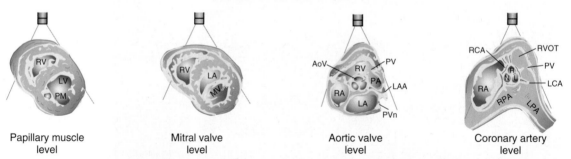

Papillary muscle   Mitral valve   Aortic valve   Coronary artery
     level   level   level   level

Figure 5.7   Anatomy of the heart demonstrated in the parasternal long-axis and short-axis views.   *Ao,* aorta; *AoV,* aortic valve (with right, left, and neutral cusps); *DAo,* descending aorta; *LA,* left atrium; *LAA,* left atrial appendage; *LCA,* left coronary artery; *LPA,* left pulmonary artery; *LV,* left ventricle; *MV,* mitral valve; *PA,* pulmonary artery; *PM,* papillary muscle; *PV,* pulmonic valve; *PVn,* pulmonary vein; *RA,* right atrium; *RCA,* right coronary artery; *RPA,* right pulmonary artery; *RV,* right ventricle; *RVOT,* right ventricular outflow tract.

situations dilates the coronary arteries and increases blood flow to the myocardium. In patients with coronary artery disease, atherosclerosis impairs the ability of blood vessels to dilate during increased metabolic demand. Coupled with vessel narrowing by the atherosclerotic plaque, blood flow to the myocardium cannot increase, and as a result, that part of the heart does not contract normally. Therefore, the cardiologist assesses for altered contractility of the heart as an indirect sign of coronary artery disease.

Radioisotope Studies

Radioisotope studies are performed primarily to evaluate cardiac perfusion and function. Radioisotopes such as thallium 201 and technetium 99m sestamibi are injected intravenously, and myocardial perfusion is recorded as a series of images. Myocardial perfusion

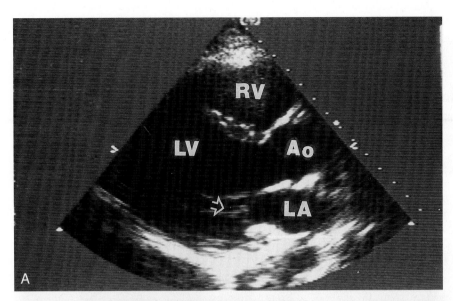

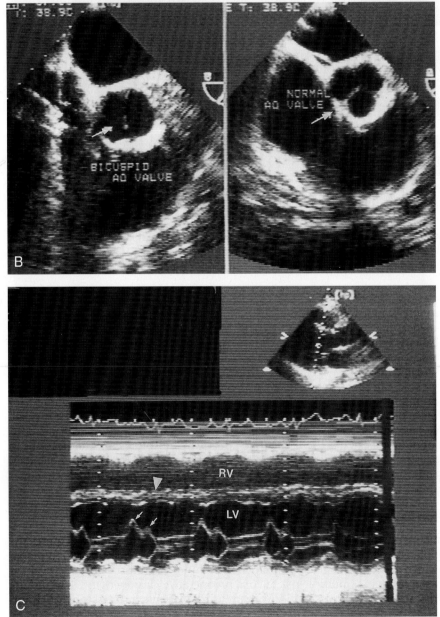

Figure 5.8   Normal echocardiographic anatomy.   A. Two-dimensional parasternal view showing the normal right ventricle (*RV*), left ventricle (*LV*), ascending aorta (*Ao*), and left atrium (*LA*). The aortic valve is open in this view made in systole. The mitral valve is closed (*arrow*). **B.** Aortic valve variations showing a bicuspid valve in the left panel and a normal tricuspid valve in the right panel (*arrows*). **C.** M-mode parasternal view shows a normal right ventricle (*RV*), interventricular septum (*arrowhead*), mitral valve (*small arrows*), and left ventricle (*LV*).

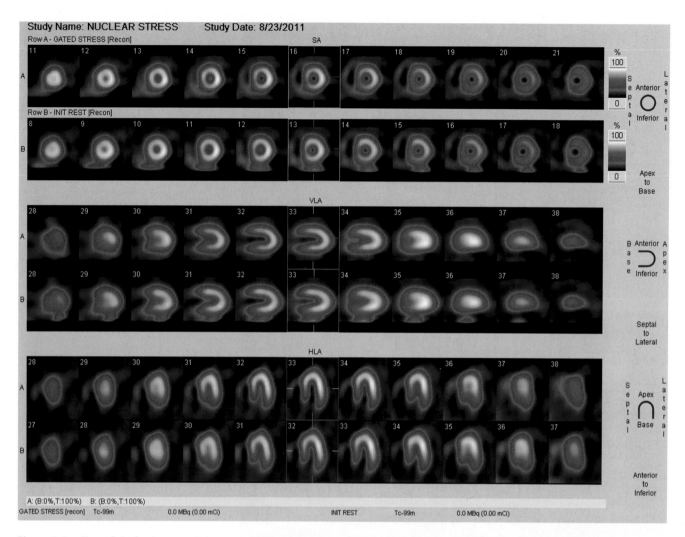

Figure 5.9 **Normal single photon emission computed tomography nuclear sestamibi scan with stress and rest testing.** Distribution of blood flow is uniform over the left ventricle, as evidenced by the uniform distribution of the isotope between rest and stress. First row, short-axis stress; second row, short-axis rest; third row, vertical long-axis stress; fourth row, vertical long-axis rest; fifth row, horizontal long-axis stress; sixth row, horizontal long-axis rest.

images are usually obtained with stress and rest (Fig. 5.9). The hallmark of ischemic heart disease is a myocardial perfusion defect with stress that reverses or normalizes with rest (Fig. 5.10). Patients typically walk on a treadmill to stress the heart. If the patient cannot walk or exercise, pharmacological stress can also be performed with intravenous adenosine. Adenosine is a vasodilator agent that simulates the effects of exercise on the coronary arteries. Adenosine can also induce bronchospasm in patients with asthma or chronic obstructive pulmonary disease. Therefore, any patient should be closely monitored for the signs of bronchospasm, and bronchodilators should be available and ready if needed. Dipyridamole has similar effects as adenosine and can be substituted. As with echocardiography, dobutamine can also be used. There are several absolute contraindications to cardiac stress testing: recent myocardial infarction, unstable angina, severe aortic stenosis, pulmonary embolism, acute pericarditis, aortic dissection, and hemodynamically significant arrhythmias (ventricular tachycardia).

Single Photon Emission Computed Tomography

Exams are obtained with a technique called *SPECT*, where a gamma camera acquires the data in multiple circular rotations around the patient. This is more accurate than planar acquisition which has been largely replaced. This technique is most useful for evaluating clinically stable angina, multiple risk factors, preoperative clearance, and determining subsequent risk stratification for significant future cardiac events in the setting of abnormal findings (Fig. 5.10).

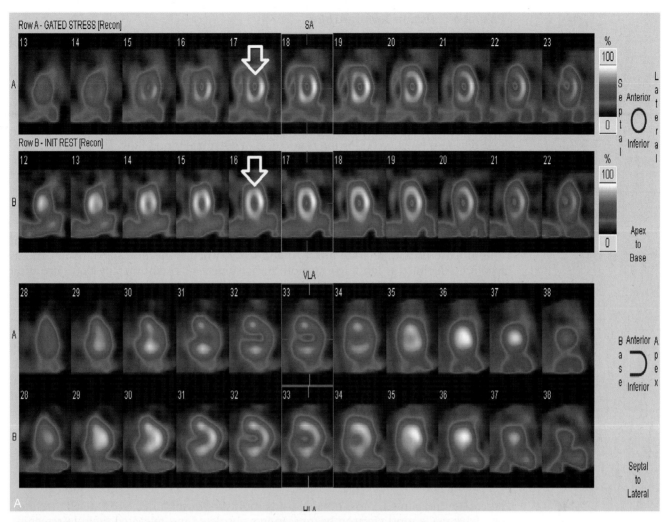

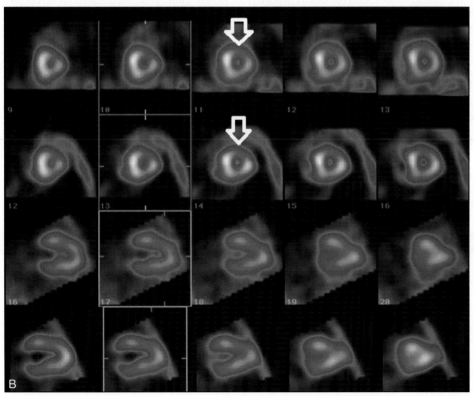

Figure 5.10 Abnormal single photon emission computed tomography nuclear stress. A. Reversible perfusion defect or ischemia shows decreased tracer activity or perfusion of the distal anterior wall with stress (top row, *arrow*) that fills in on stress images (second row, *arrow*). **B.** Different patient. Infarcted area of the anterior left ventricular wall, as demonstrated by a photopenic area during stress and rest (*arrows*).

Positron Emission Tomography

PET studies with F 18 fluoro-2-deoxyglucose are used to assess the viability of myocardial tissue, especially when coronary artery bypass surgery is being considered. Exams are commonly combined with rubidium 82 or nitrogen 13 to assess myocardial perfusion as well. The advantage of PET is its ability to assess both perfusion and viability in one setting. While SPECT imaging can identify ischemic heart tissue, it cannot distinguish a myocardial infarct from chronically ischemic or hibernating myocardium. However, both PET and MRI can make that critical distinction. Hibernating myocardium is still viable that may return to function following restoration of adequate blood flow. Therefore, PET and MRI are important modalities that can help predict the success of coronary revascularization. Given its higher photon energy and less soft tissue attenuation, PET is also more accurate than SPECT in obese patients.

Radioisotope Ventriculography

Lastly, radioisotope ventriculography studies with technetium 99m–tagged red blood cells are also used to analyze the right and left ventricular ejection fractions in patients who are scheduled to undergo cardiothoracic surgery or chemotherapy that may affect cardiac function.

Computed Tomography

Dramatic advances in CT technology in the last 15 years allow for accurate noninvasive assessment of the heart. Previously, CT evaluation of heart disease was difficult given the rapid motion of the heart during the cardiac cycle. *Electron beam CT*, a variation of conventional CT, was originally designed for this purpose given its fast temporal resolution. Examinations were performed without intravenous contrast to calculate the amount of calcium in the coronary arteries and to estimate the risk of the patient experiencing a myocardial event in the next 5 years. However, electron beam CT suffered from poor contrast resolution, low generator capacities, and high cost limiting its ability to perform accurate contrast-enhanced coronary artery imaging.

Computed Tomography Advances

Recent advances in CT, most notably using multislice or multidetector (MDCT) technology, have made most electron beam scanners obsolete (and relegated them to screening baggage at airports). Not only can MDCT now produce accurate calcium scoring exams like electron beam CT, but coronary artery imaging with intravenous contrast has also dramatically improved. The introduction of 64 or higher slice MDCT technology has dramatically expanded the applications of cardiac CT. Coupled with faster gantry rotation and electrocardiographic gating, CT images the relatively small coronary arteries with excellent anatomic detail and no motion artifact. CT can distinguish between a calcified and soft plaque (Fig. 5.11), which is not possible with cardiac catheterization. This imaging technology also allows the reconstruction of three-dimensional images displaying the anatomic relationships of the coronary arteries (Fig. 5.12). Its superior ability to assess the anatomic relationships of the coronary arteries with adjacent cardiovascular structures such as the aorta and main pulmonary artery now make cardiac CT the gold standard for the evaluation of congenital anomalies of the coronary artery (Figs. 5.13 and 5.14). The radiation dose from a cardiac CT is similar to nuclear medicine thallium or sestamibi scans, although radiation doses have fallen recently due to recent dose reduction techniques.

In addition, cardiac CT is also used to evaluate the patency of coronary artery bypass grafts, to depict the size and morphology of left ventricular aneurysms and neoplasms, to evaluate aneurysms and dissections of the thoracic aorta (Fig. 5.15), to characterize certain congenital abnormalities such as coarctation of the aorta and anomalous venous connections, and to characterize pericardial effusions and pericardial disease. Multiple phases of the cardiac cycle can be reconstructed to create a contracting or dynamic video allowing for wall motion abnormalities and calculation of the ejection fraction.

In summary, cardiac CT offers several advantages over invasive angiography:

- It is noninvasive and thus without the complications of traditional angiography.
- A CT scan of the entire heart may be performed in less than 10 seconds.
- There is no need for a hospital stay.
- It is cost-effective.
- It gives better depiction of coronary anomalies.

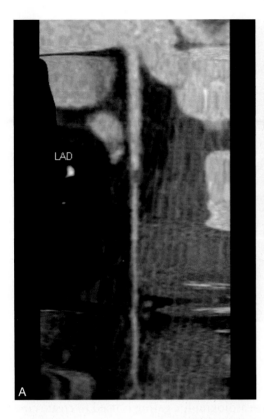

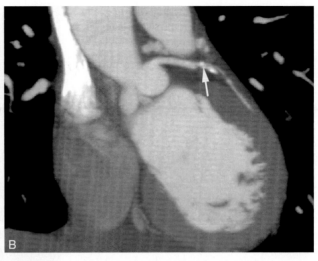

Figure 5.11   **A.** CT curved planar reformats (CPR) of the left anterior descending (*LAD*) artery shows soft plaque narrowing the proximal artery by more than 70%. Result was confirmed with coronary angiography. **B.** CPR of the LAD artery in a different patient shows a calcified plaque (*arrow*).

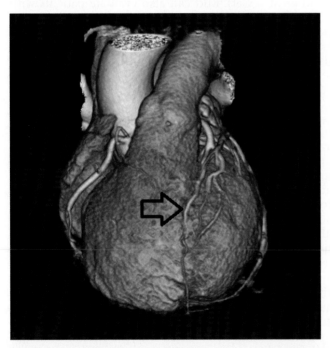

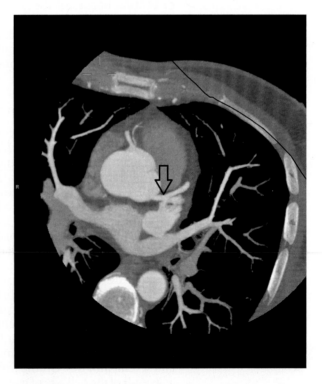

Figure 5.12   Volume-rendering technique image from a cardiac CT angiogram performed on a 64-row multidetector CT scanner.   The left main coronary artery arises from the root of the aorta beneath the left atrial appendage. The left anterior descending coronary artery (*arrow*) is in the interventricular groove.

Figure 5.13   Maximum intensity projection CT image.   This image shows the normal left main coronary artery (*arrow*) arising from the left cusp and the right coronary artery arising from the right cusp.

○ It provides clear demonstration of calcium deposits and plaque morphology.
○ It allows "one-stop shop" analysis of the coronary arteries, aorta, and pulmonary arteries in patients with acute chest pain, otherwise known as the triple rule out.
○ It allows three-dimensional volume-rendered images.

Figure 5.14   Maximum intensity projection CT image.
The left main coronary artery arises from a common trunk with the right coronary artery. The vessel then courses between the aorta and the pulmonary artery (*arrow*). This anatomic variant can lead to sudden death.

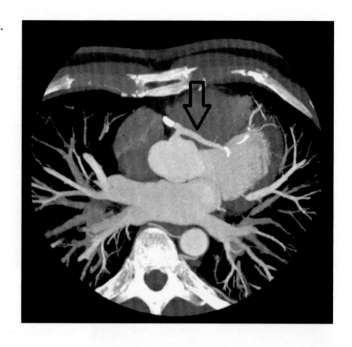

Magnetic Resonance Imaging

MRI has different advantages over CT. Electrocardiographic gating is used to create cine or beating images of the heart and great vessels. MRI can also evaluate patients with aortic dissections (Fig. 5.15) and aortic coarctation (Fig. 5.16), although MDCT is more commonly used for the evaluation of aortic disease in patients who do not have a contraindication to the use of contrast. In addition, *magnetic resonance angiography (MRA)* is used as a noninvasive method for evaluating aneurysms or stenotic disease (Figs. 5.17 and 5.18).

Indications and Limitations

The best indication for cardiac magnetic resonance (MR) is distinguishing viable or hibernating myocardium (chronically ischemic) from nonviable or infarcted myocardium. Although PET can also make the same distinction, MR has better spatial resolution allowing it to assess both transmural and subendocardial diseases. Early or mild ischemic heart disease typically involves subendocardial myocardial tissue or the portion of the heart muscle directly beneath the endocardium. This is the area of the heart at greatest risk for infarction following coronary artery occlusion or narrowing. Severe ischemic heart disease is usually transmural involving the entire thickness of the myocardium. Therefore, MR is theoretically more sensitive than PET for characterizing ischemic heart disease. However, MR cannot currently be performed with pacemaker or automatic intracardiac defibrillator devices (AICDs), which are commonly necessary in patients with ischemic heart disease. MRI requires a regular sinus rhythm and arrhythmias (including atrial fibrillation and frequent premature ventricular contractions) may not permit adequate imaging. PET is also a better option for obese patients.

Cardiac MR for ischemic heart disease should be obtained with gadolinium enhancement. Images are obtained immediately following contrast injection (first-pass perfusion) and several minutes. On the first-pass perfusion images, normal myocardium turns bright as a result of the delivery of gadolinium to the myocardium (Fig. 5.19). Infarcted or severely ischemic myocardium will not immediately perfuse with gadolinium. Tissue viability can be determined by obtaining delayed images. A special pulsing sequence is chosen to make normal myocardium dark. Contrast will slowly diffuse into infarcted myocardium creating a bright signal on the delayed images, otherwise known as delayed enhancement. The contrast washes out of the normal myocardium (Fig. 5.20). If the thickness of the brightly enhancing myocardium involves more than 50% of the total myocardial wall, the tissue is felt to be infarcted and not amenable to revascularization. If the thickness of the enhancing myocardium is less than 50% of the myocardial wall, the tissue is considered ischemic

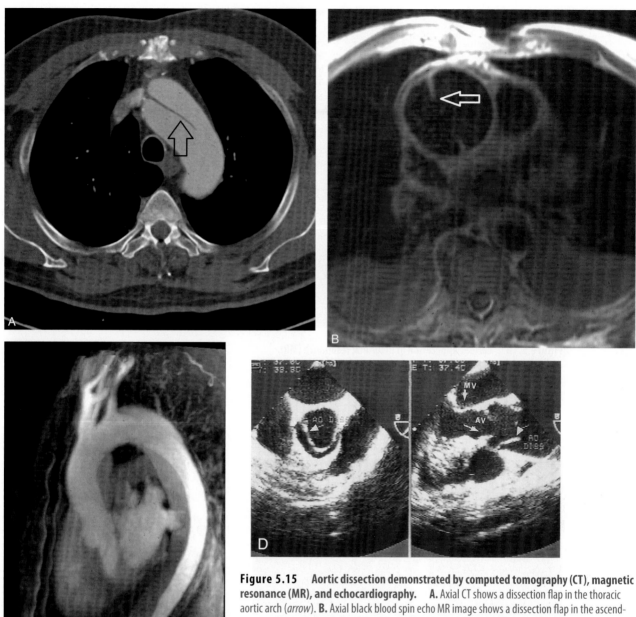

Figure 5.15 **Aortic dissection demonstrated by computed tomography (CT), magnetic resonance (MR), and echocardiography.** **A.** Axial CT shows a dissection flap in the thoracic aortic arch (*arrow*). **B.** Axial black blood spin echo MR image shows a dissection flap in the ascending aorta (*arrow*). **C. Sagittal maximum intensity projection MR imaging.** This shows the extent of the dissection throughout the entire aorta. **D.** Echocardiogram. Left panel is a short-axis image of the aortic root and shows the intimal flap (*arrowhead*) of the dissection with the crescent false lumen beyond. Right panel shows a long-axis image of the aortic root with the intimal flap of the dissection (*arrowhead*). The mitral valve (*MV, short arrow*) is closed and the aortic valve (*AV, long arrow*) is open.

and should respond to revascularization. Keep in mind that gadolinium should not be injected in patients with chronic renal disease with a glomerular filtration rate less than 30 to 60 mL/minute due to the risk of nephrogenic systemic fibrosis (NSF).

 ▶ Gadolinium compounds should not be injected in patients with chronic renal disease due to the risk of NSF.

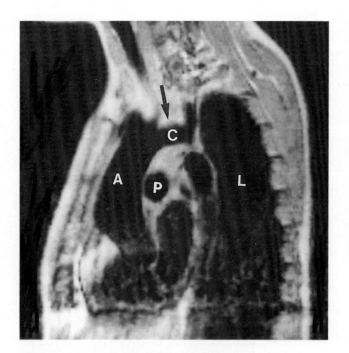

Figure 5.16   Cardiac application of magnetic resonance (MR) imaging.   Parasagittal MR image showing coarctation of the aorta (*arrow*). Note the following landmarks: *A,* ascending aorta; *C,* coarctation; *P,* pulmonary artery; *L,* lung.

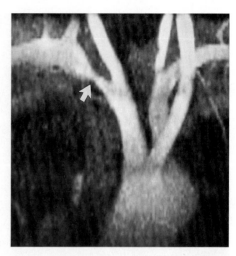

Figure 5.17   Magnetic resonance angiograms (MRA).   MRA of the great vessels in a patient with subclavian steal syndrome. Note the stenosis of the right subclavian artery (*arrow*) and poststenotic dilatation. Compare with the left.

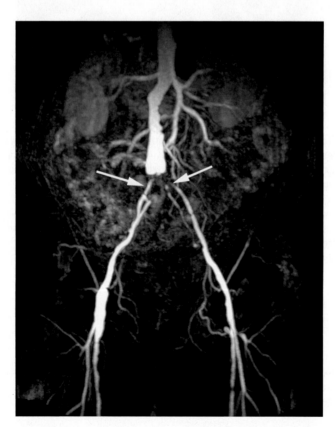

Figure 5.18   Magnetic resonance angiograms (MRAs).   MRA of aortoiliac runoff. There is stenosis of both common iliac arteries (*arrows*). Note the plaque in the distal aorta.

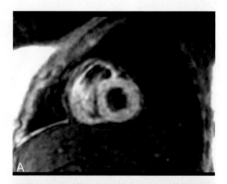
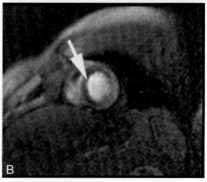

Figure 5.19   Normal and abnormal first-pass perfusion on cardiac magnetic resonance.   A. Short-axis image shows bright signal in the entire myocardium following gadolinium injection. **B.** Another patient with ischemia shows the anterior and septal walls are not bright and do not enhance (*arrow*). (Courtesy of Carl Fuhrman, MD, Department of Radiology, University of Pittsburgh School of Medicine.)

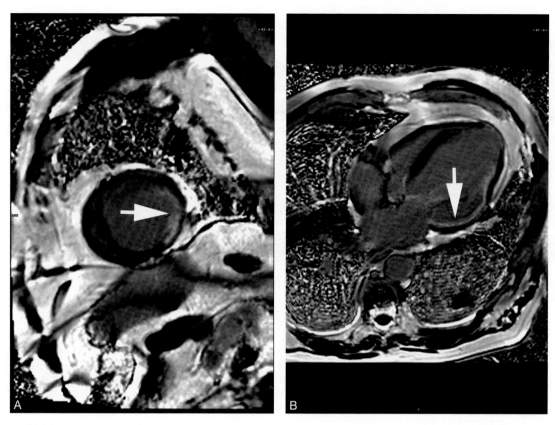

Figure 5.20   Cardiac magnetic resonance imaging with delayed enhancement series.   A. Short-axis image demonstrates abnormally high signal (*arrow*) involving the lateral basilar wall. **B.** Four-chamber view (horizontal long axis) showing same finding in a different plane (*arrow*). Note the signal involves nearly the entire thickness of the myocardium consistent with infarcted tissue. Also note the septal myocardium is dark which is normal.

Other Indications for Magnetic Resonance Imaging

Other uses for MRI are in evaluating cardiac anatomy and morphology, assessing global and regional myocardial function, quantifying valvular heart disease, and calculating shunt fractions in patients with an intracardiac shunt (atrial septal or ventricular septal defects). MRI is very useful in the evaluation of cardiac masses and tumors and can often be useful in separating thrombus from tumor in the heart chambers (Fig. 5.21). MR can usually differentiate between constrictive pericardial disease and restrictive

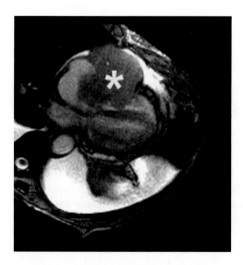

Figure 5.21   Cardiac plasmacytoma (*asterisk*) involving the right atrium and right ventricle.   (Courtesy of Carl Fuhrman, MD, Department of Radiology, University of Pittsburgh School of Medicine.)

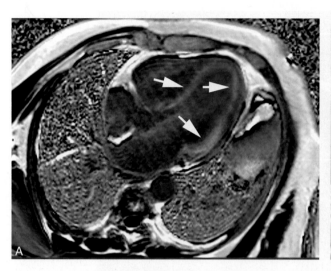
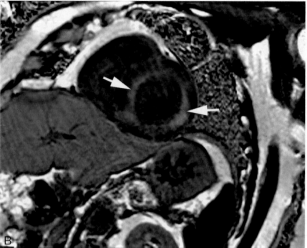

Figure 5.22   Cardiac amyloidosis.   A. Four-chamber view shows diffuse subendocardial hyperenhancement (*arrows*) typical for amyloidosis.
B. Short-axis view shows the same finding in a different plane.

myocardial disease, which have similar clinical presentations. MRI is very useful for evaluating pericardial disease, including pericardial effusions and thickening, although it cannot detect pericardial calcification, a finding characteristic for constrictive pericarditis. Infiltrative diseases of the myocardium such as sarcoidosis, hemochromatosis, and amyloidosis create a very rigid and stiff myocardium, which prevents adequate myocardial filling or a restrictive cardiomyopathy (Fig. 5.22). MR can detect fatty and fibrous infiltration of the right ventricle making it the gold standard for a rare but potentially lethal disease called *arrhythmogenic right ventricular dysplasia.* Research is continuing into the use of MR for coronary artery imaging, although it is limited for routine clinical use at the present time.

Anatomic Considerations

To appreciate the anatomic relationships of the heart and its chambers on a chest x-ray, you need to think in three-dimensional terms. The following sections examine the position of the cardiac chambers, the great vessels, and the aortic and mitral valves, as seen on PA and lateral radiographs in Figure 5.23. Anatomic considerations for the other cardiac imaging modalities are beyond the scope of this chapter and will not be discussed.

Structures

- Cardiac chambers
- Pulmonary vasculature
- Aortic arch

Cardiac Chambers

Posterior–Anterior View

On the *PA view* (see Fig. 5.23A), most of the cardiac silhouette is made up almost exclusively of the right side of the heart; the left ventricle forms the left cardiac border. The right atrium forms the right border of the heart, merging imperceptibly into the image of the superior vena cava. The left atrium is not seen in this view under normal circumstances. However, a small portion of the left border of the heart just beneath the pulmonary trunk is represented by the left atrial appendage. In this view, the aortic valve is positioned obliquely, with its lower end oriented to the right approximately in the midline just below the waist of the cardiovascular silhouette. The mitral valve, which is oriented on a similar plane in this view, lies just below the aortic valve area and to the left. Occasionally, calcification of these valves or their annuli will be seen on this view (Fig. 5.24).

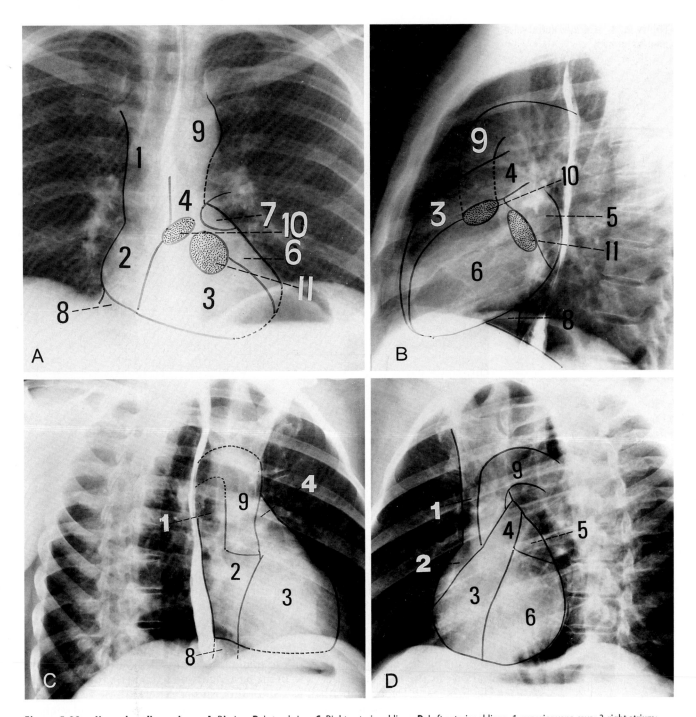

Figure 5.23 Normal cardiac series. **A.** PA view. **B.** Lateral view. **C.** Right anterior oblique. **D.** Left anterior oblique. *1,* superior vena cava; *2,* right atrium; *3,* right ventricle; *4,* pulmonary outflow tract; *5,* left atrium; *6,* left ventricle; *7,* left atrial appendage; *8,* inferior vena cava; *9,* ascending aorta and aortic arch; *10,* aortic valve; *11,* mitral valve.

Mainstem Bronchi

One additional useful anatomic relationship to note is that of the *mainstem bronchi* to the heart. The trachea bifurcates below the aortic arch. The bronchi continue downward and branch from this point. The left mainstem bronchus, however, has a close relationship with the left atrium. Consequently, enlargement of the left atrium may result in elevation of the left mainstem bronchus and widening of the normal carinal angle to greater than 75° in adults, otherwise known as "splaying of the carina." Greater angulation is allowed for infants and children.

Figure 5.24 Calcified mitral valve annulus (*arrows*).

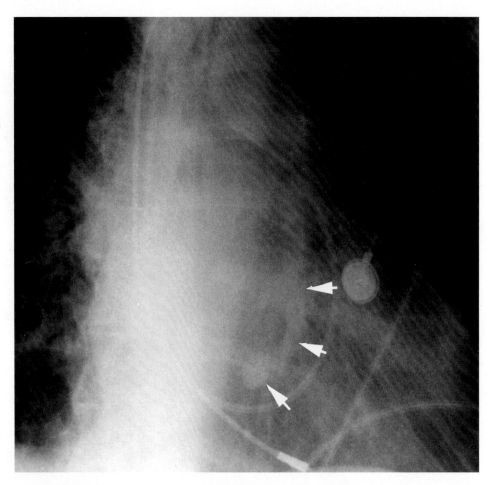

Normal Lateral View

In the *normal lateral view* (see Fig. 5.23**B**), the anterior border of the cardiac silhouette consists of the right ventricle. The posterior cardiac border is that of the left atrium with the left ventricle more inferior and anterior. The image of the inferior vena cava superimposes on the posteroinferior border of the left ventricle, occasionally extending just posterior to the left ventricular outline. Frequently, the pulmonary artery is observed arching up from the right ventricle and passing inferiorly to the arch of the aorta, which is also visible on the lateral film. In this view, the aortic valve lies almost horizontally just below the narrow waist of the cardiovascular pedicle. As indicated in Figure 5.23**B**, the mitral valve ring lies in an oblique plane, inferior and posterior to that of the aortic valve. Valvular or annular calcification can also be seen in this view. In the past, right and left anterior oblique views (see Fig. 5.23**C** and **D**) were obtained as part of the "cardiac series." These views are no longer performed since cardiac ultrasound is now used to determine the size and configuration of the heart chambers.

Pulmonary Vasculature

The pulmonary arteries and veins account for the lung markings seen on a chest radiograph. It is sometimes difficult to differentiate between arteries and veins on a radiograph. However, a useful method is by analyzing the *direction* of the vessels to determine whether they are arterial or venous. Normally, the pulmonary arteries radiate from the hilar region in a fairly uniform, fanlike appearance (Fig. 5.25A). The veins, on the other hand, follow a different course because of the lower location of the left atrium, into which they must terminate. The upper lobe veins assume an obliquely downward course, in some instances almost vertical, as they "dive" for the left atrium; the lower lobe veins assume a more horizontal course, located almost directly opposite the level of the left atrium (Fig. 5.25B). It is important to be able to differentiate arteries from veins because the proposed approach for diagnosis is based on analysis of the pulmonary vasculature.

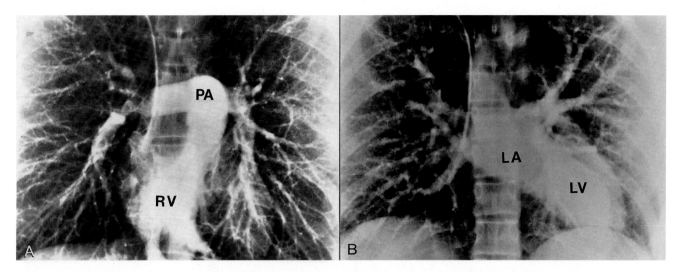

Figure 5.25 Normal pulmonary arteriogram. A. Arterial phase. Injection was made into the right ventricle (*RV*). Contrast material passes through the pulmonary outflow tract into the pulmonary arteries (*PA*). **B.** Venous phase. Contrast material passes from the pulmonary veins into the left atrium (*LA*) and then into the left ventricle (*LV*). Note the difference in orientation between the pulmonary arteries and pulmonary veins.

▶ The pulmonary arteries radiate from the hilar region in a fairly uniform, fanlike appearance.
▶ The pulmonary veins follow a different course; the upper lobe veins assume an obliquely downward course, in some instances almost vertical, as they "dive" for the left atrium; the lower lobe veins assume a more horizontal course, located almost directly opposite the level of the left atrium.

In a normal heart, the vascularity of the lower lobes is more prominent than that of the upper lobes. This relationship is altered in a normal person in the recumbent position, where gravity results in greater flow to the cephalic regions.

Aortic Arch

Finally, it is important to observe the side on which the aortic arch is located and the position of the gastric air bubble. Under normal circumstances, the aortic arch is on the left. However, there are anomalies of this vessel in which the arch is on the right (Fig. 5.26). The gastric air bubble is also ordinarily on the left. However, in patients with

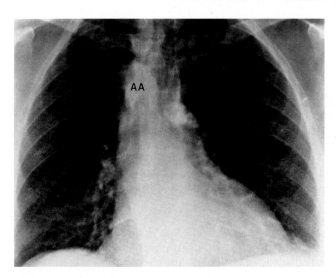

Figure 5.26 Right aortic arch (*AA*) in an elderly patient with no evidence of heart disease.

Figure 5.27   Situs inversus and dextrocardia in a patient who suffered a gunshot wound to the *left* axilla.   The radiograph is oriented in the customary viewing position. If one were in doubt about the laterality, the easiest way to solve the dilemma would be to examine the patient! Note the marker (*arrow*).

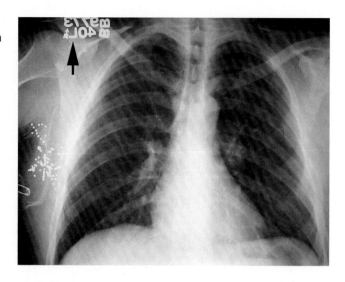

certain forms of *situs inversus* and *dextrocardia* (Fig. 5.27), the gastric bubble is on the right. Always check the image orientation and markings carefully to avoid the pitfall this condition engenders.

Pathologic Considerations

This discussion focuses on the radiographic evaluation of patients with heart disease. Although chest x-rays usually cannot make a specific cardiac diagnosis, most patients with heart disease will have an abnormal radiograph. Therefore, it is a valuable screening tool for suspected heart disease. More advanced cardiovascular imaging studies can be ordered, including echocardiography, angiography, cardiac CT, or MR imaging, to make a specific diagnosis. The chest x-ray can also diagnose various pulmonary and vascular diseases. It is also a valuable triage tool for patients with chest pain or dyspnea. Finally, the chest radiograph can assess the status of patients with established heart disease and its complications.

The following entities will be discussed:

- Pulmonary edema
- Pleural effusion
- Pulmonary hypertension
- Chamber enlargement
- Cardiac and aortic calcifications
- Pericardial effusion
- Trauma
- Postoperative appearances
- Congenital abnormalities

Pulmonary Edema

The most important diagnosis to make on a chest x-ray in an adult with suspected or known heart disease is pulmonary edema. Pulmonary edema is a complication of congestive heart failure or fluid overload where fluid extravasates into the pulmonary interstitial tissues and alveolar spaces when pulmonary venous pressures overwhelm the pulmonary lymphatics. Since pulmonary edema is frequently misdiagnosed on chest radiograph, you must follow a systematic approach to maximize the chances of reaching the correct diagnosis.

First, assess the heart size. As discussed in the chest section, heart size can only be accurately estimated on a full inspiratory PA film. Heart size is frequently overestimated on expiratory PA, AP, or portable radiographs. Avoid falling into the "cardiomegaly trap" when interpreting portable chest images. Most patients with congestive heart failure will have an enlarged cardiac silhouette on the frontal view exceeding more than 50% on the width of the lower chest at the rib margins. An enlarged heart is a clue that the patient has ischemic heart disease, valvular heart disease, or a dilated cardiomyopathy.

▶ An enlarged heart implies ischemic heart disease, valvular heart disease, or a dilated cardiomyopathy.

Finally, examine the lungs. There are many chest x-ray findings of pulmonary edema. The most specific finding of pulmonary edema is the presence of Kerley B or septal lines. These lines are a manifestation of distended pulmonary lymphatics from pulmonary venous hypertension. These lines are much easier to see on a PA radiograph and almost impossible to perceive on a portable study (Fig. 5.28). Other signs of lymphatic distention include thickening of the fissures on both projections and thickening of the posterior trachea on the lateral projection. Another fairly specific finding of pulmonary edema is ill-defined (fuzzy) pulmonary vessels due to fluid leaking into the adjacent pulmonary interstitium. Cephalization or enlarged pulmonary veins in the upper lobes is a well-known sign of early pulmonary edema. This finding should only be called on an upright view and preferably a PA projection. However, this sign is frequently misinterpreted and overcalled. Therefore, only experienced chest x-ray readers should rely on this finding.

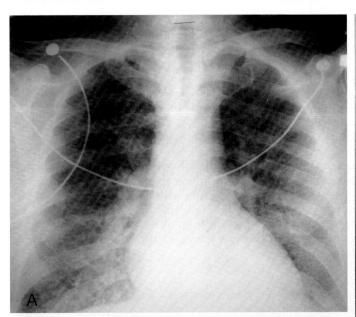

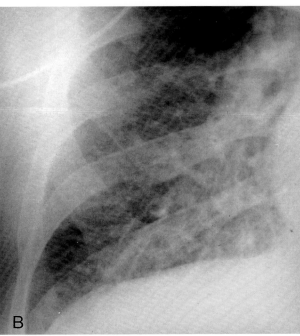

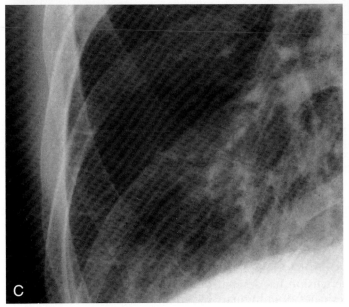

Figure 5.28   Kerley lines in two patients with congestive heart failure.   A. Frontal radiograph shows pulmonary edema is present. Note the prominent interlobular septa (Kerley lines) throughout both lungs. **B.** Magnified view of the right lower lung in the same patient. **C.** Magnified view of the right lower lung in another patient shows the linear and peripheral Kerley B lines to advantage.

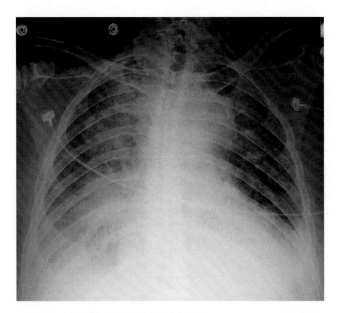

Figure 5.29   Alveolar pulmonary edema.   The edema in this patient is primarily central. Note the bilateral pleural effusions creating a haziness in the lower lungs. Patient also has an aortic aneurysm.

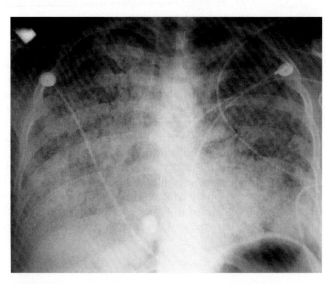

Figure 5.30   Alveolar and interstitial pulmonary edema.   Note the fluffiness of the densities, the indistinctness of the cardiac border, and the combination of findings that indicate alveolar and interstitial abnormalities.

Other less specific clues to pulmonary edema include bilateral perihilar infiltrates or consolidation, otherwise known as the "bat wing" sign (Fig. 5.29). However, this may also occur with atypical pneumonia and an inflammatory pneumonitis. Any acute air space disease consolidation may represent pulmonary edema, especially when it is bilateral and symmetric (Fig. 5.30). However, acute airspace disease is also seen with pneumonia, acute respiratory distress syndrome, and pulmonary hemorrhage. Nevertheless, the onset and clearing is faster with pulmonary edema and much slower with pneumonia. Alveolar pulmonary edema may be asymmetric if the patient has been lying on one side before having the radiograph. Furthermore, edema may be present from another (noncardiac) source, such as heroin intoxication, inhalation of noxious fumes, or drowning. In these conditions, the heart is usually normal in size.

   ▶ Pulmonary edema may be present from a noncardiac source. When this occurs, the heart is usually normal in size.

Mediastinal widening may be a sign of an enlarged cava or pulmonary veins from pulmonary venous hypertension. However, mediastinal widening is frequently a normal finding in obese patients and can be seen with mediastinal hemorrhage, tumors, and aneurysms.

Pleural Effusion

The next abnormality to look for is the presence or absence of pleural effusions. Most patients in congestive heart failure or fluid overload will have bilateral pleural effusions. One of the most sensitive exams for a pleural effusion is the lateral projection with fluid pooling in the posterior costophrenic sulcus (Fig. 5.31). Most small pleural effusions will not be demonstrated on a portable radiograph. This is yet another reason to order a two-view chest x-ray rather than a portable study in patients with suspected heart disease. Pleural effusions are easily demonstrated on chest CT examinations (see Fig. 4.60).

Pulmonary Hypertension

Pulmonary hypertension is defined as an average pulmonary artery pressure exceeding 25 mm Hg. Pulmonary hypertension has several causes. One easy method to remember many of the different etiologies of pulmonary hypertension is to use the anatomic

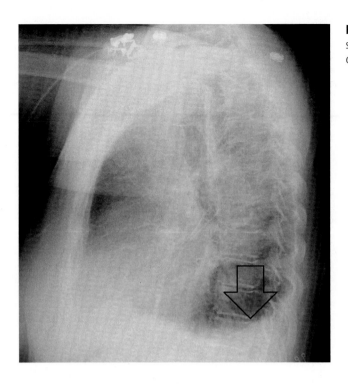

Figure 5.31 Small pleural effusions. Lateral view shows small bilateral pleural effusions blunting both posterior costophrenic angles (*arrow*).

model. Divide the pulmonary vasculature into three categories as blood enters and exits: precapillary, capillary, and postcapillary. Precapillary diseases include chronic pulmonary embolism or intracardiac shunts. Capillary diseases include diseases that impair oxygen exchange, including emphysema, pulmonary fibrosis, obesity, and obstructive sleep apnea. The final category is postcapillary disease, which includes diseases of the left heart and pulmonary veins. Abnormalities in this category leading to pulmonary hypertension include ischemic heart disease, valvular heart disease, and cardiomyopathies as well as more unusual diseases that narrow the pulmonary veins like fibrosing mediastinitis (Fig. 5.32).

Over time, elevated pulmonary pressures will enlarge the pulmonary arteries and right heart. On a chest x-ray, patients will have large central pulmonary arteries that rapidly taper in the periphery of the lung, otherwise known as pruning. *Main pulmonary artery enlargement* produces bulging of the central pulmonary artery segment along the left cardiac border. In addition, prominent right main pulmonary arteries may also be observed (Fig. 5.33). Also look for an enlarged right heart (see below).

Keep one caveat in mind. Young adult women will commonly have main pulmonary artery bulging on the frontal view. This is frequently a normal finding in this patient population. When in doubt, look for other signs of pulmonary hypertension such as right heart enlargement and pruning.

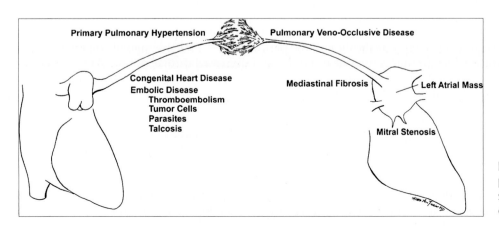

Figure 5.32 Anatomic model for pulmonary hypertension. Diagram showing the anatomic model for the causes of pulmonary hypertension.

Figure 5.33   Pulmonary hypertension.
Frontal view shows an enlarged main pulmonary artery (*white arrow*) and right pulmonary artery (*black arrow*).

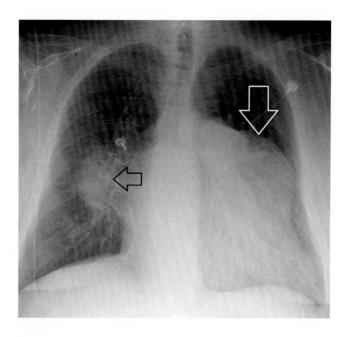

Chamber Enlargement

Determining cardiac chamber enlargement is very useful. *Right ventricular* enlargement is better demonstrated on the lateral radiograph where there is loss of the retrosternal clear space. Normally, the right heart should occupy the inferior third of the vertical distance in the anterior chest. Right-sided cardiac enlargement will occupy one-half or two-thirds of the anterior chest (Fig. 5.34). *Right atrial enlargement* as an isolated finding is rare. It usually accompanies enlargement of the right ventricle and pulmonary arteries. Right atrial enlargement is suggested by prominence of the right cardiac border. Enormous right atrial enlargement will create a boxlike appearance, as in *Ebstein anomaly* which is a form of congenital heart disease where the right atrium protrudes into the right ventricle (Fig. 5.35). *Left ventricular enlargement* produces a downward and left bulge of the cardiac apex on the frontal radiograph. However, this can be difficult to distinguish from global cardiomegaly. *Left atrial enlargement* will create a double density on the frontal view with splaying of the carina. On the lateral projection, draw an imaginary vertical line along the posterior tracheal margin into the inferior chest. If the heart intersects this line, the left atrium is enlarged (Fig. 5.36).

Cardiac and Aortic Calcifications

Cardiac calcifications are also useful to recognize. Calcification of the coronary arteries can be seen on a chest x-ray in patients with severe coronary artery disease or diabetes (Fig. 5.37). Aortic valvular calcification is a reliable sign of aortic stenosis. This is easier to see on the lateral view in the expected location of the aortic valve (Fig. 5.38). This condition is closely associated with an ascending aortic aneurysm, which is better seen on the frontal projection. This produces a convexity along the right cardiomediastinal border, but the lateral view is rarely helpful. The more common mitral annular calcifications are associated with mitral valve disease but can also be age related in patients with a normal mitral valve (see Fig. 5.24). Calcification of the pericardium is a reliable sign of constrictive pericarditis which produces right heart failure and decreased cardiac output (Fig. 5.39). Cardiac aneurysms particularly in the apex can calcify signifying prior myocardial infarction (Fig. 5.40). Cardiac neoplasms rarely calcify.

    ▶ Aortic valvular calcification is a reliable sign of aortic stenosis.

Calcification of the aorta is usually best seen at the aortic knob on the frontal view and in the aortic arch and descending aorta on the lateral view. The amount of calcification

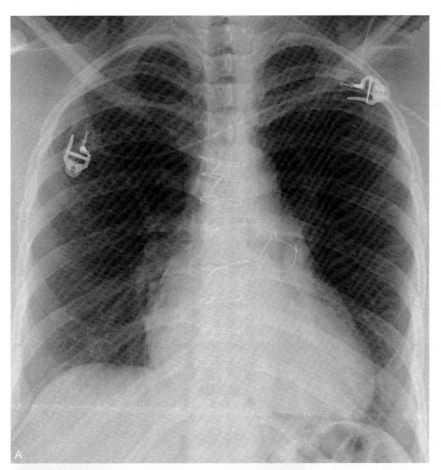

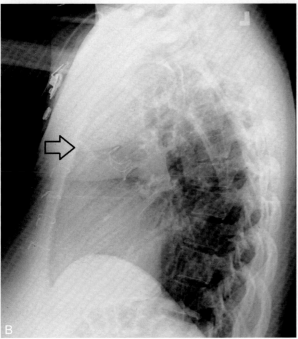

Figure 5.34   Enlarged right ventricle.   A. Frontal view demonstrates a borderline enlarged cardiac silhouette occupying about 50% of the width of the chest. **B.** Lateral view is markedly abnormal with obliteration of the retrosternal clear space (*arrow*). This is a reliable sign of right ventricular enlargement.

increases with age. However, some research suggests that patients with a calcified aorta have an increased risk of a cardiovascular event. A tortuous or "snake-like" descending aorta is commonly seen as a sign of chronic hypertension (Fig. 5.41). An abnormally dilated thoracic aorta usually indicates an aortic aneurysm or aortic dissection (Fig 5.42).

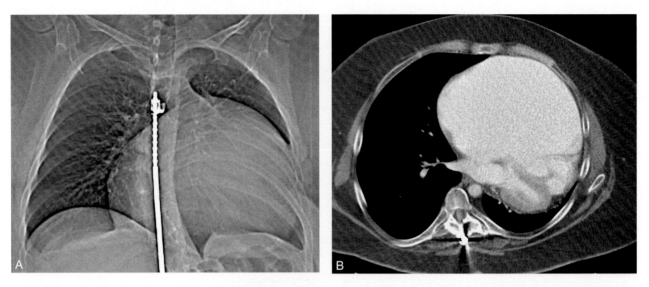

Figure 5.35   Ebstein anomaly.   CT topogram **(A)** and axial CT image **(B)** show massive right atrial enlargement.

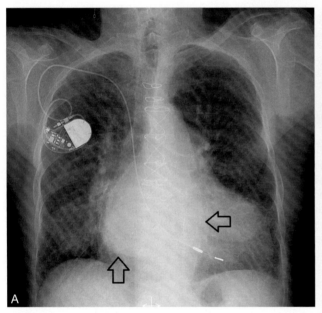

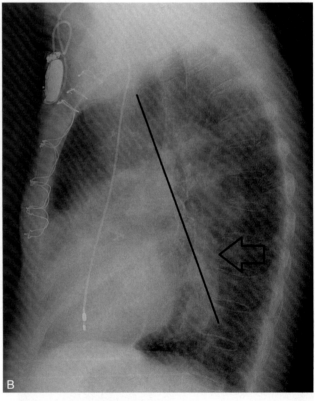

Figure 5.36   Left atrial enlargement.   A. Frontal view demonstrates a hyperdense mass behind the heart, otherwise known as the "double density" (*arrows*). **B.** The anterior tracheal line intersects the posterior heart or left atrium on the lateral view also consistent with left atrial enlargement (*arrow*).

▶ An abnormally dilated thoracic aorta usually indicates an aortic aneurysm or aortic dissection.

Pericardial Effusion

Pericardial effusion must always be considered when evaluating a patient with an enlarged heart. The heart will have a "water bottle" appearance (Fig. 5.43). Occasionally, the pericardium is demonstrated in normal patients as a thin, dense line separated by layers of subepicardial and mediastinal fat. In patients with pericardial effusion, this line is

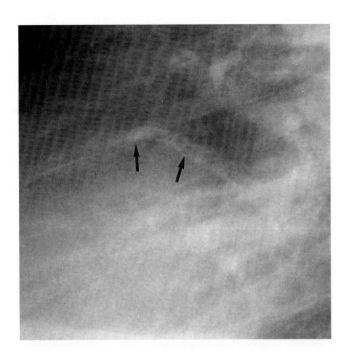

Figure 5.37 Coronary artery calcification (*arrows*) in an elderly man.

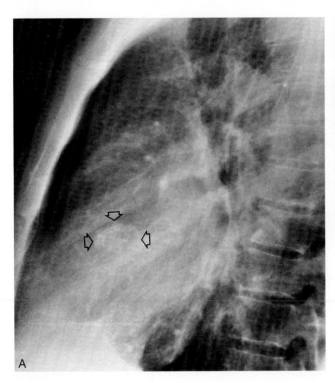

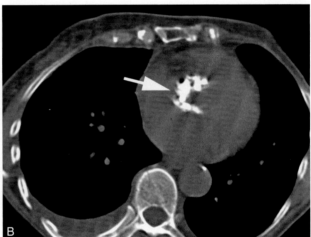

Figure 5.38 **Aortic valve calcification.** **A.** Lateral chest view shows aortic valve calcification (*arrows*). Once these calcifications are seen on chest x-ray, the aortic stenosis is usually severe. Compare with the mitral annular calcification shown in Figure 5.24. **B.** Axial CT image with same finding (*arrow*).

thickened, otherwise known as the "Oreo cookie" or the "stripe" sign (Fig. 5.44). CT and MRI may be also used to diagnose pericardial effusion. The fluid will encircle the heart. CT and MR can also differentiate simple effusions from complex effusions by the density of the fluid. Water or serous fluid has CT Hounsfield units less than 20 where blood or protein will be greater than 20 Hounsfield units. A pericardial effusion can also be further characterized based on different signal intensities on black blood and bright blood MR images (Fig. 5.45). Lastly, if the pericardium enhances, an exudative pericardial effusion is present. Acute pericarditis should be considered in this situation. Echocardiography commonly detects and easily characterizes a pericardial effusion. Ultrasonic shadows reflected off the pericardial and myocardial surfaces will demonstrate an abnormal collection of fluid in the pericardial sac (Fig. 5.46).

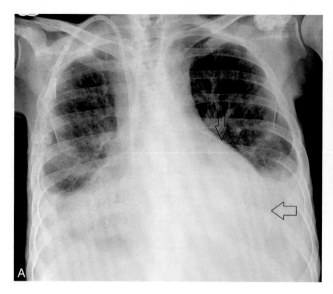

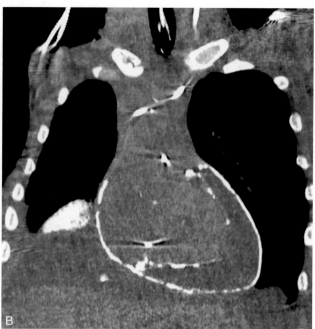

Figure 5.39   Uremic constrictive pericarditis.   A. Frontal view shows thick calcification of the pericardium (*arrow*). **B.** Coronal CT reformatted image shows calcification of the visceral and parietal pericardium.

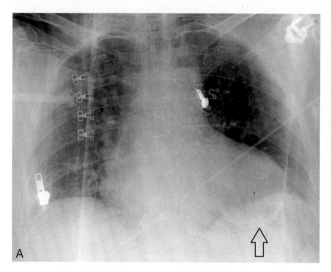

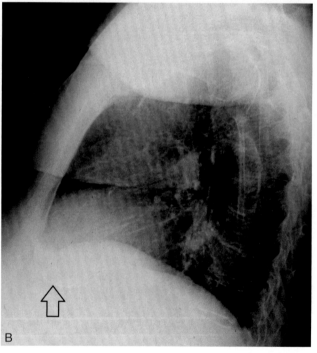

Figure 5.40   Calcified left ventricular apical aneurysm.
A. Frontal view shows a round calcification overlying the left ventricular apex (*arrow*). **B.** Lateral view shows same finding in the anterior chest (*arrow*). Note the calcification does not conform to the margin of the cardiac silhouette. This allows differentiation from pericardial calcification and constrictive pericarditis (see Fig. 5.39).

Trauma

Patients who have suffered severe thoracic trauma may have an injury to the heart or great vessels. The most common mechanism is the result of the chest of an unrestrained driver of a motor vehicle striking the steering wheel. Radiographically, the most common finding is a widened superior mediastinum (Fig. 5.47). You should be careful, as a supine radiograph in a large patient commonly shows a widened mediastinum. Therefore, the altered "fuzzy" contour and increased density of the mediastinal borders is more specific for an acute aortic injury. CT of the thorax is now used routinely on patients with suspected injury to the great vessels to look for evidence of mediastinal hemorrhage (Fig. 5.48).

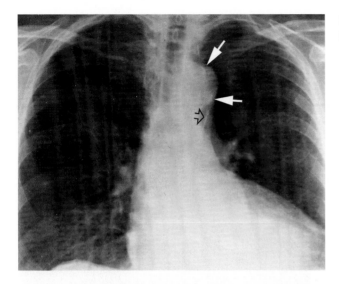

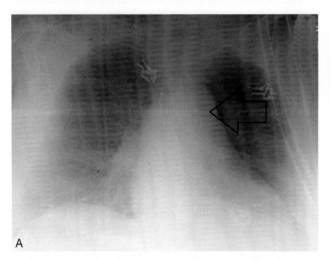

Figure 5.41 Calcification of the aortic arch (*white arrows*) and descending aorta (*open black arrow*).

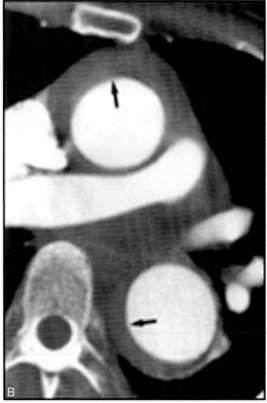

Figure 5.42 Aortic dissection. A. Portable frontal chest x-ray shows thickening of the aortic knob and medial displacement of the calcified intima suspicious for an aortic dissection (*arrow*). **B.** Axial CT shows an intramural hematoma in the aortic wall (*arrows*).

The study is performed after intravenous injection of iodinated contrast. CT has replaced the aortogram (Fig. 5.49) for diagnostic purposes in trauma centers in the United States. However, aortography is valuable for inserting an endograft stent device to treat the torn aorta without the need for an emergent and invasive cardiovascular operation.

Postoperative Appearances

Cardiac surgery produces many characteristic radiographic changes. Many patients with valvular or ischemic heart disease have sternotomy wires from prior cardiac surgery.

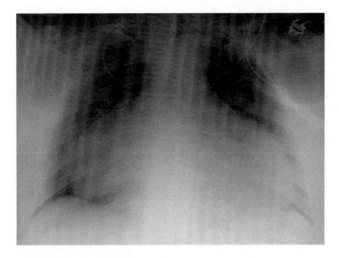

Figure 5.43   Pericardial effusion.   Portable chest film shows massive enlargement of the patient's cardiac silhouette or the "water bottle" heart.

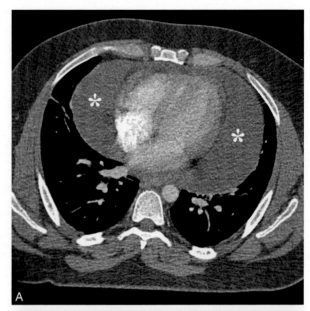

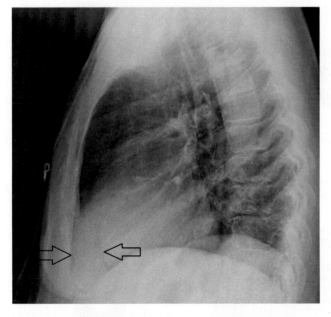

Figure 5.44   Pericardial effusion.   Lateral chest view shows the "Oreo cookie" sign with outer black stripes and the central white stripe which represents the pericardial effusion (*arrows*). This sign is very specific but not very sensitive for a pericardial effusion.

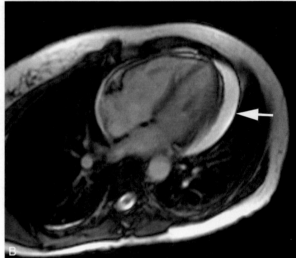

Figure 5.45   Pericardial effusion.   **A.** Axial CT image shows a serous fluid collection (*asterisk*) encircling the heart. **B.** Axial bright blood gradient echo magnetic resonance image shows bright serous fluid (*arrow*) surrounding the heart.

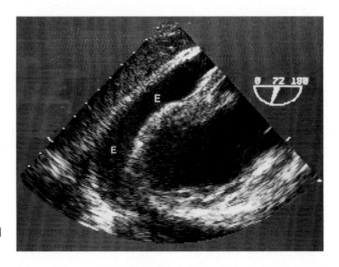

Figure 5.46   Pericardial effusion (*E*) demonstrated on a parasternal long-axis echocardiogram image.

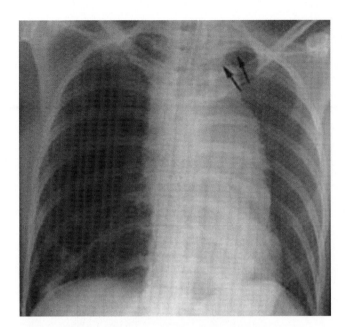

Figure 5.47   Widened mediastinum.   Frontal chest film shows a widened mediastinum with loss of the aortic knob shadow and left apical pleural thickening (*arrows*).

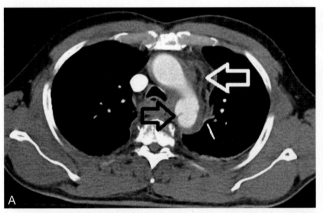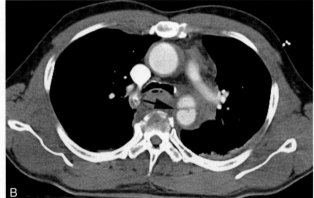

Figure 5.48   Acute aortic injury on CT.   A and **B.** Axial CT images demonstrate an intimal flap in the descending aorta (*black arrows*). Note the mediastinal fat stranding and soft tissue attenuation consistent with hemorrhage (*white arrow*). This produces the mediastinal widening seen on chest x-ray.

If the patient has a valve prosthesis, determine its location. The lateral view is very helpful. Draw an imaginary straight line from the apex of the heart to the hilum. If the prosthesis is above this line, the aortic valve has been replaced. If the prosthesis is below this line, the mitral valve has been replaced (Fig. 5.50). Rarely, the pulmonic or tricuspid valves are replaced. Here the frontal view is more helpful. A pulmonic valve replacement has a superior location below the main pulmonary artery along the left heart border (Fig. 5.51). A tricuspid valve replacement is the only valve that overlies the right side of the cardiac silhouette on the frontal projection. The valve is anteriorly positioned on the lateral projection (Fig. 5.52).

▶ Regarding prosthetic cardiac valves, draw an imaginary straight line from the apex of the heart to the hilum on a lateral radiograph. If the prosthetic valve is above this line, it is aortic; if below, it is mitral.

▶ Regarding prosthetic cardiac valves on the frontal radiograph, a pulmonic valve replacement is located below the main pulmonary artery along the left heart border; a tricuspid valve replacement overlies the right side of the cardiac silhouette; on the lateral view, it is anteriorly placed.

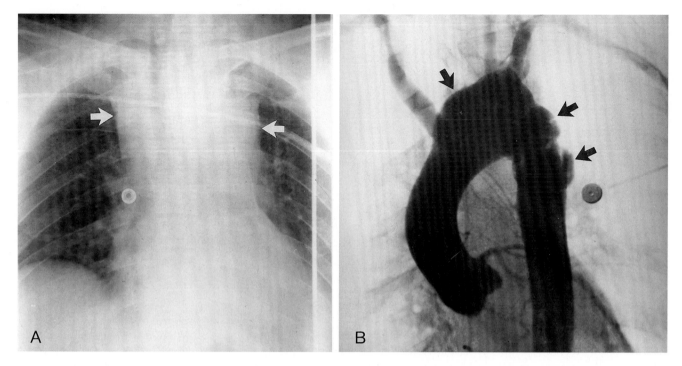

Figure 5.49   Posttraumatic aortic tear in an unrestrained driver.   A. Frontal radiograph shows widening of the superior mediastinum (*arrows*). Note the tracheal deviation to the right. **B.** Arteriogram shows the pseudoaneurysm (*arrows*). Note the irregular contour of the aortic arch.

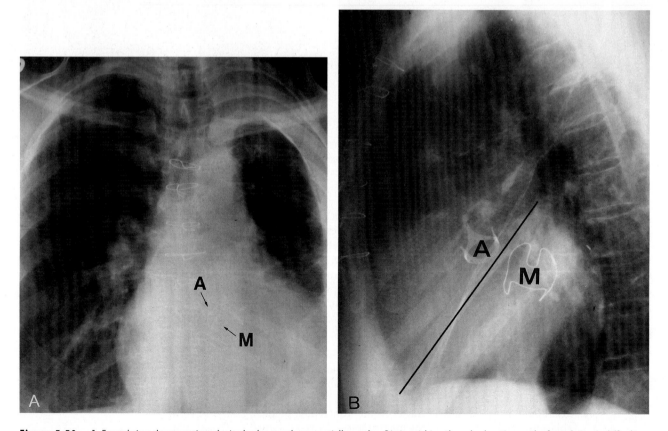

Figure 5.50   A. Frontal view shows aortic and mitral valve prostheses partially overlap. Distinguishing the valve location on the frontal view is difficult. **B.** Lateral view shows an imaginary line from the apex of the heart to the hilum. Note the aortic valve (A) lies above the line and the mitral valve (M) lies below the line.

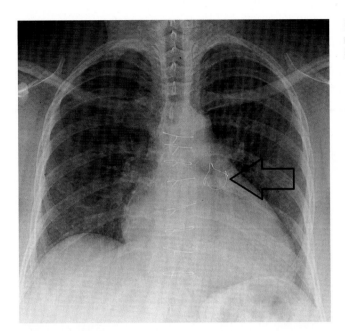

Figure 5.51 Frontal view shows the pulmonary valve replacement superiorly located along the left side of the heart (*arrow*).

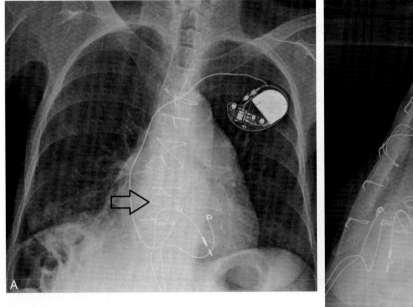
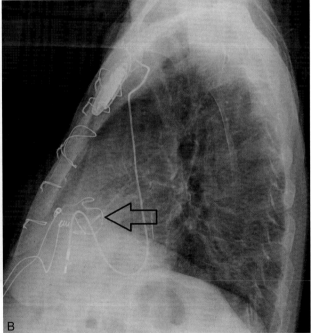

Figure 5.52 **A.** Frontal view shows the tricuspid valve replacement overlying the right heart in a patient with a pacemaker device (arrow). **B.** Lateral view shows the anterior position of the tricuspid valve (*arrow*).

Patients with prior coronary artery bypass grafting surgery (CABG) will have mediastinal surgical clips and sternotomy wires. If the left internal mammary artery has been harvested, surgical clips will overlie the left heart border. Some cardiac surgeons place circular markers on the aorta for each saphenous vein graft tied into the ascending aorta (Fig. 5.53). These make future coronary angiograms easier to perform because the openings of the grafts are easily visible on the fluoroscopic screen. The number of bypass grafts can also be estimated. However, this surgical technique is not universally performed. A variation, known as minimally invasive coronary bypass surgery, is performed using a

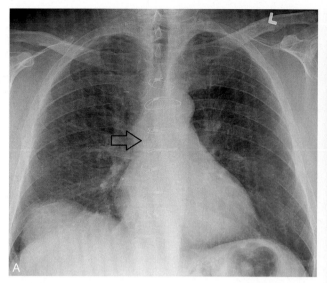

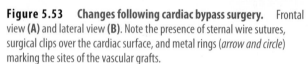

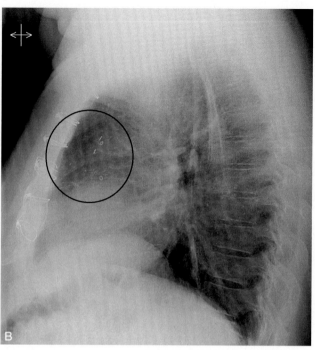

Figure 5.53   Changes following cardiac bypass surgery.   Frontal view **(A)** and lateral view **(B)**. Note the presence of sternal wire sutures, surgical clips over the cardiac surface, and metal rings (*arrow and circle*) marking the sites of the vascular grafts.

thoracoscope through small incisions in the chest wall ("keyhole procedure"). This type of surgery leaves no telltale sternal wires, but the surgical clips near the grafts are visible on radiographs.

Coronary artery stents are frequently seen on chest x-rays. These have the radiographic appearance of a tubular structure with a chicken-wire mesh (Fig. 5.54). All stents are visible on CT, but stent patency can only be demonstrated with a gated cardiac CT exam or

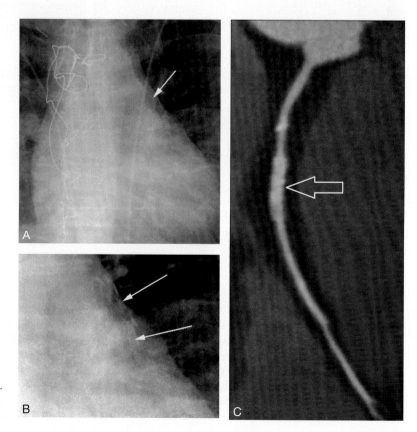

Figure 5.54   Coronary artery stents (*arrows*).
A. Detail of chest radiograph shows a stent along the left cardiac border. **B.** Magnified view shows several stents in place. **C.** Curved planar reformatted CT image shows a patent stent in the right coronary artery.

on an angiogram. Knowing a patient has had CABG surgery or stent insertion tells you that the patient has significant ischemic heart disease placing the patient at risk for myocardial infarction and congestive heart failure.

Patients with heart disease commonly have *pacemakers* in place. The intracardiac variety is usually of three types: *unipolar* with a single lead in the right ventricle, *bipolar* with one lead in the right ventricle and the other in the coronary sinus portion of the right atrium, and *biventricular* with leads in the right atrium, right ventricle, and coronary sinus (Fig. 5.55). Another device seen in heart patients is the automatic implantable cardiac defibrillator (AICD) (Fig. 5.56). The two defibrillating coils along the lead are in the superior vena cava and the right ventricle. Often an AICD is combined with a pacemaker.

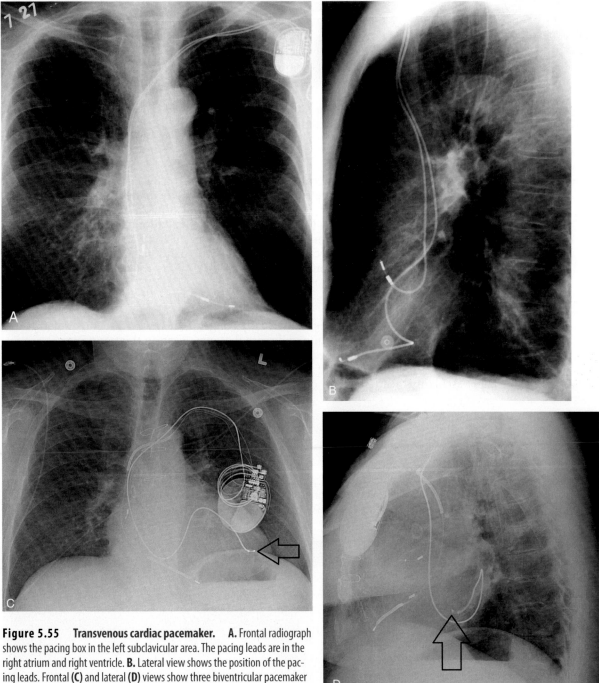

Figure 5.55   Transvenous cardiac pacemaker.   A. Frontal radiograph shows the pacing box in the left subclavicular area. The pacing leads are in the right atrium and right ventricle. **B.** Lateral view shows the position of the pacing leads. Frontal **(C)** and lateral **(D)** views show three biventricular pacemaker leads in the right atrium, right ventricle, and coronary sinus (*arrow*).

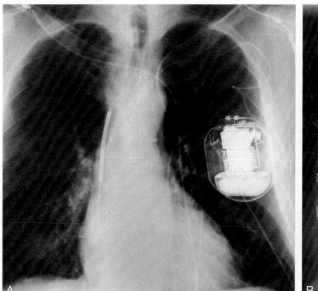
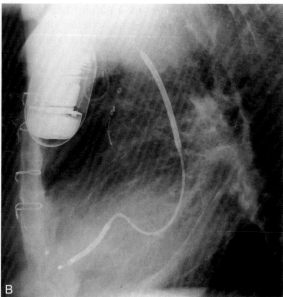

Figure 5.56   Automated implantable cardiac defibrillator (AICD).   Single AICD lead has two thick coiled springs incorporated into it to defibrillate the patient out of dangerous arrhythmias. Both leads are better demonstrated on the lateral **(B)** view.

Many cardiologists or critical care physicians will insert a Swan-Ganz catheter into the pulmonary artery to measure pressures and quickly assess the patient's cardiovascular status. At many cardiovascular hospitals, physicians will also insert an intra-aortic balloon pump into the descending aorta (Fig. 5.57). The pulsating balloon augments cardiac output when the balloon deflates and increases coronary perfusion when the balloon inflates. Any patient with a Swan-Ganz catheter or intra-aortic balloon pump should be closely scrutinized for the presence of pulmonary edema.

Congenital Abnormalities

Cardiac disease in pediatric patients is usually congenital. However, rheumatic heart disease is an important form of acquired disease that may occur in this age group.

Traditionally, experienced pediatric radiologists often suggest a specific diagnosis or a short differential diagnosis of congenital heart disease based on the type of pulmonary vascularity, heart size and configuration, and a limited history. However, modern

Figure 5.57   Swan-Ganz catheter and intra-aortic balloon pump.   *Black arrow* shows position of Swan-Ganz catheter tip in the main pulmonary artery. *White arrow* shows only tip of the intra-aortic balloon pump in the mid-descending thoracic aorta. Frequently, only the tip of the balloon pump is demonstrated on chest x-ray.

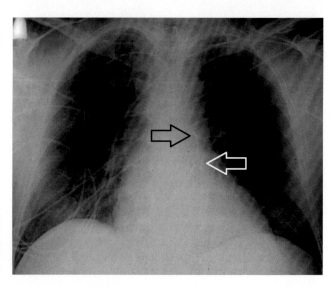

imaging, including echocardiography, CT, MRI, and cardiac catheterization, is more accurate and widely accessible at most children's hospitals. Therefore, the pediatric radiologist is no longer relied upon to make a specific diagnosis. Nevertheless, the chest radiograph is an important screening tool for symptomatic neonates and toddlers with suspected congenital heart disease. Therefore, it is very important to recognize an abnormal pulmonary vascular pattern, heart, or other chest abnormality as a clue that the patient may have congenital heart disease, and additional testing should be ordered. A thorough radiographic approach to congenital heart disease is beyond the scope of this book. However, the authors' approach is outlined in the supplemental web-based material.

Pulmonary Vascularity

The pulmonary circulation can be abnormal in several different ways. First, like adults, pulmonary edema may be present as a result of pulmonary venous hypertension and congestive heart failure. This is otherwise known as "passive" congestion. The pulmonary arteries are ill defined with leakage of fluid into the adjacent interstitial tissues (Fig. 5.58). Additional signs of failure include a large heart, pleural effusions, and symmetric bilateral infiltrates. Pulmonary edema in children also has cardiac and noncardiac causes. Cardiac causes include left-sided heart disease such as hypoplastic left heart, patent ductus arteriosus, aortic coarctation, and mitral/aortic valve disease.

The pulmonary circulation can also be altered by abnormally increased or decreased circulation of blood through the pulmonary vessels. If the caliber of the pulmonary arteries is larger than normal but they remain well defined, the pulmonary vascularity is increased (Fig. 5.59). This is otherwise known as "active" congestion or *shunt vascularity*. This is commonly seen with intracardiac shunts such as ventricular septal and atrial septal defects. Generally, the amount of blood through the pulmonary vessels needs to be more than double than the aorta for this finding to be seen on a chest x-ray. If the pulmonary vessels are small, then the pulmonary vascularity is decreased. This is a valuable clue and signifies obstructive right heart disease with decreased pulmonary blood flow such as pulmonic/tricuspid valve atresia and tetralogy of Fallot (Fig. 5.60). These patients are commonly cyanotic.

Considerations of the Newborn

Heart Size and Configuration

Accurately estimating heart size with a newborn or toddler chest x-ray is difficult and frequently incorrect. These studies are usually obtained with an AP or portable technique,

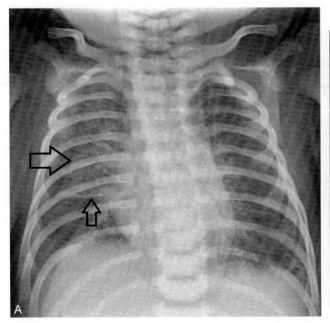 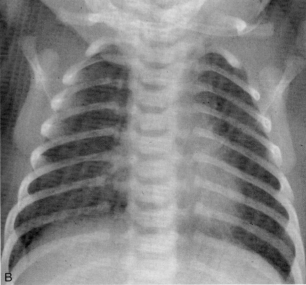

Figure 5.58   Pediatric pulmonary edema or "passive" congestion in two patients.   *Arrows* in **(A)** indicate normal thymus.

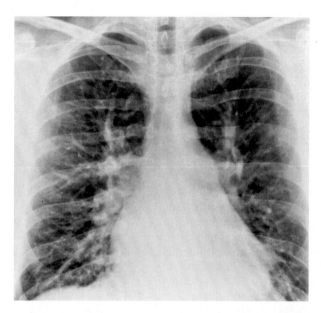

Figure 5.59   Shunt vascularity.   Frontal chest film shows enlargement of the central and peripheral pulmonary arteries, which are well defined consistent with excessive circulation of blood in the pulmonary arteries, usually from an intracardiac shunt. This is otherwise known as "active" congestion.

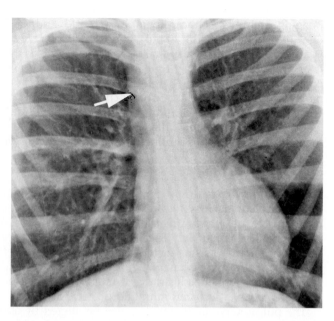

Figure 5.60   Tetralogy of Fallot.   The heart size is normal but has a boot shape. The pulmonary vascularity, however, is diminished. Note the right aortic arch (*arrow*).

which overestimates the size of anterior structures in the chest, including the heart. Furthermore, most of the studies on younger children are obtained when the patients are crying. Crying produces images in expiration and with the Valsalva effect, both of which make the cardiac silhouette appear larger. Some authorities have suggested increasing the cardiothoracic threshold for cardiac enlargement from 50% to 60%. However, that can also be erroneous. Therefore, the interpretation should be supplemented with an assessment of cardiac configuration and position. Is the heart in its normal anatomical position in the left chest? Abnormal position of the heart in the right chest (dextrocardia) can be a sign of congenital heart disease. Also observe the position of the aortic arch. Right-sided aortic arch is associated with tetralogy of Fallot, truncus arteriosus, and transposition of the great vessels. Is there evidence for specific chamber enlargement? A lateral view is helpful to assess for left atrial and right ventricular enlargement. If the left margin of the cardiac silhouette is boot shaped or curves upward, this is a sign of right ventricular hypertrophy, commonly seen with tetralogy of Fallot (see Fig. 5.60). If the heart looks like it is tipped on its side with a narrow mediastinum or what is referred to as an "egg on a string," then that is a sign of transposition of the great vessels. If the cardiomediastinal silhouette and superior mediastinum are both widened or show what is known as the "figure 8" sign, the patient should be suspected of having total anomalous pulmonary venous return. There are additional but rare radiographic signs of congenital heart disease. Given the superiority of modern cross-sectional imaging (CT and MRI) in defining the abnormal cardiac anatomy, the radiographic diagnosis of specific congenital heart disease is no longer necessary and is now an intellectual curiosity. There are noncardiac chest findings that can indicate the presence of congenital heart disease. The aortic knob that has an indented or lobulated appearance is seen with aortic coarctation. This is otherwise known as the "figure 3" sign. Rib notching on the undersurface of the ribs is a manifestation of collateral arteries in the chest wall with coarctation, but does not usually develop on chest radiographs until adolescence or adulthood (Fig. 5.61). Some patients have other vascular abnormalities that can indent or narrow the trachea like a vascular ring from a double aortic arch (Fig. 5.62) or an aberrant course of the pulmonary artery otherwise known as a "pulmonary sling." Many patients with congenital heart disease have other congenital abnormalities such as spinal or rib deformities or abnormal position of the abdominal organs or situs inversus.

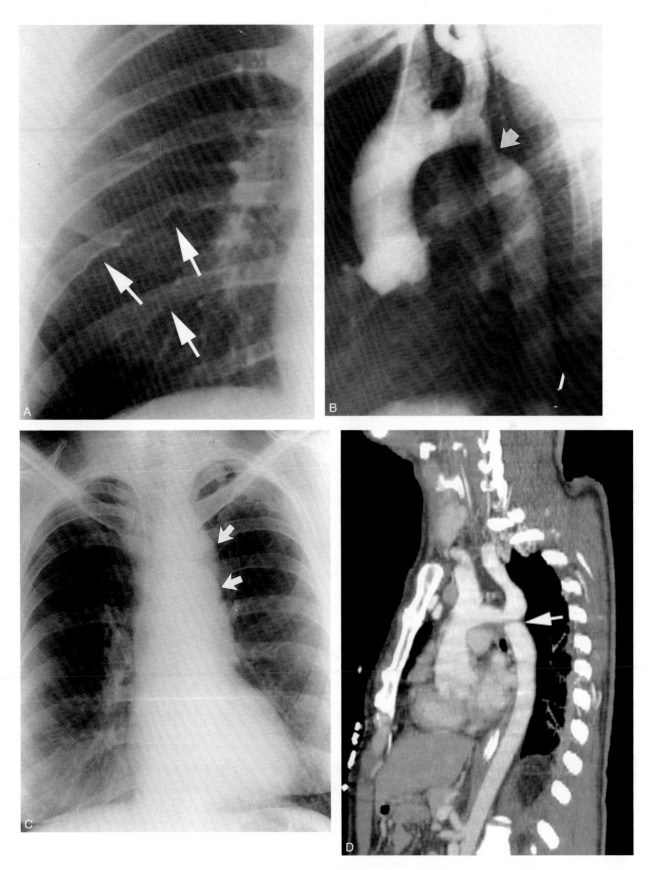

Figure 5.61 **Aortic coarctation.** **A.** Coned down frontal view shows rib notching on the undersurface of the ribs (*arrows*) produced by the enlarged intercostal arteries providing collateral circulation to the lower extremities. **B.** Aortogram shows the coarctation (*arrow*). **C.** Frontal view in another patient demonstrates the lobulated contour of the aortic arch, otherwise known as the "figure 3" sign. **D.** Sagittal CT shows narrowing of the proximal descending thoracic aorta (*arrow*).

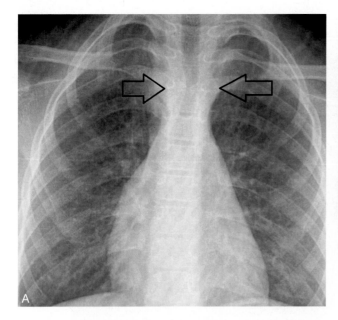

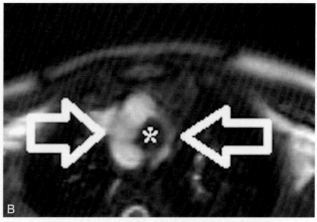

Figure 5.62   Double aortic arch vascular ring.   A. Frontal view shows a double aortic arch indenting and narrowing the trachea from both sides (*arrows*). **B.** Axial bright blood gradient echo magnetic resonance image shows bright double aortic arch (*arrows*) encircling the trachea (*asterisk*). Note the right arch is larger than the left arch.

Summary and Key Points

▶ Radiography remains the initial screening imaging study for most patients with suspected heart disease.

▶ CT, MR, SPECT, and PET imaging are playing a greater role in assessing disease of the coronary arteries, structural heart disease, and congenital heart disease.

▶ Pulmonary edema, pulmonary hypertension, cardiomegaly, and pleural effusion are common complications of heart disease easily diagnosed on plain film.

▶ Chamber enlargements, congestive heart failure, pericardial effusion, and trauma all produce characteristic changes on chest radiographs.

▶ Radiography can detect congenital heart disease, but echocardiography, CT, and MRI are more accurate at defining the abnormal cardiovascular anatomy.

Suggested Additional Reading

American College of Radiology Manual on Contrast Media, Version 8. www.acr.org.

Armstrong WF, Ryan T. Feigenbaum's Echocardiography. 7th Ed. Philadelphia, PA: Lippincott Williams and Wilkins, 2010.

Baron MG. Plain film diagnosis of common cardiac anomalies in the adult. Radiol Clin N Am 1999;37:401–420.

Baron MG, Book WM. Congenital heart disease in the adult: 2004. Radiol Clin N Am 2004;42:675–690.

Bonow RO, Mann DL, Zipes DP, Libby, eds. Braunwald's Heart Disease: A Textbook of Cardiovascular Medicine. 9th Ed. Philadelphia, PA: Saunders Elsevier, 2012.

Chen JTT, Capp MP, Johnsrude IS, et al. Roentgen appearance of pulmonary vascularity in the diagnosis of heart disease. AJR 1971;112:559–570.

Crean A, Dutka D, Coulden R. Cardiac imaging using nuclear medicine and positron emission tomography. Radiol Clin N Am 2004;42:619–634.

Fuster V, Walsh R, Harrington R, eds. Hurst's the Heart. 13th Ed. New York: McGraw-Hill, 2010.

Hagen-Ansert SL. Textbook of Diagnostic Ultrasonography. 7th Ed. St. Louis, MO: Mosby-Year Book, 2012.

Lipton MJ, Boxt LM. How to approach cardiac diagnosis from the chest radiograph. Radiol Clin N Am 2004;42:487–495.

Manning WJ, Pennell DJ. Cardiovascular Magnetic Resonance. 2nd Ed. Philadelphia, PA: Saunders Elsevier, 2010.

Miller SW, Abbara S, Boxt L. Cardiac Imaging: The Requisites. 3rd Ed. Philadelphia, PA: Mosby Elsevier, 2009.

Poutschi-Amin M, Gutierrez FR, Brown JJ, et al. How to plan and perform a cardiac MR imaging examination. Radiol Clin N Am 2004;42:497–514.

Schoepf UJ, Becker CR, Hofmann LK, Yucel EK. Multidetector-row CT of the heart. Radiol Clin N Am 2004;42:635–649.

chapter 6

Breast Imaging

Nilima Dash   Richard H. Daffner

Breast cancer is the second most common cause of death from malignancy in American women. The American Cancer Society estimates that one of every eight women will get cancer of the breast in her lifetime. Fortunately, breast cancer can be diagnosed at an early and highly curable stage by the appropriate use of mammography. In recent years, breast cancer mortality has decreased because of a rise in the frequency of early diagnosis and better treatment options (chemotherapeutic agents). Indeed, patients with screening-detected breast cancer have a survival rate at least 33% greater than symptomatic patients.

The following are guidelines established by the American Cancer Society and endorsed by the American College of Radiology (ACR) regarding screening for breast cancer and the appropriate use of mammography.

> Breast cancer can be diagnosed at an early and highly curable stage by the appropriate use of mammography. In recent years, breast cancer mortality has decreased because of a rise in the frequency of early diagnosis and better treatment options.

Asymptomatic Women

- Women 20 years of age and older should perform breast self-examination monthly.
- Women age 20 to 40 should, in addition, have a physical examination of the breasts every 3 years.
- Women at age 40 should have a baseline mammogram.
- Women 40 years of age and older should have a mammogram and a physical examination of the breasts every year.

Symptomatic Women

- Symptomatic women with a dominant breast mass, persistent discomfort, skin dimpling, or nipple discharge should have a thorough breast examination that includes mammography and any other diagnostic study (ultrasound and sometimes MRI) to determine if cancer is present. These studies should be performed regardless of the patient's age.

Further Recommendations

- The ACR and the Food and Drug Administration further recommend that the mammographic technique used produce the greatest anatomic detail and resolution possible.

○ These tests are to be provided with the lowest possible radiation dose needed to produce high-quality images. Mammography should be performed and interpreted by experienced, well-trained individuals using modern, carefully monitored equipment. All practices certified by the ACR conform to these high standards. The mammographic findings should be correlated carefully with thorough physical examination.

○ However, there are limitations of mammography and clinicians must be aware of them. They should remember that the mammogram, physical exam, and ultrasound of the breast are complementary.

○ Patients with palpable masses and an unremarkable mammogram should undergo ultrasound examination of the breast.

The largest breast cancer screening project was performed by the American Cancer Society in conjunction with the National Cancer Institute in the 1970s under the Breast Cancer Detection Demonstration Project. In this study, more than 275,000 female volunteers were evaluated by physical examination and mammography at 27 centers nationwide. The results supported the value of mammography as a screening tool as well as a diagnostic method for detecting early breast cancer. Almost immediately after the study began, controversy developed regarding the safety of mammography because of the radiation dose involved. The controversy was based on several studies of women who had received extremely high doses of radiation to the breast in early childhood and who belonged to three separate populations: women exposed to the atom bombs at Hiroshima and Nagasaki, those with tuberculosis who received repeated chest radiographs and fluoroscopic examinations, and a group of women who were treated with radiation for postpartum mastitis. The controversy spurred the development of improved equipment and improved screen and film products (low dose) to further decrease the radiation dose. As a result, mammography is a safe diagnostic procedure when used by experienced personnel. For a more in-depth discussion on aspects of breast cancer, its detection, and the issue of radiation carcinogenesis, refer to the text by Kopans.

▶ The results of the Breast Cancer Detection Demonstration Project supported the value of mammography as a screening tool as well as a diagnostic method for detecting early breast cancer.

▶ Mammography is a safe diagnostic procedure when used by experienced personnel.

Technical Considerations

Modern mammograms use either low-dose analog (film-screen) technology or digital radiography (Fig. 6.1), which lowers the dose even further. Mammography is also used to localize a mass for surgical excision (Fig. 6.2). Diagnostic ultrasound is used once a mass is detected to determine if it is cystic or solid (Fig. 6.3). Ultrasound is also used to localize breast lesions for percutaneous biopsy. Lesions that are seen only on a mammogram undergo biopsy using stereotactic techniques (Fig. 6.4).

▶ Diagnostic ultrasound is used once a mass is detected to determine if it is cystic or solid.

The basic imaging techniques used for imaging the breast are

○ x-ray mammography,
○ digital mammography,
○ ultrasound,
○ magnetic resonance imaging.

X-Ray Mammography

X-ray mammography is performed using a radiographic film and screen combination that provides high detail with a relatively low radiation dose. The diagnostic accuracy is

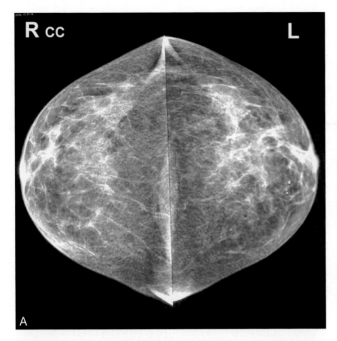

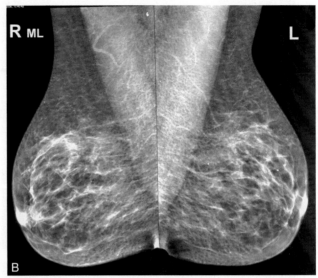

Figure 6.1   Normal digital mammogram of a 63-year-old woman.   A. Craniocaudal (CC) view. **B.** Mediolateral oblique (MLO) view. Note the exquisite detail the digital image provides.

identical to that of xerography, a technique used extensively in the 1970s and early 1980s. Although xerography provided exquisite soft tissue detail, it is no longer used today because of the high radiation dose required to produce the images.

Digital Mammography

Digital mammography (see Fig. 6.1) is replacing conventional film-screen mammography in most departments. The greatest advantage of digital mammography is its ability to provide improved image quality. In addition, the digital images can be electronically manipulated, which has resulted in fewer repeat images being required for technical reasons. In addition, digital mammography allows images to be sent via teleradiology, facilitating mammography services in areas that do not have radiologists. Finally, digitization allows computer-aided diagnosis. A recent study comparing film-screen and digital mammography showed both to be similar in the overall diagnostic accuracy. However, digital mammography was more accurate in women under the age of 50 and in women with dense breasts.

Ultrasound

Ultrasound is used for both diagnostic and interventional purposes in patients with breast diseases. First and foremost, ultrasound is used to study all breast masses detected on mammograms to determine whether the lesion is cystic (see Fig. 6.3) or solid (Fig. 6.5). Furthermore, ultrasound is used for imaging guidance in the performance of breast biopsies.

Magnetic Resonance Imaging

Magnetic resonance imaging (MRI) is also used to evaluate breast lesions. MRI is used to find occult breast carcinoma in patients with malignant axillary nodes, to evaluate the extent of disease in recently diagnosed breast cancer patients, to diagnose chest wall involvement by the tumor, and to monitor the response of a tumor to preoperative chemotherapy. MRI of the breast is also indicated in asymptomatic, high-risk women who are gene-positive, have a personal history of breast cancer, or have multiple first-degree relatives with breast cancer.

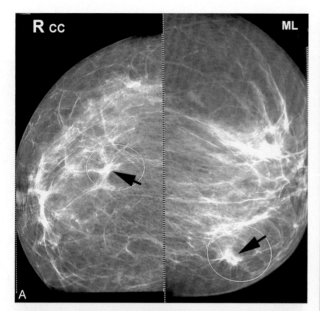

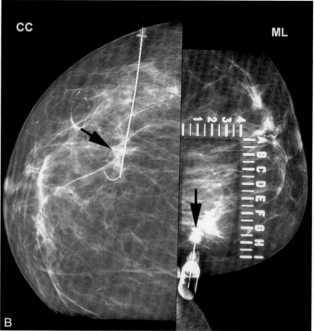

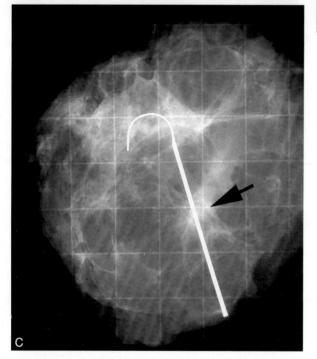

Figure 6.2   Use of mammography for needle localization.
A. Craniocaudal (CC) and mediolateral (ML) digital mammograms show a spiculated mass with microcalcifications (*arrows*). **B.** Needle localization image shows the needle and wire in position through the mass (*arrows*). **C.** Specimen radiograph shows the mass and microcalcifications transfixed by the needle and wire. Diagnosis: ductal carcinoma in situ.

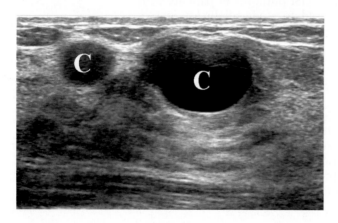

Figure 6.3   Breast sonography, simple cysts.   Note two sonolucent masses representing cysts (*C*) with posterior acoustic enhancement.

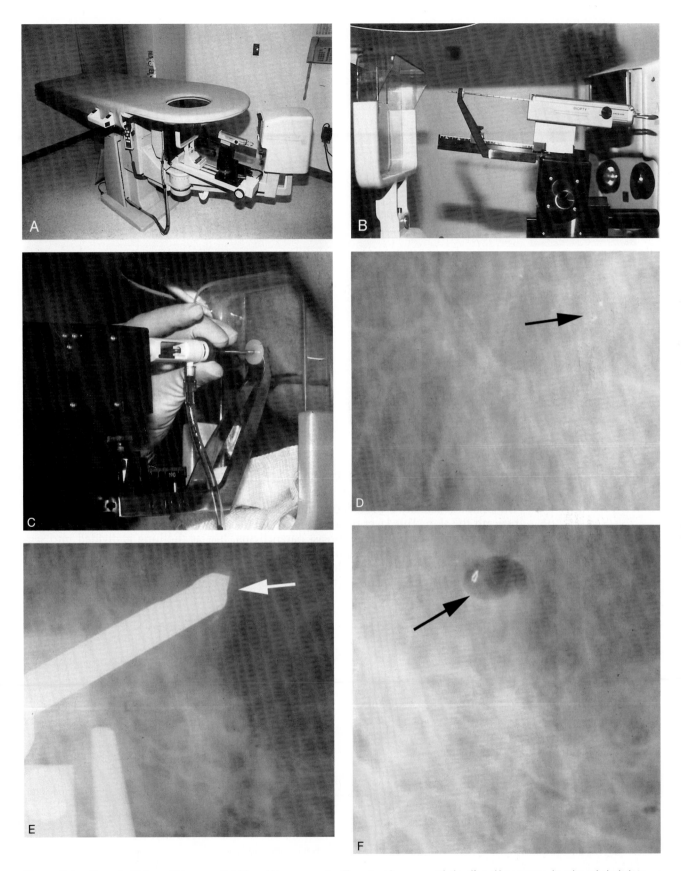

Figure 6.4 Stereotactic breast biopsy. **A.** Table and biopsy apparatus. The patient lies prone with the affected breast protruding through the hole in the tabletop. **B.** View of the biopsy apparatus fixed in front of a mammography tube and compression device. **C.** Mammographer guides the biopsy needle into place. **D.** Detail of a mammogram showing microcalcifications in a small mass (*arrow*). **E.** Placement of the core biopsy needle into the lesion (*arrow*). **F.** Following biopsy, the mass and calcifications are gone and a small surgical clip is present at the excision site (*arrow*).

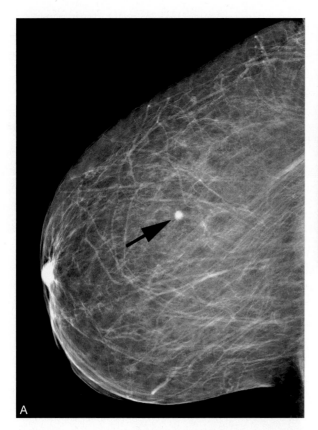

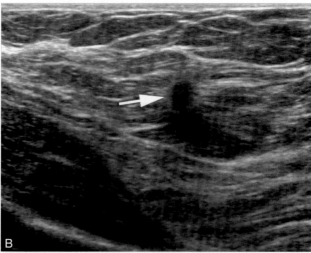

Figure 6.5   Small 5-mm carcinoma.   A. Mediolateral oblique (MLO) view. **B.** Ultrasound. Note although the nodule appears to have smooth margin on mammogram (*arrow*), ultrasound shows irregular margin (*arrow*), taller than wide, suspicious for malignancy. Biopsy showed invasive ductal carcinoma.

Anatomic and Physiologic Considerations

The breast is actually a modified skin gland derived from the superficial layer of fascia beneath the skin. This layer divides into a superficial layer and a deep layer that form a fibrous capsule containing the breast parenchyma. Just as the lung is divided into segments beginning at the bronchus, the breast is divided into segments. Each segment is drained by a major lactiferous duct that terminates at its orifice in the nipple (Fig. 6.6). The ducts branch into a series of terminal lobules that contain glandular lactiferous acini.

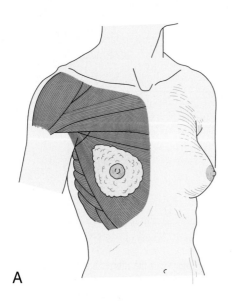

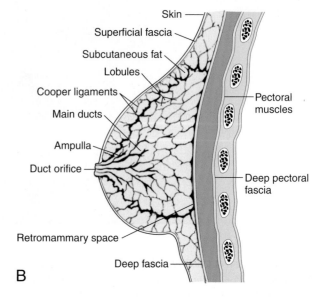

Figure 6.6   Breast anatomy.   A. Position of the breast on the pectoral muscles. **B.** Breast anatomy in longitudinal section.

The organization of segments is somewhat random and heterogeneous, making it difficult to precisely locate a lesion in a particular segment. Fortunately, this does not affect diagnostic accuracy.

Structures

The glandular tissue is supported by a crisscrossing network of fibrous tissue. Its fibrous stroma joins the superficial layer of fascia. Because of the malleable nature of the breast, imaging of the entire breast is complicated by the location of this cone-shaped structure on the cylindrical support of the chest wall. Breast tissue may be found as far medially as the sternal margin, laterally extending high into the axilla, and inferiorly into the inframammary fold. As a result, breast images are never completely free of chest wall structures—a distinct disadvantage to two-dimensional imaging. Although the standard mammogram relies on two views, craniocaudal (CC) and mediolateral oblique (MO), additional views in selected cases are sometimes necessary to fully image the breast.

Normal Anatomic Variants and Anomalies

Imaging the breast is further complicated by the physiologic changes that occur in relationship to the patient's age and stage in the menstrual cycle. The breast in a young woman is extremely dense and consists mostly of glandular tissue. This glandular tissue is denser in a lactating woman. The tissue also increases in density and size during the later part of the menstrual cycle. As a woman ages, the glandular tissue is slowly replaced by fat. Because breast cancer is more common in older women whose breasts contain larger amounts of fat, the lesions are easier to detect than in younger women, in whom the dense glandular material often masks a tumor.

Pathologic Considerations

The American College of Radiology has developed the Breast Imaging Reporting and Data System or BI-RADS. This is a quality assurance tool published and trademarked by the ACR. The BI-RADS assessment categories are

- 0: Incomplete
- 1: Negative
- 2: Benign finding(s)
- 3: Probably benign
- 4: Suspicious abnormality
- 5: Highly suggestive of malignancy
- 6: Known biopsy-proven malignancy.

All mammogram reports list the BI-RADS category at the end.

Benign Lesions

A large variety of benign histologic changes occurs in the breast. Many of these changes likely represent variations of normal parenchyma relating to hormonal status. The term *fibrocystic disease* is a catchall category of changes that include the presence of cysts, benign fibrous tissue, and dilated ducts in various configurations. The anatomy of the breast is such that a clinician palpating what is believed to be either a cyst or mass may, in fact, be feeling normal glandular tissue or fat surrounded by the fibrous stroma.

> ▶ *Fibrocystic disease* is a catchall category of changes that include the presence of cysts, benign fibrous tissue, and dilated ducts in various configurations.

As a rule, benign lesions are round with smooth, well-defined margins (Figs. 6.7 and 6.8) and usually do not distort the normal breast architecture. They are often multiple and bilateral. Benign calcifications are usually coarse and are easily detectable with the unaided eye (Fig. 6.9). Macrocysts are cystic dilatations of the lactiferous duct. They are increasingly common in women in their mid-to-late 30s and are most commonly found

Figure 6.7   Breast sonography, fibroadenoma (*FA*) in a 17-year-old patient.   Note smooth border, but internal echo indicating a solid mass.

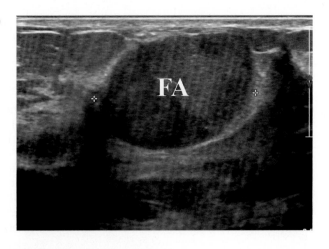

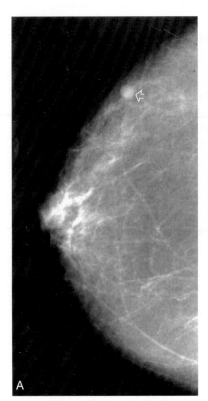

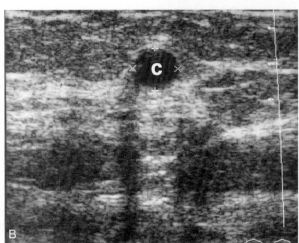

Figure 6.8   Benign breast cyst. A. Craniocaudal view shows a well-defined mass with smooth margins (*arrow*). **B.** Ultrasound shows the sonolucent cyst (*C*) with posterior acoustic enhancement and no internal echoes.

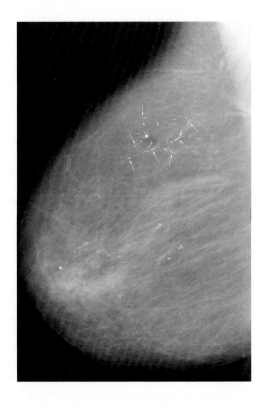

Figure 6.9   Benign duct calcifications (*arrows*). Linear calcifications are present in a branching pattern. Note their smooth margins.

in the premenopausal years. They generally regress after menopause. Cysts are usually distinguishable from solid tumors by ultrasound (see Fig. 6.8**B**). The fluid within the cysts varies in color, being clear, brown, green, or even black.

> ▶ Benign lesions are round with smooth, well-defined margins and usually do not distort the normal breast architecture.

Fibroadenoma

The most common solid benign tumor of the breast is the *fibroadenoma* (Fig. 6.7). These tumors are hormonally sensitive and are found more commonly in young women. They are the solid lesions of the breast that undergo biopsy most frequently in women up to the mid-30s. The reason for their frequent biopsy is that they cannot be distinguished from well-circumscribed carcinomas, either by physical examination or imaging methods. Involution of fibroadenomas in postmenopausal women often produces coarse calcifications.

> ▶ The most common solid benign tumor of the breast is the *fibroadenoma*.

Malignant Lesions

Ninety percent of breast cancer begins in the ductal epithelium, 10% begins in the lobule. Although the carcinoma may be confined within the ductal tissue, ultimately it will invade through the duct wall and spread via the lymphatic and vascular systems with resultant lymphatic and hematogenous metastases. The most common areas of lymphatic spread are to the axillary and internal mammary lymph nodes. If, at the time of detection, the axillary lymphatics are uninvolved, the 5-year survival is given as approximately 95%. This survival decreases to approximately 75% if axillary lymph nodes are involved and to approximately 20% if distant metastases are present.

> ▶ Ninety percent of breast cancer begins in the ductal epithelium, 10% begins in the lobule.

The radiographic findings of malignancy are those of a mass with ill-defined or irregular margins (Fig. 6.10). Other signs include a lobulated margin (Fig. 6.11), distortion and invasion of surrounding parenchyma (Fig. 6.12), clustered microcalcifications (Fig. 6.13), asymmetric density, asymmetric dilated ducts, and nipple retraction. Skin thickening and retraction are frequently found late in the disease and result from the desmoplastic effect of the tumor on the ligamentous support of the breast. Finally, enlargement of axillary lymph nodes may also be detected in a patient whose carcinoma has spread beyond the breast.

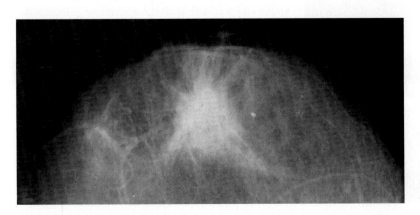

Figure 6.10   Breast carcinoma showing classic spiculated, irregular margins.   Craniocaudal view shows distortion of normal breast parenchyma.

Figure 6.11   Breast carcinoma.   Lobular margins and spiculated borders. Again, note the distortion of breast parenchyma anteriorly. The dense dot adjacent to the lesion is a marker placed by the technologist at the site of palpable lump.

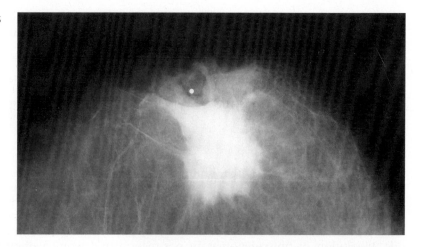

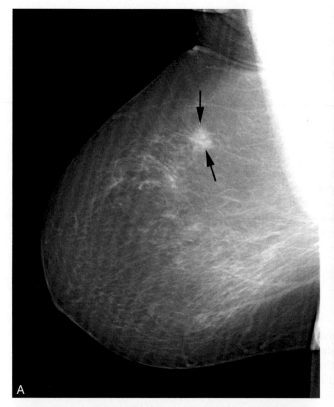

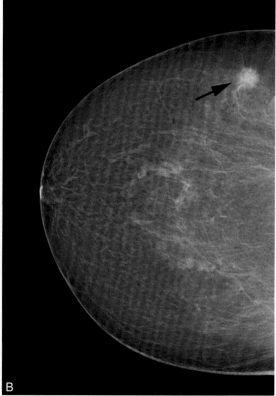

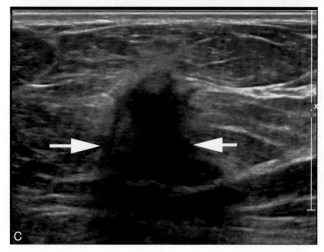

Figure 6.12   Breast carcinoma.   Mediolateral oblique **(A)** and craniocaudal **(B)** mammograms of right breast in a 62-year-old female showing carcinoma, upper outer quadrant with spiculated margin (*arrows*). **C.** Ultrasound image in same patient. Note spiculated margin and posterior shadowing (*arrows*).

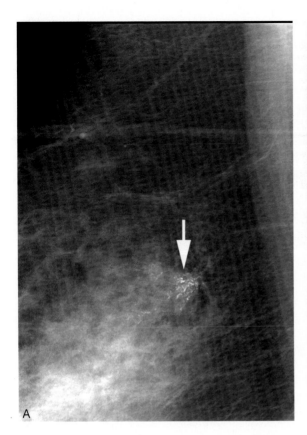 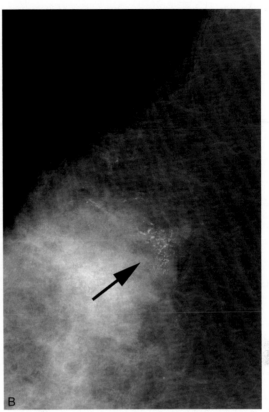

Figure 6.13   Magnification.   Mediolateral oblique **(A)** and craniocaudal **(B)** views of typical malignant calcifications (*arrows*). Note different size, shape, and density of individual calcification.

 ▶ The radiographic findings of malignancy are those of a mass with ill-defined or irregular margins. Other signs include a lobulated margin, distortion and invasion of surrounding parenchyma, clustered microcalcifications, asymmetric density, asymmetric dilated ducts, and nipple retraction.

Summary and Key Points

▶ Breast cancer is one of the most common malignancies in women.
▶ The mortality may be diminished by self-examination, clinical examination, and screening mammography.
▶ A baseline mammogram should be obtained on all asymptomatic women at age 40. Women of age 40 and older should have a yearly mammogram according to the most recent guidelines by the American Cancer Society and the ACR.
▶ Mammography should be performed only by skilled technologists under the supervision of an equally qualified radiologist to produce an examination of high diagnostic quality with a low radiation dose.
▶ Ultrasound and/or MRI of the breast is indicated in a selected group of patients.

Suggested Additional Reading

American College of Radiology. ACR Practice Guideline for Performance of Screening and Diagnostic Mammography. Reston, VA: American College of Radiology, 2008.
American College of Radiology. ACR Practice Guideline for Performance of Contrast-enhanced Magnetic Resonance Imaging (MRI) of the Breast. Reston, VA: American College of Radiology, 2008.

American College of Radiology. ACR Practice Guideline for Performance of Stereotactically Guided Breast Interventional Procedures. Reston, VA: American College of Radiology, 2009.

American College of Radiology. ACR Standard Practice Guideline for the Performance of Ultrasound-Guided Percutaneous Breast Interventional Procedures. Reston, VA: American College of Radiology, 2009.

American College of Radiology. ACR Practice Guideline for Magnetic Resonance Image-guided Breast Interventional Procedures. Reston, VA: American College of Radiology, 2011.

American College of Radiology. ACR Appropriateness Criteria® on:

Breast Microcalcifications, 2011;

Nonpalpable Mammographic Findings, 2010;

Palpable Breast Masses, 2011;

Stage I Breast Cancer, 2011.

Reston, VA: American College of Radiology. www.acr.org

Bassett LW, Mahoney M, Apple S, D'orsi C. Breast Imaging. Philadelphia, PA: Saunders Elsevier, 2011.

IKEDA DM. Breast Imaging: The Requisites. 2nd ed. St. Louis, MO: Elsevier Mosby, 2011.

Kopans DB. Breast Imaging. 3rd Ed. Philadelphia, PA: Lippincott Williams & Wilkins, 2006.

Morris EA, Liberman L, eds. Breast MRI: Diagnosis and Intervention. New York: Springer, 2005.

National Cancer Institute at the National Institutes of Health. Breast cancer screening (PDQ®). 2011. www.cancer.gov/cancertopics/pdq/screening/breast/

Stavros AT. Breast Ultrasound. Philadelphia: Lippincott Williams & Wilkins, 2003.

chapter 7

Abdominal Radiographs

Matthew S. Hartman   Richard H. Daffner

Computed tomography (CT) of the abdomen is used extensively for diagnosing acute abdominal disorders. However, the abdominal radiograph is still an important examination for evaluating patients with suspected intraabdominal disease. The lack of significant contrast among the abdominal viscera is considered by some a disadvantage in diagnosing disease (compared with the natural contrast occurring in the chest). This relatively unsophisticated imaging technique is highly sensitive and still provides a wealth of information from single or multiple abdominal radiographs, provided you know the anatomy and applied pathophysiology. Furthermore, the abdominal radiograph involves much less radiation exposure than does CT and costs considerably less than other studies.

There are certain principles that may help you to make a correct diagnosis in a patient with suspected abdominal disease and may guide you to perform additional diagnostic studies. As with any imaging study, you should always consider the diagnostic possibilities before ordering an abdominal radiograph. Remember the **DOTDAM** principle:

- Don't
- Order
- Tests that
- Don't
- Alter
- Management

Radiographic abnormalities are rare in patients with known or suspected bleeding from esophageal varices, peptic ulcers, or the colon. In these instances, endoscopic or contrast examination is required to make the diagnosis. However, abdominal radiographs will, for example, provide diagnostic information concerning free air, obstructions, gallstones, renal calculi, appendicoliths, and foreign bodies.

Technical Considerations

A basic law of physics is that hot air rises. We use this *"law of burps and farts"* to our advantage with abdominal radiographs. Free intraperitoneal air and air in obstructed loops of bowel will have a different appearance depending on how the study was performed—supine, erect, or laterally.

Common abdominal imaging procedures include

- Supine radiograph (KUB)
- Upright radiograph
- Abdominal CT
- Ultrasonography

Abdominal Radiograph

The standard abdominal radiograph, or *KUB* (an image showing the **k**idneys, **u**reters, and **b**ladder), consists of a *supine* view, the so-called *flat plate*. Please note that you will not see air-fluid levels on a supine radiograph—remember the law of burps and farts. Free air will rise to the top of the abdomen on a supine radiograph and may be difficult to detect if one does not know where to look.

Upright Radiograph

For many patients suspected of having acute abdominal disease, an *upright* radiograph of the abdomen and chest will also be obtained as part of the acute abdomen series. The purpose of this view is twofold: to identify the presence of free intraperitoneal air and to detect the presence of intestinal air-fluid levels, which can be a finding of obstruction.

Upright views are obtained by having the patient stand or sit. The principle involves the use of a horizontal x-ray beam. If the patient cannot stand or sit, a horizontal beam study may be performed by placing the patient in the left lateral decubitus position (frontal image with the left side down, right side up). Free air will rise beneath the diaphragm in the upright position and above the liver edge on the left lateral decubitus radiograph (Fig. 7.1). This study is especially useful in severely ill patients who are suspected of having free intraperitoneal air. It is important that the patient be placed on the left side for several minutes to allow free air to rise over the dome of the liver. This technique can detect as little as 1 mL of free air. Once again, because of the horizontal beam, intestinal air-fluid levels may be detected.

▶ Free air will rise beneath the diaphragm in the upright position and above the liver edge on the left lateral decubitus radiograph.

Please note that an upright chest radiograph is often included in the acute abdomen series. Remember to look for air under the diaphragm as well as airspace disease. Pneumonia, especially in the lower lobes, is an important and often forgotten cause of abdominal pain (Fig. 7.2).

Abdominal Computed Tomography

Abdominal CT is one of the best technical advances for making a diagnosis of intraabdominal disease. Multidetector CT can be performed in under 1 minute with or without intravenous and oral contrast. As mentioned previously, the lack of sufficient tissue contrast between the various abdominal organs is a handicap to routine radiographic diagnosis.

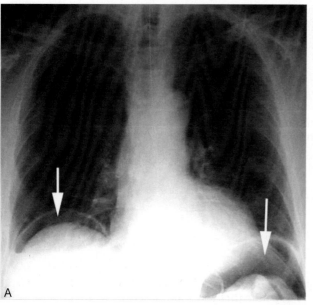

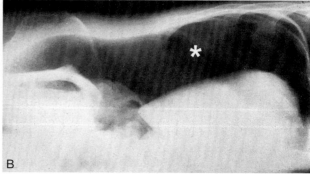

Figure 7.1   Best radiographic views for free air.   A. Upright radiograph with air under the diaphragm (*arrows*). **B.** Left lateral decubitus with air located between the liver edge and abdominal wall (*asterisk*).

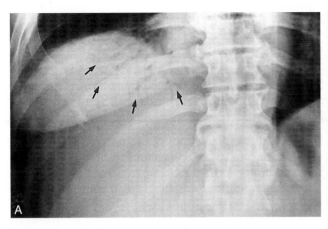

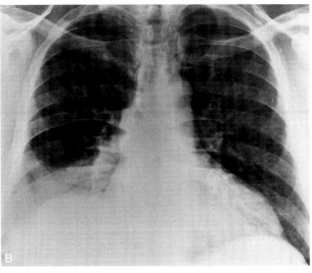

Figure 7.2 **Right lower lobe pneumonia seen on an abdominal radiograph.** **A.** Abdominal radiograph detail shows multiple air-bronchograms (*arrows*) behind the liver image. **B.** Chest radiograph shows the consolidation in the right lower lobe.

However, the abdominal CT scan differentiates organ densities better than radiographs, can outline these organs, and can detect subtle abnormalities that may escape diagnosis on abdominal radiographs. This is discussed further in Chapters 8 and 9. We include many CT and radiographic correlations in this chapter.

Ultrasonography

Ultrasonography is another important adjunct in the evaluation of abdominal disease and does not require any ionizing radiation. It can be used in the pediatric population for diagnosis of intussusceptions and pyloric stenosis. Ultrasound can identify large fluid collections in the chest and abdomen to aid with paracentesis and thoracentesis. Ultrasound is also used as a first line screening tool by ER physicians and trauma surgeons to detect free intraperitoneal blood. Ultrasound is also useful for evaluating masses and aortic aneurysms (Fig. 7.3), and in patients with renal failure for whom intravenous contrast may be a contraindication. Ultrasound also excels in differentiating cystic from solid renal masses, in hydronephrosis and biliary problems such as acute cholecystitis.

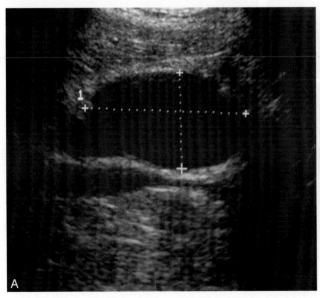

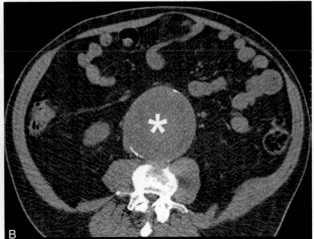

Figure 7.3 **Abdominal aortic aneurysm.** **A.** Longitudinal sonographic image demonstrates a large saccular abdominal aortic aneurysm. **B.** Axial CT shows the aneurysm (asterisk).

Anatomic and Physiologic Considerations

As with any other radiologic study, you should first examine the images for proper iden-tification and technical quality. A radiograph that is too light or too dark is of little diag-nostic value. Motion obscures soft tissue images and blurs the outline of gas-filled bowel, calcifications, and other structures. As a rule, portable radiographs are helpful in detecting only gross intraabdominal abnormalities such as postsurgical foreign bodies (Fig. 7.4). Abdominal radiographs can also help answer the question of whether an enteric feeding tube is properly placed or if it is malpositioned and will put the patient at risk for a life-threatening emergency (Fig. 7.5).

Figure 7.6 shows a normal supine abdominal radiograph and Figure 7.7 shows a nor-mal upright radiograph. Note the air-fluid level in the stomach, which confirms that the study was taken in the upright view.

Structures

Identifying the stomach and distinguishing the small bowel can be accomplished using several tricks. The first is anatomy. With the exception of congenital anomalies, mass effect, or surgical repositioning, the gastric fundus will always be located in the left upper quadrant and will have an air-fluid level on upright radiographs. The colon is located peripherally, and has *haustra*. The more central small bowel can be distinguished by its vertical *valvulae conniventes* and its smaller caliber (<3 cm) (Fig. 7.8). The normal small bowel valvulae conniventes and colonic haustra should not exceed 3 mm in thickness when outlined by air. The *rule of 3's* is useful for remembering normal bowel anatomy:

- No more than **3** air-fluid levels should be present on an upright radiograph;
- <3 mm for bowel wall thickness;
- <3 cm for small bowel diameter;
- <3 cm for large bowel diameter;
- <9 cm (3 × 3) for cecal diameter;

The properitoneal flank or fat stripe outlines the margins of the abdomen lateral to the ascending and descending colon. This stripe appears as a lucent line separating the soft

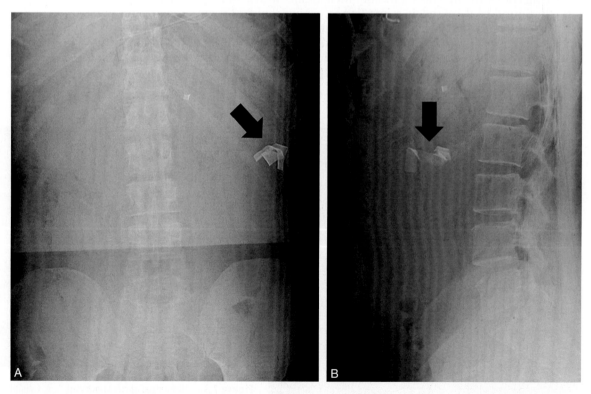

Figure 7.4   Retained sponge in a postoperative patient.   The missing sponge (*arrows*) is identified on both the supine (**A**) and lateral (**B**) radiographs.

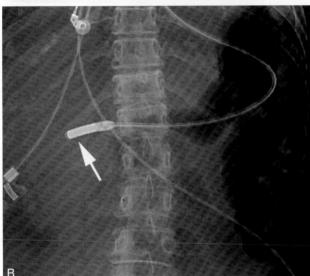

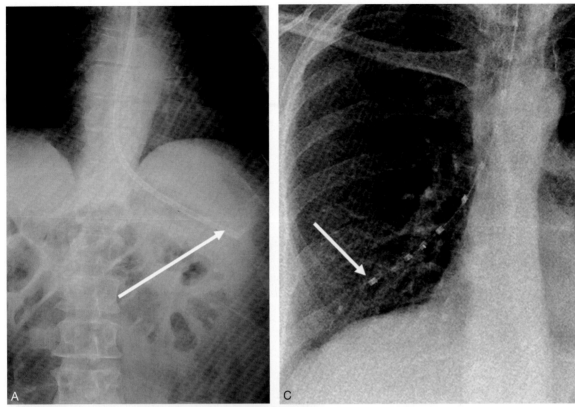

Figure 7.5   Feeding tube placement.   A. Abdominal radiograph demonstrates proper positioning of an enteric tube with its tip below the diaphragm and in the stomach (*arrow*). **B.** Abdominal radiograph demonstrates a Dobbhoff feeding catheter (note the radiopaque terminus) with tip (*arrow*) in the duodenal bulb. **C.** Chest radiograph demonstrates a pH probe with tip (*arrow*) in the right mainstem bronchus.

tissues of the skin from the abdominal cavity. The line is often obliterated in inflammatory conditions of the abdomen (appendicitis, peritonitis, etc.). There should be no gas between this stripe and the cecum on the right or the descending colon on the left.

 ▶ There should be no gas between the properitoneal fat stripe and the cecum on the right or the descending colon on the left.

Under normal circumstances, gas patterns should change over a period of several minutes when serial radiographs are obtained. This indicates normal peristaltic activity. Absence of this activity, particularly when there is absolutely no change in the appearance of the bowel, is strongly suggestive of bowel infarction or ileus.

Figure 7.6   Normal supine abdomen (KUB).   The bowel gas pattern is unremarkable. The following soft tissue shadows are visible: (*1*) kidneys, (*2*) spleen, (*3*) liver margin, (*4*) psoas muscles, (*5*) bladder, and (*6*) uterus. There are no abnormal calcifications.

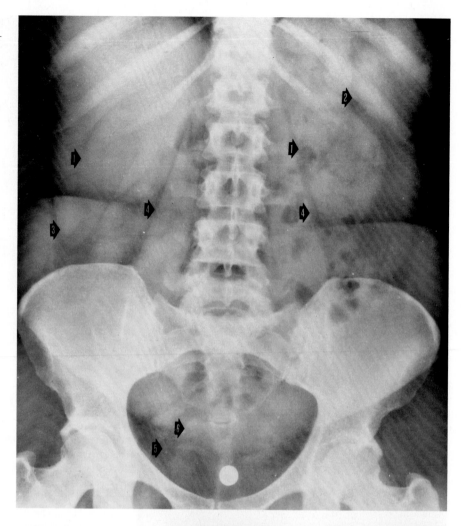

Figure 7.7   Normal upright view from an acute abdominal series.   Note the air-fluid level in the stomach (*black arrow*), which confirms that the radiograph was taken with the patient in the upright position.

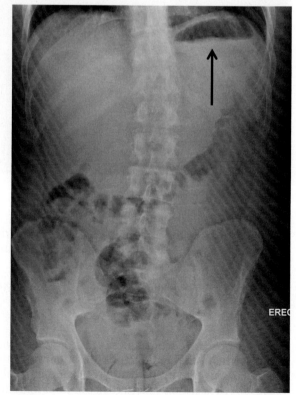

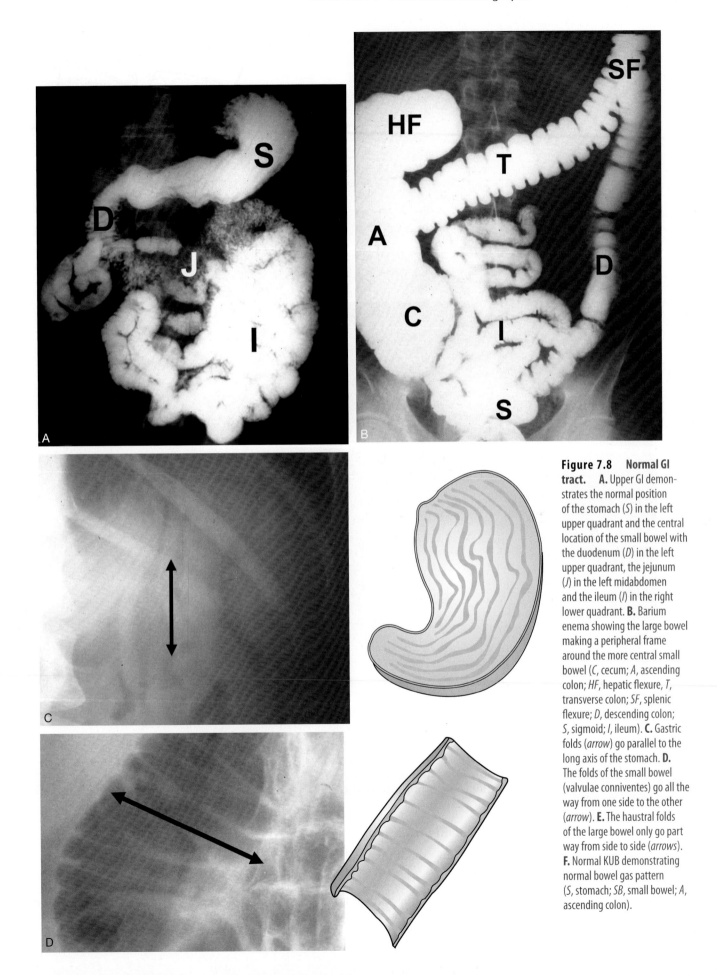

Figure 7.8   Normal GI tract.   A. Upper GI demonstrates the normal position of the stomach (*S*) in the left upper quadrant and the central location of the small bowel with the duodenum (*D*) in the left upper quadrant, the jejunum (*J*) in the left midabdomen and the ileum (*I*) in the right lower quadrant. **B.** Barium enema showing the large bowel making a peripheral frame around the more central small bowel (*C*, cecum; *A*, ascending colon; *HF*, hepatic flexure, *T*, transverse colon; *SF*, splenic flexure; *D*, descending colon; *S*, sigmoid; *I*, ileum). **C.** Gastric folds (*arrow*) go parallel to the long axis of the stomach. **D.** The folds of the small bowel (valvulae conniventes) go all the way from one side to the other (*arrow*). **E.** The haustral folds of the large bowel only go part way from side to side (*arrows*). **F.** Normal KUB demonstrating normal bowel gas pattern (*S*, stomach; *SB*, small bowel; *A*, ascending colon).

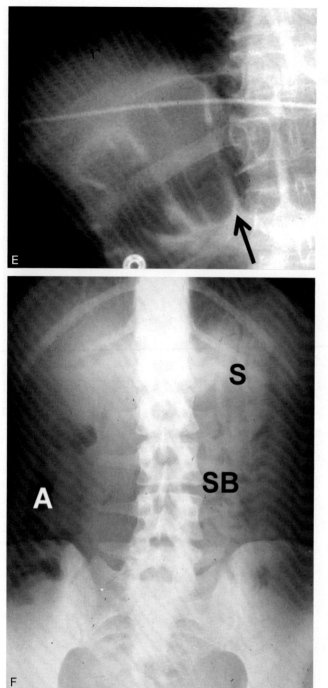

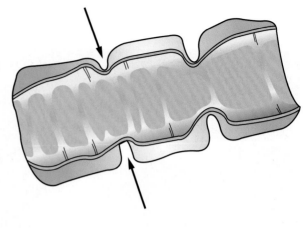

Figure 7.8   *(Continued)*

Finally, one should be aware that there is a significant amount of the lower lobe of each lung visible on abdominal radiographs. It is not uncommon for pneumonia to occur in these extreme basal portions of the lungs (see Fig. 7.2) and to present as acute abdominal pain, particularly in a child.

Normal Abdominal Radiograph

When interpreting abdominal radiographs it is important to have a standard approach, similar to that used for looking at any diagnostic study. As with chest radiographs, start with lines and tubes (see Fig. 7.5). A useful mnemonic that covers all of the important aspects of an abdominal radiograph is *Gas, Mass, Stones, and Bones.* Figure 7.6 shows a normal supine abdominal radiograph of a young woman. There are no lines or tubes. The abdominal **gas** pattern is normal. There are no findings of free air or obstruction. The caliber of the air-filled bowel is normal. There are no findings of abdominal **mass** or mass effect. There are no abnormal radiopaque densities (or **stones**). The **bones** are normal in appearance without findings of fracture or pathologic process.

▶ A useful mnemonic for things to look for on abdominal radiographs is Gas, Mass, Stones, and Bones.

Keeping this prototypical normal abdominal radiograph in your mind, we discuss different abnormalities that can be identified on an abdominal series.

Pathologic Considerations

Abdominal Gas

As previously mentioned, to correctly interpret abdominal radiographs and to be able to distinguish upright from supine radiographs when they are not labeled, one must remember the law of burps and farts: hot air rises. An upright radiograph should have several air-fluid levels. A good place to look is the stomach where there is almost always an air-fluid level (see Fig. 7.7). Air-fluid levels can be "balanced" where they occur at the same level or can resemble a staircase with the two ends residing at different levels (Fig. 7.9).

Free air (pneumoperitoneum) and obstructions can be life-threatening emergencies. These abnormalities will look different on supine and upright radiographs. The correct radiographic interpretation can be made if one knows where to look and which study to order. Before we discuss bowel gas pathologies, let us take a look at the normal bowel gas pattern on both supine and upright radiographs.

Intraluminal Gas

The gas demonstrated on abdominal radiographs is either intraluminal or extraluminal. The abnormalities produced by intraluminal gas include distension or dilation of one or more bowel loops, the presence of air-fluid levels (see Fig. 7.9), and the presence

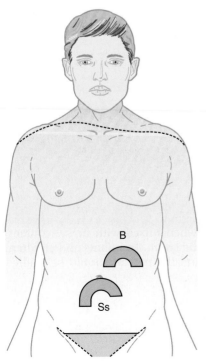

Figure 7.9   Air-fluid levels come in two varieties: Balanced (*B*), where the two ends are at the same level, and the stair-step (*Ss*) appearance, which can be a finding of obstruction.

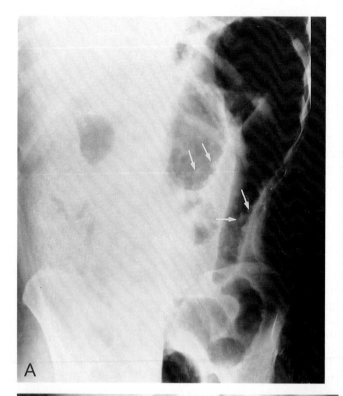

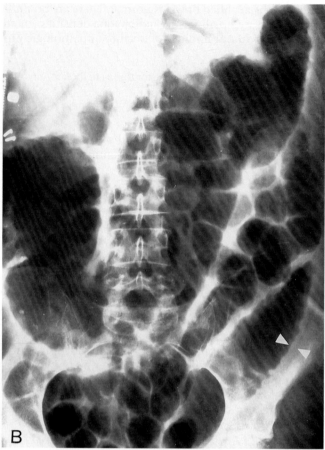

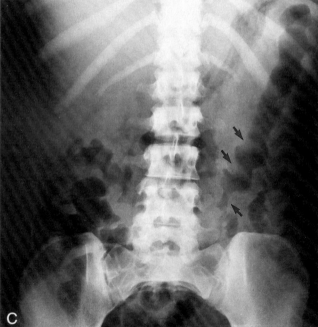

Figure 7.10   Mucosal thickening in three patients with ulcerative colitis.   A. Pseudopolyps representing areas of preserved mucosa are present throughout the bowel (*arrows*). **B.** Note the thickened bowel wall on the left side (*arrowheads*). **C.** The thick mucosa has the appearance of "thumb-prints" (*arrows*). Note the loss of haustral markings more proximally.

of mucosal thickening (Fig. 7.10). Intraluminal gas, when mixed with bowel content, frequently gives a bubbly appearance, particularly in the colon. In infants and children, however, this "adult stool pattern" is never normal, and the patient should be studied further to determine the source of the abnormality.

 ▶ The "adult stool pattern" is always abnormal in abdominal radiographs of infants and children.

How do we deal with studies that are not conclusive for the presence or absence of abdominal obstruction? A term that is frequently used for those studies is *"nonspecific abdominal gas pattern."* This term should be abandoned because it gives little information regarding what is actually present on the radiograph. Maglinte has suggested that the term be replaced by something more descriptive of the various intestinal gas patterns encountered. He has four categories: (1) *normal*, defined as either absence of small bowel gas or presence of gas within not more than four variably shaped loops of small intestine that are also less than 2.5 cm in diameter; (2) *mild bowel stasis*, defined as multiple slightly dilated (2.5–3 cm) loops with three or more air-fluid levels, without disproportionate distension of the small bowel relative to the colon; (3) *probable obstructive pattern*, defined as unequivocal dilation of multiple gas or fluid-filled loops of bowel, with multiple air-fluid levels but an element of uncertainty of the diagnosis of obstruction; and (4) *definite obstructive pattern*, in which the diagnosis is unequivocal. For small bowel obstruction, gaseous distension of the small bowel is disproportionate to that in the colon.

The Rule of 3's

Having stated the principles above, how can you, the clinician, determine whether a loop or multiple loops of bowel are dilated? No firm answers or numerical limits are listed in references but you can use the Rule of 3's as an initial reference. Two other rules of thumb may help you decide: (1) a single air-filled loop of small bowel or colon that is distinctly much larger than the others on serial radiographs may represent local dilation, and (2) multiple air-filled loops of small bowel or colon that give the abdomen a distinctive "gas bag" appearance usually represent ileus or obstruction.

Distended or Dilated Bowel

Distended or dilated bowel may occur under a variety of circumstances. Most often this is the result of an adynamic ileus, in which peristalsis is markedly diminished. The typical appearance shows gaseous distension of both the colon and small bowel (Fig. 7.11). Air-fluid levels may also be present in these patients, occurring in both the large and small bowels in what has been termed a "balanced" (even-distribution) pattern. Ileus occurs most commonly in patients following trauma (including surgery), with peritonitis,

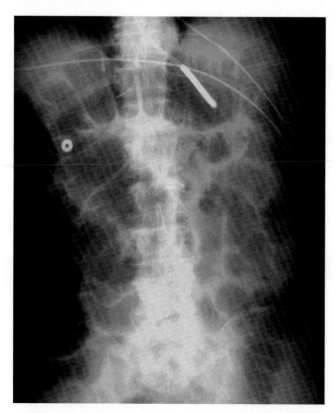

Figure 7.11 Adynamic ileus.
Supine radiograph demonstrates a Dobbhoff type catheter in the stomach. Small and large bowel loops are dilated with air. Patient did not have any bowel sounds and was on large-dose opioids for pain control.

as a manifestation of medicines such as opioids which decrease peristalsis, in bowel ischemia, and in chronically ill, bedridden patients. Clinically, patients with an adynamic ileus will have a distended abdomen with absent bowel sounds as opposed to a small bowel obstruction where bowel sounds can be hyperactive. A localized ileus that persists on serial studies is referred to as a *sentinel loop*. Its presence suggests an adjacent area of inflammation such as pancreatitis (Fig. 7.12), appendicitis, or cholecystitis.

Obstruction

Obstruction, on the other hand, results in dilated loops of bowel proximal to the obstruction and a paucity of gas distal to the obstruction. The appearance of an obstruction will appear differently on upright and supine radiographs (Fig. 7.13). The bowel loops frequently have a stepwise or hairpin (180° turn) appearance on upright views. Loops of small bowel may also be dilated in the supine view; however, there will be no air-fluid levels. The presence of gas within the rectum does not rule out bowel obstruction. Colonic gas may be present in an early or partial obstruction. Gas may be introduced into the rectum by digital examination, colonoscopy, rectal temperature determination, and enemas. In an early obstruction, the characteristic pattern may not be well developed. However, serial examinations will show the development of the characteristic loops.

 ▶ Gas within the rectum does not rule out bowel obstruction.

The causes of a mechanical obstruction vary, depending on whether the patient is an adult or a child. In the adult, common causes include adhesions (see Fig. 7.13), inflammation (often from Crohn disease), inguinal hernia (Fig. 7.14) that can become incarcerated, and appendicitis (Fig. 7.15). Small bowel tumors are very rare (as opposed to colon cancer) but can occasionally serve as a lead point for a small bowel obstruction.

Considerations of the Newborn

In the newborn with bilious vomiting, congenital abnormalities such as malrotation or duodenal atresia should be suspected. Each of these conditions has characteristic radiographic and fluoroscopic (discussed in the next chapter) findings that, when present,

Figure 7.12   Small bowel sentinel loop in a patient with pancreatitis of the tail of the pancreas.   A single dilated loop of jejunum (*arrow*) measuring 4 cm in diameter is present. Note the increased distance between the jejunum and the contrast-filled stomach as the result of pancreatic phlegmon.

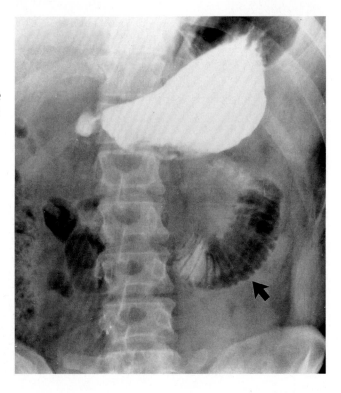

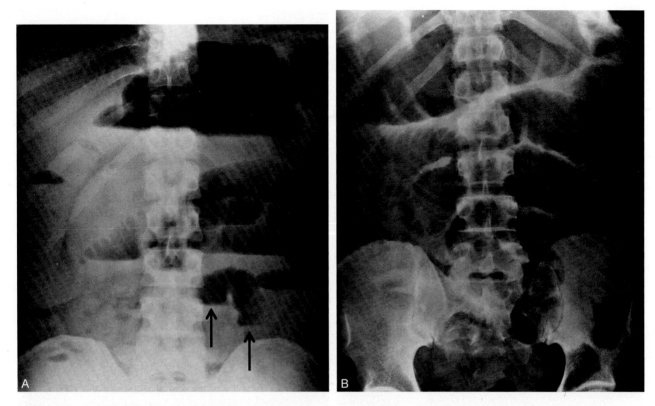

Figure 7.13 Small bowel obstruction secondary to adhesions. A. Upright view demonstrates multiple air-fluid levels including stair-steps (*arrows*) in a patient with small bowel obstruction. **B.** Supine radiograph demonstrates dilated loops (*arrow*) of small bowel proximal to the obstruction.

should allow you to make a correct diagnosis. Duodenal atresia is the most common site of intestinal atresia. Two variants occur: membranous and stenosis. The abdominal radiograph typically demonstrates gaseous dilatation of the stomach and duodenal bulb without distal gas. The appearance has been termed the "double-bubble" sign (Fig. 7.16).

Special Pediatric Considerations

In infants and children, *intussusception* (Fig. 7.17) is a common cause of obstruction and classically presents with "currant jelly stool." As mentioned earlier, ultrasonography can be used in the pediatric population to make this diagnosis. *Intussusception* occurs when a segment of intestine (the *intussusceptum*) invaginates or "telescopes" into the contiguous distal segment (the *intussuscipiens*). This produces mechanical obstruction and, if left untreated, ischemia. Approximately 90% of intussusceptions are ileocolic; the remainder are (in decreasing order of frequency) ileoileocolic, ileoileal, and colocolic. Unlike adults, in whom intussusceptions are typically caused by mesenteric neoplasms, those in the pediatric age group are idiopathic. Radiographic findings, when present, include a mass effect, target-like lucencies in the mass (representing mesenteric fat trapped in the intussusception), and a crescent or streaks of air outlining the trapped bowel. The intussusception can often be reduced with an air enema under fluoroscopy thus sparing the patient from surgery (see Fig. 7.17C).

Causes of Small and Large Bowel Obstructions

There is some overlap with the etiologies for small and large bowel obstruction: hernias can involve loops of small and or large bowel, which can become incarcerated. In the adult population, diverticulitis, colon cancer, and colonic volvuli are important causes of large bowel obstruction (Fig. 7.18). Only portions of the colon that have a mesentery are affected including the sigmoid colon, cecum, and transverse colon. The correct diagnosis of volvulus can often be made on radiographs. When the cecum twists there is dilation up to the point of twisting, which is usually located in the left mid or upper abdomen (Fig. 7.19). If the sigmoid twists and undergoes volvulus, it dilates and usually is located in

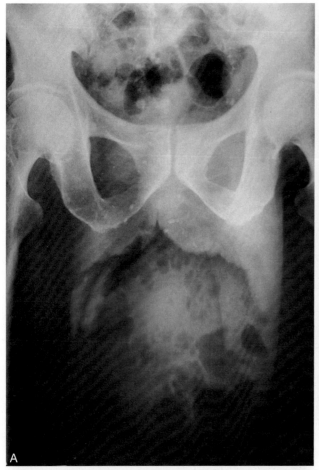

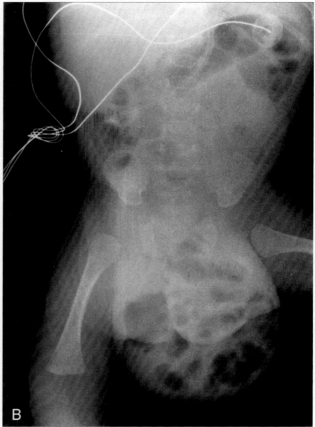

Figure 7.14   Inguinal hernia.   **In both an adult **(A) and a newborn **(B)**, loops of bowel fill the scrotum. **C.** A barium study confirms the presence of large bowel within the inguinal hernia in a third patient.

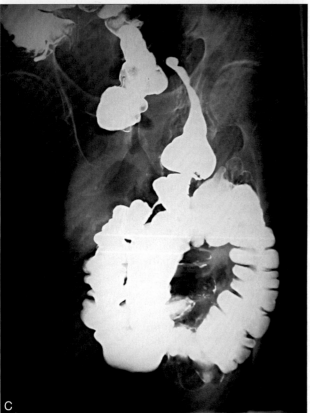

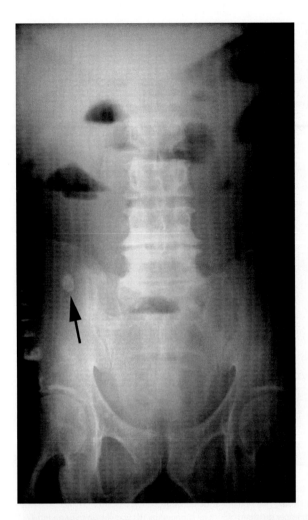

Figure 7.15   Small bowel obstruction secondary to appendicitis.   Upright radiograph demonstrates multiple air fluid levels with a calcified appendicolith in the right lower quadrant (*black arrow*). At surgery patient had a perforated appendix with an abscess that was causing the small bowel obstruction.

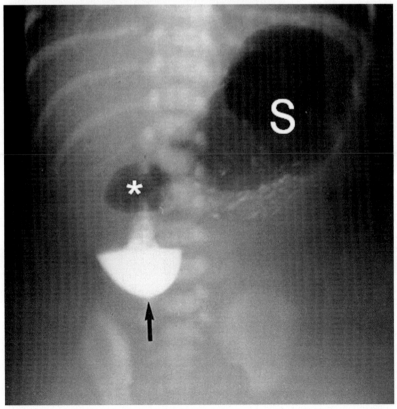

Figure 7.16   Duodenal atresia.   Supine radiograph demonstrates the "double bubble" of air trapped in the stomach (*S*) and the duodenal bulb (*asterisk*). Note the absence of other gas in the abdomen. The white density beneath the duodenal air is barium in the descending duodenum. Note the abrupt termination of this loop at the level of the atresia (*arrow*).

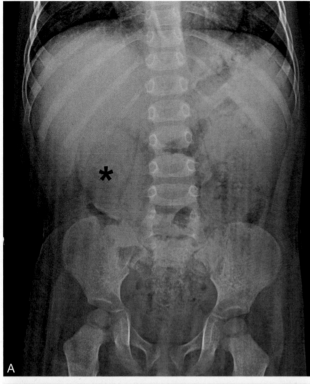

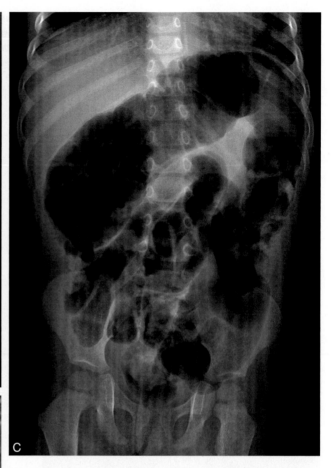

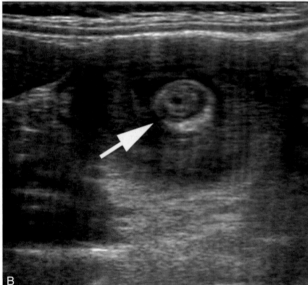

Figure 7.17   Intussusception in a 3-year-old with bloody diarrhea.   A. First image demonstrates a soft tissue mass (*asterisk*) in the right upper quadrant, which on sonography (**B**) was shown to be an intussusception. Note the "bullseye" appearance (*arrow*). **C.** The intussusception was successfully reduced with an air enema and the resultant radiograph demonstrates an air filled small and large bowel.

the right upper quadrant (Fig. 7.20). A volvulus can be confirmed with CT or fluoroscopy. As with small bowel obstructions, there will be disproportionate dilation of the bowel loops proximal to the obstruction and relative decompression distal to the obstruction.

> ▶ With cecal volvulus, the dilated bowel is located in the left upper quadrant of the abdomen.
> ▶ With sigmoid volvulus, the dilated bowel is located in the right upper quadrant.

Special Pediatric Considerations

Distal colonic obstructions in children occur with colonic atresias, meconium plugs, meconium ileus (often seen in newborns with cystic fibrosis), and Hirschsprung disease. *Hirschsprung disease* is the result of congenital absence of the intramural ganglion cells

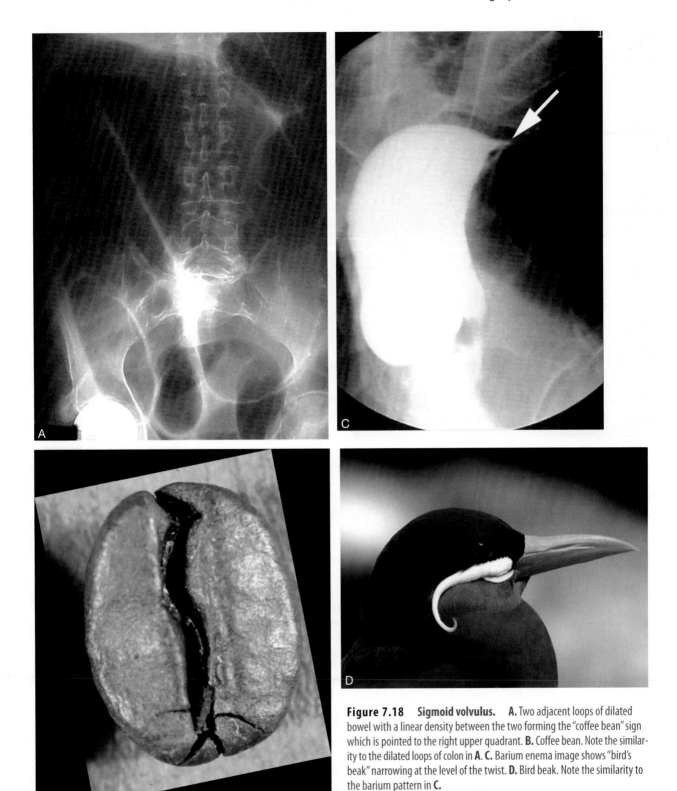

Figure 7.18 Sigmoid volvulus. A. Two adjacent loops of dilated bowel with a linear density between the two forming the "coffee bean" sign which is pointed to the right upper quadrant. **B.** Coffee bean. Note the similarity to the dilated loops of colon in **A**. **C.** Barium enema image shows "bird's beak" narrowing at the level of the twist. **D.** Bird beak. Note the similarity to the barium pattern in **C**.

in the distal bowel and can result in a spectrum of disease from a newborn who has not passed meconium with a high-grade obstruction to an older child or adult with chronic constipation (chapter 8).

Gasless Abdomen

Finally, one should be aware that one additional possibility exists: the *gasless abdomen*. Small and large bowel that is entirely fluid filled may be dilated or nondilated (obstructed

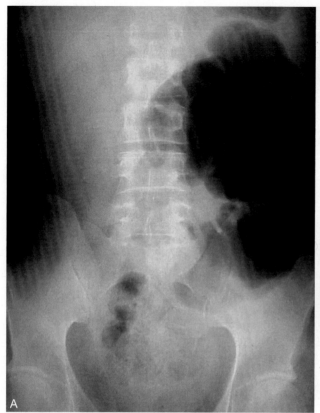

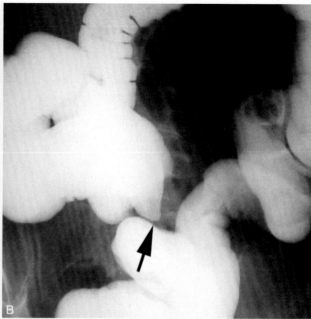

Figure 7.19   Cecal volvulus.   A. Supine radiograph demonstrates a dilated loop of large bowel in the left upper quadrant. **B.** Barium enema shows "bird's beak" narrowing in the cecum (*arrow*) corresponding with the area of twist in this cecal volvulus.

or nonobstructed); however, the lack of inherent contrast will preclude an accurate diagnosis. CT can be helpful in these cases to better define the bowel loops and pathology.

Extraluminal Gas

Extraluminal gas may be either free (pneumoperitoneum) or contained within an abscess cavity, the retroperitoneum, the bowel wall, or the biliary or portal venous systems of the liver. Free intraperitoneal air in the absence of immediate previous surgery or intervention (i.e., paracentesis, peritoneal dialysis, placement of a gastrostomy tube) suggests a perforated viscus. The most common cause is a perforated peptic ulcer or a colonic diverticulum. Penetrating trauma is another important cause. If the perforation is intraperitoneal, gas will be seen under the diaphragm on an upright radiograph (Fig. 7.21**A**). Furthermore, decubitus positioning may also demonstrate free intraperitoneal air (see Fig. 7.1**B**). However, it is possible to make the diagnosis of pneumoperitoneum on a supine film from the *"double wall sign" or Rigler sign*, which results when air on both sides of the bowel outlines that structure rather distinctly (Fig. 7.21**B**). Under normal circumstances, the serosal surface of bowel is not visible because of its water density. Air within the peritoneal cavity, however, changes the radiographic density that outlines the bowel wall.

Special Pediatric Considerations

In infants, who are usually examined in the supine position, free intraperitoneal air may outline the falciform ligament (Fig. 7.22). The *"football sign"* can be seen especially in children, in which there is an overall lucency to the abdomen. The faliciform ligament, when surrounded by free air on either side, can appear as a sharp line with the ribs running perpendicular much like football laces.

▶ Air outlining both sides of the bowel wall is known as the "double wall sign" or "Rigler sign."

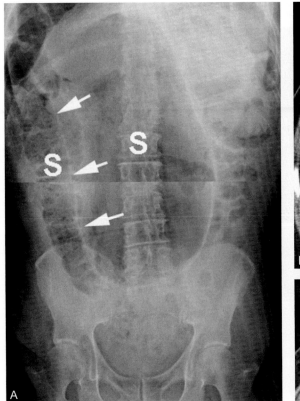

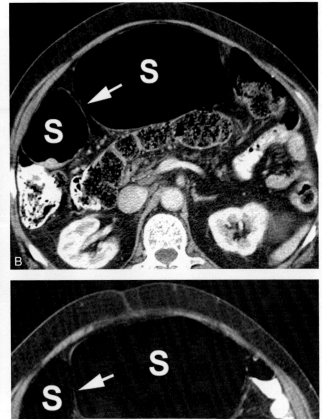

Figure 7.20   Sigmoid volvulus.   A. The sigmoid colon (*S*) is dilated. The dense white line (*arrows*) that runs obliquely from the right upper abdomen into the pelvis represents two adjacent walls of the colon. **B** and **C.** Axial CT images show the sigmoid (*S*) is massively dilated. The dense white line seen on the KUB is formed by the two adjacent walls of the colon (*white arrows*). The mesentery tapers (*black arrow* in **C**) at the point of the twist.

Miscellaneous Extraluminal Air Collections - Where to Look

Retroperitoneal air, particularly from a perforated duodenal ulcer or ruptured duodenum secondary to trauma, often manifests as air outlining the psoas muscle, the kidney, or adrenal margin or air adjacent to the properitoneal fat stripe. This diagnosis may be difficult to make based on radiographs. However, on a CT scan, the presence of retroperitoneal air is easily detected. Loculated gas within the abdomen generally indicates the presence of an abscess. The air may be confined to a known anatomic space (such as air within Morrison's pouch beneath the liver), to an emphysematous gallbladder (Fig. 7.23), to the renal capsule (Fig. 7.24), to the lesser sac, or within an organ (Fig. 7.25A), or it may be free within the abdominal cavity. Please note that air within the Morrison's pouch or the lesser sac is intraperitoneal. The gas may be a small localized collection or, more commonly, may have a mottled bubbly appearance. Frequently, it is necessary to do a CT examination with oral or rectal contrast to determine the location of normal loops of bowel and to rule out the presence of an aberrant loop of bowel being responsible for the abnormal shadow. The CT scan is also the most reliable study for the diagnosis of abscesses (Fig. 7.25**B**).

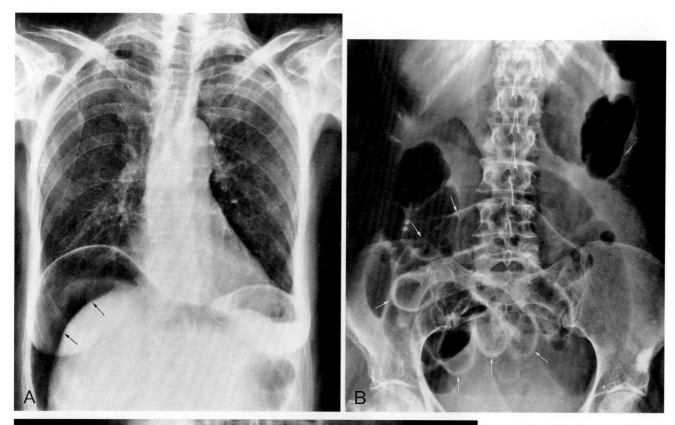

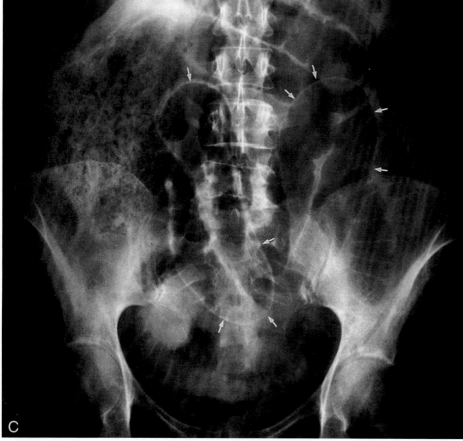

Figure 7.21   Pneumoperitoneum.
A. Chest radiograph shows air beneath the diaphragm. The liver margin is outlined by air (*arrows*). **B.** Supine abdominal radiograph of this massive pneumoperitoneum shows air on both sides of the bowel wall (Rigler sign) (*arrows*). **C.** Supine radiograph in another patient also shows air on both sides of the bowel wall. The serosal surfaces are clearly defined (*arrows*).

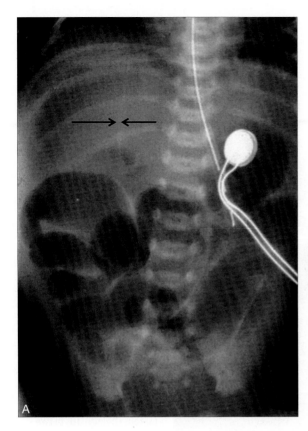

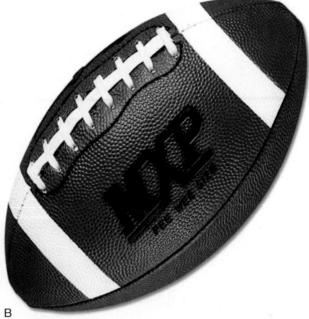

Figure 7.22 **Pneumoperitoneum in an infant.** **A.** The free air in the abdomen overlies the liver with air on either side of the falciform ligament (*arrows*) representing the laces of a football. **B.** Football. Note the similarity to the gas pattern in A.

Intramural Gas

Intramural gas (*pneumatosis intestinalis*) may be found in a variety of benign and pathologic conditions. Common causes of pneumatosis in older adults are ischemia and microperforation of a diverticulum. Gas appears as streaky densities surrounding the bowel (Fig. 7.26). CT easily demonstrates intramural gas. Intramural gas may also be found in bowel infarction in older patients and particularly in premature newborn children with necrotizing enterocolitis (Fig. 7.27). In both types of patients with intestinal ischemia, gas may track into the portal system of the liver (Fig. 7.28) via the mesenteric veins. Occasionally, a giant air cyst will occur.

Gas in the biliary tree may occur following endoscopic papillotomy (Fig. 7.29), penetrating trauma to the gallbladder, with a gallstone ileus where a fistulous tract is formed between the bowel and biliary system, following surgery in which the common bile duct is anastomosed to the small bowel, or in infection. Portal gas is usually located in the periphery, whereas biliary gas in seen more centrally. Correlation with the clinical findings is necessary to properly interpret this observation.

 ▶ Portal venous gas is usually located in the periphery; biliary gas is seen more centrally.

Mucosal Patterns

The natural contrast between the soft tissues, the mucosa, and the air within the bowel allows evaluation of that bowel. A thickened bowel wall is always abnormal. Mucosal thickening is generally present when the valvulae conniventes of the small intestine or the colonic haustra are thicker than 3 mm (remember the Rule of 3's). If the bowel is distended with air, the actual (edematous) wall may be identified by air on one side and increased soft tissue density on the other. Thickened mucosa are most often encountered in inflammatory bowel disease (Fig. 7.30), neoplasms including lymphoma and bowel

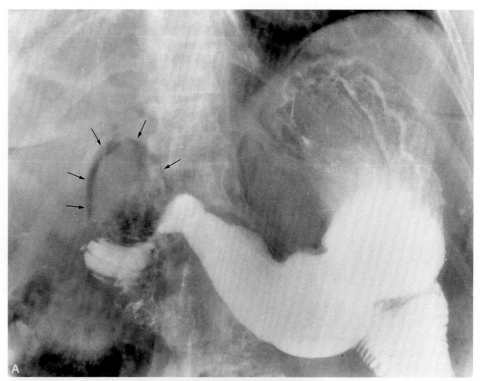

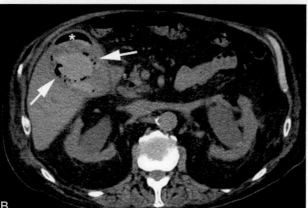

Figure 7.23   Emphysematous cholecystitis in two diabetic patients.
A. Gas outlines the gallbladder (*arrows*) in the abdominal radiograph. **B.** CT image of another patient shows abnormal pockets of gas within the gallbladder wall (*arrows*) and lumen (*asterisk*).

Figure 7.24.   Emphysematous pyelonephritis in a diabetic patient.
A large collection of gas outlines the right kidney (*arrows*. The psoas margin on the right is lost.

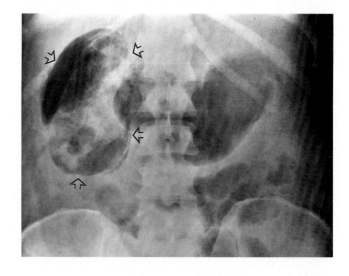

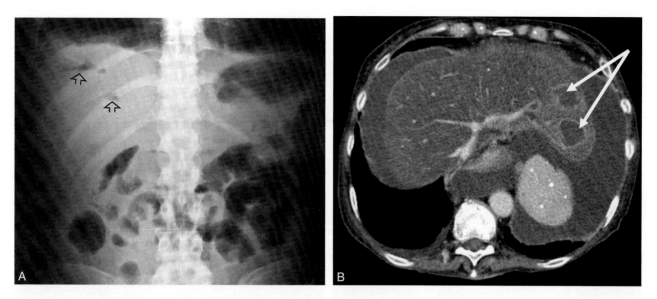

Figure 7.25   Liver abscess.   A. Radiograph shows collections of gas within the liver (*arrows*). **B.** CT image demonstrates additional abscesses within the left hepatic lobe (*arrows*) with peripherally enhancing walls.

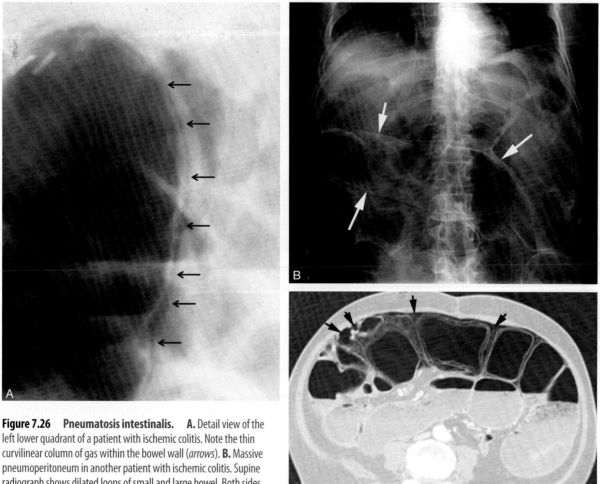

Figure 7.26   Pneumatosis intestinalis.   A. Detail view of the left lower quadrant of a patient with ischemic colitis. Note the thin curvilinear column of gas within the bowel wall (*arrows*). **B.** Massive pneumoperitoneum in another patient with ischemic colitis. Supine radiograph shows dilated loops of small and large bowel. Both sides of the bowel wall can be seen (*arrows*). **C.** Axial CT image shows the abnormal gas collection is within the wall of the bowel (*arrows*).

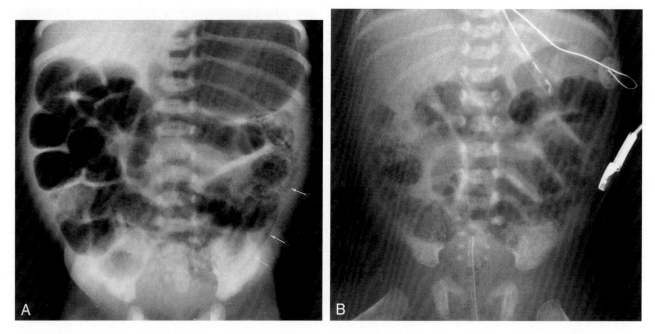

Figure 7.27   Necrotizing enterocolitis in a premature newborn.   A. Pneumatosis intestinalis is on the left side (*arrows*). **B.** A similar pattern appears bilaterally in another patient. The adult stool pattern is always abnormal in an infant.

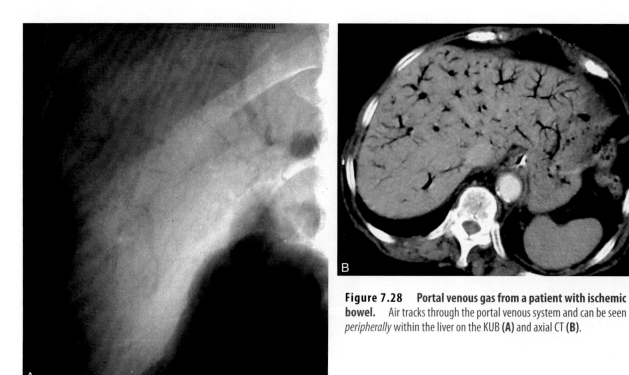

Figure 7.28   Portal venous gas from a patient with ischemic bowel.   Air tracks through the portal venous system and can be seen *peripherally* within the liver on the KUB **(A)** and axial CT **(B)**.

carcinoma, bowel edema in hypoproteinemic and malabsorption states, submucosal hemorrhage of any cause, and ischemia. These last two conditions often produce two interesting patterns of mucosal thickening: thumblike indentations in the gas-filled bowel (*"thumbprinting"*) and a picket fence appearance of the valvulae in the small bowel (the *"stacked coin"* appearance). The exact cause of the thickening cannot be determined without applying important history and physical examination findings. For example, a patient with a history of sudden onset of abdominal pain accompanied by blood-streaked diarrhea and dilated bowel on plain film is likely to have colitis.

Figure 7.29 Pneumobilia in a patient following endoscopic papillotomy. Note the air in the dilated common bile duct (*solid arrow*), common hepatic ducts, and intrahepatic ducts (*open arrow*). Surgical clips (*arrowheads*) from a previous cholecystectomy are present.

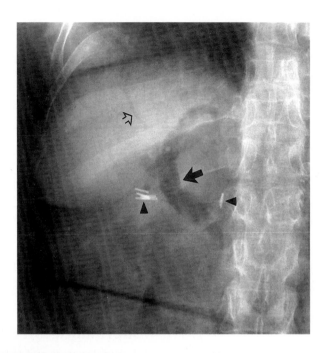

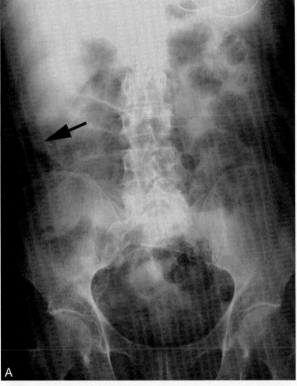

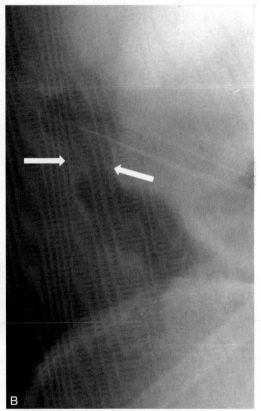

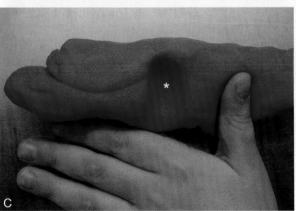

Figure 7.30 Mucosal thickening in a patient with ulcerative colitis. The thumbprint sign in the KUB **(A)** and magnified view **(B)**. The thick mucosa has the appearance of being depressed by a "thumbprint" (*arrows*). Note the loss of haustral markings more proximally. **C.** Thumbprint (*asterisk*) in clay. Note the similarity to the gas pattern in A and B.

Figure 7.31   Hepatosplenomegaly in a patient with Hodgkin disease.   Note the enlargement of the liver (*H*) and spleen (*S*). The gastric air bubble (*G*) is displaced to the right of midline.

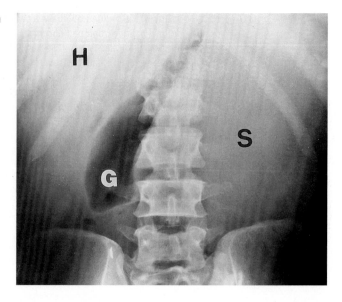

Abnormalities of Soft Tissue Images—Masses and Mass Effect

Abdominal masses and mass effect can be some of the subtlest but most important findings to appreciate on abdominal radiographs. Although CT, ultrasound, and magnetic resonance (MR) images provide more detailed information regarding these abnormalities, radiographs can detect many of them—if one knows where to look.

Organ Enlargement

Enlargement of the abdominal organs may cause displacement of other organs. For example, splenomegaly will displace the gastric air shadow medially (Fig. 7.31). Hepatomegaly is suspected when its inferior margin extends below the iliac crest on the supine radiograph. The kidney may be displaced inferiorly by an enlarged adrenal gland or tumor and laterally by enlarged paraspinal lymph nodes.

Displacement or Distortion of Viscera

Abdominal masses are frequently revealed by the displacement or distortion of normal viscera (Fig. 7.32). The loss of the margin of a soft tissue structure is a valuable sign in

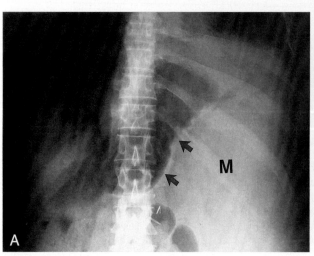
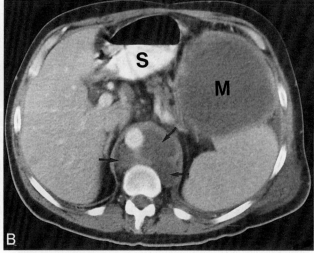

Figure 7.32   Mass effect caused by splenic metastases.   **A.** Detail of an abdominal radiograph shows a large mass (*M*) displacing and compressing the greater curvature of the stomach (*arrows*). **B.** CT image shows the necrotic mass (*M*) to be located in the anterior pole of the spleen. Note the relationship of the mass to the stomach (*S*) as well as the necrotic paraaortic lymph nodes (*arrows*).

evaluating patients with abdominal disease. The loss of a renal outline or psoas margin generally indicates an inflammatory condition in the retroperitoneum. The loss of the psoas margin accompanied by scoliosis is a nonspecific finding that may be seen in acute appendicitis, urinary calculus, or perforated viscus. As mentioned previously, the loss of the properitoneal fat line may also be seen in several inflammatory conditions, particularly appendicitis.

Abnormal Fluid—Ascites

Ascites can cause a mass effect on the bowel, which is discussed below. The classic appearance of ascites has been described as diffuse, "ground glass" density of the abdomen. Generally, by the time this has occurred, ascites is clinically apparent and need not be diagnosed by radiographic means. However, small amounts of peritoneal fluid (ascites or blood) may appear in a subtle manner. The accumulation of several hundred milliliters of ascitic fluid may be apparent on the supine radiograph as a collection of water-density material overlying the sacrum above the bladder. This occurs because the fluid collects posteriorly in the pelvis. With increasing volume, however, the ascites extends superolaterally out of the pelvis, producing bilateral collections on either side of the main fluid bulk, giving the appearance of "dog ears." Further increase in the amount of fluid (to more than 500 mL) will extend up along the lateral gutters, displacing the colon medially from the radiolucent flank stripes. As the amount of fluid increases, the liver and spleen are displaced from the body wall. Finally, floating loops of small bowel may be seen in the "sea of ascites." CT and ultrasound are much more sensitive in diagnosing ascites (Fig. 7.33) and planning treatment via paracentesis.

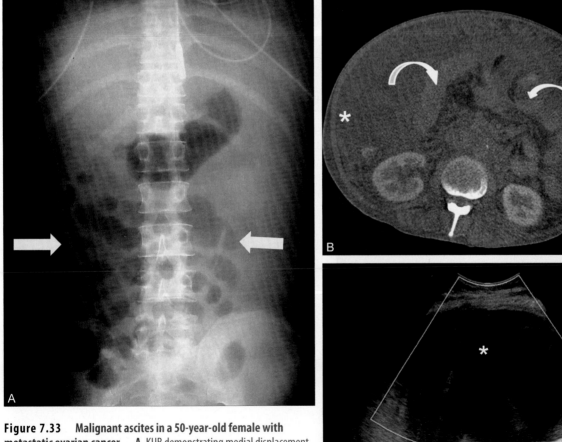

Figure 7.33   Malignant ascites in a 50-year-old female with metastatic ovarian cancer.   A. KUB demonstrating medial displacement of the small bowel loops (*arrows*) with bulging of the flanks. **B.** CT image shows the massive ascites (*asterisk*) displacing the bowel loops (*curved arrows*) centrally. **C.** Ultrasound demonstrates a large pocket of fluid (*asterisk*) that was safely drained.

Calcifications

The list of calcifications that may be found on abdominal radiographs is long and beyond the scope of this text. However, certain physiologic conditions frequently produce calcifications seen on abdominal studies. These include

- ○ costal cartilages,
- ○ vascular calcifications (such as phleboliths in the pelvic venous plexus),
- ○ atherosclerotic plaques of the aortoiliac vessels,
- ○ prostatic calcifications,
- ○ calcified granulomas of spleen and lymph nodes.

Several of these are illustrated in (Fig. 7.34).

Abnormal calcifications include biliary (Fig. 7.35) and urinary calculi (Fig. 7.36), calcified aneurysms (Fig. 7.37), pancreatic calcifications (Fig. 7.38), calcified uterine fibroids,

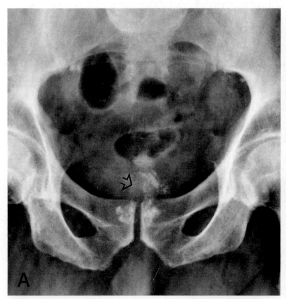

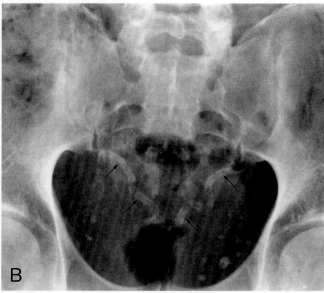

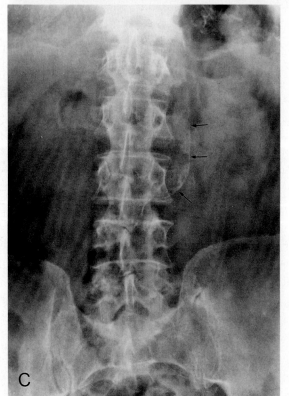

Figure 7.34   Abdominal calcifications   A. Prostate (*arrow*) **B.** Vas deferens (*arrows*) in a diabetic man. **C.** Abdominal aortic aneurysm (*arrows*).

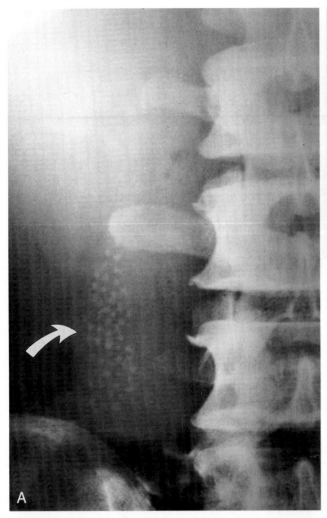

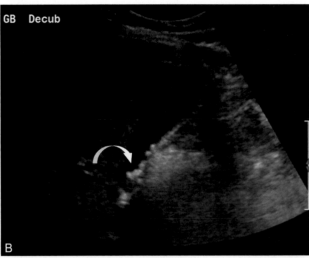

Figure 7.35 Multiple calcified gallstones (*arrows*) on a magnified KUB in A and ultrasound on B.

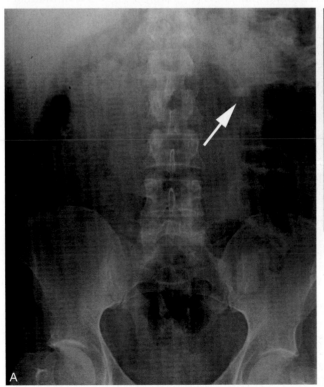

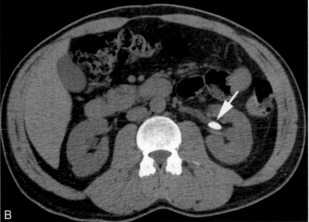

Figure 7.36 Left ureteropelvic junction renal calculus (*arrows*) on KUB (A) and axial CT (B).

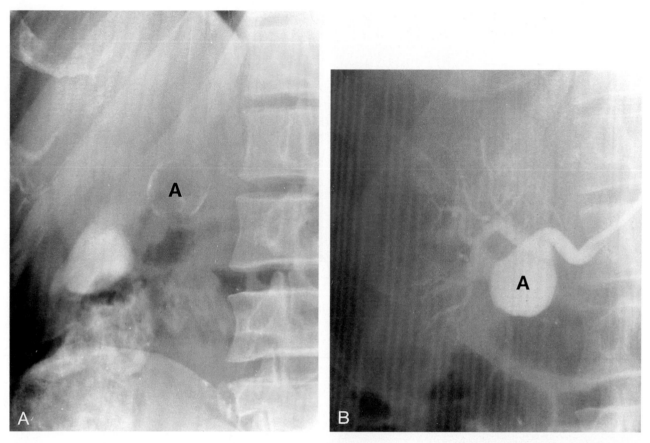

Figure 7.37   Renal artery aneurysm.   A. Radiograph shows the peripherally calcified aneurysm (*A*). **B**. Renal arteriogram shows the aneurysm (*A*) to advantage.

and calcified appendiceal fecaliths (see Fig. 7.15). In addition, foreign bodies may often be seen. These may include ingested foreign materials (e.g., tablets; Fig. 7.39) or traumatic foreign bodies (e.g., bullets, buckshot, or shrapnel). You may, on occasion, see a patient with a self-introduced rectal foreign body (Fig. 7.40).

Postoperative Changes in the Abdomen

It is important to recognize the signs of previous surgery in the abdomen. Wire sutures or surgical clips in the abdomen are typical indicators. In this era of laparoscopic surgery, metallic clips may be the only evidence that a surgical procedure has been performed. The position of the sutures or staples frequently can give an idea of what type of surgery was performed. For example, wire sutures extending obliquely from the midline toward the right flank may indicate that the patient has had traditional (not laparoscopic) biliary surgery. Metallic clips in the region of the esophagogastric junction indicate previous vagotomy: those in the right upper quadrant indicate cholecystectomy. Multiple surgical clips in the pelvis indicate gynecologic surgery in a woman or prostate surgery in a man. Ostomy devices and dialysis catheters are easily identified. Radiographs are often taken in the operating room when "the sponge count is off" and there is a suspected missing sponge or surgical instrument (see Fig. 7.4). Finally, displacement of surgical clips or a foreign body such as a bullet may provide clues to the diagnosis of recurrent tumor (Fig. 7.41) or an intraabdominal abscess, respectively. Scarring and fibrosis result in the clips moving together.

Bone and Joint Abnormalities

The bony structures encountered on an abdominal radiograph include the lower thoracic and lumbar vertebrae, sacrum, lower ribs, pelvis, and hips. Frequently, degenerative

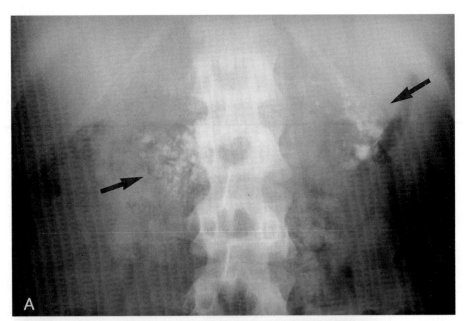

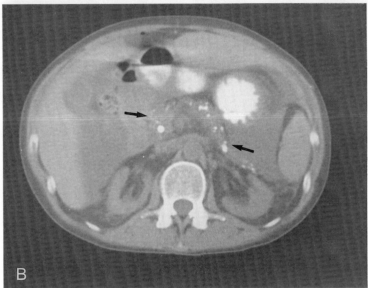

Figure 7.38 Pancreatic calcifications (*arrows*). **A.** Detail of a radiograph. **B.** CT image.

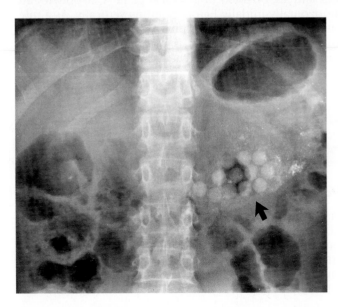

Figure 7.39 Ferrous sulfate tablets in the stomach (*arrow***).**

Figure 7.40   Rectal foreign body.   The patient was "delighted" following removal.

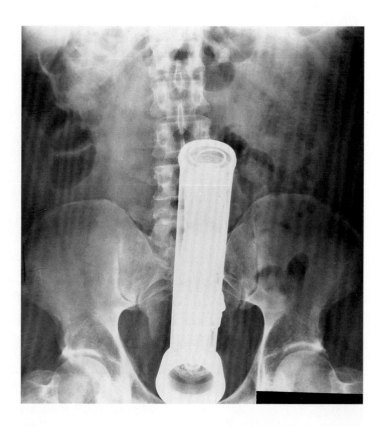

changes are present in the spines of older individuals. Fractures, metastases (Fig. 7.42), and spondyloarthropathies can easily be missed if one does not include bony structures as part of the search pattern.

Skeletal Manifestations

Many intraabdominal disorders have well-recognized skeletal manifestations. Furthermore, inflammatory bowel disease (regional enteritis, ulcerative colitis) may have an associated spondyloarthropathy that affects the lumbar vertebrae and the sacroiliac joints. In these patients, asymmetric syndesmophyte formations may occur along the vertebral end plates. Syndesmophytes are distinguished from the more common osteophytes by the direction in which the spurring points. Syndesmophytes represent ossification of Sharpey fibers of the disc annulus and are oriented in a vertical plane. Osteophytes are simple bone spurs that extend horizontally initially before pointing vertically. As a rule, syndesmophytes are more delicate and thinner than osteophytes. Another manifestation of the spondyloarthropathy of inflammatory bowel disease is sacroiliitis that may be symmetric or asymmetric. In many instances, bowel mucosal changes may be appreciated in addition to the bony changes (Fig. 7.43).

> Syndesmophytes and osteophytes are distinguished from each other by the direction the spurs point. Syndesmophytes are oriented vertically; osteophytes are initially oriented horizontally.

Other Musculoskeletal Manifestations

Other musculoskeletal manifestations include osteolytic or osteoblastic metastatic lesions from a variety of malignancies. Large lytic lesions suggest renal carcinoma or myeloma; blastic lesions suggest prostate carcinoma in a man and breast cancer in a woman (Breast cancer can result in lytic or blastic bony lesions). Dense bones with smudged, thickened trabeculae are characteristic of renal osteodystrophy. In such an instance, look for evidence of dialysis catheters or of a renal transplant (Fig. 7.44).

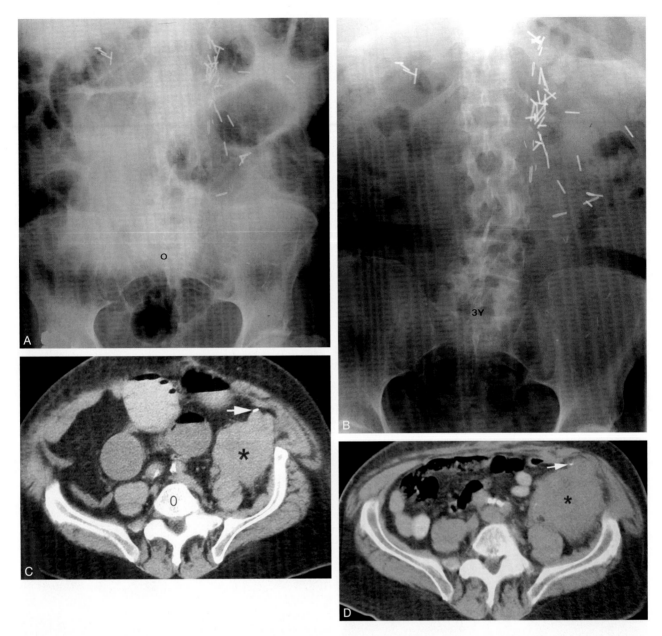

Figure 7.41 Recurrent tumor. A. Radiograph shows surgical clips in the left flank. **B.** Follow-up radiograph 3 years later shows the clips have become splayed apart. **C.** CT image made at the same time as radiograph in **A** shows a mass (*asterisk*). Note the position of the surgical clip (*arrow*). **D.** CT image made at the same time as radiograph in **B** shows the mass (*asterisk*) to have enlarged. Note the shift of the clip (*arrow*) anteriorly.

Diagnosis

When deciding what study to order, you must determine the clinical questions you are trying to answer. Radiographic studies have diagnostic limitations and have associated radiation and monetary costs. With respect to the abdomen, KUBs are the least expensive, have less radiation, and are excellent for confirmation of tube placement or foreign body. If the question is free air, an upright or decubitus radiograph will usually answer the question (see Fig. 7.1). If the question is obstruction or other cause of pain (abscess, bleed), CT is the modality of choice especially in the emergency setting. The ACR Appropriateness Criteria® (www.acr.org) can also offer guidance as to which study to order for certain conditions. Finally, when reviewing any CT study always look at the scout view. Many significant abnormalities will be visible on abdose miniature digital images (Fig. 7.45).

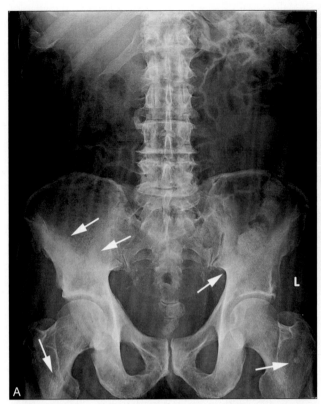

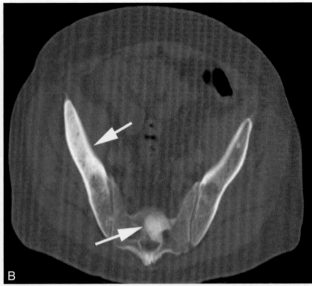

Figure 7.42   Osteoblastic metastases (*arrows*) on KUB (A) and CT (B) from prostate carcinoma.

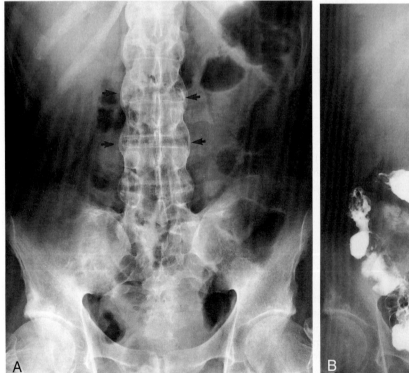

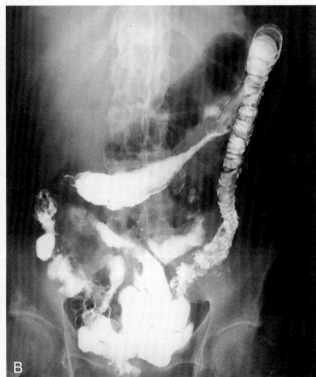

Figure 7.43   Spondyloarthropathy of inflammatory bowel (Crohn) disease.   A. Abdominal radiograph shows ankylosis of the sacroiliac joints. There are also syndesmophytes bridging the vertebral discs (*arrows*). **B.** Barium enema shows loss of haustra and irregularity of the transverse colon and terminal ileum, typical of Crohn disease (see Chapter 8).

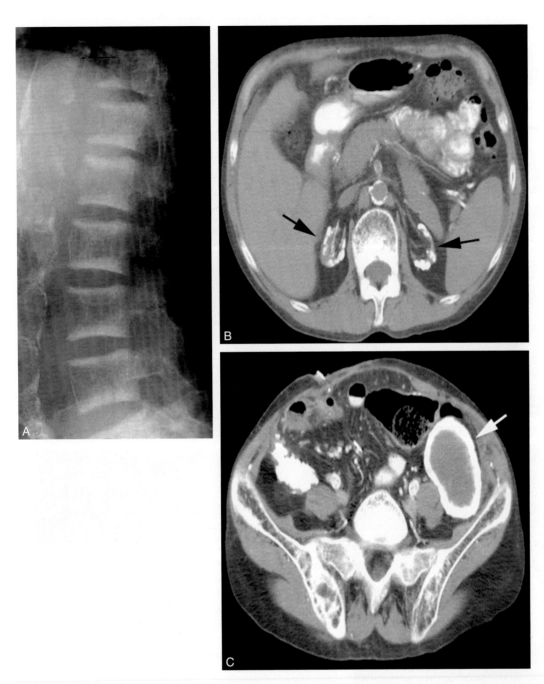

Figure 7.44   Renal osteodystrophy.   A. Lateral view of the lumbar spine demonstrates the "rugger jersey" spine with alternating horizontal bands of osteoporosis centrally with osteosclerosis along the vertebral end plates. **B.** Axial CT demonstrates calcified atrophic native kidneys (*arrows*). **C.** Axial CT of the pelvis demonstrates cortical calcification of a left lower quadrant renal allograft (*arrow*) that has failed. Note the sclerotic bone in the pelvis.

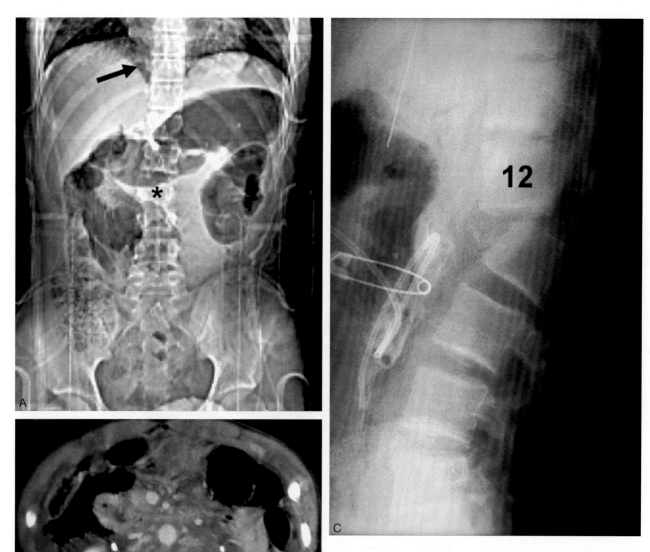

Figure 7.45   Value of CT scout views.   16-year-old with abdominal pain following motor vehicle crash. History of wearing a lap-type seat belt. **A.** Scout view of an abdominal CT shows pneumoperitoneum (*arrow*). Note the distraction of the posterior elements at T12-L1 (*asterisk*). **B.** CT image shows absent posterior elements (*asterisk*) with "naked" facets at T12 as a result of the distraction dislocation. The spine abnormality was not recognized on either the scout view or the axial images. The patient underwent laparotomy where a duodenal tear was repaired. After surgery he became paraplegic. **C.** Lateral radiograph made after the patient became paraplegic shows the dislocation of T12 on L1.

Summary and Key Points

▶ Abdominal radiographs are sensitive for detecting certain acute and chronic abnormalities.

▶ It is imperative to know how the film was taken: upright, supine, or decubitus as free air and obstructions will present differently on abdominal radiographs.

▶ It is important to have a systematic approach to abdominal radiographs. Do not fail to account for all lines and tubes. Gas, mass, stones, and bones is a useful mnemonic to help your search pattern.

▶ In general if patient is sick enough CT should be obtained instead.

▶ Never forget to look at the scout view on all CT studies.

▶ The follow-up of suspected lesions in the gastrointestinal and urinary tracts are discussed in Chapters 8 and 9, respectively.

Suggested Additional Reading

Brant WE, Helms CA. Fundamentals of Diagnostic Radiology. 4th Ed. Philadelphia, PA: Lippincott Williams & Wilkins, 2012:Chapter 25.

Buonomo C, Taylor GA, Share JC, et al. Gastrointestinal tract. In: Kirks DR, Griscom NT, eds. Practical Pediatric Imaging: Diagnostic Radiology of Infants and Children. 3rd Ed. Philadelphia, PA: Lippincott-Raven, 1998:821–1007.

Federle M, Jeffrey R, Anne V. Diagnostic Imaging: Abdomen. Philadelphia, PA: WB Saunders, 2005.

Frimann-Dahl J. Roentgen Examinations in Acute Abdominal Diseases. 3rd Ed. Springfield, IL: Charles C. Thomas, 1974.

Maglinte DDT. Nonspecific abdominal gas pattern: an interpretation whose time is gone. Appl Radiol 1997;26:5–8.

Margulis AR, Burhenne HJ, eds. Alimentary Tract Radiology. 5th Ed. St. Louis, MO: Mosby-Year Book, 1997.

Meyers MA, Charnsangavej C, Oliphant M. Dynamic Radiology of the Abdomen: Normal and Pathologic Anatomy. 6th Ed. New York: Springer, 2011.

Silva AC, Pimenta M, Guimarães LS. Small bowel obstruction: what to look for. Radiographics 2009;29:423–439.

chapter 8

Gastrointestinal Imaging

Rishi K. Maheshwary   Matthew S. Hartman   Richard H. Daffner

Gastroenterology, like radiology, has undergone significant technical and therapeutic changes in the past 30 years. As often happens, technical advances in one specialty radically change another. Five such developments have changed the way physicians evaluate the gastrointestinal (GI) system and how radiology has adapted to improving technology and played a pivotal role in the diagnosis of GI disorders.

The first of these developments was the perfection of and improvements in *flexible fiberoptic endoscopy* for evaluation of the stomach, duodenum, and colon. The use of double-contrast fluoroscopy has dramatically decreased as the use of endoscopy has increased despite barium studies and endoscopy having similar sensitivities in detecting diseases of the GI tract. Further advances of video endoscopy and double-balloon endoscopy to evaluate small bowel pathology have also decreased the use of fluoroscopy, especially the small bowel follow-through. Endoscopy has become the standard diagnostic modality for several reasons. First, clinicians now refer their patients directly to gastroenterologists for colon cancer screening and for diagnosis of other GI abnormalities. Second, improvements in endoscopy training and equipment have made the procedure safer. Third, if an abnormality, such as a colon polyp, is found on a barium study, the patient will be referred for endoscopic biopsy and/or excision and likewise for upper GI cases with the diagnosis of peptic ulcer or polyp.

Endoscopy is not without risks. Most of these studies are performed using conscious sedation. In addition, there is always the risk of perforation of the bowel during the procedure.

The issue of cost efficiency must also be addressed. Cost effectiveness is determined by the total cost of obtaining a diagnosis in the shortest period of time. A normal double-contrast barium enema is relatively less expensive than a colonoscopy. However, an abnormal barium study always results in a colonoscopic examination, which increases the cost of finding the polyp or carcinoma. It should be noted that in many parts of the world where endoscopy is not or cannot be performed, barium examinations remain the main investigative modality for suspected diseases of the GI tract. Thus, despite the decrease in number of fluoroscopic examinations for the diagnosis of disease, it is still important for a radiologist to understand and identify fluoroscopic findings of common GI disorders as well as the postoperative appearance of patients, which has led to a growing role for fluoroscopy.

The second advance in gastroenterology was the emergence of *computed tomography* (CT). This allowed noninvasive detection of traumatic solid visceral rupture (Fig. 8.1) and evaluation of inflammatory and neoplastic processes throughout the abdomen and pelvis (Fig. 8.2). The speed of modern multidetector CT scanners now allows a complete examination of the abdomen to be performed in a few seconds. The speed and ease of access of CT has also led to a dramatic increase in the number of CT scans performed, particularly in the emergency room setting. Image-guided biopsies and drainages are often performed using CT (Fig. 8.3) with less risk and morbidity than an open surgical procedure.

The third development was related to improvement in *diagnostic ultrasound* (US) technology that allowed better detection of different diseases and remains the diagnostic test

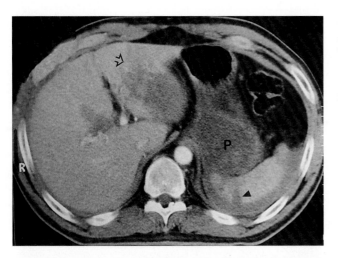

Figure 8.1 Hepatic (*open arrow*) and splenic (*arrowhead*) fractures in a trauma patient. In addition, there is a large hematoma in the tail of the pancreas (*P*). Note the fluid (blood) surrounding the spleen.

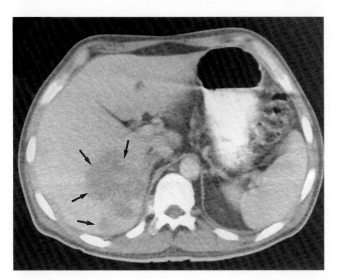

Figure 8.2 Liver metastases. Patient with rectal carcinoma. There are multiple lucent areas within the right lobe of the liver (*arrows*).

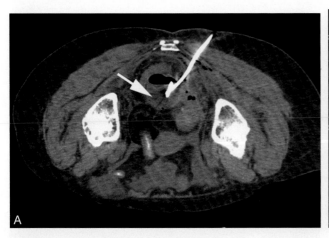

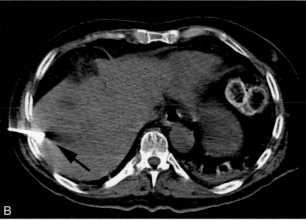

Figure 8.3 CT-guided abscess drainage and biopsy. **A.** A catheter has been placed into an abscess (*arrow*) secondary to sigmoid diverticulitis with the patient in the prone position. **B.** A biopsy needle has been placed into a right hepatic lobe lesion (*arrow*) that was proven metastatic colon cancer.

of choice for finding gallstones and other biliary pathology. US also provides the benefit of not using ionizing radiation, a factor that has become more important as the use of CT has markedly increased. US is also the primary choice for pediatric patients (Fig. 8.4). US also permits real-time imaging of organs and its ease of use has allowed emergency medicine and trauma physicians to use it at bedside. New techniques have developed with

Figure 8.4   Ultrasound appearance of appendicitis.   Blind ending tubular structure representing the appendix (*A*) in the right lower quadrant in a patient with pain. The appendix is mildly dilated (distance between the +'s), has a thick- ened wall (*x*), and does not compress, find- ings consistent with acute appendicitis.

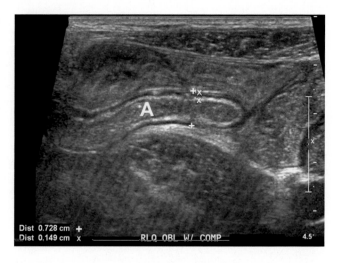

improving technology to help identify bowel pathology that was previously not detect- able. US also allows for safe and accurate ways to perform percutaneous biopsy and drain- age procedures (Fig. 8.5).

The fourth technical advance is *magnetic resonance (MR) imaging* that is now used to investigate many GI disorders, including those of the hepatobiliary system. Many organ- specific MR techniques have been developed to help identify lesions detected by other modalities because MR offers better tissue characterization. MR also has the benefit of no radiation risk which is especially important in younger patients. MR enterography is an accurate way for surveillance of patients with Crohn disease which is most often seen in young patients (Fig. 8.6). *Magnetic resonance cholangiopancreatography (MRCP)* is now being performed for suspected biliary obstruction (Fig. 8.7). Its accuracy approaches that of *endoscopic retrograde cholangiopancreatography (ERCP)*, a procedure performed by gas- troenterologists. However, MRCP is entirely noninvasive and, therefore, is without the complication rate of ERCP.

The final technical advance is *"virtual colonoscopy"*, a type of CT examination in which a sophisticated computer program produces three-dimensional images of the interior of the colon (Fig. 8.8). Accuracy rates have been similar to colonoscopy and in some studies

Figure 8.5   Ultrasound-guided biopsy.   Needle (*arrow*) being placed into one of two hypoechoic lesions (*asterisks*) in a patient with metastatic breast cancer.

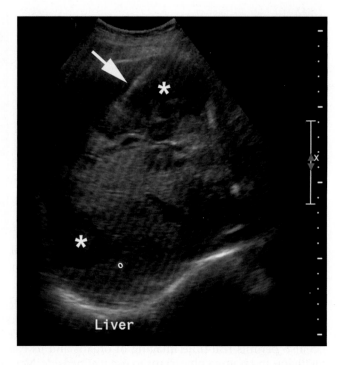

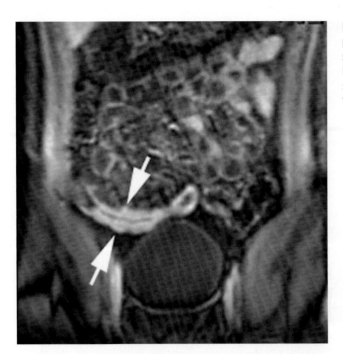

Figure 8.6 MR enterography of a patient with Crohn disease demonstrating thickening (*arrows*), mucosal hyperenhancement (brightness), and string-like luminal narrowing through the terminal ileum.

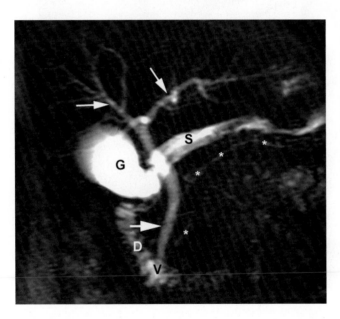

Figure 8.7 Normal MRCP. Maximum intensity projection (MIP) image showing the biliary system. Normal caliber intrahepatic ducts (*small arrows*) forming the common bile duct (*large arrow*). The pancreatic duct (*asterisks*) is thin and normal in caliber and inserts along with the common bile duct at the ampulla of Vater (*V*). Gallbladder (*G*), duodenum (*D*), and stomach (*S*) are also seen as there is fluid within all of these structures as well.

show promise. Also, there are decreased complication risks since there is no need for sedation and patients tolerate the exam with less discomfort. Virtual colonoscopy still has not become widespread but a few institutions are using it as initial screening for colon cancer, while others use it as an adjunct in the setting of an incomplete colonoscopy in place of a traditional barium enema.

The advances in imaging have led to many specialized protocols for the evaluation of certain disorders. As discussed, CT/MR enterography has been developed and in many circumstances replaced previous radiologic procedures performed traditionally by fluoroscopy.

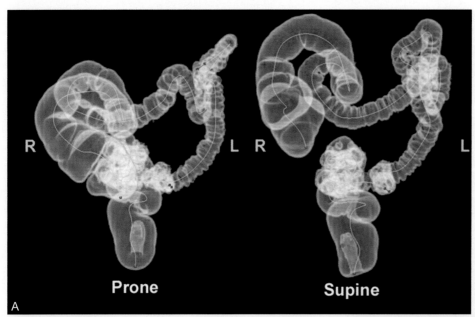

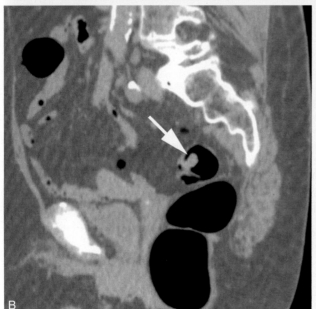

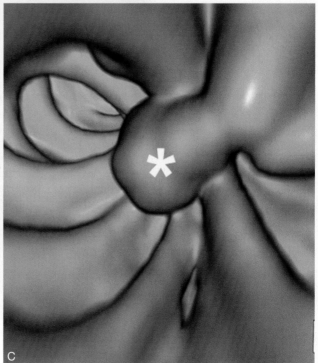

Figure 8.8   **CT colonoscopy is performed in both supine and prone position with computer algorithm allowing for reconstructed images. A.** Shows the track detected by the software in both the prone and supine positions. **B.** Shows a pedunculated polyp (*arrow*) in the source image. **C.** The endoluminal view after reconstructing data collected during CT colonography to simulate an endoscopic view of the colon showing the polyp (*asterisk*).

Impact of New Imaging Technology

The real impact of newer imaging forms can best be appreciated in light of how many intra-abdominal lesions were evaluated as little as 30 years ago. Although intrinsic lesions of the GI tract have always been evaluated by contrast examinations and subsequently by endoscopy, suspected intraabdominal masses were evaluated by studies that showed the effect of the mass on surrounding organs by detecting their displacement when filled with barium or some other contrast. Furthermore, once a mass was detected, angiography was often employed to determine if there were any parameters that suggested malignancy. Diagnostic US, CT, and MR imaging now afford us the opportunity to directly identify the masses themselves. The appearances on the different modalities along with the contrast enhancement pattern allow many lesions to be characterized as benign or malignant, thus saving unnecessary procedures or surgery.

Chapter 7 showed that abdominal radiographs are valuable as preliminary diagnostic studies. However, it is necessary to opacify the GI tract with contrast material to determine the presence of intrinsic abnormalities and/or perform cross-sectional imaging (US/CT/MR) to better evaluate and diagnose abdominal disorders. Choosing the correct study often is the most crucial decision in making the correct diagnosis. Understanding basic principles and the advantages of each modality will help in obtaining the correct test.

Technical Considerations

Common GI radiographic procedures include the following:

- Fluoroscopy
- US
- CT
- MRI
- Angiography
- Percutaneous cholangiography
- ERCP
- GI bleeding localization
- Technetium 99m pertechnetate scan

Fluoroscopic Examination

Although there has been a decline in the number of studies performed, fluoroscopy is still utilized today in the primary diagnosis of multiple GI disorders as well as in the evaluation of postoperative patients. Fluoroscopic evaluation allows direct visualization of motility and dysmotility through the GI tract: a big advantage over endoscopy.

In general, fluoroscopic examination is best for evaluation of the esophagus, stomach, and duodenum with CT as an adjunct for staging purposes. Similarly the small bowel and colon traditionally were evaluated by fluoroscopic exams (small bowel follow-through and barium enema). However, this is becoming less frequent with the increased use of colonoscopy and CT colonography and for small bowel pathology with the use of video capsule and other modalities such as CT/MR enterography. Fluoroscopic evaluation has always been and continues to have a key role in the postoperative setting, for evaluation of motility, and for evaluation of leaks.

Under normal circumstances, two modes of radiographic recording are used: fluoroscopy and radiography. Fluoroscopic examination is important to determine the swallowing mechanism and the motility of the GI tract (peristalsis), which is a distinct advantage over endoscopy.

A source of confusion for many clinicians and students is the difference between a modified swallow and an esophagram. A modified swallow is done in conjunction with a speech pathologist who will administer various liquid and solid substances to a patient with dysphagia who is at risk for aspiration (often a patient who has had a stroke). The radiologist will record the examination and evaluate the images with the speech pathologist to determine the type of oral diet, if any, that can be safely tolerated by the patient (Fig. 8.9). A regular esophagram is performed for patients with dysphagia who are not at risk for aspiration and may have a pathologic process intrinsic to the esophagus (Fig. 8.10).

You may hear the terms single- (oral/rectal contrast only) and double-contrast studies (oral/rectal contrast and air) with respect to GI fluoroscopy. The preferred method for routine study is to use a thick preparation of barium to coat the mucosa and to distend the GI tract with gas (double/air contrast study). When studying the upper GI tract, a gas-releasing preparation of effervescent crystals is ingested with the oral barium. When evaluating the lower GI tract, air is introduced through the rectal tube and distends the colon. The resulting study portrays the mucosa in detail and is usually sufficient to reveal subtle abnormalities. If the patient is unable to tolerate a double-contrast examination because of comorbidities, a single-contrast examination can be performed without the introduction of air.

Bowel Preparation and Contraindications

The optimal way to study any hollow viscus filled with contrast material is to have that organ completely empty of any other content. For a study of the upper GI tract and small

Figure 8.9   Modified barium swallow showing aspiration (*arrow*) of barium entering the trachea (*T*) seen anterior and the posterior to the esophagus (*E*).

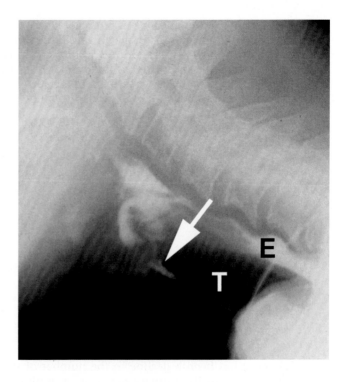

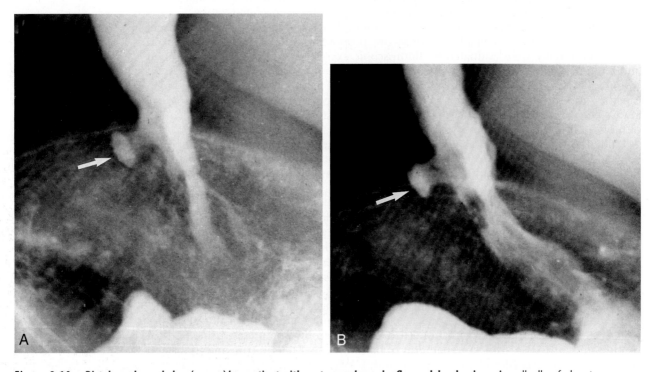

Figure 8.10   **Distal esophageal ulcer (*arrows*) in a patient with gastroesophageal reflux and dysphagia.**   A small collar of edematous mucosa leads up to the ulcer crater.

bowel follow-through, an overnight fast is usually sufficient. For a barium enema, there are many preparations using combinations of laxatives, enemas, and flushing by ingestion of massive quantities of fluids. These should be used with special precautions for dialysis patients who are prone to dehydration. It is not necessary to vigorously cleanse the colon in children because usually the clinician is not looking for the small mucosal lesions that are found in adults. Each institution has different protocols for bowel preparation. The quality of the preparation will be determined by a scout radiograph prior to the procedure. An incomplete preparation may result in a postponement of the procedure.

Contraindications

There are few contraindications from using barium as discussed in Chapter 2. Patients who have had recent surgeries/biopsies or at are at high risk for perforation should be initially studied with water-soluble contrast and not barium which could result in a desmoplastic reaction if it spills into the peritoneum. Patients who are suspected of having toxic megacolon, acute ulcerative colitis, or obstruction should not have cleansing enemas and should be studied directly by colonoscopy.

 ▶ Patients who are suspected of having toxic megacolon, acute ulcerative colitis, or obstruction should not have cleansing enemas and should be studied directly by colonoscopy.

Fasting

Overnight fasting or fasting for at least 4 hours is essential for evaluation of the hepatobiliary system under US. Fasting limits the amount of excess gas as well as optimizes distension of the gallbladder. Technical limitations include body habitus and excessive bowel gas that cause sound attenuation that limits the field of view since the US beams are unable to penetrate to see deeper structures.

Information Exchange

It is important for the clinician to give as much *clinical information* as possible to the referring radiologist. The request should always contain pertinent information and a tentative diagnosis. The radiologist should also question the patient and ask about symptoms necessitating the examination. It is not unusual, however, for a patient to go for an examination without understanding the reason for the study or with few or no complaints referable to the area of the body under examination. Pediatricians should inform the parents that they will probably be allowed to be in the room while their child is examined. In some instances, they may even assist in holding the child and giving reassurance.

The patient should also be informed that the clinician, after receiving the results of the examination from the radiologist, will notify him/her of the findings. This removes the onus from the radiologists of having to report serious findings such as colon cancer to patients they may not know well. Radiologists should make it a practice to inform a patient when a study is normal, however, because most patients are apprehensive about the condition for which they are studied. Quite often, the patient will not see the referring physician for several hours or perhaps days or weeks following the examination. To make a patient worry about a diagnosis of cancer or some other serious illness when the study is normal is simply not in anybody's best interests.

Ultrasound

Ultrasound should be the first imaging choice for patients with suspected biliary disease. It is often used initially for patients with abnormal liver function tests to exclude biliary dilation and diffuse hepatocellular disease. It also is a good initial study to evaluate the visceral organs and has the added benefits of nonionizing radiation. CT and/or MR imaging are often used as supplements to help delineate or access abnormalities detected by US. MRCP is often used to help delineate biliary tree that may not be answered by US alone.

Computed Tomography

CT is often used initially in the workup of abdominal pain in the emergency setting especially with history of trauma. CT is the preferred modality for patients with clinical suspicion of appendicitis except in pediatric and pregnant population where US and MR play an important role. Evaluation of bowel obstruction is now performed by CT with better detection of the cause and location of transition point as well as complications including ischemia and perforation. CT in many ways replaced the small bowel follow-through. CT angiography was developed to help detect small bowel tumors, source for suspected GI bleeds, and evaluation of mesenteric ischemia. CT enterography is used for evaluation of patients with suspected inflammatory bowel disease. CT is also used for staging malignancies of the GI tract because it can demonstrate local invasion as well as abnormal lymph node metastases. Positron emission tomography (PET) CT (Fig. 8.11) improves sensitivity and specificity.

 ▶ Evaluation of bowel obstruction is now best performed by CT because of better detection of the cause and location of transition point as well as complications such as ischemia and perforation.

MRI has the advantage of increased contrast resolution and lack of ionizing radiation. As mentioned earlier, MR excels with respect to evaluation of the biliary tree, cystic pancreatic lesions, and in pregnant or pediatric patients where radiation is a concern. Most institutions have a preferred protocol to evaluate patients with suspected liver or pancreatic lesion and discussion with a radiologist can be helpful.

Limitations

With respect to CT, intravenous (IV) contrast is used in most cases of trauma and inflammation to better opacify the blood vessels and organs. Remember from Chapter 2 that patients with suspected renal calculi or retroperitoneal hematomas do not need to receive IV contrast. This is a good time to review the precautions with IV contrast with regard to renal insufficiency and allergies as discussed in Chapter 2 for CT and MRI. Contraindications for MRI include pacemaker devices and certain metallic devices (older vascular coils and stents).

The final limitation for CT and MRI is large body habitus because the scanners have weight limits as well as limitations of body width due to the bore of an MRI scanner. Additionally MRI is sensitive to respiratory motion which can cause significant artifact limiting the quality of the study. Alternatively, CT does not have that limitation given the speed of new scanners today.

Angiography

Angiography is used to evaluate the GI tract primarily for diagnosis and therapy in patients with acute GI hemorrhage. The bleeding site may be localized by selective catheterization of celiac or mesenteric branches and a vasopressor infused to control or stop the bleeding (Fig. 8.12). Angiography is also used to evaluate patients with portal hypertension before a contemplated transjugular intrahepatic portosystemic shunt (TIPS) procedure (*see* Chapter 3) or shunt surgery, and in mapping hepatic metastases if partial hepatectomy or infusion chemotherapy is being considered.

Percutaneous Cholangiography

Percutaneous cholangiography with the thin-walled (Chiba) needle is used by radiologists to study patients with obstructive jaundice. Contrast material injected through the needle, which has been placed in a dilated biliary duct, is used to localize the site of the obstruction (Fig. 8.13). Following this, a catheter may be inserted for percutaneous decompression and drainage, or a stent may be introduced, as mentioned in Chapter 3.

Endoscopic Retrograde Cholangiopancreatography (ERCP)

ERCP is a procedure in which the ampulla of Vater is cannulated under direct endoscopic control. The examination takes a skilled endoscopist, most often a gastroenterologist. After cannulation, contrast material is injected into the ductal system, and fluoroscopic spot and overhead radiographs are made. A stent or drainage catheter may be left in place as part of this procedure. The endoscopist also can perform a papillotomy. ERCP is being supplanted in some institutions by MRCP (*see* Fig. 8.7) because the latter procedure is noninvasive.

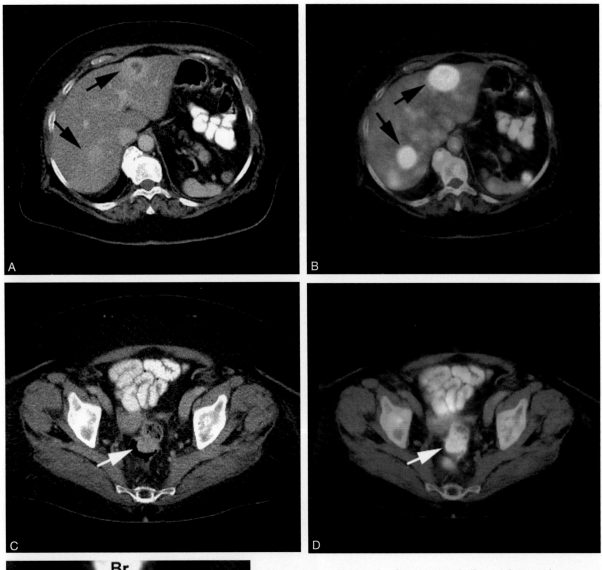

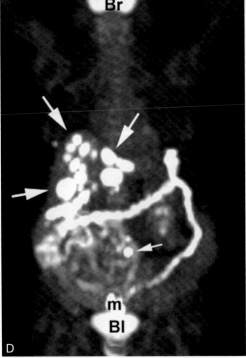

Figure 8.11 **Metastatic colon cancer.** **A.** CT image shows two hepatic metastases (*arrows*) with peripheral enhancement. **B.** Corresponding PET CT fused image shows FDG uptake in the same areas (*arrows*). CT image **(C)** and corresponding PET CT fused image **(D)** show the colonic neoplasm in the rectosigmoid junction (*arrows*). **E.** MIP image from PET portion showing multiple hepatic metastases (*large arrows*), left-sided periaortic lymph node (*small arrow*) as well as rectosigmoid mass (*M*) just above the bladder (*Bl*). Note the physiologic activity within the brain (*Br*), collecting system, and bladder with some excretion into the bowel, particularly the colon.

Figure 8.12   Mesenteric arteriogram in a patient with lower gastrointestinal bleeding.   Delayed image shows a "stain" of contrast (*arrow*) at the site of a bleeding diverticulum in the descending colon.

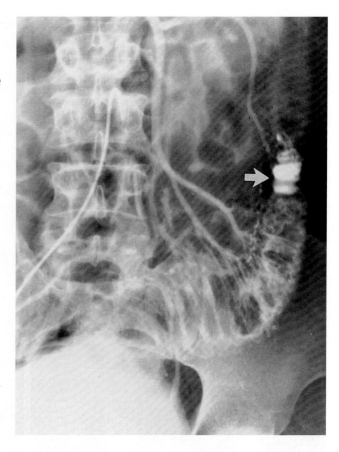

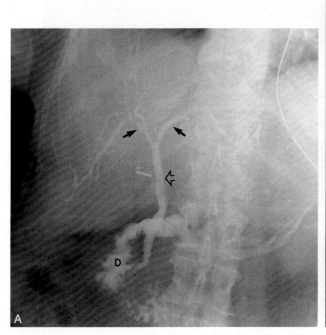

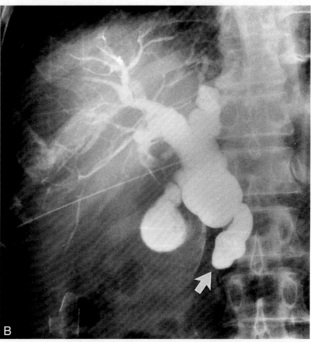

Figure 8.13   Cholangiograms.   A. Intraoperative examination demonstrates normal-sized hepatic (*small arrows*) and common bile (*open arrow*) ducts. Contrast flows freely into the duodenum (*D*) and refluxes into the stomach. **B.** Percutaneous transhepatic cholangiogram shows massive dilation of the common bile duct and hepatic ducts in this patient with obstruction near the distal common bile duct (*arrow*). This was subsequently percutaneously decompressed with a catheter.

Hepatobiliary Nuclear Imaging

Two commonly used nuclear imaging studies to investigate abnormalities of the GI tract are hepatobiliary imaging and GI bleeding localization. The biliary scan uses technetium 99m–labeled mebrofenin and iminodiacetic acid derivatives to investigate uptake and excretion physiology of the liver as well as kinesis of radio-labeled bile in the extrahepatic biliary tree. The radiotracer is administered intravenously and then removed from the blood by the liver and concentrated in the bile. Under normal circumstances, the agent can be detected in the gallbladder within 10 to 15 minutes of administration (Fig. 8.14). It is excreted through the common bile duct into the duodenum within 30 to 45 minutes. An obstruction of the cystic duct will prevent the passive filling of the gallbladder (Fig. 8.15), thus allowing a diagnosis of acute cholecystitis. In the setting of acute

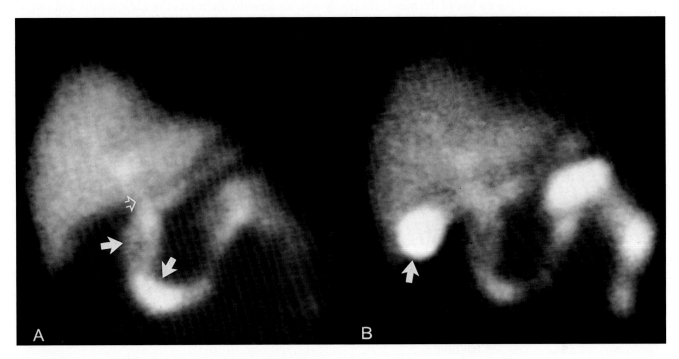

Figure 8.14   Normal technetium 99m–labeled mebrofenin scan.   A. Thirty minutes after injection, the isotope is being excreted by the liver through the common bile duct (*open arrow*) into the duodenum (*closed arrows*). **B.** At 60 minutes, the isotope fills the gallbladder (*arrow*).

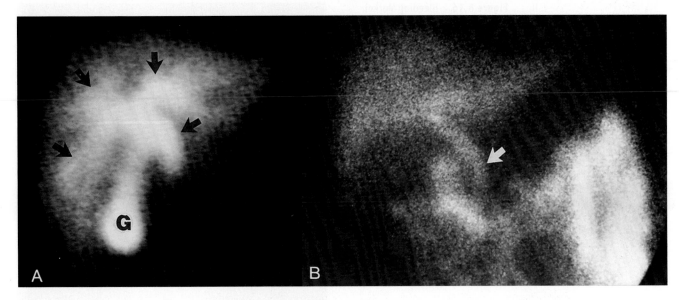

Figure 8.15   Abnormal technetium 99m–labeled hepatobiliary scans.   A. Patient with a common duct stone. Ninety minutes after injection, the isotope is in the liver and gallbladder (*G*). There is no excretion into the duodenum, and the biliary tree is dilated (*arrows*). **B.** Patient with acute cholecystitis from cystic duct stone. No gallbladder filling occurs at 60 minutes. The isotope passes freely into the duodenum through the common bile duct (*arrow*).

cholecystitis, a hepatobiliary imaging study has a 95% positive and negative predictive value. The predictive value of this study is improved by concordant US imaging of the right upper quadrant for anatomic correlation. Hepatobiliary imaging is also useful in the setting of biliary surgery or trauma to diagnose intraperitoneal biliary leaks. Finally, hepatobiliary imaging with additional chemical challenges using cholecystokinin can help in the diagnosis of biliary dyskinesia or acalculous cholecystitis.

Gastrointestinal Bleeding Localization

Technetium 99m–tagged autologous red blood cells are used to investigate active GI bleeding. In patients who have lower GI bleeding in an acute setting along with some hemodynamic instability, a nuclear medicine bleeding scan is very helpful in localization of the site of the bleed. This study is more sensitive than invasive angiography and can, in fact, help plan the therapeutic angiography if necessary. A GI bleeding scan will detect as little as 0.1 mL/min of active extravasation into the GI lumen compared with the 1 mL/min flow usually cited for angiographic evaluation.

Technetium 99m Pertechnetate Scan

A technetium 99m pertechnetate scan, also known as a Meckel scan, is used primarily in the pediatric setting for diagnosis of a Meckel diverticulum, a common congenital malformation of the ileocecal region (Fig. 8.16). Although most of these diverticula are asymptomatic, some contain gastric mucosa, which may occasionally result in lower GI bleeding. In pediatric patients who present with intermittent lower intestinal bleeding manifesting as "currant jelly" stools, a bleeding scan is very helpful. The "free" technetium 99m pertechnetate is excreted in the gastric mucosa. Using this physiology, localization of an abnormal gastric mucosal site in the right lower quadrant is easily achieved.

Anatomic and Physiologic Considerations

Structures

- Esophagus
- Stomach
- Duodenum
- Jejunum
- Colon

Figure 8.16   Bleeding Meckel diverticulum.   Increased isotope concentration in the ileocecal region (*arrow*) is caused by bleeding. *B*, bladder.

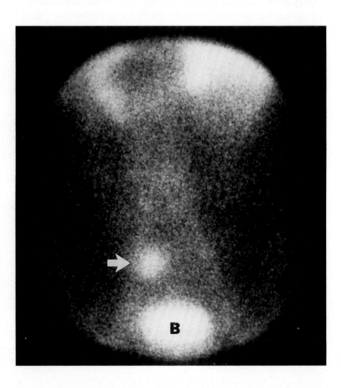

Esophagus

It is important to recognize the normal anatomy of the GI tract and the variations that may occur. For example, six indentations may be seen on the esophagus as it courses from the pharynx into the abdomen. The uppermost is the indentation of the cricopharyngeus muscle posteriorly at the level of C6. Other indentations occur at the thoracic inlet, at the aortic arch at the level of T4 to T5, at the left mainstem bronchus, proximal to the diaphragmatic hiatus by the descending aorta, and at the esophagogastric junction (Fig. 8.17).

Stomach

The stomach may assume various positions, lying either vertically or horizontally within the abdomen. This depends mainly on the patient's body habitus. The radiologic anatomy of the normal stomach includes the fundus, body, antrum, prepyloric region, and pylorus (Fig. 8.18). The gastric mucosa (*rugae*) appears as linear parallel folds extending along the length of the stomach (Fig. 8.19). There is wide variation in the size of the rugae.

Duodenum

The duodenum begins at the pylorus. The first portion is the *bulb*, which appears as a triangular-shaped structure with the base toward the pylorus. The duodenum then sweeps

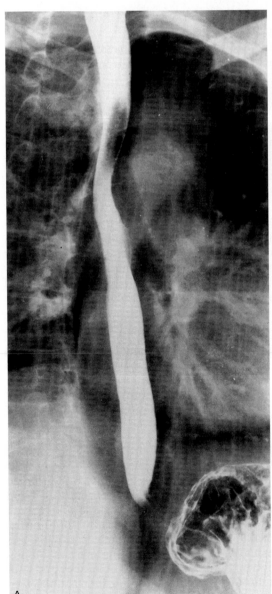

A

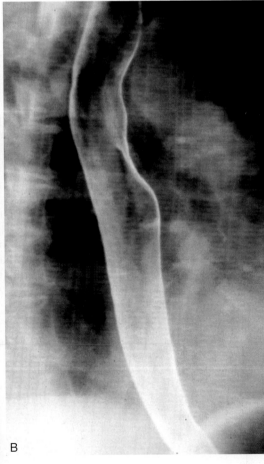

B

Figure 8.17 Esophagram. A. Normal single-contrast esophagus. A small amount of air is present in the upper esophagus. Note the indentation at the level of the aortic arch. **B.** Double-contrast evaluation of the esophagus after the administration of effervescent crystals that distends the esophagus with air and barium which coats the mucosa. Note the fine mucosal detail that one can achieve with double-contrast technique.

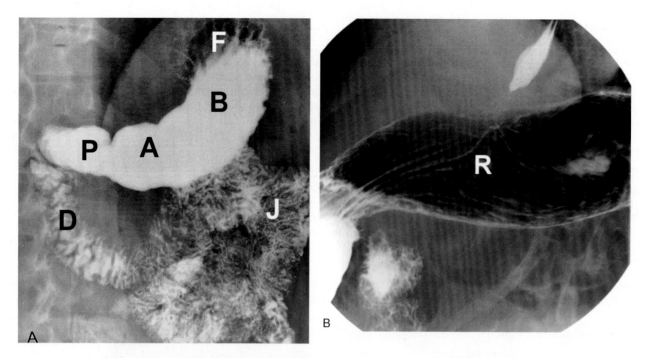

Figure 8.18   Stomach.   **A.** Predominantly single-contrast appearance of the stomach. *F*, fundus; *B*, body; *A*, antrum; *P*, pylorus; *D*, duodenum; *J*, jejunum. Note how the duodenum passes to the left of the ligament of Treitz and the jejunal loops are located in the left upper quadrant. **B.** Normal double-contrast appearance of the stomach. Note the rugae (*R*).

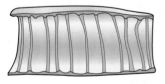

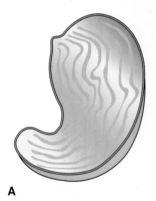

Figure 8.19   Normal mucosal patterns.   A. Stomach showing rugae. **B.** Small intestine showing valvulae conniventes. **C.** Colon showing haustra.

downward (the second or descending portion), curves medially (third portion), and twists back upward (fourth portion), terminating at the *ligament of Treitz*. Occasionally, on a normal duodenal examination, a small indentation representing the ampulla of Vater may be observed along the medial border of the descending portion.

Jejunum and Ileum

The jejunum begins at the ligament of Treitz, gradually merging with the ileum, which enters the cecum via the ileocecal valve. It is usually possible to differentiate the jejunum from the ileum by the mucosal pattern. In normal people, the cecum is in the right lower quadrant of the abdomen. The wormlike (*vermiform*) appendix typically projects downward from the cecum. In some people, however, it may be oriented cranially (*retrocecal appendix*). Usually, the ileocecal valve is on the medial aspect of the cecum.

Colon

The colon ascends, forming two loop-like structures in the right and left upper quadrants known as the *hepatic and splenic flexures*, respectively. The descending colon terminates in the sigmoid colon that is often quite redundant, particularly in older patients. The sigmoid colon continues on to the rectum (Fig. 8.20). Under normal circumstances, the rectum can be distended with barium greater than half the distance between the walls of the pelvis.

Physiology

In addition to assessing the anatomy of the GI tract, the clinician must also be concerned with its physiology—that is, its motility. The causes of motility disorders are varied and complex. Suffice it to say that in the normal esophagus, a stripping wave should be seen propagating a bolus of barium in a smooth, progressive motion. Peristalsis continues in the stomach from the fundus extending down to the pylorus. In the duodenum, peristalsis is slightly different: the stripping motion found in the esophagus and stomach is not present. Instead, there is distension of the duodenal bulb, which opens at its apex and contracts forcibly as a unit moving the bolus through. Propulsive contractions are observed throughout the small intestine and colon.

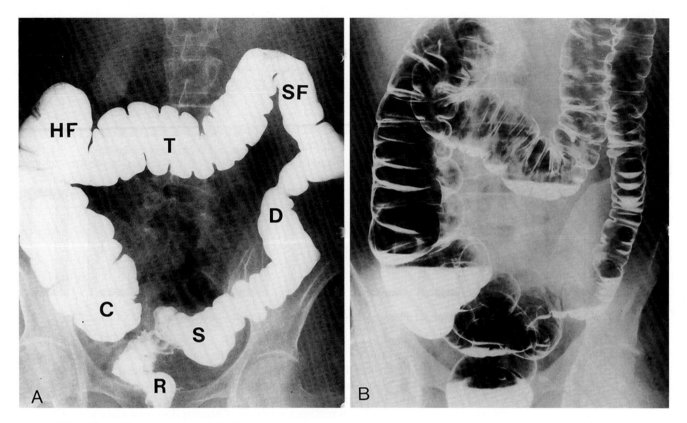

Figure 8.20 Normal barium enema. A. Single contrast. *C*, cecum; *HF*, hepatic flexure; *T*, transverse colon; *SF*, splenic flexure; *D*, descending colon; *S*, sigmoid colon; *R*, rectum; **B.** Double contrast. Note the finer mucosal detail.

Pathologic Considerations

Six Patterns of Pathology

The GI tract can be thought of as a hollow tube from mouth to anus. There are six pathologic alterations that can affect the tube: narrowing, dilation, filling defect (*innie*), outpouching (*outie*), displacement (external compression), and wall thickening (Fig. 8.21). These patterns of pathology are not necessarily mutually exclusive and assigning an abnormality to one of these categories combined with the location will provide a short differential. Pathologic alterations found in one segment appear identical when encountered in any other segment. For example, a mucosal tumor of the esophagus has an appearance identical to a similar-sized tumor of the stomach, small intestine, or colon. The incidence of these lesions varies from location to location, and you must learn the common locations of these lesions in each segment. However, remember that for practical purposes, these lesions all have a similar appearance, no matter where they occur. (Using the same concept, a broad generalization may be made that similar-appearing lesions are also found in other tubular structures such as the urinary tract, bronchi, and blood vessels.)

▷ There are six pathologic alterations that can affect any tubular structure: narrowing, dilation, filling defect ("innie"—polyp, mass, foreign body), outpouching ("outie"—ulcer, diverticulum), displacement (external compression), and wall thickening.

▷ In a tubular structure such as the GI tract, all lesions due to a particular etiology have a similar appearance, no matter where they are located.

Narrowing and Dilation

Let's practice this pattern approach. The first two patterns, narrowing and dilation often occur together. Narrowing can be benign or malignant and often is preceded by upstream

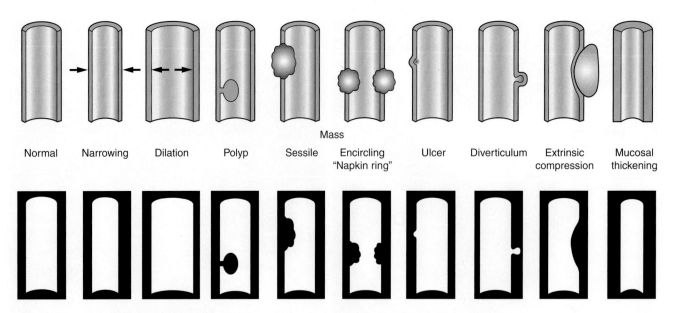

| Normal | Narrowing | Dilation | Polyp | Sessile | Mass
Encircling
"Napkin ring" | Ulcer | Diverticulum | Extrinsic
compression | Mucosal
thickening |

Figure 8.21   The patterns of disease and the radiographic appearances that can affect tubular structures.

(proximal) dilation of the GI tract. A benign stricture appears as a concentric or eccentric narrowing of the lumen. Dilation is most often caused by a distal obstruction as in achalasia (Fig. 8.22). There are both benign and malignant causes of small bowel dilation including adhesions, strictures from prior inflammation or infection such as Crohn disease or diverticulitis, or from malignant lesions. Dilation does not always have a distal obstruction as in toxic megacolon seen in patients with ulcerative colitis or toxoplasmosis.

Filling Defects

Filling defects ("innies") appear as small, rounded, filling defects in the lumen. They may be broad based (*sessile*, Fig. 8.23) or on a stalk (*pedunculated*, Fig. 8.24). They can occur in any portion of the wall. Mucosal and submucosal lesions tend to have acute angles at the wall whereas extrinsic lesions have obtuse angles with smooth contour. Evaluating the margins whether irregular or smooth, unicentric or lobulated, and well defined or ill defined also plays an important role in determining the diagnosis. Size, multiplicity, and ulceration are also key characteristics to identify.

> Mucosal and submucosal lesions tend to have acute angles at the wall whereas extrinsic lesions have obtuse angles with smooth contours.

Mucosal masses frequently begin as small polyps. As a polyp enlarges, its surface may become irregular. Puckering may occur near the base of the lesion. There is an abrupt change of the mucosa from normal to tumor (Fig. 8.25). This frequently produces a "shoulder" of tumor at the mucosal transition point. Further growth results in encasement as the tumor grows completely around the lumen, producing the classic "napkin ring" or "apple core" appearance (Fig. 8.26). Mucosal masses, especially if they are malignant, may ulcerate (Fig. 8.27) which is our next pattern: outpouchings.

Outpouchings

Contrast can be located outside of the expected lumen ("outies") secondary to diverticula, perforations, ulcerations, or fistulae. Diverticula are benign outpouchings of the wall of the GI tract that are covered by *all* layers of the bowel wall. They can occur anywhere in the GI tract (Fig. 8.28). We saw an example of a perforation in Chapter 2—remember to use water-soluble contrast in these patients.

> Diverticula are benign outpouchings of the wall of the GI tract that are covered by *all* layers of bowel wall.

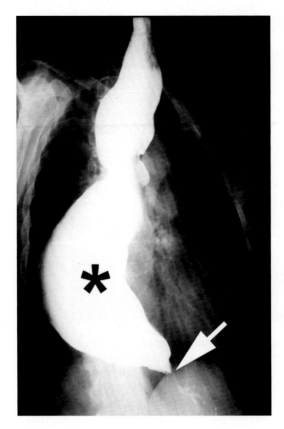

Figure 8.22   Achalasia. A single-contrast esophagram demonstrates bird's beak narrowing at the gastroesophageal junction (*black arrow*) and upstream dilation of the esophagus (*asterisk*). Please refer to Figure 8.17 for a normal example of the esophagus.

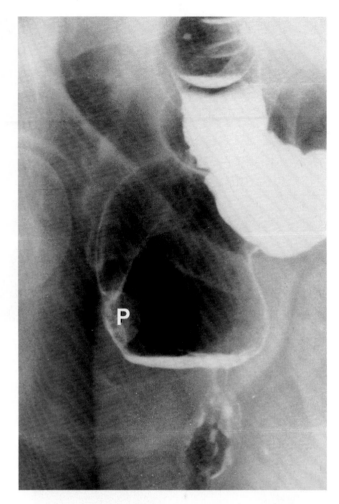

Figure 8.23   Sessile polyp (*P*) of the rectum.

Ulcers of the GI tract are most likely to be diagnosed by endoscopy today. However, from a radiologic standpoint ulceration of the GI tract produces another type of "outie" in which a collection of barium is found outside the normal lumen. Frequently, the ulcer crater is surrounded by an edematous ulcer collar or mound, which is a finding of benign ulcers. In the stomach mucosal folds may be observed radiating into a benign ulcer crater (Fig. 8.29). Ulcerations of the GI tract are seen with less frequency with the advent of proton pump inhibitors and increased awareness of gastroesophageal reflux disease (GERD). Reflux and problems with esophageal motility can be seen real-time under fluoroscopy: a distinct advantage over endoscopy.

You should remember that there are no malignant ulcers; there are ulcerating malignancies. We have seen several examples of mucosal masses that had an ulcerative component (*see* Fig. 8.27). There are certain radiographic features that can suggest malignancy within an ulcer. Ulcerating malignancies will often have an irregular nodular shape and an eccentric location of the ulcer within the mass. The intraluminal crater is often located between abrupt points of transition in contrast to the intraluminal crater in a mound of even edematous surrounding tissue. Patients with multiple or recurrent ulcers should be studied for *Zollinger-Ellison syndrome* to search for gastrin-producing tumors. If there is any doubt that an ulcer is benign or malignant, the patient will be referred for definitive diagnosis with endoscopy.

⦆ There are no malignant ulcers; there are ulcerating malignancies.
⦆ Patients with multiple or recurrent peptic ulcers should be studied for Zollinger-Ellison syndrome to search for gastrin-producing tumors.

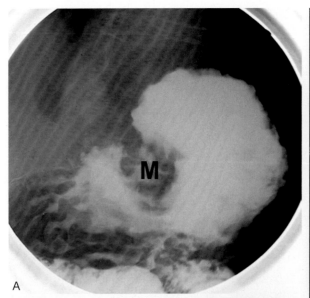

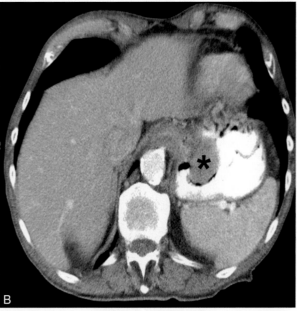

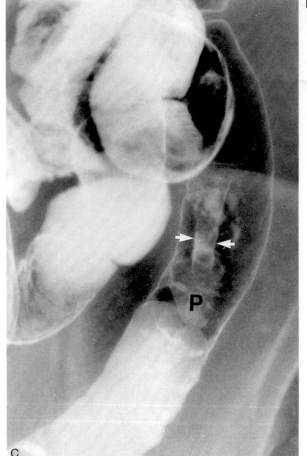

Figure 8.24   Pedunculated melanoma metastasis growing into the lesser curvature of the stomach.   A. Fluoroscopic evaluation shows a mass (*M*) growing into the lesser curvature of the stomach. **B.** The mass (*asterisk*) that resembles a mushroom is easier to appreciate on CT where it is seen protruding into the lumen. **C.** Pedunculated polyp (*P*) of the descending colon. Note the stalk of the polyp (*arrows*).

Displacement

The next pattern is displacement that is usually caused by visceral structures causing compression on the GI tract. Extrinsic compression (Fig. 8.30) appears as a smooth indentation of the bowel wall with gradually tapering margins. Herniations (Fig. 8.31) and congenital abnormalities such as malrotation can also result in bowel displacement.

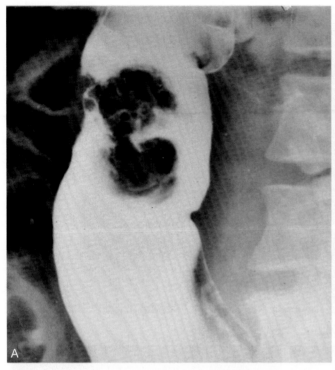

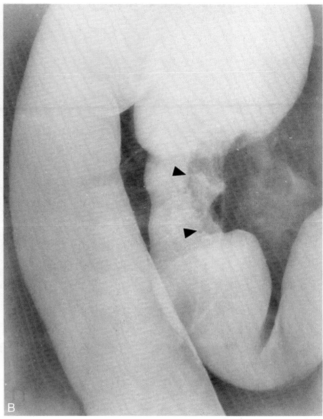

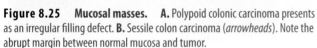

Figure 8.25   Mucosal masses.   A. Polypoid colonic carcinoma presents as an irregular filling defect. **B.** Sessile colon carcinoma (*arrowheads*). Note the abrupt margin between normal mucosa and tumor.

Wall Thickening

The last pattern, wall thickening, which often results in luminal narrowing, can be one of the hardest patterns to recognize on fluoroscopy. It is not until one does a cross-sectional exam that one realizes that bowel wall thickening is the cause (Fig. 8.32). Bowel wall thickening can be focal or diffuse (Fig. 8.33).

This pattern approach can be helpful in your approach to GI radiology. Remember that there is also overlap on how diseases can present, for instance gastric carcinoma can appear as a filling defect with or without ulceration, wall thickening, or narrowing.

Inflammatory Bowel Disease

We can apply the pattern approach to inflammatory bowel disease which is a term that is applied to both ulcerative colitis and Crohn disease (*regional enteritis*) of the bowel. Both diseases produce a spectrum of pathologic changes, including ulceration, obstruction, and formation of pseudopolyps, strictures, and fistulas. In addition, chronic ulcerative colitis is prone to undergo malignant change. Both chronic inflammatory bowel conditions are of unknown origin. However, they share many clinical, epidemiologic, pathologic, radiographic, and even immunologic features. Some authorities feel that each entity represents a different pathologic response to a common cause; others believe both diseases represent different parts of the spectrum of a single disease process. The definitive diagnosis of both diseases is best made by endoscopy with or without biopsy. Nevertheless, classic radiographic findings have been described for each of these diseases and are briefly contrasted here.

Ulcerative Colitis

The typical case of ulcerative colitis has radiographic findings that directly reflect the pathologic manifestations, including exudative inflammation involving primarily the bowel mucosa and submucosa. Classically, the muscularis is spared. Edema of the bowel wall gives the impression of thickened bowel (see Fig. 8.33A). Ulcerations are shallow and coalescent (Fig. 8.34), often isolating islands of normal mucosa that are termed

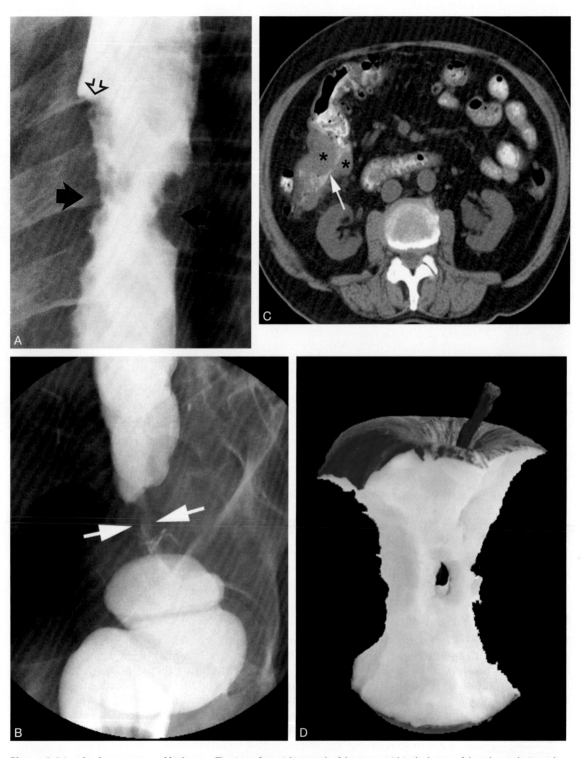

Figure 8.26   Apple-core mucosal lesions.   The circumferential ingrowth of the tumor within the lumen of the tube results in apple-core type narrowing. **A.** Esophageal carcinoma shows the constricting lesion (*solid arrows*) with abrupt mucosal margins, termed a "tumor shoulder" (*open arrow*). **B.** Single-contrast barium enema demonstrating an annular colon carcinoma resulting in an apple-core narrowing of the lumen (*arrows*). **C.** CT shows annular type growth through the hepatic flexure of the colon (*asterisks*) demonstrating apple-core narrowing of the lumen (*arrow*). **D.** Note the resemblance of the lesions in **A–C** to an apple core.

pseudopolyps (Fig. 8.35). In the acute stages, spasm and irritability are evident fluoroscopically. Edema results in smudging and haziness of the mucosal folds. The disease characteristically involves the entire colon. Occasionally, the terminal ileum is involved (*backwash ileitis*); however, this more commonly occurs in Crohn disease.

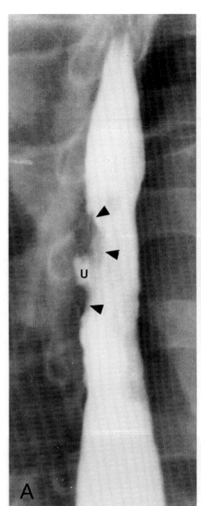

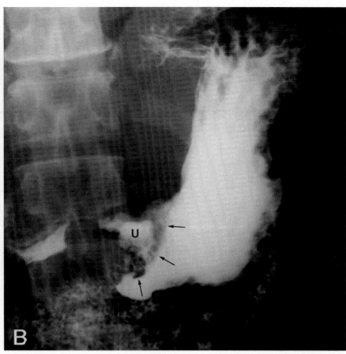

Figure 8.27 Ulcerating malignancies. A. Ulcerating esophageal carcinoma. An ulcer crater (*U*) is present within the mucosal mass (*arrowheads*). **B.** Ulcerating malignancy of the gastric antrum. The ulcer (*U*) is within the mucosal mass (*arrows*).

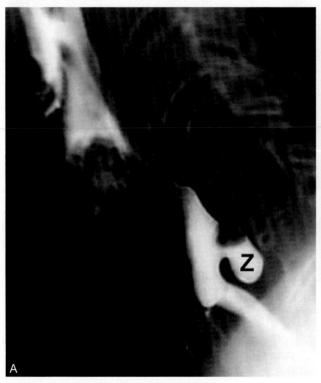

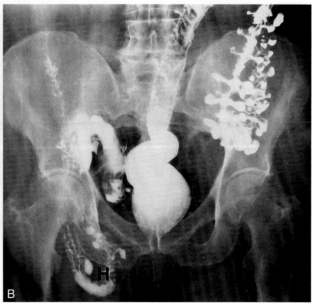

Figure 8.28 Diverticula within the GI tract. A. Zenker diverticulum (*Z*) of the cervical esophagus. **B.** Colonic diverticulosis most prominent in the descending colon with too numerous to count diverticula. Note the inguinal hernia (*H*) on the right, which is an example of displacement.

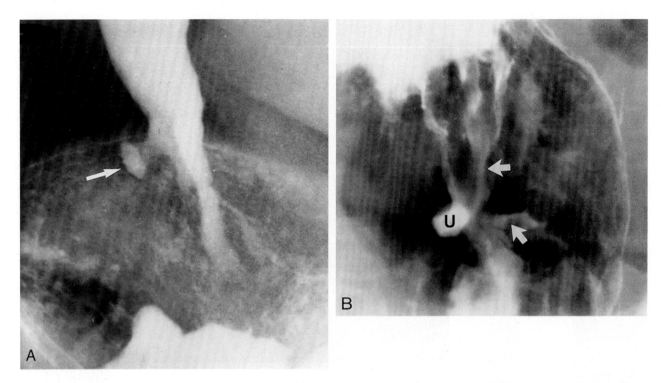

Figure 8.29   Ulcers   A. Distal esophageal ulcer (*arrow*) in a patient with gastroesophageal reflux. Note the small collar of edematous mucosa that leads up to the ulcer crater. **B.** Benign gastric ulcer (*U*). Regular folds radiate into the ulcer crater, a radiographic sign of a benign ulcer.

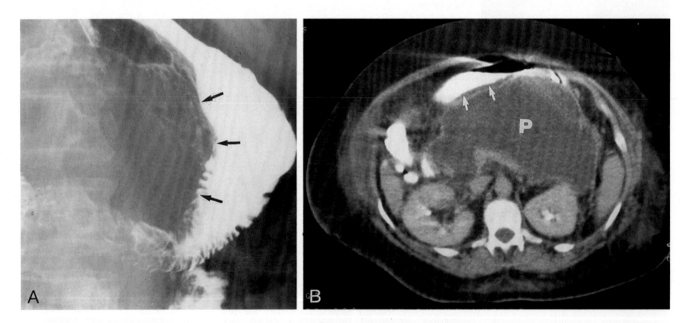

Figure 8.30   Pancreatic pseudocyst causing mass effect and displacing the stomach.   A. A spot image from an upper GI examination shows extrinsic compression of the stomach by a large pancreatic pseudocyst (*arrows*). **B.** CT image shows the pseudocyst (*P*). Note the compression of the contrast-filled stomach (*arrows*).

> ▶ In ulcerative colitis the mucosa and submucosa are involved; the muscularis is spared.
> ▶ Ulcerative colitis typically involves the entire colon.

Long-standing disease results in the chronic or "burned-out" stage, which produces foreshortening of the colon and narrowing of the lumen. The barium enema reveals a very tubular ("pipestem") appearance of the colon with a loss of normal haustral markings

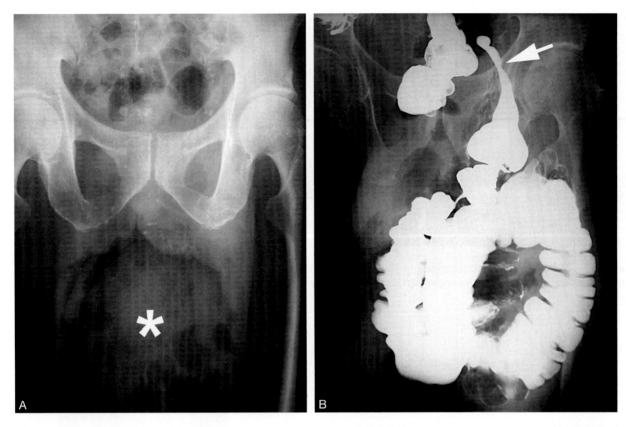

Figure 8.31   Scrotal hernias in two patients.   A. Radiograph shows massive enlargement of the scrotum (*asterisk*), which contains air-filled loops of bowel. **B.** Barium enema in another patient shows colon herniated into the scrotum. The neck of the hernia is shown as narrowing in the inguinal region (*arrow*).

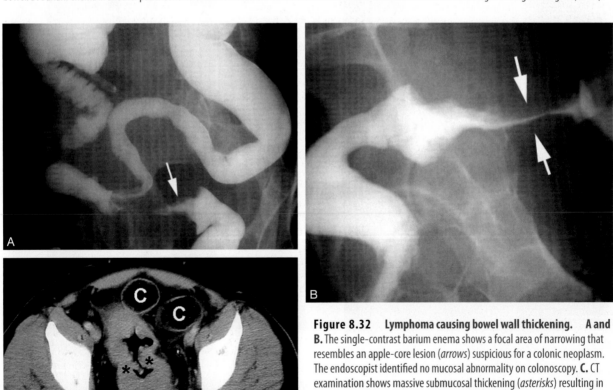

Figure 8.32   Lymphoma causing bowel wall thickening.   A and B. The single-contrast barium enema shows a focal area of narrowing that resembles an apple-core lesion (*arrows*) suspicious for a colonic neoplasm. The endoscopist identified no mucosal abnormality on colonoscopy. **C.** CT examination shows massive submucosal thickening (*asterisks*) resulting in the luminal narrowing. Note the more normal caliber colon anteriorly (*C*) whose wall is paper thin and measures less than 3 mm. A biopsy through the submucosa of the involved thickened segment revealed lymphoma.

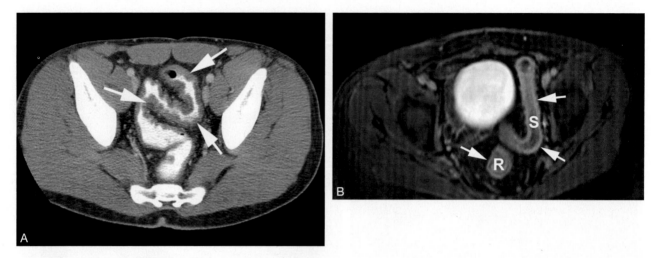

Figure 8.33   Ulcerative Colitis   A. CT examination demonstrates diffuse thickening through the sigmoid colon (*arrows*). **B.** MR enterography demonstrates diffuse thickening and hyperenhancement (*arrows*) through the sigmoid colon (*S*) and rectum (*R*).

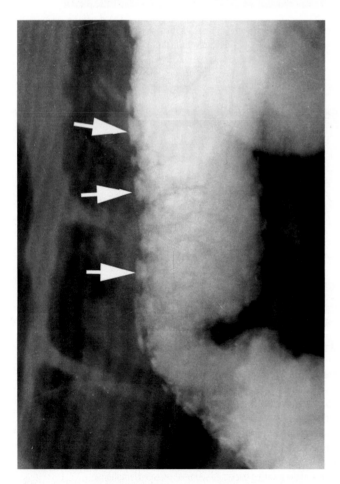

Figure 8.34   Barium enema demonstrates "collar button" ulcers (*arrows*) in a patient with ulcerative colitis.

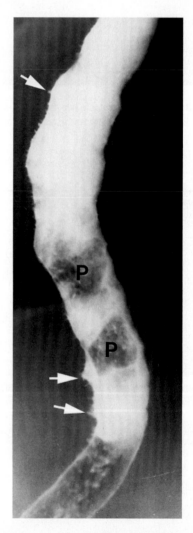

Figure 8.35   Pseudopolyps (*P*) in a patient with ulcerative colitis present as multiple intraluminal masses.   Pseudopolyps represent islands of normal mucosa. Note the irregular ulcers along the mucosal margin (*arrows*).

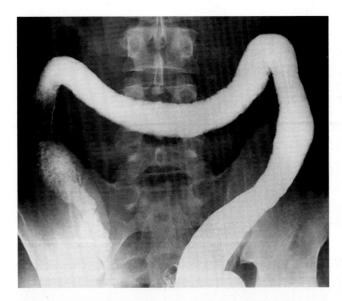

Figure 8.36   Appearance of the colon in long-standing ulcerative colitis.   The colon is fairly rigid, devoid of haustral markings, and is foreshortened.

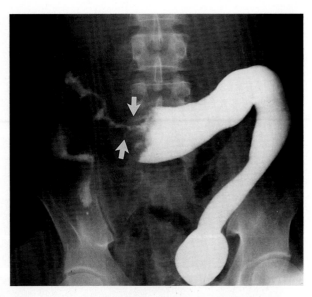

Figure 8.37   Colon carcinoma in a patient with long-standing ulcerative colitis.   (This is the same patient as in Fig. 8.36, 7 years later. An apple-core lesion is present in the mid transverse colon (*arrows*).

(Fig. 8.36). Colon carcinoma may develop in as many as 5% of patients with long-standing ulcerative colitis (Fig. 8.37).

Crohn Disease

Crohn disease of the colon (*granulomatous colitis*) is identical to regional enteritis that occurs elsewhere in the GI tract. Crohn disease classically involves *all* layers of the bowel wall. This results in strictures and obstruction as well as enteroenteric, enterocutaneous, and enterovertebral fistulas (Fig. 8.38).

 ▶ Crohn disease typically involves *all* layers of the bowel wall.

The radiographic manifestations in most instances are distinct from those of ulcerative colitis. The barium enema generally demonstrates patches of involved bowel with normal intervening mucosa—the so-called skip lesions (Fig. 8.39). Typically, the rectum is spared but the right colon is more severely involved. The terminal ileum is involved in almost every instance, producing a pattern often referred to as the "string sign" (Fig. 8.40). Fistulous tracts are often demonstrable. Unlike ulcerative colitis, development of colon carcinoma is unusual.

Table 8.1 contrasts the two diseases.

 ▶ Patients with ulcerative colitis are susceptible to the development of colon carcinoma. Carcinoma is unusual in Crohn disease.

Although these patterns were first used to help the radiologist identify and differentiate disease with fluoroscopy, the same patterns are now applied to CT and MR enterography that have, in many circumstances, replaced fluoroscopic examinations (*see* Figs. 8.38–8.40) to identify and characterize inflammatory bowel disease. These new modalities detect strictures, dilation, and ulceration and now have the added bonus of demonstrating additional findings such as hyperemia of the mesentery, hyperenhancing mucosa consistent with acute inflammation, mesenteric lymphadenopathy, and developing abscesses/fistula among other complications and associations seen with inflammatory bowel disease.

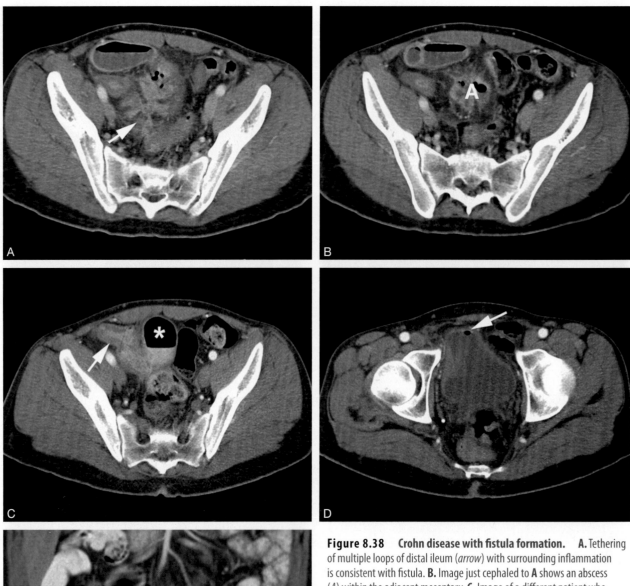

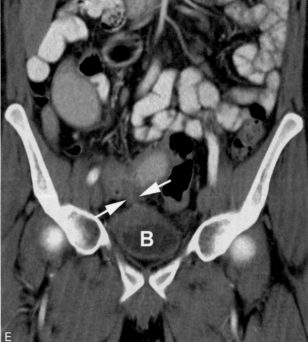

Figure 8.38   Crohn disease with fistula formation.   A. Tethering of multiple loops of distal ileum (*arrow*) with surrounding inflammation is consistent with fistula. **B.** Image just cephaled to **A** shows an abscess (*A*) within the adjacent mesentary. **C.** Image of a different patient who developed an enterovesicular fistula between a loop of distal ileum and the bladder. Note the loop of ileum with diffuse bowel wall thickening (*arrow*). The proximal bowel is dilated with an air fluid level (*asterisk*). **D.** There a focus of gas (*arrow*) within the bladder lumen with no history of recent instrumentation. **E.** Coronal image shows the enhancing tract (*arrows*) from the loop of ileum to the bladder dome (*B*). There is associated thickening of the bladder dome.

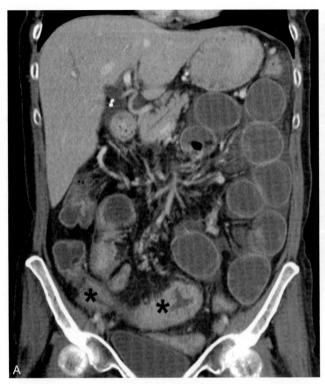

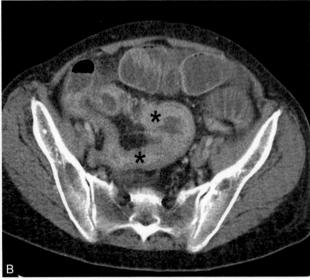

Figure 8.39 Crohn disease with skip lesions. A. Coronal and **B.** Axial CT enterography images show noncontinuous areas of thickened (*asterisks*) small bowel. Note the dilated proximal bowel loops.

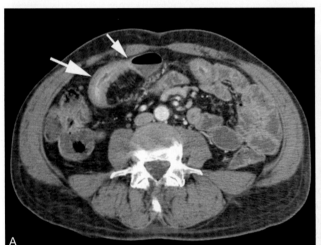

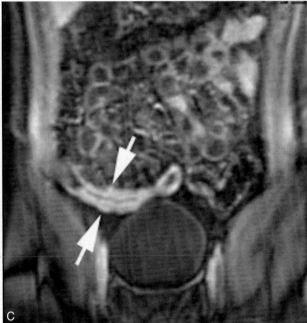

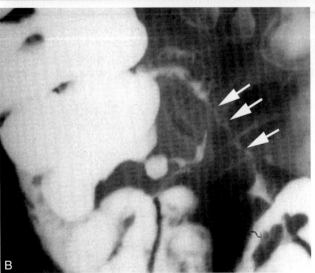

Figure 8.40 A. Crohn disease with bowel wall thickening and hyperenhancement of the mucosa (*large arrow*) with resultant luminal narrowing (*small arrow*). B. Small bowel follow-through in another patient demonstrates string-like narrowing of the terminal ileum (*arrows*). **C.** MR enterography demonstrating thickening, mucosal hyperenhancement, and string-like luminal narrowing through the terminal ileum (*arrows*).

Table 8.1 COMPARISON OF ULCERATIVE COLITIS AND CROHN DISEASE

Feature	Ulcerative Colitis	Crohn Disease
Clinical		
Fever, malaise	+	++
Rectal bleeding	++	±
Tenderness	±	++
Diarrhea	+++	+++
Abdominal mass	−	+++
Abdominal pain	−	+++
Fistulas	−	+++
Endoscopic		
Rectal disease	+++	+
Linear ulcers	−	+
Continuous disease	+++	−
Skip lesions	−	+++
Radiographic		
Continuous disease	+++	−
Skip lesions	−	+++
Ileal involvement	+	+++
Strictures	−	+
Fistulas	−	++
Carcinoma	+++	−
Pseudopolyps	+++	−
"Collar button" ulcers	+++	+
"Cobblestone" pattern	−	+++

+, finding present; the more pluses, the more common the finding; −, finding not present; ±, finding may or may not be present.

Postoperative Appearance of the Gastrointestinal Tract

Surgical procedures alter the appearance of the GI tract in several ways. As discussed previously, fluoroscopic examination is the preferred modality to look for postoperative complications such as anastomotic leaks and fistulae. Not surprisingly, most patients seen in fluoroscopic exam rooms today are examined for these reasons. Understanding the surgery performed is a crucial step in determining if an exam is normal or abnormal. Talking with patients, reviewing operative notes, and in some circumstances direct communication with the surgeon is necessary for complete understanding of the postsurgical anatomy. It is also important to remember that in a patient who is immediately postoperative or in whom there is concern of a potential leak, using water-soluble contrast first is most important and if necessary this can be followed by barium as discussed in Chapter 2.

Esophageal Bypass Surgery

Esophageal bypass surgery for carcinoma or stricture is done primarily using gastro-esophagostomy. In this procedure, sometimes called an esophagogastrectomy, the stomach is mobilized, preserving its blood supply, and is brought into the chest where it is anastomosed with the resected end of the esophagus. On a chest radiograph or esophagram, this appears as a soft tissue density that may contain air or mottled fluid just to the right of the cardiac silhouette (Fig. 8.41). Frequently, the gastric rugae identify this structure. On the lateral view, the transposed stomach is in an anterior position. In some instances, a segment of transverse colon may be used. Another palliative procedure for this disease is the use of stents in an attempt to keep the esophageal lumen open (Fig. 8.42).

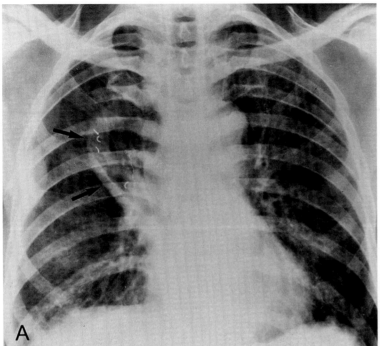

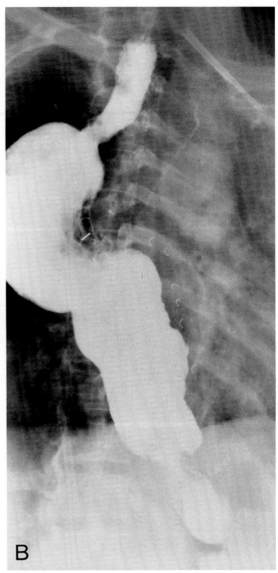

Figure 8.41 **Appearance after esophageal bypass surgery (gastroesophagostomy).** **A.** Frontal chest radiograph shows an air-containing mass in the right paratracheal region (*arrows*). Surgical clips are evident. **B.** Esophagram shows that the "mass" is the result of the transposed stomach.

Laparoscopic Procedures for Esophageal Reflux

A number of procedures, many of which are performed through a laparoscope, have been designed to treat esophageal reflux with or without a hiatal hernia. Most of these (Belsey, Thal, Nissen) involve fundoplication, in which the gastric fundus is sutured around the esophagus to create a tighter sphincter. This results in the radiographic appearance of a mass with smooth, intact mucosa near the esophagogastric junction (Fig. 8.43). This finding should alert the fluoroscopist to the type of procedure performed. There are usually surgical clips in the vicinity of the esophagogastric junction.

Bariatric Surgery

Surgical procedures developed for treating morbid obesity (*bariatric surgery*) involve gastric bypasses and have evolved over the past decade with many types of procedures being performed to make a small stomach/pouch for the patient. Two procedures are commonly used. The first is the Roux-en-Y gastric bypass, which can be performed laparoscopically, in which a small stomach is made from the patient's native stomach which then drains into a portion of the jejunum that is pulled up. The remaining stomach is excluded (Fig. 8.44). The second procedure is called the laparoscopic adjustable gastric band ("lap band"), in which the stomach is not cut but an adjustable band is placed around the proximal portion of the stomach, thus limiting the amount of food that one

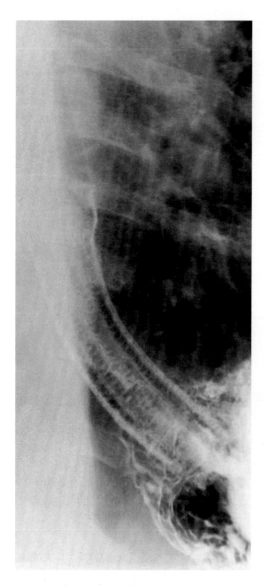

Figure 8.42   Esophageal stent placed for carcinoma.

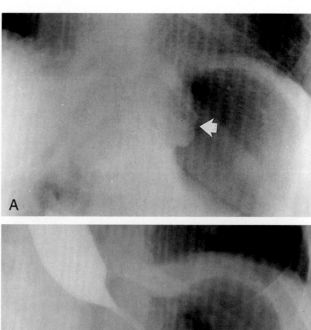

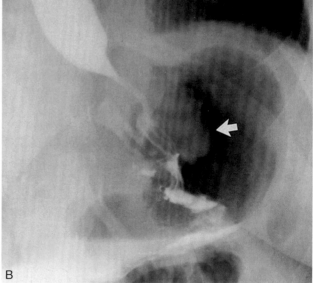

Figure 8.43   Appearance after Nissen fundoplication procedure for esophageal reflux.   A. Close-up view of epigastric region of a chest radiograph shows a mass (*arrow*) in the gastric fundus. **B.** Upper GI examination shows narrowing of the esophagogastric junction and the mass (*arrow*) representing the plicated portion of the gastric fundus.

can eat (Fig. 8.45). Older procedures include gastric stapling or gastric banding, in which the overall volume of the stomach is made smaller by closing off a portion of the fundus and body. The type of procedure may be recognized by the location of surgical staple lines located at the anastomotic or operative sites. A careful history from the patient is usually sufficient to determine if the patient has had one of these procedures. Complications of these procedures include anastomotic leaks (Fig. 8.46), fistula, and obstruction, all of which may be demonstrated with the appropriate contrast examinations. Additionally, Roux-en-Y bypass surgery can develop internal hernias and lap band bypass can develop malpositioned bands (Fig. 8.47) that can occur weeks, months, or even years after surgery.

Indications for Computed Tomography

CT is used extensively to evaluate patients after surgery. The prime indications for this procedure are for detecting infections and abscesses, for recurrence or local spread of a known malignancy (Fig. 8.48), and for metastases (Fig. 8.49). As mentioned earlier, CT is often performed in conjunction with PET imaging.

Accessory Digestive Organs

The accessory digestive organs are the gallbladder, liver, and pancreas. These organs are best evaluated by diagnostic US, CT, and occasionally by MR imaging. As previously

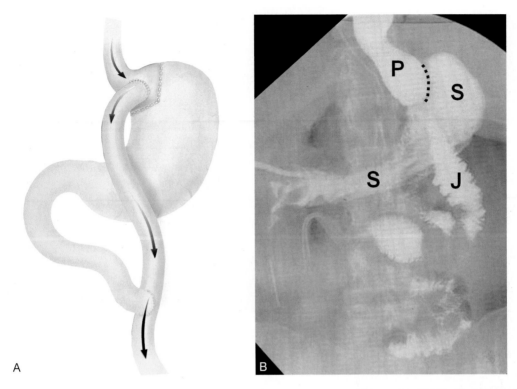

Figure 8.44   Roux-en-Y bypass.   A. Drawing showing the surgical anastomoses of ileum to gastric fundus and duodenum to ileum. The fundus has also been stapled to form a pouch. **B.** Fluoroscopic spot image shows the bypass. The contrast flows from the gastric pouch (P) across the gastrojejunal anastamosis (dotted line) into the jejunum (J). Patient had a gastrostomy tube and the bypassed stomach (S) was opacified to better understand the anatomy. Please note that the bypassed stomach does not normally opacify with contrast unless there is a leak.

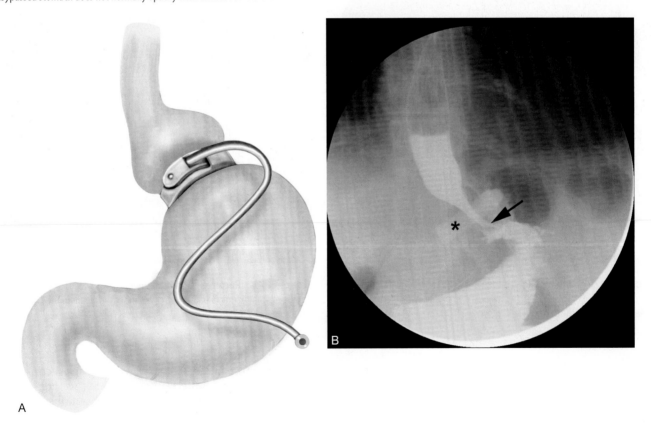

Figure 8.45   Lap band.   A. Drawing showing the band in place over the fundus. Saline injected into the reservoir port fills the adjustable band, creating a neostomach with a stoma emptying into the remainder of the stomach. Patients experience feelings of early satiety when the stoma is adjusted to 3–4 mm in diameter. **B.** Fluoroscopic spot image shows the constriction due to the band (*asterisk*) and the stoma (*arrow*).

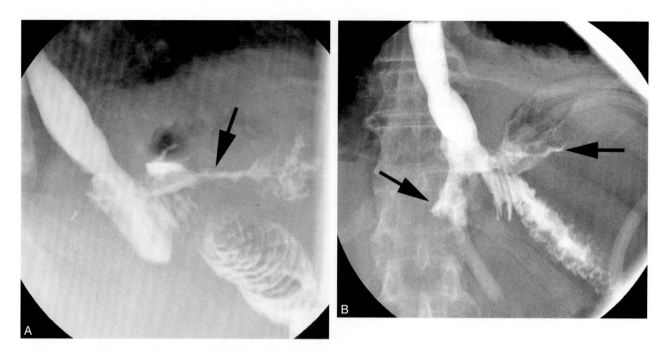

Figure 8.46   Anastomotic leak following bariatric surgery.   A and B. Fluoroscopic spot images show the leakage of contrast (*arrows*).

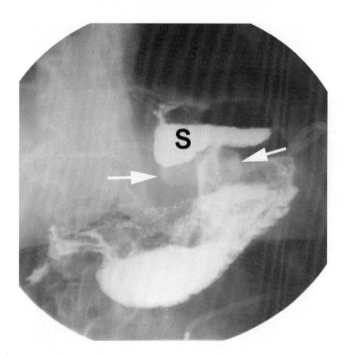

Figure 8.47   Band slippage.   Fluoroscopic image obtained following administration of oral contrast shows enlargement of the neostomach (*S*) with inferior slippage of the gastric band (*arrows*).

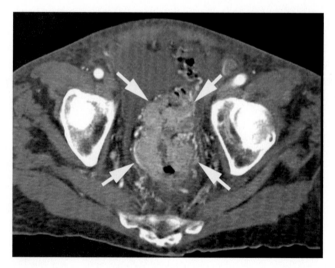

Figure 8.48   Recurrent colon carcinoma.   CT image of the pelvis shows recurrent perirectal masses (*arrows*). The tissue planes in the area are indistinct owing to local invasion.

mentioned, the biliary tract may be visualized either by US or CT/MR. The most common abnormalities encountered in the biliary tract are cholecystitis (Fig. 8.50; *see* Fig. 8.15), cholelithiasis (Fig. 8.51), and choledocholithiasis (Fig. 8.52) with or without obstruction.

Liver Abnormalities

The most common clinical significant abnormalities encountered in the liver are obstructive jaundice and metastases (Fig. 8.53 **A–D**, *see* Fig. 8.49) and patients with underlying

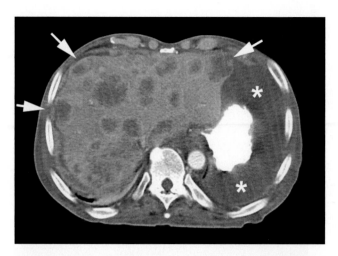

Figure 8.49   Metastases from colon carcinoma. (This is the same patient as in Fig. 8.48.) CT image through the liver demonstrates multiple round and irregular areas of low density, representing metastases. The patient also has peritoneal carcinomatosis with ascites (*asterisks*) in the left upper quadrant and deposits causing scalloping of the liver margin (*arrows*).

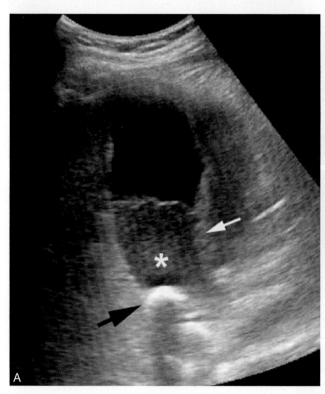

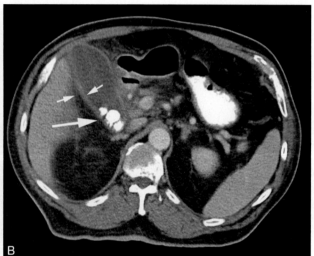

Figure 8.50   Cholecystitis. A. Ultrasound shows thickening of the gallbladder wall (*white arrow*) with many internal echoes representing "sludge" (*asterisk*). A large stone is present (*black arrow*). Note the shadowing beneath the stone. The obstructing calculus is not demonstrated in this study. **B.** CT image shows the thickened gallbladder wall (*small arrows*) and multiple stones (*large arrow*).

hepatic disease, hepatocellular carcinoma (Fig. 8.53**E–G**). US and CT may evaluate both of these. The CT scan, however, is often the first modality used for metastatic workup and can make the diagnosis with the benefit of evaluation of all the visceral organs. MR imaging is particularly useful in evaluating patients with liver lesions that are indeterminate or lesions detected incidentally on other modalities including US and CT (Fig. 8.54). Both US and CT can be used in biopsy of liver lesions and are operator dependent as to the preferred modality. MR is the preferred modality for patients with diffuse liver disease such as hemochromatosis of the liver by demonstrating the iron-laden liver as having a low signal on both T1- and T2-weighted images (Fig. 8.55) or hepatic steatosis (Fig. 8.56).

Pancreatic Diseases

The pancreas was one of the most elusive organs to image in the past. Although pancreatitis and pancreatic pseudocysts make themselves clinically apparent at a relatively early stage of the disease, pancreatic carcinoma often does not. Once the patient with pancreatic carcinoma becomes symptomatic, he/she is usually beyond cure from either surgery

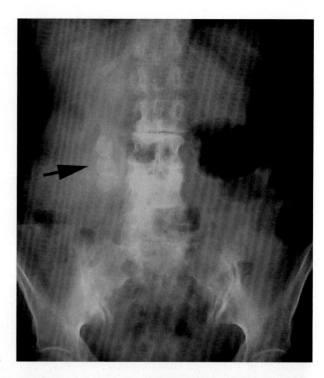

Figure 8.51   Cholelithiasis.

Figure 8.52 Choledocholithiasis.   A. Ultrasound image shows cholelithiasis (*small arrows*) as well as choledocholithiasis (*large arrow*). **B.** CT image of the same patient shows cholelithiasis (*small arrow*) as well as a stone within the distal common bile duct (*large arrow*). **C.** MIP image from an MRCP in another patient shows a filling defect from a stone (*arrow*) within the common bile duct. Note the proximal dilated duct. **D.** Image from an ERCP in another patient with the same finding (*arrow*).

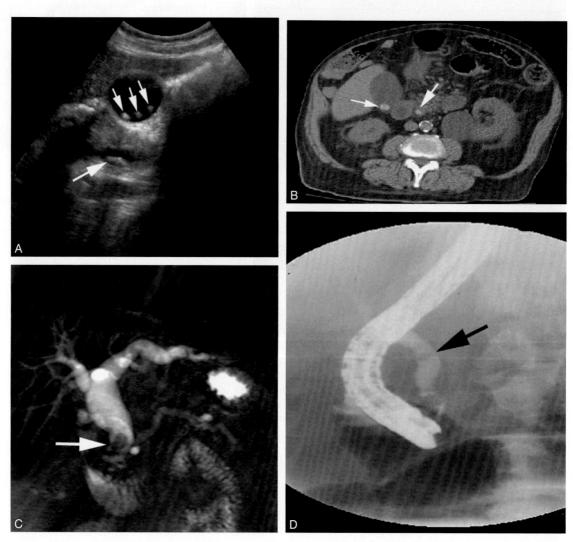

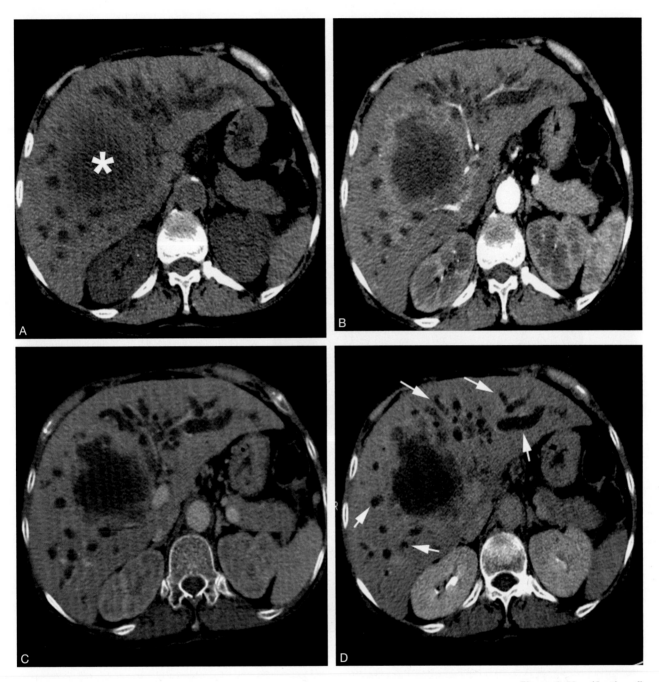

Figure 8.53 (Continued)

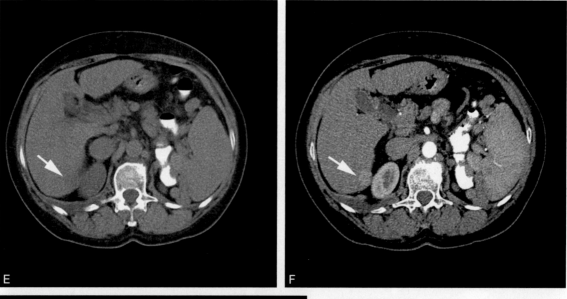

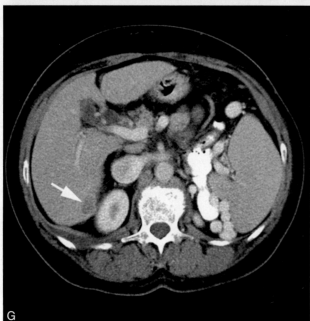

Figure 8.53   Hepatic neoplasms.   A–D. Patient with obstructive jaundice later due to cholangiocarcinoma. Multiple CT images in different phases of contrast administration: without **(A)**, arterial **(B)**, portal venous **(C)**, and delayed **(D)** show a large mass (*asterisk*) within the central portion of the liver causing left- and right-sided intrahepatic biliary dilatation (*arrows* in **D**) typical of cholangiocarcinoma. **E–G.** CT images in different phases in a patient with hepatitis with a low-density lesion (*arrows*) on the noncontrast image **(E)** that demonstrates brisk arterial enhancement **(F)** with washout of contrast **(G)** typical of hepatocellular carcinoma.

or radiation therapy. Direct pancreatic imaging, therefore, has become one of the major advances in medical diagnosis in the last three decades. CT is the preferred modality for studying pancreatic pathology (Figs. 8.57–8.59) as well as for staging and surgical resectability of carcinoma (Fig. 8.60).

Appendicitis and Intraabdominal Abscess

The evaluation of appendicitis (Figs. 8.61 and 8.62) and intraabdominal abscess from any cause has been greatly facilitated by the development of CT. Both etiologies are easier to diagnose with IV and oral contrast administration. Although most abdominal abscesses demonstrate abnormalities on abdominal radiographs, a definitive diagnosis may be made by CT examination (Fig. 8.63). Furthermore, CT-guided drainage is now possible (*see* Fig. 8.3) and US-guided drainage is becoming increasingly utilized for this same purpose. US can also be used in evaluation of appendicitis especially in the pediatric population and pregnant patients and is often the first choice followed by CT or MR.

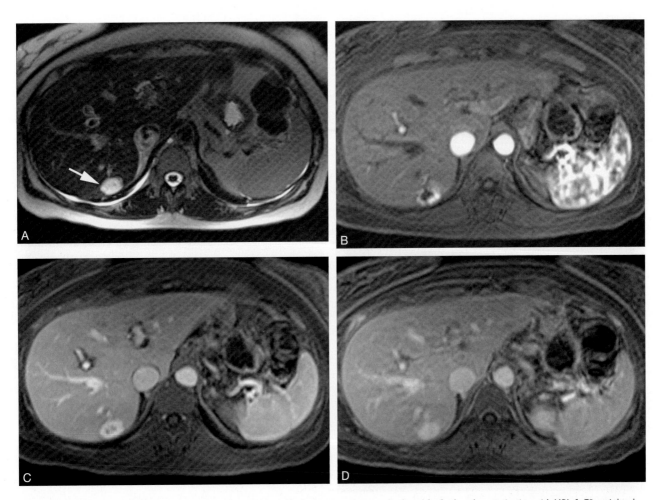

Figure 8.54   MRI hemangioma.   Patient with an incidental lesion seen on ultrasound referred for further characterization with MRI. **A.** T2-weighted hyperintense lesion within the posterior right hepatic lobe (*arrow*) that shows peripheral nodular enhancement on arterial phase **(B)** with progressive filling in of contrast on the further portal venous **(C)** phase and finally complete filling in of contrast on the delayed images **(D)**. This is diagnostic of hemangioma and saves the patient from unnecessary biopsy.

Trauma and Other Emergencies

Finally, CT has made it easier to diagnose traumatic injuries to the liver, spleen, and pancreas (*see* Fig. 8.1). Modern CT machines are able to scan the abdomen in 10 to 20 seconds, making it possible for most patients to cooperate by holding their breath to obtain an ideal study. The speed of CT with its ability to access multiple organs makes it ideal for patients with acute onset of pain within the emergency department (Figs. 8.64–8.67).

Special Pediatric Considerations

A large variety of disorders affects the GI tract and accessory organs of digestion in the pediatric age group. A complete description would be beyond the aim and scope of this text. However, several disorders occur in sufficient frequency as to merit special mention. These are esophageal foreign body, malrotation, pyloric stenosis, Hirschsprung disease, and intussusception. Each has characteristic imaging features that should be easily recognizable.

Foreign Objects

Infants and small children frequently put objects in their mouths and all too often end up swallowing them. In most instances, the object (coins are most common) readily passes through the GI tract without incident. Occasionally, the object lodges within the

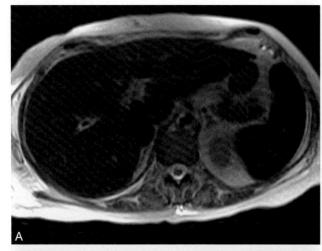

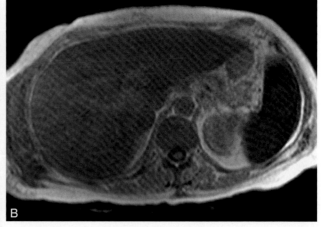

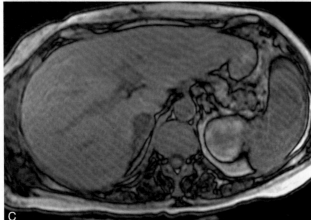

Figure 8.55   Hemochromatosis.   A. T2-W imaging showing a patient with very low signal in both the liver and spleen with loss of signal seen on T1-W imaging out of phase **(B)** versus in phase **(C)** secondary to heavy metal toxicity from repeat transfusions in this patient with secondary hemochromatosis.

esophagus, usually at the level of the thoracic inlet (Fig. 8.68). Irregular and sharp foreign bodies are more likely to cause complications, such as perforation. The radiographic evaluation of every patient suspected of swallowing a foreign object should include radiographs of the chest and abdomen. Small children can usually be studied with a single image.

Bilious Vomiting

Bilious vomiting in the newborn can be a surgical emergency and results from obstruction distal to the ampulla of Vater. A congenital abnormality such as malrotation or duodenal atresia (*see* Fig. 7.16) is a diagnosis of exclusion. After an initial abdominal radiograph, an upper GI series to define the intestinal anatomy is the study of choice. Normal embryonic rotation of bowel results in a long, fixed base that keeps the small bowel mesentery from twisting. If there is malrotated bowel, there is abnormal fixation that results in a short mesenteric base, predisposing to midgut volvulus (Fig. 8.69). This is a surgical emergency that requires prompt diagnosis and treatment to prevent intestinal ischemia. On fluoroscopic evaluation, the radiologist must demonstrate that the third portion of the duodenum crosses midline from right to left and crosses the ligament of Treitz. The duodenojejunal junction should be to the left of the spine and at the same level or higher than the duodenal bulb.

Persistent Nonbilious Vomiting

On the other hand, persistent, nonbilious, and often projectile vomiting in an infant who is several months old often results from *hypertrophic pyloric stenosis* in which there is hypertrophy and hyperplasia of the circular muscle layer of the pylorus. Although the

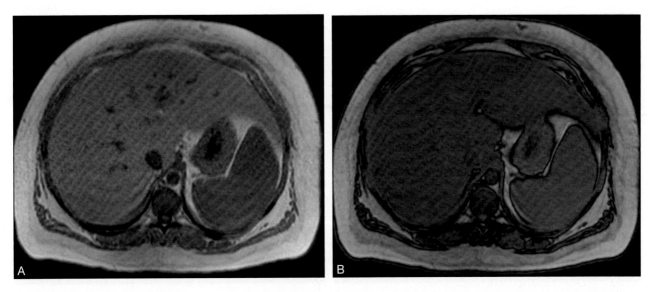

Figure 8.56 Diffuse hepatic steatosis. The reverse of heavy metal toxicity with loss of signal on T1-W out of phase imaging with the liver **(A)** in comparison to T1-W in phase **(B)** consistent with microscopic fat seen in hepatic steatosis.

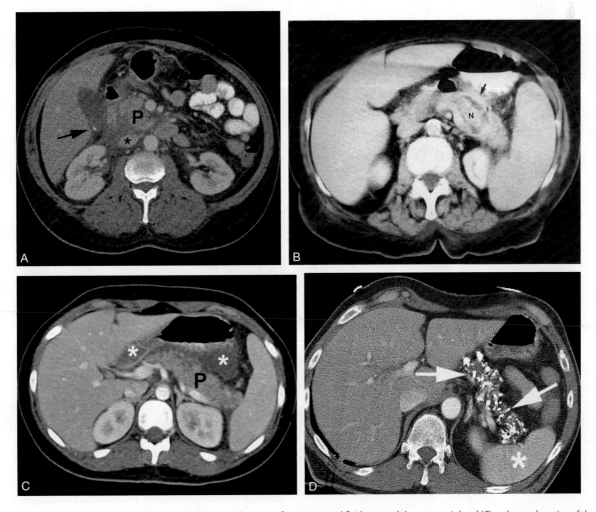

Figure 8.57 Pancreatitis in four patients. **A.** CT image showing inflammation and fluid surround the pancreatic head (*P*) and second portion of the duodenum with fluid in the retroperitoneum just anterior and lateral to the inferior vena cava (*asterisk*). Also note the cause of this patient's pancreatitis with a gallstone (*arrow*) in the gallbladder. **B.** CT image shows enlargement of the pancreas (*arrow*) and a necrotic focus (*N*) in the central portion. **C.** CT image shows enlargement of the pancreas (*P*) and fluid collections (*asterisks*) anteriorly. **D.** CT image of a patient with chronic pancreatitis shows multiple calcifications in the pancreas. Note how the tail of the pancreas ends in the hilum of the spleen (*asterisk*).

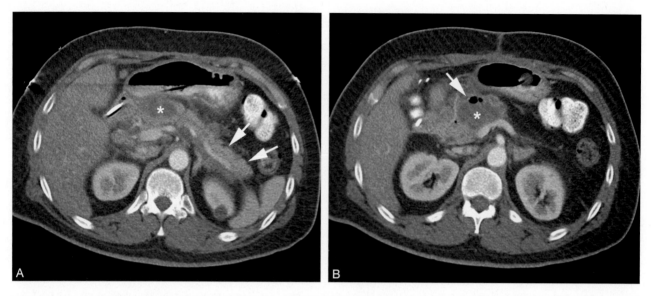

Figure 8.58   Pancreatitis with abscess.   A. CT image shows inflammation surrounding the pancreas most pronounced around the tail (*arrows*). There is an abscess in the head (asterisk). **B.** Image just below **A** shows the fluid collection (*asterisk*) in the region of the pancreatic neck that contains gas (*arrow*) consistent with an abscess.

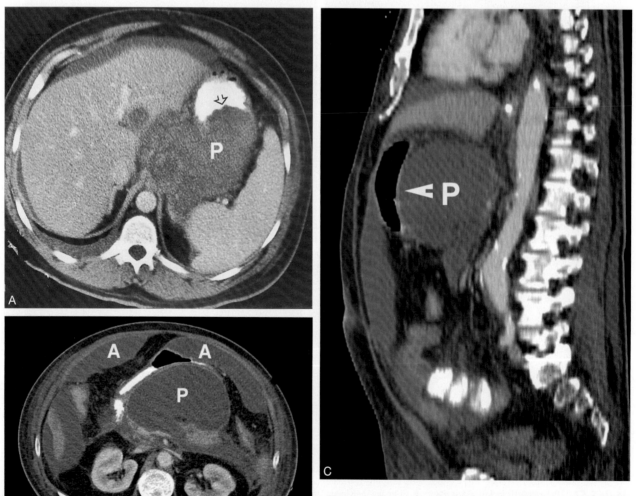

Figure 8.59   Pancreatic pseudocysts.   A. CT image shows a large pseudocyst compressing the posterior gastric wall (*arrow*). **B.** Pseudocyst (*P*) in another patient with ascites (*A*). **C.** Sagittal CT image shows the pseudocyst compressing the stomach (*arrowhead*).

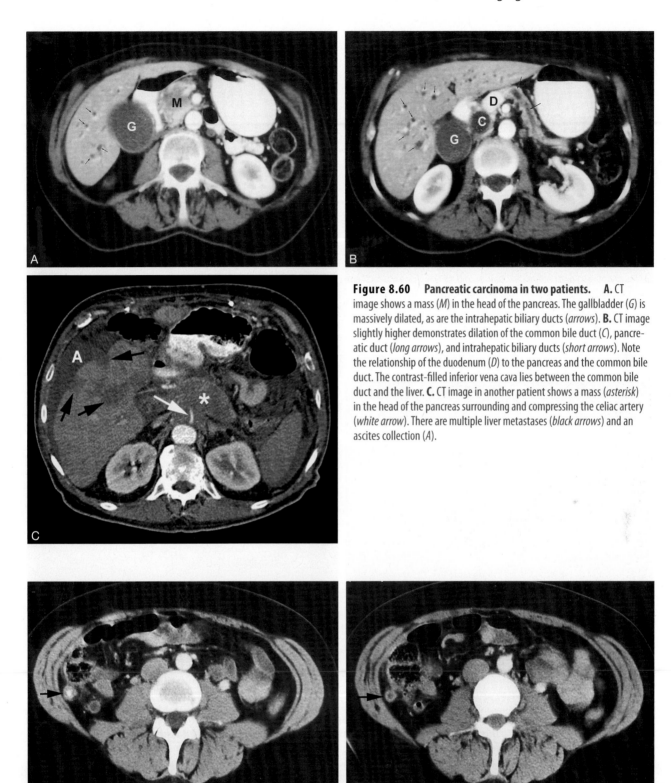

Figure 8.60   Pancreatic carcinoma in two patients.   A. CT image shows a mass (*M*) in the head of the pancreas. The gallbladder (*G*) is massively dilated, as are the intrahepatic biliary ducts (*arrows*). **B.** CT image slightly higher demonstrates dilation of the common bile duct (*C*), pancreatic duct (*long arrows*), and intrahepatic biliary ducts (*short arrows*). Note the relationship of the duodenum (*D*) to the pancreas and the common bile duct. The contrast-filled inferior vena cava lies between the common bile duct and the liver. **C.** CT image in another patient shows a mass (*asterisk*) in the head of the pancreas surrounding and compressing the celiac artery (*white arrow*). There are multiple liver metastases (*black arrows*) and an ascites collection (*A*).

Figure 8.61   Appendicitis.   A. CT image shows a fecalith in a thickened appendix (*arrow*). **B.** Image slightly higher shows the thickened appendiceal wall (*arrow*).

diagnosis is made primarily on clinical grounds, US and barium studies are used to confirm the diagnosis demonstrating elongation and thickening of the pylorus (Fig. 8.70). A barium study can sometimes be performed in equivocal cases but has the disadvantage of ionizing radiation.

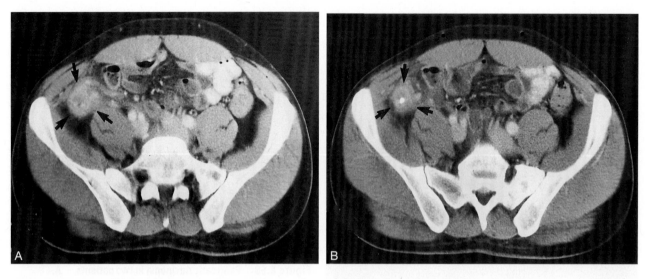

Figure 8.62   Appendicitis with abscess.   A. CT image shows a soft tissue inflammatory mass in the right lower quadrant (*arrows*). **B.** Image slightly lower shows a calcified fecalith within the thickened appendix (*arrows*).

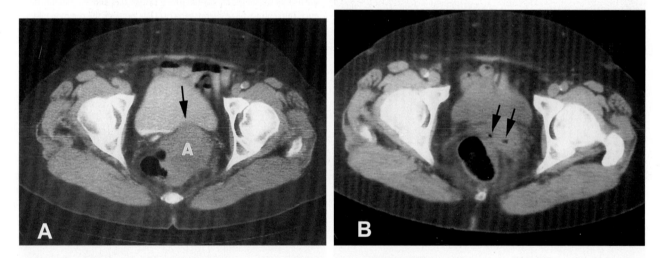

Figure 8.63   Perirectal abscess.   A. CT image shows a large abscess (*A*) compressing the floor of the bladder (*arrow*). **B.** Slightly lower, the abscess contains gas (*arrows*).

Intussusception

Intussusception occurs when a segment of the intestine (the *intussusceptum*) invaginates or "telescopes" into the contiguous distal segment (the *intussuscipiens*). This produces mechanical obstruction and, if left untreated, ischemia. The majority (approximately 90%) of intussusceptions are ileocolic. The remainder are (in decreasing order of frequency) ileoileocolic, ileoileal, and colocolic. Unlike intussusceptions in adults, which are caused by mesenteric neoplasms, those in the pediatric age group are idiopathic. Radiographic findings, when present, include a mass effect, target-like lucencies in the mass (representing mesenteric fat trapped in the intussusception), and a crescent or streaks of air outlining the trapped bowel (*see* Fig. 7.17). If there is no evidence for either pneumoperitoneum or peritonitis, an air or barium enema may be performed for diagnostic purposes as well as to reduce the intussusception. Current practices prefer the air enema to reduce the likelihood of barium-induced peritonitis in the setting of possible colonic rupture as an adverse outcome of an attempted intussusception reduction. Using fluoroscopic guidance and a pressure valve-equipped catheter, air is instilled into the colon progressively until the obstructing component of the intestine or small bowel is pushed back and reduced into the anatomically normal location.

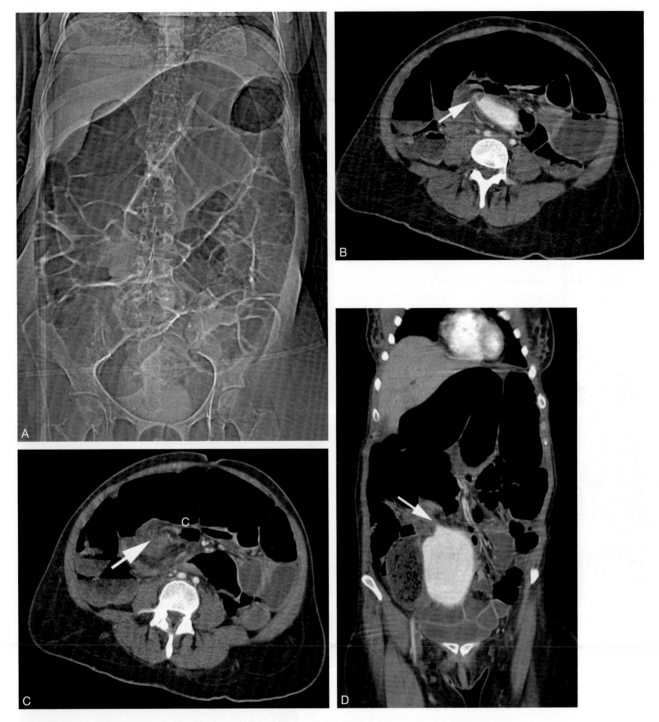

Figure 8.64 Sigmoid volvulus. A. Scout view from CT shows the dilated loops of bowel, mostly large bowel. Axial images **(B and C)** along with a coronal image **(D)** show contrast in the rectum from a rectal tube given by emergency department prior to CT with an abrupt cut off "birds beak" (*arrows* **B** and **D**). There is twisting of the mesentery producing a "swirl sign" (*arrow*) seen on **C**. Patient subsequently went to flexible sigmoidoscopy for reduction of the volvulus.

Hirschsprung Disease

Hirschsprung disease is the result of congenital absence of the intramural ganglion cells in the distal bowel. It is more common in boys than in girls. The absence of the distal ganglion cells results in the inability of the peristaltic wave to pass through the abnormal bowel segment and thus produces an obstructive clinical picture, manifested primarily as chronic constipation. Radiography is beneficial in making the diagnosis. Abdominal radiographs reveal an obstructive pattern in infants and evidence of fecal impaction in older children (Fig. 8.71A). A barium enema may demonstrate the atonic bowel segment as an area of abrupt tapering of the lumen (Fig. 8.71B).

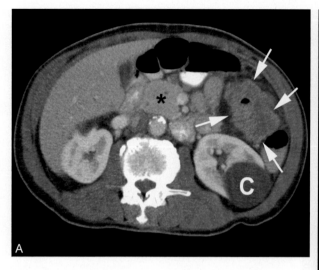

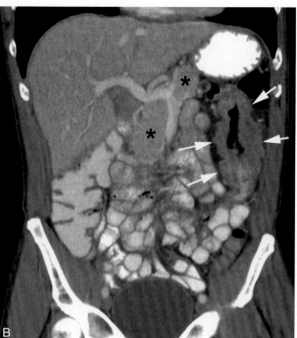

Figure 8.65   Colon cancer.   Patient with a history of weight loss presented with left upper quadrant pain. Axial **(A)** and coronal **(B)** CT images show circumferential thickening of the proximal descending colon (*arrows*) and narrowing of the lumen consistent with colon carcinoma and classic "apple-core lesion." Note the metastatic deposits in the lymph nodes (*asterisks*), and renal cyst (*C*) in the left kidney on the axial image.

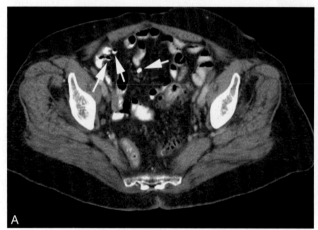

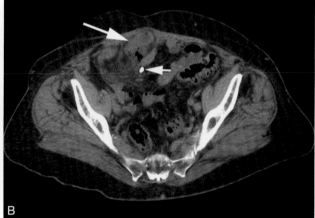

Figure 8.66   Small bowel diverticulitis.   **A.** CT image shows multiple small bowel diverticula (*arrows*). **B.** Follow-up CT of the same patient who came to the emergency department with right lower quadrant pain shows inflammation and gas (*large arrow*) around the same diverticulum with high density within its lumen (*small arrow*) consistent with small bowel diverticulitis.

Figure 8.67   Perforated duodenal ulcer.   Patient came into the emergency department with acute onset of epigastric pain. CT scan shows oral contrast in the duodenal bulb (*D*) with contrast spilling out laterally and surrounding the liver (*small arrows*). There is also a small amount of pneumoperitoneum (*large arrow*) consistent with perforated ulcer.

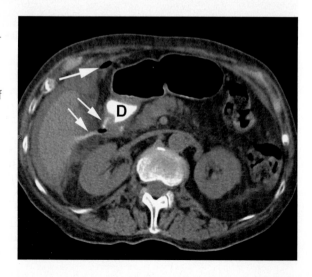

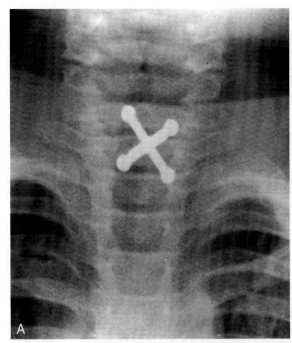

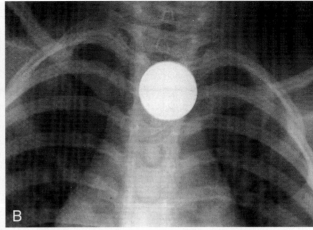

Figure 8.68 Esophageal foreign bodies. A. Jack. **B.** Coin.

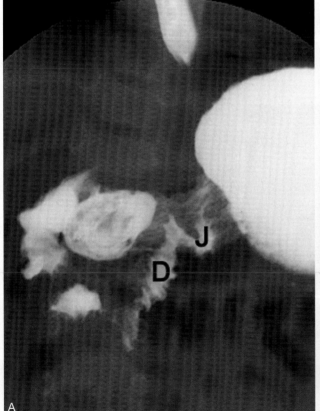

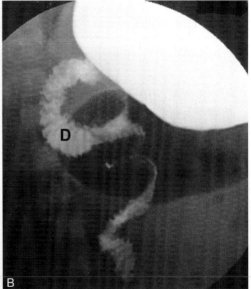

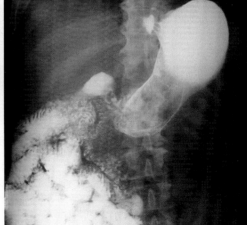

Figure 8.69 Malrotation. A. Fluoroscopic spot image in a newborn with bilious vomiting demonstrates a corkscrew appearance of the jejunum (*J*). The third portion of the duodenum (*D*) does not cross the ligament of Treitz as it does in this normal newborn patient in **B**. The duodenojejunal junction should be to the left of spine and at the same level or higher than the duodenal bulb with conventional anatomy. **C.** Companion case showing malrotation that was detected incidentally in an asymptomatic 30-year-old patient. Note that the duodenum does not cross the ligament of Treitz and the jejunal loops are located in the right midabdomen and not in the left upper quadrant. Using our pattern approach, this is an example of displacement.

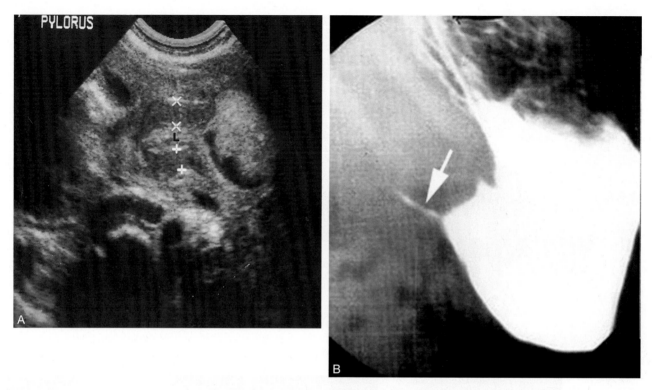

Figure 8.70   Pyloric stenosis.   A. Ultrasound examination of the pyloric region shows a narrowed lumen (*L*) and thickening of the wall of the pylorus (sonolucent area between the white x's and +'s). **B.** Upper GI showing string-like narrowing through the pyloric region (*arrows*) caused by the thickened pylorus. Ultrasound is the study of choice to diagnose pyloric stenosis because of the lack of ionizing radiation.

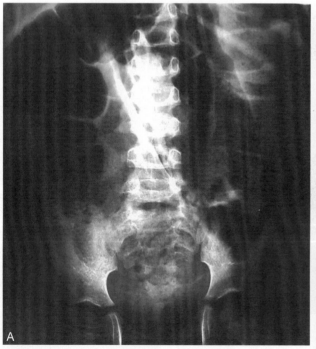

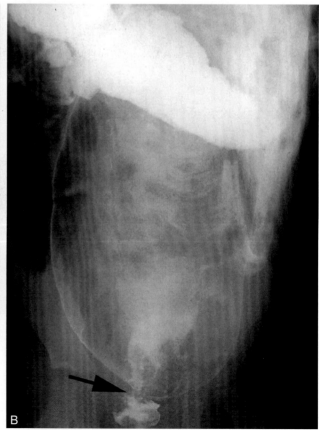

Figure 8.71   Hirschsprung disease.   A. Abdominal radiograph demonstrates massive dilatation of large and small bowel. **B.** Frontal image from a barium enema images demonstrate dilated colon ending in a small, tapered, atonic segment at the rectum (*arrow*).

Summary and Key Points

▶ The GI tract is a tubular structure that allows recognition of patterns of disease that may occur in any portion.

▶ Typical abnormalities include polypoid lesions, mucosal tumors, ulcerations, diverticula, extrinsic compression, and benign strictures.

▶ Although the appearance of these lesions is quite similar from segment to segment, the incidence varies depending on the disease.

▶ Special imaging procedures and their applications to the GI tract were also discussed.

▶ Endoscopy has largely replaced conventional barium imaging in the United States.

Suggested Additional Reading

Blickman JG, Parker BR, Barnes PD. Pediatric Radiology: The Requisites. 3rd Ed. St. Louis, MO: Mosby/Elsevier, 2009.

Brant WE, Helms CA. Fundamentals of Diagnostic Radiology. 4th Ed. Philadelphia, PA: Lippincott Williams & Wilkins, 2012:670–795.

Buonomo C, Taylor GA, Share JC, et al. Gastrointestinal tract. In: Kirks DR, Griscom NT, eds. Practical Pediatric Imaging: Diagnostic Radiology of Infants and Children. 3rd Ed. Philadelphia, PA: Lippincott-Raven, 1998:821–1007.

Donnelley LF, Jones BV, Merrow C, O'Hara S, et al. Diagnostic Imaging: Pediatrics. 2nd Ed. Salt Lake City, UT: Amirsys, 2011.

Federle MP, Jeffrey RB, Woodward PJ. Diagnostic Imaging: Abdomen. 2nd Ed. Salt Lake City, UT: Amirsys, 2011.

Gore RM, Levine MS. Textbook of Gastrointestinal Radiology. 3rd Ed. Philadelphia, PA: WB Saunders/Elsevier, 2008.

Ziessman HA, O'Malley JP, Thrall JH. Nuclear Medicine: The Requisites. 3rd Ed. St. Louis, MO: Mosby, 2006.

chapter 9

Urinary Tract Imaging

Matthew T. Heller   Richard H. Daffner

Urinary tract imaging has undergone tremendous evolution during the past few decades due to advances in imaging equipment, information technology, and contrast materials. Previously, intravenous urography (IVU) was the primary imaging modality of the urinary tract but that has been supplanted by ultrasound (US), computed tomography (CT), and magnetic resonance imaging (MRI). These technical advances have facilitated the evaluation of the two basic types of abnormalities affecting the urinary tract: physiologic and morphologic. *Physiologic abnormalities* typically affect the glomeruli, tubules, and interstitial tissues and are often referred to as the *"medical nephropathies."* The initial imaging findings of nephropathies are often nonspecific or absent and a diagnosis is best established by image-guided renal biopsy. Advanced nephropathy is manifest as renal atrophy and reduced parenchymal enhancement and excretion during imaging studies using intravenous (IV) contrast. Conversely, pathologic processes resulting in *morphologic abnormalities* constitute a heterogeneous group of diseases for which imaging is more helpful in establishing a diagnosis and a treatment plan. These diseases are discussed in the "Pathologic Considerations" section.

Technical Considerations

In general, 10 types of imaging examinations can be used to evaluate the urinary tract and are listed in Table 9.1.

Currently, US, CT, and MRI, as mentioned above, are the modalities most frequently used to assess the urinary tract. While several of the listed imaging modalities do not require the use of IV contrast material to produce a diagnostic examination, its use during CT and MRI is often quite helpful for the proper characterization of pathologic conditions such as masses. In all patients, allergies and renal function should be reviewed prior to the administration of IV contrast. If a history of a true contrast allergy is elicited, the radiologist and referring physician must decide whether an alternative, noncontrast study can be substituted or if the patient can be successfully premedicated with a standard regimen of oral steroids (prednisone) and antihistamines (diphenhydramine). Iodinated IV contrast should not be injected in any patient with a history of anaphylaxis induced by IV contrast or with current evidence of renal failure and who is not on dialysis.

▶ Iodinated IV contrast should not be injected in any patient with a history of anaphylaxis induced by IV contrast or with current evidence of renal failure and who is not on dialysis. Please review Chapter 2 and the online supplement for a more complete discussion about contrast.

Table 9.1 COMPARISON OF URINARY TRACT IMAGING EXAMINATIONS

Examination	Ionizing Radiation	Intravenous Contrast Required	Catheter Required
US	No	No	No
CT	Yes	No[a]	No
MRI	No	No[a]	No
Intravenous urogram (IVU)	Yes	Yes	No
Retrograde urogram (RUG)	Yes	No	Yes
Cystogram	Yes	No	Yes
Voiding cystourethrogram (VCUG)	Yes	No	Yes
Nephrostogram	Yes	No	Yes
Isotope studies[b]	Yes	No	No
Angiogram	Yes	Yes	No

[a]IV contrast is often preferred, especially for evaluation of potential mass lesions.
[b]Examples include renal scintigraphy and positron emission tomography (PET).

Computed Tomography

Contrast-enhanced CT, which can be performed during the renal parenchymal and excretory phases (CT urogram), has almost entirely replaced the traditional IVU for most renal and ureteral applications. Additionally, US, MRI, and MR urography are radiation-free alternatives which are effectively used to evaluate the entire genitourinary tract.

Intravenous Urography

IVU, also known as intravenous pyelography (IVP), is rarely performed in the United States due to the better multiplanar anatomic detail afforded by CT and its ability to evaluate the entire abdomen. The IVU provides information regarding relative renal function, excretion, and obstruction, and also allows morphologic assessment of kidneys, ureters, and bladder. The IVU begins with an abdominal radiograph to evaluate for renal calculi that may be obscured by the excretion of contrast material and to determine the degree of bowel cleanliness. Bowel preparation is necessary to eliminate overlying gas and fecal material that may obscure small renal masses, calculi, and proper renal measurements.

After injection of IV contrast, the IVU consists of a series of radiographs of the abdomen and pelvis during various phases of contrast uptake and secretion by the kidneys. Several tomographic radiographs are obtained at specified depths to elucidate the renal contours that may otherwise be obscured by overlying bowel gas or stool (Fig. 9.1).

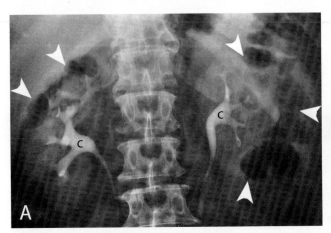
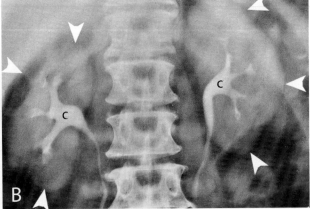

Figure 9.1   Intravenous urography with nephrotomogram.   A. Anteroposterior (AP) radiograph of the kidneys shows excretion of contrast into the renal collecting systems (C) and proximal ureters. Overlying bowel gas obscures portions of the renal borders (*arrowheads*). **B.** A subsequent renal tomogram obtained at a specific depth has excluded most of the overlying bowel gas and shows the smooth, normal-appearing renal borders (*arrowheads*).

Retrograde Examinations

Retrograde examinations are performed to evaluate the urethra, bladder, ureters, and renal collecting systems by instilling water-soluble contrast via a small caliber catheter under fluoroscopic observation. The *urethrogram* is primarily used to evaluate for strictures, diverticula, or trauma to the male urethra. Urethrography can be performed in the trauma bay and allows rapid grading of male urethral injuries to guide the surgeon during operative repair. Similarly, the cystogram is often performed to determine the integrity of the urinary bladder, as well as to evaluate for *vesicoureteral reflux*. A retrograde study of the ureters and the renal collecting system—*retrograde ureteropyelogram* (Fig. 9.2)—is performed by urologists in the operating room in cases of clinically suspected obstruction or tumor, or prior to ureteral stent placement.

Voiding Cystourethrogram

The *voiding cystourethrogram (VCUG)* is commonly used to evaluate for vesicoureteral reflux, especially in children. During VCUG, the bladder is filled with contrast that is instilled via a Foley catheter and the patient is asked to void during fluoroscopic observation. The VCUG is also used to assess morphology and excretory function in patients with recurrent urinary tract infections, hydroureteronephrosis, hematuria, potential diverticula, and complex genitourinary anomalies.

Nephrostograms

Nephrostograms are performed to diagnose obstruction or extravasation following placement of a percutaneous nephrostomy catheter. Contrast injected into the indwelling nephrostomy catheter is monitored fluoroscopically and spot radiographs are obtained at various intervals.

Ultrasound

US allows detailed morphologic assessment of the kidneys and bladder and has replaced the IVU as the initial study of choice for evaluating the renal parenchyma, size, and shape (Fig. 9.3). US is useful in characterizing renal masses by determining if they are solid or cystic based on the quality of internal echoes, within the masses. Simple renal cysts contain only fluid, have no internal echoes and appear homogeneously black on US and are referred to as *anechoic* (Fig. 9.4). Conversely, tumors frequently show internal echoes,

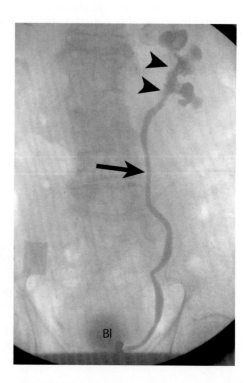

Figure 9.2   Retrograde ureteropyelogram.   Intraoperative fluoroscopic image obtained during cannulation of the left ureter shows retrograde opacification of the left ureter (*arrow*) and the renal collecting system (*arrowheads*). Note the irregularity of the collecting system due to transitional cell carcinoma. *Bl* = bladder.

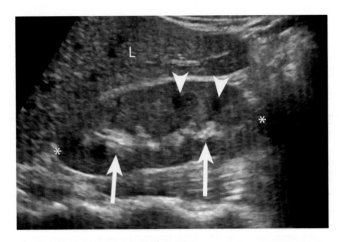

Figure 9.3   Normal renal ultrasound, sagittal (longitudinal) view.
The kidney has an ovoid shape and smooth borders. Centrally, fat in the
renal hilum is bright, or echogenic (*arrows*). Some of the renal pyramids
(*arrowheads*) are shown and appear darker, or hypoechoic, compared to the
remainder of the kidney. *Asterisks* mark the superior and inferior poles of the
kidney. *L* = liver.

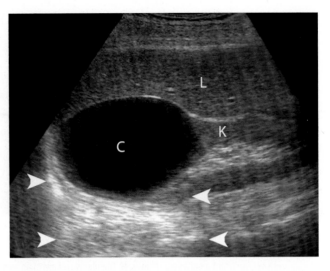

Figure 9.4   Simple renal cyst.   Sagittal US image shows the anechoic
cyst (*C*). Note the increased brightness, or "through transmission" (*arrowheads*),
posterior to the cyst. *L* = liver, *K* = kidney.

indicating their solid nature (Fig. 9.5). Doppler US is used to assess renal parenchymal
blood flow, determine lesion vascularity, evaluate renal transplant vasculature, and screen
for renal artery stenosis in patients with hypertension (Fig. 9.6).

US is also used to evaluate the prostate gland. The development of the transrectal US
transducer makes it possible to study the internal anatomy of the prostate (Fig. 9.7). While
US can often differentiate benign prostatic hypertrophy from carcinoma (Fig. 9.8), its main
strength is its ability to facilitate biopsies with a transrectal US biopsy device. These techniques hold promise to reduce the morbidity and mortality rate of prostatic carcinoma.

Computed Tomography

While US has many uses in evaluation of the kidneys, CT is the preferred modality in cases
of suspected renal trauma (Fig. 9.9). Abdominal CT scanning is also used to detect and

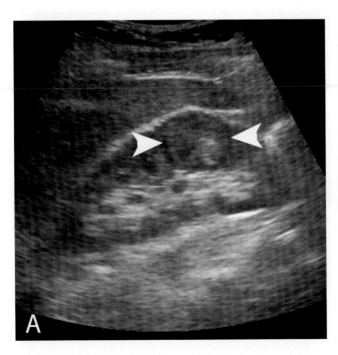

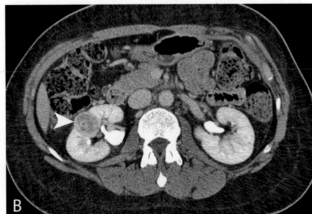

Figure 9.5   Renal cell carcinoma.   A. Sagittal US image shows a solid
mass (*arrowheads*) in the mid portion of the right kidney. Note the internal echoes in the tumor compared with the anechoic cyst in Fig. 9.4. **B.** Corresponding
contrast-enhanced CT image shows the rounded, heterogeneously enhancing
mass (*arrowhead*) in the mid portion of the right kidney.

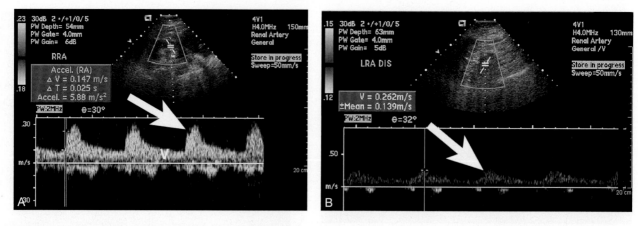

Figure 9.6   Doppler US of the renal arteries.   A. Doppler US images show a normal waveform of an arcuate branch of the right renal artery. The slope (*arrow*) of the brisk systolic upstroke (>3 m/sec²) is normal. Peak systolic velocities (*V*) in the right renal artery are normal (<180 cm/sec), consistent with no significant renal artery stenosis. **B.** Doppler waveform of an arcuate branch of the left renal artery in the same patient shows slow blunted systolic upstroke and delay to peak velocity (parvus-tardus morphology) (*arrow*) distal to a significant stenosis.

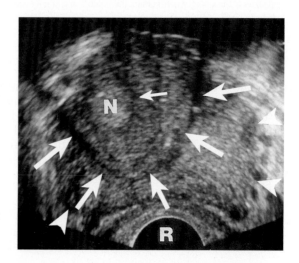

Figure 9.7   "Normal" prostate US in an elderly man.   A transrectal US image depicts two distinct regions of the prostate. The peripheral zone is the area immediately adjacent to the rectum (*R*) surrounded by the true capsule (*arrowheads*). The transitional zone is outlined by the surgical capsule (*large arrows*). Within this zone are the urethra (*small arrow*) and a few, thin septations. An echogenic adenomatous nodule (*N*) is present.

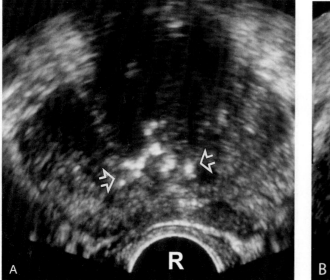

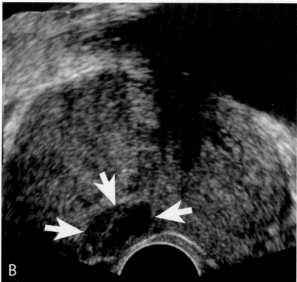

Figure 9.8   Prostate pathology.   A. Benign prostatic hypertrophy (BPH). In BPH, the prostate gland enlarges, especially in the transitional zone. Incidental central calcifications (*arrows*) are echogenic. *R* = rectum. **B.** Adenocarcinoma. Most prostate cancers occur in the peripheral zone and are solid, hypoechoic lesions (arrows). Hypoechoic nodules are nonspecific findings and require US-guided biopsy for diagnosis. Approximately 25% turn out to be cancerous.

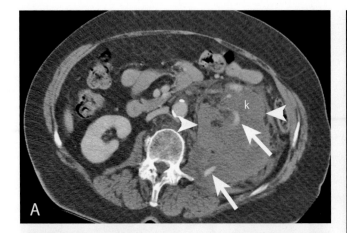

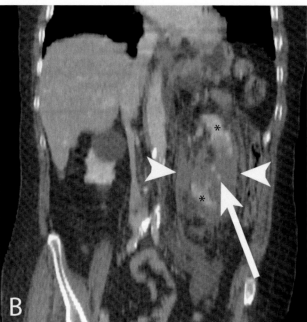

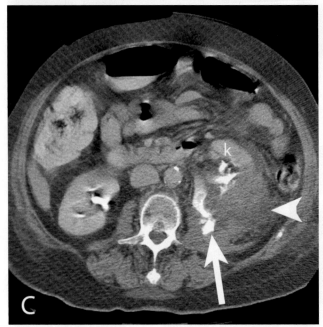

Figure 9.9   Renal trauma.   A. Axial contrast-enhanced CT image shows a large hematoma (*arrowheads*), foci of active hemorrhage (*arrows*), and anterior displacement of the largely devascularized left kidney (*k*). **B.** Coronal reconstructed CT image shows the hematoma (*arrowheads*) separating the superior and inferior aspects of the left kidney (*asterisks*) and foci of active hemorrhage (*arrow*). **C.** Axial CT image obtained during the excretory phase shows the hematoma (*arrowhead*) and leakage of excreted contrast from the ureteropelvic junction (*arrow*) due to traumatic disruption. The patient required emergent nephrectomy.

characterize renal lesions and to determine the origin of extrarenal masses that distort or displace the normal urinary tract. The most common renal lesion is the simple cyst that appears as a low-density, well-marginated structure on noncontrast CT. The internal CT density, measured in Hounsfield units (HU), of a simple cyst is similar to that of urine in the renal collecting system or bladder. Following injection of IV contrast material, there is no enhancement of the cyst, which appears as a prominent "lucency" against the bright, contrast-containing parenchyma (Fig. 9.10). Most renal malignancies are typically isodense (i.e., the density or attenuation of the mass is equivalent to normal renal parenchyma) on the unenhanced scan; following injection of IV contrast, renal malignancies are generally hypervascular and show brisk, early enhancement manifested by increased density. Additionally, the use of IV contrast allows evaluation for malignant vascular invasion (Fig. 9.11) and areas of tumor necrosis (Fig. 9.12). Noncontrast CT is an effective method to evaluate the urinary tract for calculi and obstruction (Fig. 9.13). Additionally, post-contrast excretory phase CT can help to localize the ureters and exclude calculi.

Magnetic Resonance Imaging

MRI of the urinary tract can be used to evaluate renal masses, the effects of pelvic neoplasms on the bladder (Fig. 9.14) and renal transplants (Fig. 9.15). The high soft tissue contrast and multiplanar capability of MRI are useful for evaluating pathology extending to the surrounding structures, such as invasion of the renal vein or the inferior vena cava by

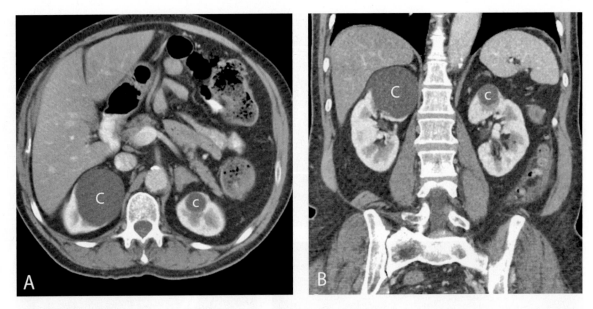

Figure 9.10   Renal cysts (same patient as in Fig. 9.4).   Axial **(A)** and coronal **(B)** reconstructed images from a contrast-enhanced CT show a low-density, homogeneous cyst (*C*) at the superior pole of the right kidney and a smaller cyst (*c*) at the superior pole of the left kidney. The attenuation measurement of these cysts was 5 Hounsfield units.

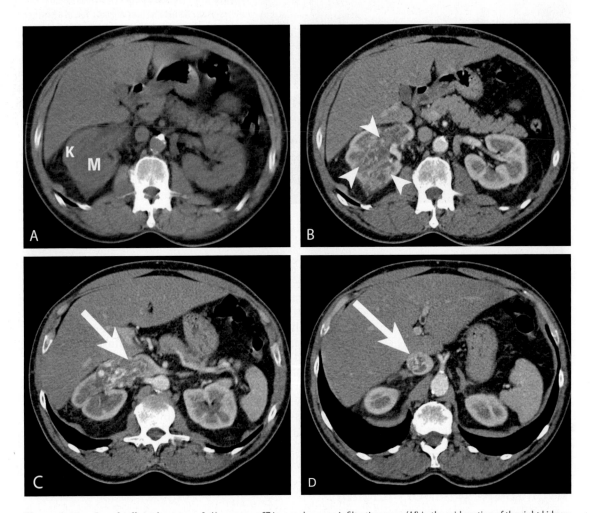

Figure 9.11   Renal cell carcinoma.   A. Noncontrast CT image shows an infiltrating mass (*M*) in the mid portion of the right kidney; note that the density of the mass is nearly equivalent to the adjacent unaffected renal parenchyma (*K*). **B.** Following injection of intrave-nous contrast, the mass shows heterogeneous hypervascularity (*arrowheads*). **C.** More inferiorly, the tumor extends into the right renal vein (*arrow*). **D.** Tumor extends into the lumen of the inferior vena cava (*arrow*).

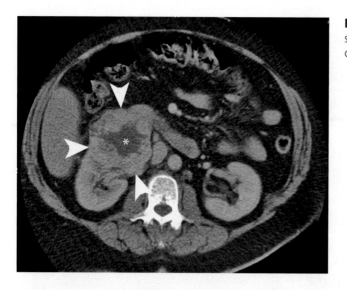

Figure 9.12   Necrotic renal cell carcinoma.   Contrast-enhanced CT shows a large mass with peripheral enhancement (*arrowheads*) and an area of central necrosis (*asterisk*).

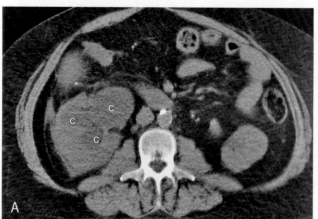

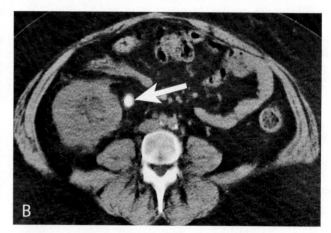

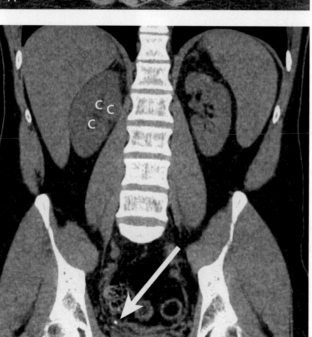

Figure 9.13   Obstructive uropathy in two patients as demonstrated by CT.   A. Noncontrast CT shows advanced dilatation of the renal collecting system (*C*). **B.** More inferiorly, there is a large obstructing stone in the ureter (*arrow*). The lower pole of the kidney is enlarged. **C.** Coronal reconstructed CT image in another patient shows mild dilatation of the right renal collecting system (*c*) and a subcentimeter stone in the distal ureter (*arrow*).

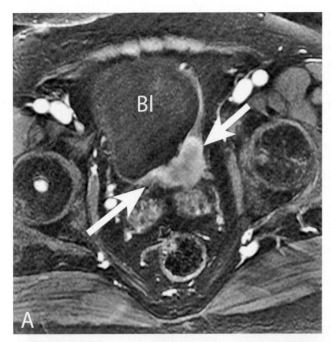

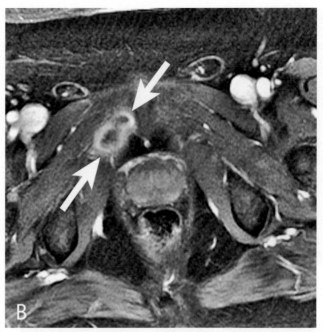

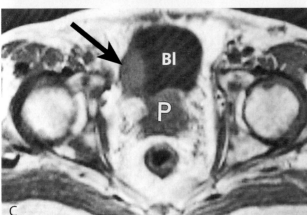

Figure 9.14   Bladder malignancy shown with MRI.   A. Contrast enhanced T1-weighted image shows an enhancing lesion (*arrows*) along the left posterolateral aspect of the bladder due to squamous cell carcinoma. **B.** More inferiorly, there is an enhancing metastasis in the right pelvic musculature (*arrows*). **C.** In another patient, a T1-weighted image shows extension of prostate carcinoma (*arrow*) into the bladder (*Bl*). *P* = prostate.

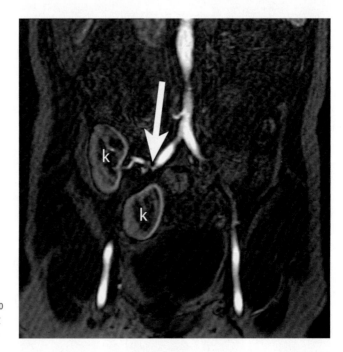

**Figure 9.15   Renal transplant complicated by stenosis at the arterial anastomosis.   **Coronal T1-weighted MRI after injection of IV contrast shows two kidney transplants (*k*) in the right lower quadrant. There is focal stenosis (*arrow*) at the arterial anastomosis between the renal artery and the right iliac artery.

renal cell carcinoma. In the past decade, MRI is being utilized more frequently to evaluate the prostate gland (Fig. 9.16). While MRI can detect prostate carcinoma and often differentiate it from other common processes, such as benign prostatic hypertrophy, the strength of prostate MRI lies in its ability to accurately stage the malignancy prior to surgery.

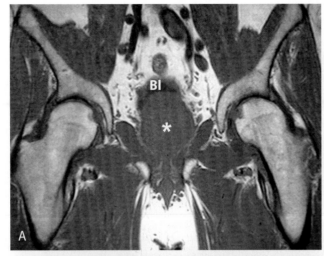

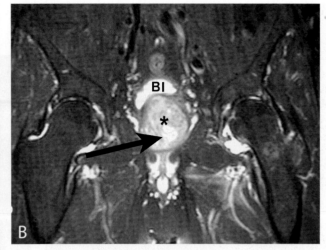

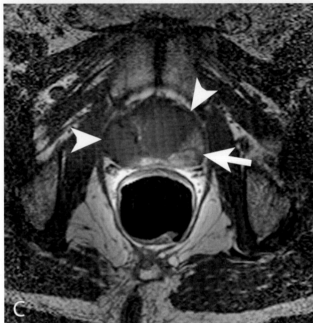

Figure 9.16   Prostate pathology shown with MRI.   T1-weighted **(A)** and T2-weighted **(B)** coronal MRI images show the enlarged prostate (*asterisk*) pressing upon the floor of the bladder (*Bl*). Note the nonspecific nodule in **B** (*arrow*). Biopsy was necessary to determine that the nodule was benign. **C.** T1-weighted axial MRI in another patient shows a large area of low signal (*arrowheads*) in the prostate, consistent with adenocarcinoma. A small region of normal prostate (*arrow*) has higher signal.

❱ The strength of prostate MRI lies in its ability to accurately stage the malignancy prior to surgery.

Renal Scintigraphy

Renal scintigraphy typically employs compounds of technetium 99m to evaluate the urinary tract in both adults and children (Fig. 9.17). Common indications for scintigraphy include detection of vesicoureteral reflux, determination of differential renal function, differentiation of hydroureteronephrosis from a nonobstructed, dilated collecting system and screening for renal artery stenosis in patients with hypertension.

Anatomic Considerations

The kidneys in a normal adult typically measure 11 to 14 cm in length. They are invested in their own fascia, with their upper poles oriented slightly posteromedially. A slight size difference between the right and left kidneys is normal; the left kidney is often 0.5 to 1.5 cm longer than the right. The collecting system consists of three to five *infundibula*, each draining one or more *calyces*. The calyx forms a sharply defined "cup" around the papilla

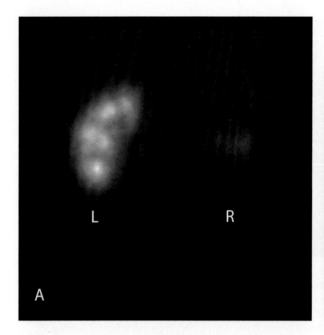

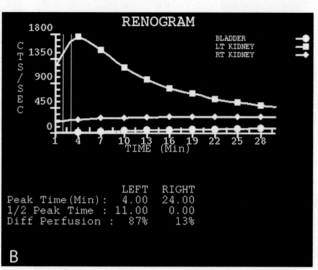

Figure 9.17   Chronic pyelonephritis shown with scintigraphy.   A. Posterior view during renal scintigraphy using the radiotracer technetium 99m MAG3 shows normal uptake in the left kidney and poor uptake in the right kidney. Poor uptake on the right was due to chronic pyelonephritis. **B.** Graph shows the normal uptake and washout of the left kidney and poor uptake with lack of washout in the right kidney. The calculated differential function indicated that the left kidney received 87% of the perfusion while the right only received 13%.

that it drains (Fig. 9.18). The calyces are easily discernible on the normal urogram as peripheral collections of contrast accumulation. The slender infundibula unite to form the renal pelvis that terminates in the ureter. The ureters course inferiorly through the retroperitoneum lateral to the vertebral column. At the level of the bony pelvis, the ureters may make a slight lateral deviation before turning medially to enter the posterolateral aspect of the bladder at the *trigone*. The ureters are not bound by fascia and are relatively mobile. The direction and degree of ureteral displacement on imaging studies is useful in the evaluation of retroperitoneal disease.

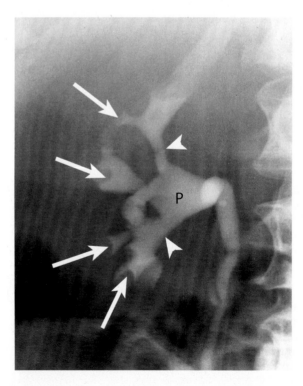

Figure 9.18   Magnified view of a normal right kidney during IVU. Note the delicate cupping of the calyces (*arrows*), the linear infundibula (*arrowheads*), and the central renal pelvis (*P*).

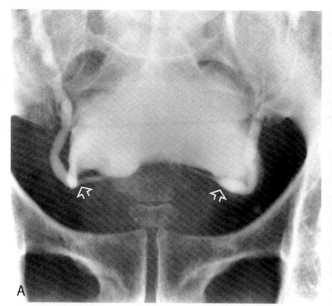

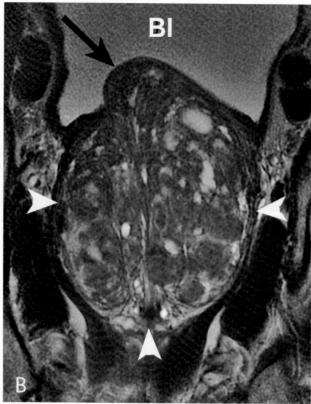

Figure 9.19   Prostate enlargement.   A. IVU shows the base of the bladder elevated by the enlarged prostate. Note the sharp angulation, or "fish hooking," of the distal ureters (*arrows*) as they enter the bladder. **B.** Coronal T2-weighted MRI shows the superior tip (*arrow*) of the massively enlarged prostate (*arrowheads*) impressing upon the base of the urinary bladder (*Bl*) due to benign prostatic hypertrophy.

The urinary bladder should have a smooth contour and ovoid shape. The bladder mucosa should be smooth without trabeculation or other mucosal lesions. Normal variations in the shape of the bladder occasionally result in a lobular configuration.

The prostate lies immediately inferior to the bladder in males and, when enlarged, may indent and elevate the floor of the bladder (Fig. 9.19). The urethra courses through the prostate. The membranous portion of the male urethra between the prostatic and bulbous urethra is fixed in the urogenital diaphragm. This area is subject to laceration from trauma to the pelvis and is a key component of urethral injury grading classifications.

The vascular supply to the kidney generally consists of a single pair of renal arteries. However, occasionally two or more arteries to each kidney are present. A single renal vein drains each kidney. On the right, the vein drains directly into the inferior vena cava without anastomosis with other veins. On the left, the renal vein communicates with the left adrenal and gonadal veins. These two communications form a collateral pathway for blood to drain the kidney in the event of renal vein thrombosis. Collateral channels in the arterial system may enlarge when there are stenotic lesions of the renal artery.

Pathologic Considerations

As previously mentioned, physiologic abnormalities uniformly result in a decrease or absence of renal function. When these occur, the only morphologic change that may be discerned is a decrease in the size of the kidneys. This discussion concentrates on diseases that produce recognizable morphologic abnormalities, including the following:

- Congenital abnormalities
- Obstructive lesions
- Infections
- Masses—cysts and tumors
- Vascular lesions
- Traumatic lesions
- Extrinsic compression
- Renal transplantation

This list is not comprehensive. It should be noted that many entities fall into a "crossover" category. For example, obstruction of the ureteropelvic junction is considered the most common congenital obstruction of the urinary tract. This entity could be categorized as both congenital and obstructive. Multicystic dysplastic kidney could be discussed with renal cystic diseases. However, the origin of this disorder is severe obstruction occurring during embryonic life. In keeping with the philosophy of this text, the discussion that follows covers the concepts of each pathologic category. For details of the specific imaging findings for a particular entity, consult one of the texts listed at the end of this chapter.

Congenital Abnormalities

The complex development of the genitourinary tract in embryonic life provides many opportunities for anomalous development to occur. Anomalies may be relatively benign, such as duplication of the collecting system (Fig. 9.20) or an uncomplicated horseshoe kidney (Fig. 9.21); or they can be severe, such as posterior urethral valves with secondary megacystis, hydroureter, and hydronephrosis in a newborn male infant. Other anomalies include ectopic kidneys and ectopic ureteroceles.

Ureterocele

Dilation of the distal portion of the ureter results in the formation of an *ureterocele*. Two types occur: simple and ectopic, depending on where they insert into the bladder. The *simple ureterocele* results from dilation of only the distalmost end of the ureter and produces a filling defect resembling a cobra-head in the contrast-filled bladder (Fig. 9.22). An *ectopic ureterocele* is the masslike, dilated submucosal distal portion of an ectopic ureter, usually resulting from a duplicated collecting system. Ectopic ureteroceles appear as sausage-shaped filling defects in the contrast-filled bladder (Fig. 9.23). On US, they have a similar appearance.

Posterior Urethral Valves

Posterior urethral valves are considered the most common cause of urethral obstruction in male children. This abnormality obstructs the flow of urine out of the bladder and frequently results in impaired renal function in as many as one-third of patients with the disorder. The disorder may be initially diagnosed with prenatal ultrasound, particularly when the obstruction is severe and results in oligohydramnios. On a VCUG or retrograde urethrogram, the classic appearance is that of dilation of the posterior urethra producing the *"spinnaker sail" sign* (Fig. 9.24).

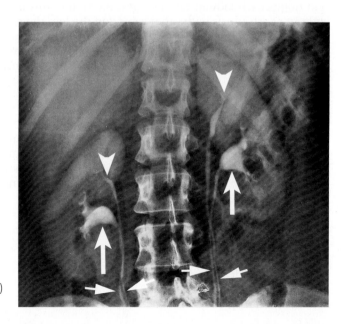

Figure 9.20   Duplication of the renal collecting system.   AP radiograph during an IVU shows two collecting systems in each kidney; in this example, the superior collecting systems (*arrowheads*) are smaller than the inferior collecting systems (*large arrows*). This duplication resulted in two ureters for each kidney that extended distally (*small arrows*) to the ureterovesical junction (not shown on this image).

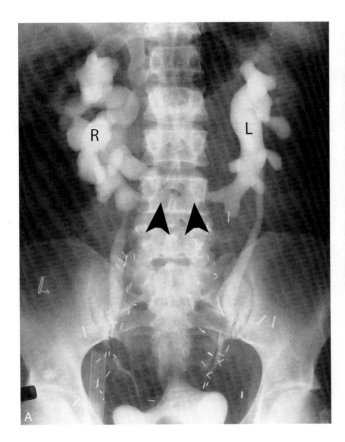

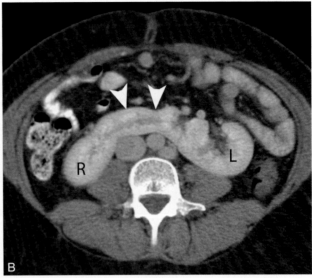

Figure 9.21   Horseshoe kidney.   A. IVU shows excreted contrast material filling the mildly distended right (*R*) and left (*L*) renal collecting systems of a horseshoe kidney. The inferior poles of the collecting systems are oriented medially and joined across midline (*arrowheads*). **B.** CT image shows the isthmus (*arrowheads*) crossing the midline and bridging the right (*R*) and left (*L*) moieties of the horseshoe kidney.

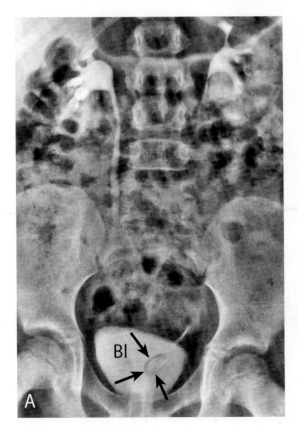

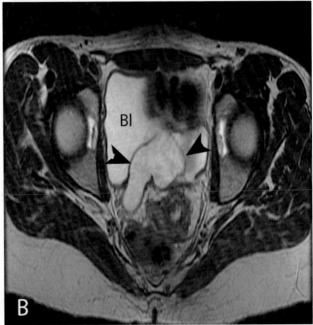

Figure 9.22   Simple ureterocele.   A. AP radiograph during an IVU shows a simple ureterocele presenting as an ovoid filling defect (*arrows*) in the left aspect of the bladder lumen (*Bl*). The kidneys are normal. **B.** MR image in a different patient shows a larger ureterocele projecting into the right aspect of the bladder (*Bl*) resembling a "cobra head."

Figure 9.23   Ectopic ureterocele.   A. Cystogram shows a large, smoothly marginated filling defect (*arrows*) in the bladder lumen (Bl). **B.** US on another patient shows a large ureterocele (*UC*) projecting into the bladder lumen (*Bl*) and a dilated left ureter (*x*).

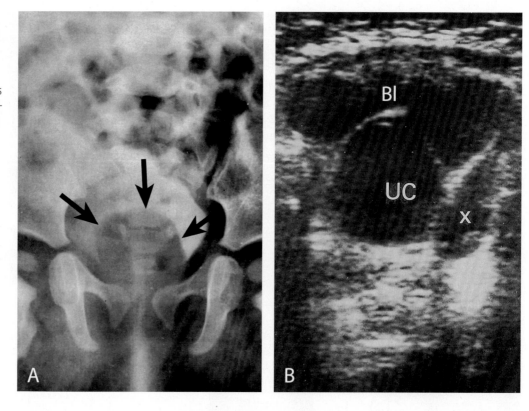

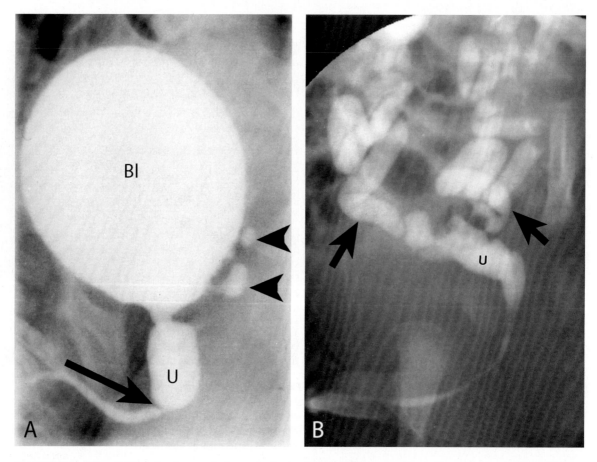

Figure 9.24   Urinary obstruction from posterior urethral valves in two patients.   A. Cystourethrogram shows the linear defect in the urethral lumen caused by the valve (*arrow*), dilated proximal urethra (*U*), and bladder diverticula (*arrowheads*). **B.** Cystourethrogram in another patient shows the dilated urethra (*U*) and dilated ureters (*arrows*).

Abnormalities of Position, Rotation, and Fusion

There are numerous congenital abnormalities of position, rotation, and fusion. *Renal ectopia* is a term used to denote the abnormal position of one kidney with regard to the other. When the affected kidney is located on the other side of the abdomen (usually beneath the normal kidney), it is termed *crossed-fused renal ectopia*. Renal malrotation is a common and not significant renal abnormality in which the renal hilus becomes directed more medially and slightly more anteriorly than normal. Ureteropelvic obstruction is the most common complication of this condition. *Horseshoe kidney* is the most common type of congenital renal fusion abnormality. The fusion occurs in the lower poles of the two kidneys across the midline, forming an isthmus of functioning renal parenchyma that lies anterior to the aorta and inferior to the vena cava. On urograms, ultrasound, and CT examinations, the fusion is easily recognized by the abnormal orientation of the renal collecting systems as well as by the isthmus itself (see Fig. 9.21). For an in-depth discussion of these and other congenital disorders, consult Dunnick's Textbook of Uroradiology.

Obstructive Lesions

Obstruction of the urinary tract may be either congenital or acquired (several of the congenital causes of obstruction were discussed previously). The acquired variety is more common and is usually the result of urinary calculi (Fig. 9.25). Other causes of

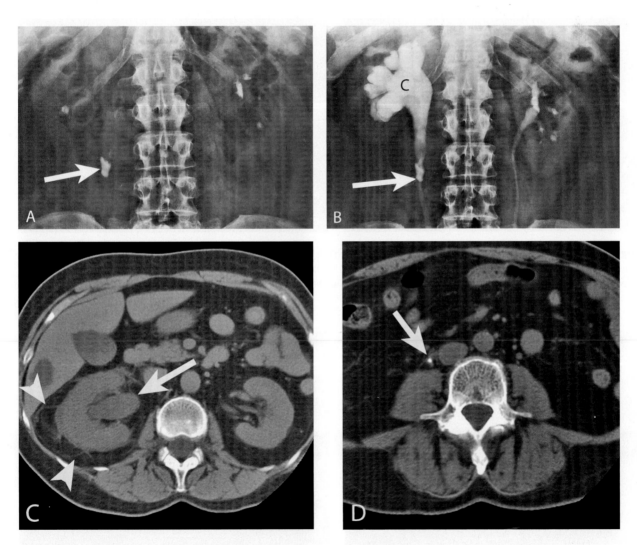

Figure 9.25   Obstructive uropathy due to urinary calculi.   A. Abdominal radiograph shows multiple renal calculi bilaterally; the largest calculus (*arrow*) lies to the right of the transverse process of L3. **B.** IVU image shows hydroureteronephrosis upstream from the large stone (*arrow*), which is located in the proximal ureter. C = renal collecting system. **C.** Noncontrast CT in a different patient shows moderate right hydronephrosis (*arrow*) and perinephric inflammation (*arrowheads*). **D.** More inferiorly, a calculus (*arrow*) is located in the mid right ureter. Note the soft tissue surrounding the calculus (the rim sign) confirming that the calcification is located within the lumen of the ureter.

obstruction include tumor (Fig. 9.26), endometriosis (Fig. 9.27), scarring, and operative manipulation. Regardless of the cause, obstruction produces a series of pathophysiologic changes that result in characteristic radiographic appearances depending on the degree of renal parenchymal destruction.

Hydronephrosis

On CT, acute obstruction results in variable degrees of *hydronephrosis*. After contrast injection, the hydronephrosis is typically accompanied by decreased enhancement ("delayed nephrogram") of the affected kidney. Most urinary stones are well depicted on noncontrast CT and are frequently the cause of hydroureter. Advanced hydronephrosis usually indicates subacute to chronic obstruction. In cases of long-standing advanced hydronephrosis, CT can depict ipsilateral renal parenchymal volume loss. Acute obstruction may also result in alternative drainage of contrast through the renal veins or lymphatics (*pyelovenous* or *pyelolymphatic transflow*, respectively).

US can also readily assess for the presence and degree of collecting system dilatation (Fig. 9.28). US is the procedure of choice for evaluating newborns and infants with palpable abdominal masses, since many such masses are caused by urinary abnormalities.

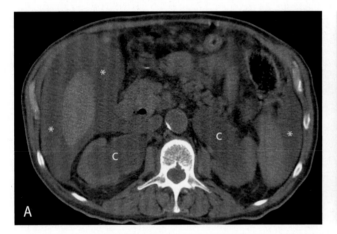
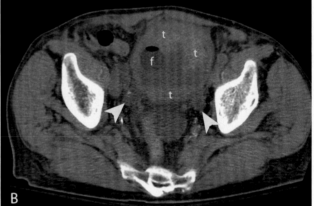

Figure 9.26   Obstructive uropathy due to bladder tumor.   A. Noncontrast CT shows dilated renal collecting systems (*C*) consistent with advanced hydronephrosis bilaterally. Incidental note is made of ascites (*asterisks*). **B.** More inferiorly, the dilated distal ureters (*arrowheads*) are obstructed by an extensive, irregular mass due to transitional cell carcinoma (*t*). A Foley catheter (*f*) is in the lumen of the bladder.

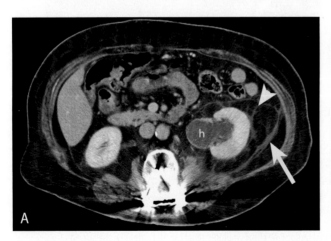
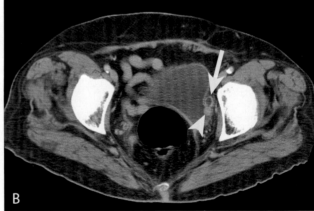

Figure 9.27   Obstructive uropathy due to endometriosis.   A. Contrast-enhanced CT shows left hydronephrosis (*h*). Note thickening of the renal fascia (*arrow*) and perinephric fat stranding (*arrowhead*) due to inflammation. **B.** More inferiorly, a focal enhancing lesion (*arrowhead*) results in obstruction of the distal ureter (*arrow*). Resection of the lesion revealed endometriosis.

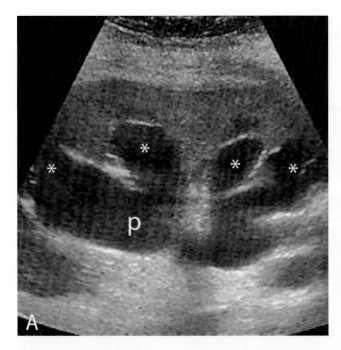
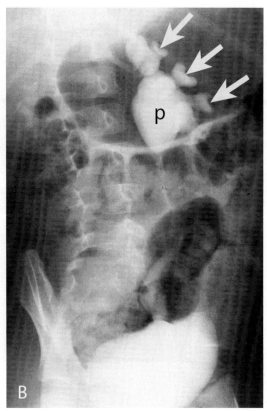

Figure 9.28   Hydronephrosis.   A. Sagittal US shows distension of the renal pelvis (*p*) and the calices (*asterisks*). **B.** In a different patient, an oblique image from an IVU shows a dilated renal pelvis (*p*) and dilated, blunted calyces (*arrows*).

Urinary Calculi

Overall, urinary calculi are the most common causes of obstruction. Even punctate radiopaque calculi are readily diagnosed with noncontrast CT. Nonopaque stones may be detected on delayed, excretory phase CT (CT-urography) as focal filling defects in the ureters. Compared to CT, US has a lower sensitivity in the detection of renal calculi and usually cannot detect ureteral stones unless they are present in the proximal ureter. Most renal calculi appear as focal, bright echogenic foci on US. If sufficiently large, renal calculi can impede transmission of the US beam and cause a "shadow," or linear dark area, in the posterior tissues. Color Doppler can also be applied to detect renal stones; when present, the calculus results in a linear beam of color referred to as *"twinkle artifact"* (Fig. 9.29).

While most renal calculi are composed of calcium oxalate, there is some regional variation. Most calculi contain a mineral deposit embedded in an inorganic matrix. This matrix has been found to be elevated in the urine of patients with hyperparathyroidism, renal infection, patients taking thiazide diuretics, and patients undergoing steroid therapy in an amount that ranges from 3 to 15 times that of normal patients. Urinary calculi may migrate from the kidneys to the ureters and the bladder. Bladder calculi are often the result of long-standing infection and/or presence of a foreign body. Large renal calculi that coalesce in hydronephrotic collecting systems are called *staghorn calculi*, due to their branched, antler-like appearance (Fig. 9.30).

Nephrocalcinosis

Urinary calculi must be differentiated from nephrocalcinosis, a pathophysiologic condition in which calcium is deposited within renal tissue. Nephrocalcinosis results from diseases that elevate the serum calcium level. Some common causes of nephrocalcinosis include medullary sponge kidney, hyperparathyroidism, renal tubular acidosis, and milk-alkali syndrome. In most instances, the calcification is limited to the distal convoluted tubules and appears as fine, stippled deposits on CT that are usually differentiated from stones by their appearance and location (Fig. 9.31). In advanced cases of nephrocalcinosis, US will show increased brightness or echogenicity of the renal medulla, sometimes appearing as numerous ringlike structures.

Figure 9.29   Renal calculus shown by US. A. Sagittal US image shows a subtle renal calculus (*arrow*) that is nearly isoechoic to the renal sinus fat. A mild degree of posterior shadowing (*arrowheads*) helps to corroborate the presence of a calculus. **B.** Same image after application of color Doppler shows a tail of disorganized color posterior to the stone (*arrowhead*), consistent with "twinkle artifact."

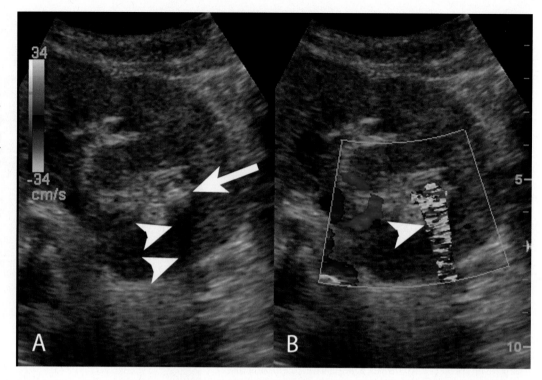

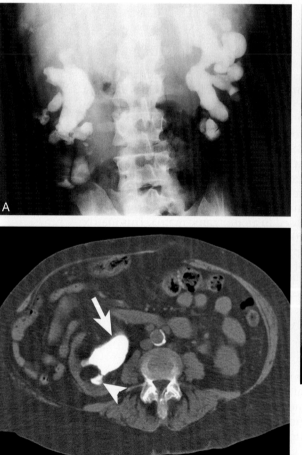

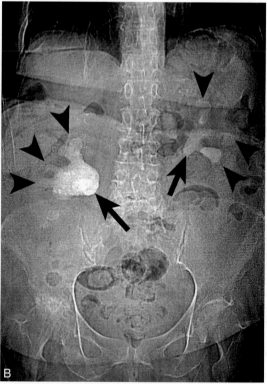

Figure 9.30   Staghorn calculi.   A. Radiograph shows bilateral staghorn calculi. **B.** CT scout radiograph on another patient shows bilateral staghorn calculi filling the renal pelvis (*arrows*) and extending into the calyces (*arrowheads*). **C.** Noncontrast CT image shows the large staghorn calculus filling the right renal pelvis (*arrow*) and extending into some of the calyces (*arrowhead*). No intravenous contrast was injected in any of these patients.

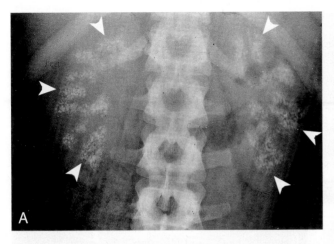
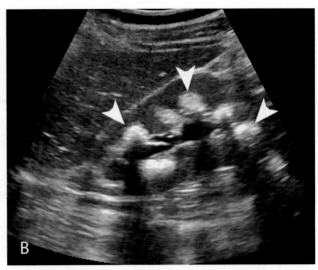

Figure 9.31   Nephrocalcinosis.   A. Radiograph shows deposition of fine calcium (*arrowheads*) within the medullary pyramids of both kidneys. **B.** Sagittal US image shows extensive calcification in the medullary pyramids often referred to as "medullary rings" (*arrowheads*) due to medullary sponge kidney.

Urinary Tract Infection

Infections of the urinary tract are common and are often encountered as a complication of obstruction. *Acute pyelonephritis* may be difficult to recognize with imaging studies because of the subtle changes it produces. Rarely, infection may be suggested on a radiograph or US if the kidney is swollen, although this is a nonspecific finding. With application of color Doppler US evaluation, regions of decreased parenchymal perfusion increase diagnostic confidence. However, in most cases of acute uncomplicated pyelonephritis, the US examination is normal. While many cases of acute pyelonephritis are diagnosed clinically, the preferred imaging modality is contrast-enhanced CT. Common CT findings include infiltration of the perinephric fat and patchy renal parenchymal enhancement, especially at the polar regions of the kidney. Additionally, CT can evaluate for the presence of a renal abscess (Fig. 9.32) and aid in planning percutaneous catheter drainage. In cases of recurrent or chronic pyelonephritis, the imaging findings include marked cortical irregularity, focal cortical scarring, clubbed irregular calyces, and loss of renal volume (Fig. 9.33). In some cases, infection can be limited to the renal collecting system referred to as *pyelitis*. In most cases, the inflammation and infection are successfully treated with antibiotics. However, complications of infection in the collecting system include *pyonephrosis*, abscess, gas collections (emphysematous infections) (Fig. 9.34), and *papillary necrosis*. The latter condition results from anoxia of the renal papilla, causing necrosis and sloughing of the papilla. While the imaging presentation can be variable, characteristic findings include a filling defect in a calyx, a ring of contrast surrounding a filling defect, an abnormal blunted calyx (Fig. 9.35), and poor excretion of contrast by the affected kidney. In addition to the kidneys, MR or CT urography allow identification of focal noncalcified filling defects in the urinary tract which raises concern for malignancy. Other differential diagnostic considerations include clot, infectious debris, and sloughed papilla.

> Urinary tract infections are common and are often the result of obstruction. In most cases of acute uncomplicated pyelonephritis, the US examination is normal.

Renal Tuberculosis

Renal tuberculosis is rare in the United States, but may be encountered in immunocompromised patients, such as those affected by acquired immune deficiency syndrome (AIDS). Initially, renal tuberculosis may produce nonspecific changes such as papillary necrosis. With progression of the disease, additional findings of stricture of an infundibulum, calyceal amputation, and cavitation may occur. Tuberculosis also causes ureteral strictures. A combination of renal and ureteral abnormalities, such as coexisting strictures,

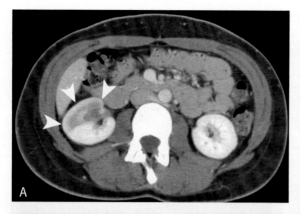

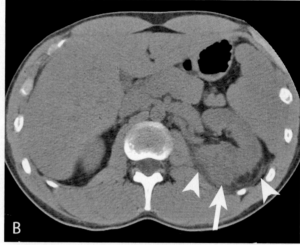

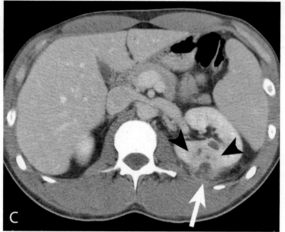

Figure 9.32   Acute bacterial pyelonephritis.   A. Contrast-enhanced CT image shows a region of poor enhancement (*arrowheads*) in the anterior aspect of the right kidney, consistent with acute pyelonephritis. **B.** In a different patient, noncontrast CT image demonstrates infiltration of the perinephric fat (*arrowheads*) and an irregular, ill-defined margin of the posterior aspect of the left kidney (*arrow*). **C.** After administration of IV contrast material, a region of poor enhancement (*arrowheads*) represents edema and inflammation from the pyelonephritis. An abscess (*arrow*) causes the renal contour abnormality. Note that there are several small abscesses in the more anterior aspect of the renal parenchyma.

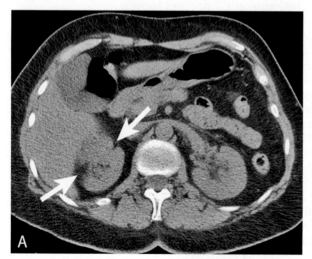

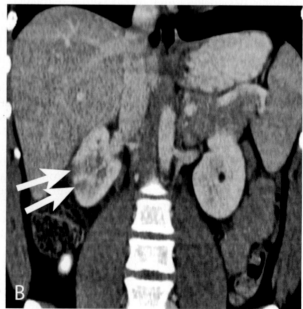

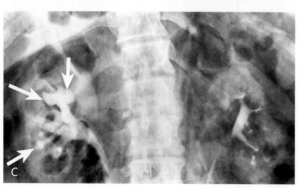

Figure 9.33   Chronic pyelonephritis in three patients.
A. Noncontrast axial CT image shows relative atrophy of the right kidney and distortion of the superior pole due to regions of scarring (*arrows*). **B.** Contrast-enhanced coronal reconstructed CT image demonstrates an atrophic right kidney with bands of poor perfusion (*arrows*) due to scarring from chronic pyelonephritis. **C.** Radiograph during IVU shows blunted, dilated calyces in the right kidney (*arrows*) due to chronic pyelonephritis.

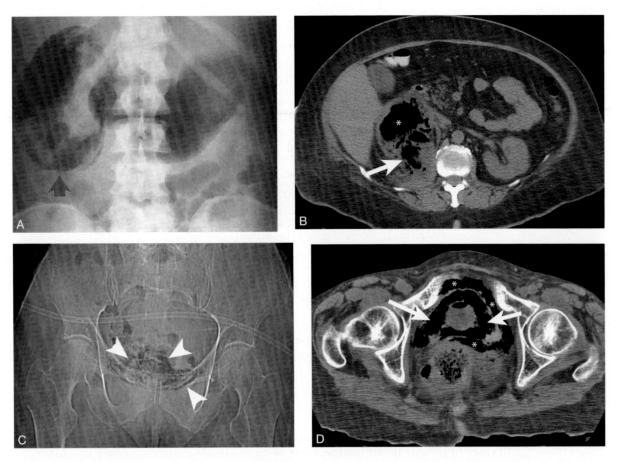

Figure 9.34   Emphysematous infections in three diabetic patients.   A. Detail of a frontal radiograph shows a reniform gas collection on the right (*arrow*). **B.** Noncontrast CT image in a different patient demonstrates extensive gas in the renal collecting system (*asterisk*) that is dissecting into the parenchyma (*arrow*). **C.** CT scout radiograph of a third patient shows an irregular gas collection in the central pelvis (*arrowheads*). **D.** Subsequent CT image reveals extensive gas within the wall of the urinary bladder (*arrows*) and extending into the space surrounding the bladder (*asterisks*).

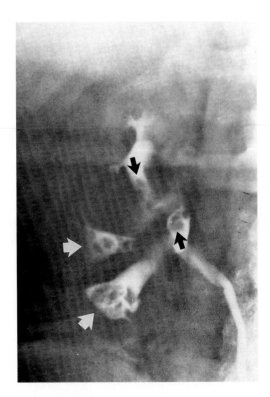

**Figure 9.35   Renal papillary necrosis.   Multiple filling defects (*arrows*) represent sloughed papillae within the collecting system.

Figure 9.36   Renal tuberculosis.   Radiograph during an IVU shows a small, nonfunctioning right kidney (*arrows*) containing calcific debris ("putty kidney") due to chronic infection with tuberculosis. Note normal enhancement and excretion in the unaffected left kidney (*arrowheads*).

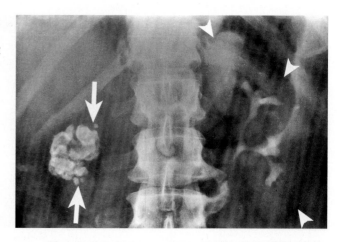

suggests the diagnosis. The end stage of renal tuberculosis is a small, shrunken, nonfunctioning kidney that often contains calcific debris, referred to as *"putty kidney"* (Fig. 9.36).

▶ The end stage of renal tuberculosis is a small, shrunken, nonfunctioning kidney referred to as "putty kidney."

Cystitis

Inflammation of the urinary bladder, referred to as *cystitis*, typically manifests as wall thickening and infiltration of the surrounding fat during US, CT, or MRI examinations. In cases of chronic inflammation, there is more extensive thickening and irregularity of the wall secondary to muscular and mucosal hypertrophy. Urinary tract obstruction and ureterovesical reflux in association with chronic cystitis may be evaluated by diuretic renal scintigraphy and radionuclide voiding cystourethrography.

Masses—Cysts and Tumors

Masses affecting the kidneys can arise from the renal parenchyma, renal collecting systems, or perinephric structures. They may result in extrinsic mass effect. Differential diagnostic considerations for masses affecting the kidneys include cysts, tumors, infection, inflammation, or fibrosis. US, CT, and MRI can all be used to detect and characterize a renal mass. Regardless of whether a mass is encountered in a symptomatic patient or as an incidental finding, the initial evaluation primarily consists of determining whether it is cystic or solid and further classifying cystic lesions as simple or complex.

Renal Cysts

Renal cysts are common in older patients and are found in a high percentage of autopsies. Renal cysts are usually asymptomatic and are frequently encountered as incidental findings on cross-sectional imaging examinations. With US, the hallmarks of a simple cyst (see Fig. 9.4) include sharp borders due to a thin, nearly imperceptible wall, a homogeneously anechoic internal composition (appearing as uniformly black), and the presence of *"through transmission"* (also sometimes referred to as "posterior enhancement") of the US beam which appears as a region of brightness beneath the cyst. The phrase "through transmission" refers to an US artifact that occurs due to the increased speed of sound through an area of low impedance, such as the water consistency of a simple cyst. This artifact is key in differentiating a cystic from a solid lesion during an US examination.

The CT appearance of a simple renal cyst includes a smooth, well-marginated, homogenously low-density (similar to water density) structure of variable size. Density measurements on CT are given in Hounsfield units (HU), and simple cysts typically have low HU ranging between 0 and 15. Renal cysts appear as spherical, near water-density lesions within the renal parenchyma or bulges along the cortical margin; frequently, a thin, beak-like collection of contrast material representing compressed parenchyma may be seen along the margin (see Fig. 9.10). Simple cysts do not enhance after IV injection of contrast material (Fig. 9.37). A cyst may also arise within, or displace, the renal collecting system, referred to as a renal sinus cyst (Fig. 9.38). On MRI, renal cysts have homogeneously low T1 signal, homogeneously high T2 signal (similar to that of water of cerebrospinal fluid), and lack enhancement after IV contrast administration. However, some of these cysts may appear dense due to internal hemorrhage or proteinaceous contents (Fig. 9.39). Renal cysts may be innumerable in some genetic disorders. In autosomal dominant *polycystic kidney disease*, renal cysts may result in nephromegaly due to near-complete replacement of the renal cortex (Fig. 9.40).

Solid Renal Tumors

A solid renal tumor has a considerably different imaging appearance (Table 9.2). With US, a solid mass has internal echoes, or variable shades of gray or degrees of brightness (Fig. 9.41 and see Fig. 9.5A). This is contrary to the anechoic composition (uniformly black) of a simple renal cyst (see Fig. 9.4). On noncontrast CT, a solid mass has higher density than a renal cyst; typically a solid mass measures between 30 and 50 HU, similar

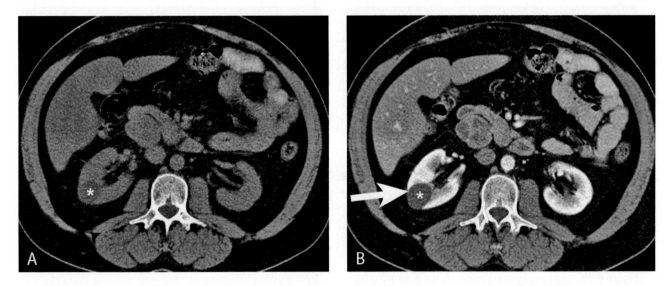

Figure 9.37 Simple renal cyst shown with CT. A. Noncontrast CT image shows a well-marginated, low-density cyst (*asterisk*) in the posterior aspect of the right kidney. **B.** After IV contrast injection, there is no contrast enhancement within the cyst (*asterisk*). Note the beaklike interface between the cyst and the renal cortex (*arrow*).

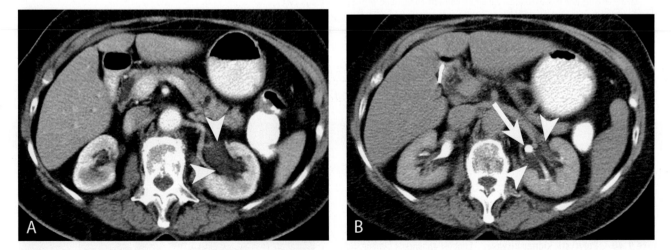

Figure 9.38 Renal sinus cysts. A. Contrast-enhanced CT image shows lobulated, low-density structures (*arrowheads*) in the left renal hilum due to renal sinus cysts; it is difficult to differentiate the cysts from hydronephrosis. **B.** Excretory phase CT image shows contrast excreted into the nondilated renal pelvis (*arrow*) and the adjacent renal sinus cysts (*arrowheads*).

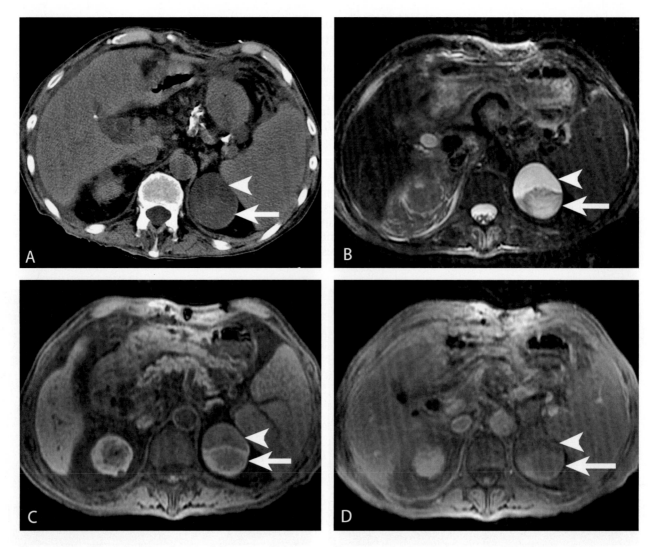

Figure 9.39   Hemorrhagic renal cyst.   A. Noncontrast CT shows a round lesion extending from the superior pole of the left kidney. The anterior component (*arrowhead*) of the lesion has low density while the posterior component (*arrow*) has higher density, approaching that of soft tissue. The patient could not receive iodinated contrast material due to a contrast allergy. **B.** T2-weighted MRI shows high signal in the anterior component (arrowhead) and heterogeneous, intermediate signal in the posterior component. **C.** T1-weighted MRI shows low signal in the anterior component (*arrowhead*) and high signal in the posterior component (*arrow*). **D.** After administration of IV gadolinium contrast material, there was no enhancement in the lesion. The signal characteristics and lack of contrast enhancement were compatible with a hemorrhagic cyst.

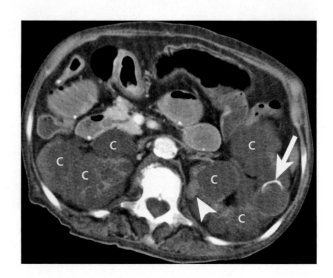

Figure 9.40   Polycystic kidney disease.   Contrast-enhanced CT image shows large kidneys with innumerable cysts (*C*) replacing the renal parenchyma. Note that some of the cysts have increased density (*arrowhead*) due to proteinaceous or hemorrhage contents while others have peripheral, curvilinear calcification (*arrow*).

Table 9.2 **COMMON IMAGING CHARACTERISTICS FOR RENAL CYST AND RENAL CELL CARCINOMA**

Examination	Renal Cyst	Renal Cell Carcinoma
Borders	Smooth, well-marginated	Ill-defined, lobular
US		
• Echogenicity	Anechoic	Internal echoes, solid
• Doppler	No flow	Usually internal flow
CT		
• Density	Low	Soft tissue, necrosis
• Enhancement	None	Heterogeneous
MRI		
• Signal intensity	Low T1, high T2	Variable, heterogeneous
• Enhancement	None	Heterogeneous

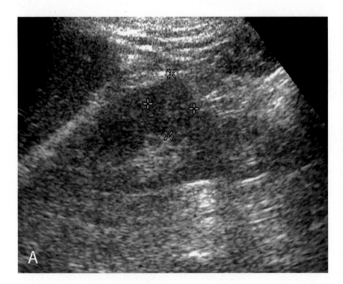 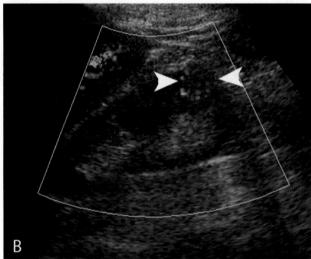

Figure 9.41 **Renal cell carcinoma shown with US.** **A.** Sagittal US image shows a solid lesion causing a contour abnormality of the midportion of the kidney. **B.** Color Doppler image shows flow within the solid lesion *arrowheads*).

to the density of soft tissue (see Fig. 9.11A). While a cyst is typically smoothly marginated, a solid mass is often lobulated or ill defined, sometimes grossly distorting or invading the renal architecture (see Figs. 9.11**B** and 9.12). Following contrast injection, many solid masses, such as renal cell carcinomas, are often hypervascular and show regions of heterogeneous enhancement (Fig. 9.42); the heterogeneity is often due to regions of necrosis, calcification, or variable tumor histologic grade. Furthermore, CT may show evidence of vascular invasion by a large tumor (see Fig. 9.11**C** and **D**).With MRI, solid renal masses have intermediate T1 signal (similar to that of skeletal muscle) and moderately increased T2 signal that is considerably less bright than that observed with simple renal cysts (Fig. 9.43). Similar to CT, MRI reveals that solid renal masses often show hypervascular, heterogeneous enhancement (Fig. 9.44) after contrast injection and potential vascular invasion.

Wilms Tumor

In adults, the overwhelming majority of solid renal masses are malignant and are due to renal cell carcinoma. Occasionally, a solid renal mass is due to a benign etiology, such as

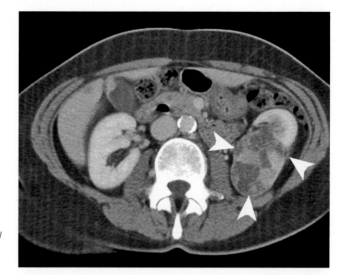

Figure 9.42   Renal cell carcinoma with necrosis.   Contrast-enhanced CT shows a heterogeneously enhancing mass (*arrowheads*) replacing the majority of the left kidney. The pathology specimen revealed several areas of necrosis in the tumor.

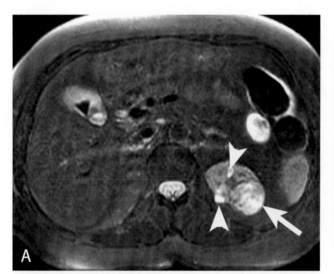

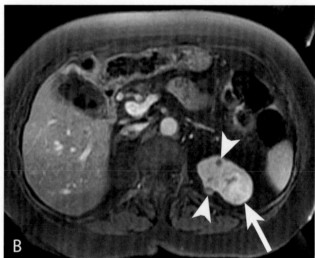

Figure 9.43   Renal cell carcinoma and cysts.   A. T2-weighted MRI with fat suppression shows strong, homogeneous signal in two simple cortical cysts (*arrowheads*) and heterogeneous, intermediate signal in a renal cell carcinoma (*arrow*) along the dorsal aspect of the left kidney. **B.** Post contrast T1-weighted MRI shows no enhancement in the cysts (*arrowheads*) and brisk enhancement in the tumor (*arrow*).

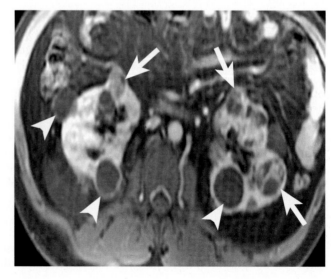

Figure 9.44   Renal cell carcinoma and cysts in a patient with tuberous sclerosis.   Contrast-enhanced T1-weighted MRI with fat suppression shows numerous cysts with homogeneously low signal and no enhancement (*arrowheads*). There are several heterogeneously enhancing lesions (*arrows*) that proved to be renal cell carcinomas at surgery.

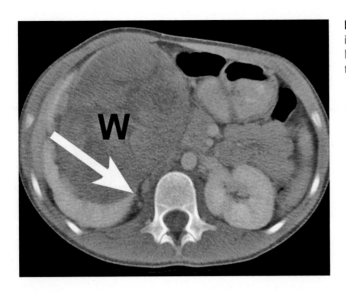

Figure 9.45   Wilms tumor. Contrast-enhanced CT image shows a large right renal mass (*W*) due to Wilms tumor. Note the "beak" of renal parenchyma at the junction of the tumor with normal kidney (*arrow*).

oncocytoma. However, most solid renal masses are treated with surgery or ablative therapy due to overlap between malignant and benign tumors. In children, Wilms tumor is the most common solid abdominal mass of early childhood and the most common renal malignant neoplasm, accounting for approximately 10% of childhood malignancies. The typical Wilms tumor manifests as a large, heterogeneously enhancing mass on CT and MRI. Due to its size, the origin of the mass may be difficult to determine. However, renal tumors result in a distinctive "beak" of parenchyma at the tumor–kidney interface. This imaging finding serves to differentiate Wilms tumor (Fig. 9.45) from extrarenal masses, such as neuroblastoma.

▶ In adults, the majority of solid renal masses are malignant.
▶ In children, Wilms tumor is the most common solid abdominal mass of early childhood and the most common malignant renal neoplasm.

Complex Cystic Renal Lesion

Not all renal lesions are able to be definitively categorized as simple cysts or solid masses. These intermediate types are generally referred to as *complex cystic renal lesions.* Complex cystic renal lesions require close imaging and clinical follow-up due to their variable risk of malignancy. In general, a complex cystic lesion can be defined as a lesion with a cystic component and a variable degree of internal septations, wall calcifications, internal echoes, or soft tissue. Typically, complex cystic lesions with an enhancing soft tissue component are treated with surgery while those with less concerning features can be followed with imaging after their risk of malignancy is stratified. Radiologists often stratify the estimated risk of malignancy for a renal lesion by using the Bosniak classification. This classification is used to triage patients for resection of suspicious renal lesions and strongly correlates imaging features with pathologic outcome. In select cases, percutaneous biopsy of a renal lesion may be needed prior to surgery or ablative therapy. Biopsies can be performed by US or CT guidance using local anesthesia or sedation in the radiology department.

Adrenals

The adrenal glands, while technically not part of the urinary tract, are briefly discussed due to their close apposition to the kidneys. Adrenal pathology is mostly due to neoplastic disease. The most common benign neoplasm is an adenoma. Most adenomas are lipid-rich and are detected as an incidental finding during abdominal or chest CT. On CT, adenomas are smoothly marginated nodules consisting of low density. During MRI, lipid-rich adenomas show signal loss on out of phase T1-weighted images (Fig. 9.46). In cases of lipid-poor adenomas, multiphase contrast-enhanced CT can be performed to calculate the contrast washout and arrive at a definitive diagnosis. Metastases from

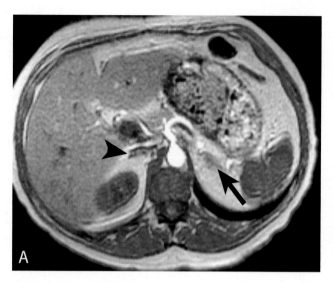

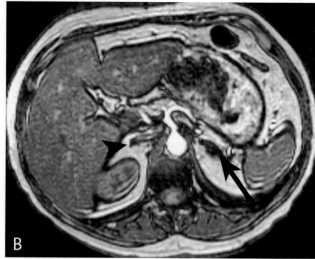

Figure 9.46   Adrenal adenoma.   A. In-phase T1-weighted MRI shows a small left adrenal nodule (*arrow*) with intermediate signal. **B.** Out-of-phase T1-weighted MRI shows loss of signal in the left adrenal nodule (*arrow*), consistent with a lipid-rich adenoma. Note that the normal right adrenal gland (*arrowheads* in **A** and **B**) maintains intermediate signal in both phases.

various primary malignancies can affect the adrenal glands. Adrenal metastases have variable imaging appearances, but typically consist of an irregularly marginated or lobular heterogeneous mass (Fig. 9.47). Metastases do not show loss of signal on out of phase images during MRI.

 ▶ The most common benign adrenal tumor is an adenoma.

Neuroblastoma

Neuroblastoma is a malignant tumor of primitive neural crest cells (neuroblasts). Neuroblastoma accounts for approximately 10% of childhood neoplasms and is second only to Wilms tumor in incidence of malignant abdominal masses in children. It may arise anywhere along the sympathetic chain or in the adrenal medulla. On CT or MRI, neuroblastoma presents as a large, heterogeneously enhancing suprarenal mass (Fig. 9.48).

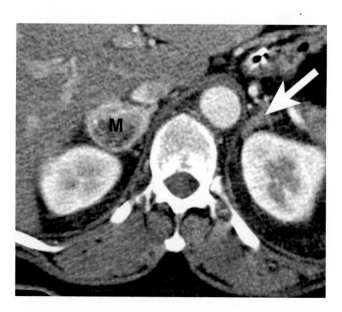

Figure 9.47   Adrenal metastasis.   Contrast-enhanced T1-weighted MRI shows a heterogeneously enhancing mass (*M*) in the right adrenal gland. Note the normal left adrenal gland (*arrow*).

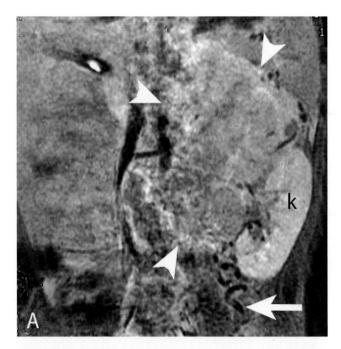

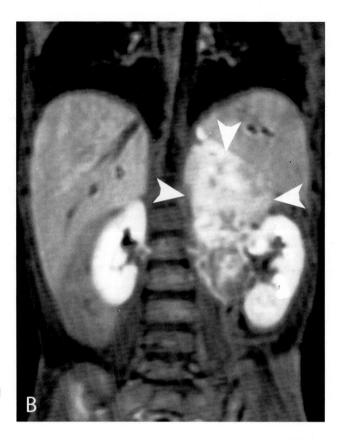

Figure 9.48   Neuroblastoma.   A. Coronal T1-weighted image shows a large left suprarenal mass (*arrowheads*) displacing the kidney (*k*) laterally. Note the serpentine dilatation of the ureteral vein (*arrow*). **B.** Contrast-enhanced coronal T1-weighted image shows the brisk enhancement of the tumor (*arrowheads*). Note the normal renal enhancement.

Neuroblastoma results in displacement of the kidney and does not cause the "beak sign" with the kidney; the imaging findings are helpful in differentiating it from Wilms tumor. Neuroblastoma results in metastases to the lungs, bones, and liver early in the disease course. After initial diagnosis, radionuclide imaging with I 123 metaiodobenzylguanidine (MIBG) is used for initial staging and restaging of neuroblastoma since MIBG imaging is specific for malignancies of neuroendocrine origin. In current practice, PET studies are also being investigated for use in imaging of neuroblastoma.

> ▶ Neuroblastoma accounts for approximately 10% of childhood tumors and is second only to Wilms tumor in incidence of malignant abdominal masses.

Vascular Lesions

Renal vascular lesions include aneurysm, pseudoaneurysm, vasculitis, stenosis, and occlusion. The imaging findings of aneurysm and pseudoaneurysm include a bulbous outpouching of contrast enhancement contiguous with the renal artery. Vasculitides affecting the renal arteries can result in luminal irregularity, wall thickening, and a beaded appearance of the vessel. Occlusion of the renal artery is rare but can be due to embolism, thrombosis, and dissection. Renal artery stenosis is an uncommon cause of hypertension, affecting approximately 1% to 4% of hypertensive patients. The most common cause of renal artery stenosis is atherosclerotic plaque occurring near the vessel origin. However, some vasculitides, such as fibromuscular dysplasia, may also result in renovascular hypertension. The primary screening examination for patients with suspected renovascular hypertension is Doppler US (see Fig. 9.6). US is noninvasive, lacks ionizing radiation, and can rapidly determine if there is compromised renal blood flow, and thereby identify the patients who require further imaging by CT or MR angiography. However, conventional US evaluation of renal artery stenosis is plagued by variable sensitivity due to artifacts, multiple renal arteries, and operator inexperience. The nuclear renogram is an alternative initial screening examination. Nuclear renography uses the chelate technetium 99m diethylenetriamine pentaacetic acid (DTPA). Scintigraphic images are obtained before and after administration of an angiotensin-converting enzyme (ACE) inhibitor such as captopril (orally) or enalapril (intravenously). These drugs enhance the discrepancy in renal uptake and excretion between the normal and abnormal kidney in patients with unilateral renal artery stenosis. In the typical radionuclide renogram, the isotopes are rapidly injected intravenously after a scintillation camera with computer-defined regions of interest has been placed over each kidney to allow for comparison. Computer-acquired data generate the renogram curves and enhance the findings. The normal curve has three phases (Fig. 9.49): a *vascular phase* with a rapid slope; a *secretory or functional phase*, usually 2.5 to 4.5 minutes; and an *excretory phase*, during which the labeled material is excreted. Generally, a plateau is reached in 20 minutes. If the initial study is normal or near normal, the ACE inhibitor is administered to the patient and the isotope study is repeated after reinjection of the radionuclides. A positive study shows prolongation of the second phase (Fig. 9.50). Other criteria include delayed peaking of counts over a kidney, delayed drainage from a kidney, and differences in renal size.

> ▶ Renal artery stenosis is an uncommon cause of hypertension, affecting approximately 1% to 4% of hypertensive patients.

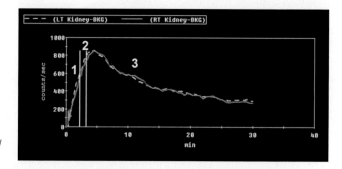

Figure 9.49   Normal radioisotope renogram.   (*1*) Vascular phase. (*2*) Secretory or functional phase. (*3*) Excretory phase. The graph for each kidney superimposes.

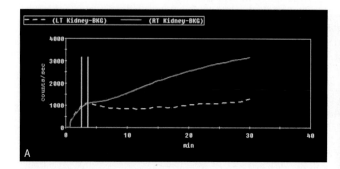

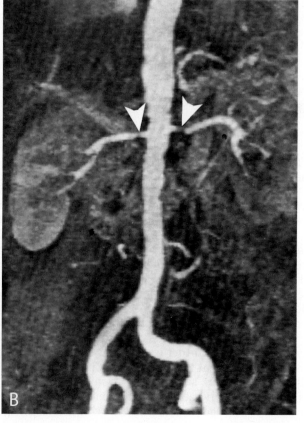

Figure 9.50   Renovascular hypertension caused by stenosis of the renal arteries.   A. Abnormal radioisotope renogram shows poor function in the right kidney (*solid line*) and no function on the left (*broken line*). **B.** MR angiogram shows stenosis in both renal arteries (*arrowheads*). The left-sided stenosis is more advanced than the right, reflecting the changes in the renogram. No IV contrast was used for this examination.

Trauma

Urinary tract trauma can be due to both blunt and penetrating injuries to the abdomen and pelvis. While the inferior ribs, spine, psoas muscles, and perinephric fat provide some protection to the kidney, sufficient force can result in a multitude of renal injuries. Examples of renal injury include parenchymal contusion, laceration, shattering, active hemorrhage, perinephric hematoma, vascular avulsion, and disruption of the ureteropelvic junction. Contrast-enhanced CT is the preferred imaging modality to evaluate for the many types of renal injury (Fig. 9.51). The kidneys and perinephric spaces should be thoroughly searched for findings of active hemorrhage, such as ill-defined regions of contrast extravasation or increasing size of a hematoma on subsequent evaluation. Additionally, perinephric fluid collections should be evaluated on a delayed, excretory phase of imaging to assess for leakage of contrast from an injured renal collecting system or ureter (see Fig. 9.9C). The urinary bladder and male urethra are frequently injured as a result of fractures of the pelvis. The proximity of those structures to the pubic bones makes them particularly vulnerable to shearing injuries or puncture by a shard of displaced bone. Fluoroscopic urethrography is used to evaluate for a traumatic urethral injury while fluoroscopic cystography (Fig. 9.52) and CT cystography are the preferred methods of evaluating the bladder.

Extrinsic Compression

Pathologic processes in adjacent organs can result in altered morphology of the urinary tract. Examples include displacement of a kidney by a suprarenal mass; displacement of a ureter by retroperitoneal adenopathy, ureteral compression, and secondary obstruction; compression of the bladder by pelvic masses; and elevation of the bladder floor by an enlarged prostate (see Fig. 9.19). CT, US, and MRI can all evaluate the degree of extrinsic mass effect upon the urinary tract; CT provides a rapid, global assessment of the morphology of the urinary tract and the origins of the extrinsic compression (Fig. 9.53).

Renal Transplantation

Renal transplantation is a common surgical procedure for patients with end-stage renal disease. US is the preferred imaging modality for evaluation of the transplanted kidney because it can quickly evaluate for hydronephrosis, parenchymal lesions, vascular stenosis,

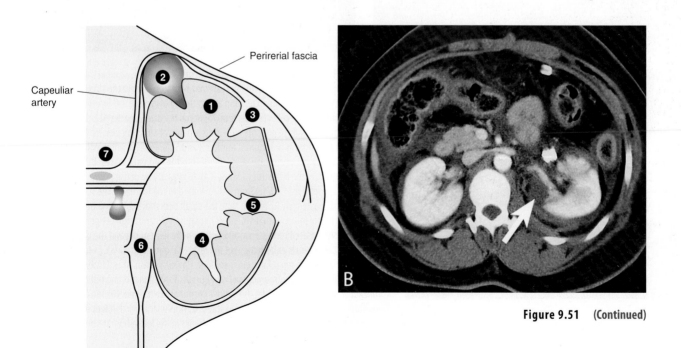

Figure 9.51 **(Continued)**

A

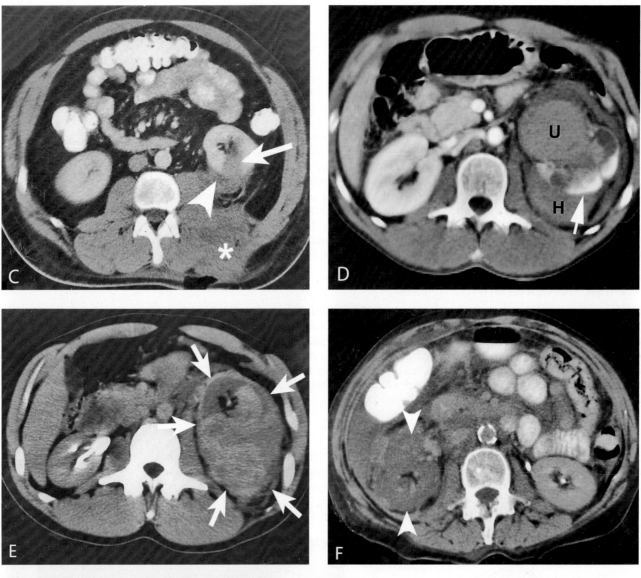

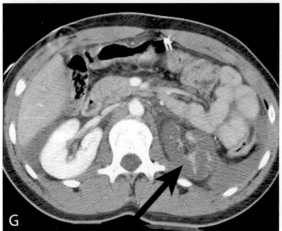

Figure 9.51   Renal trauma.   A. Drawing of various forms of renal trauma: (*1*) Renal contusion. (*2*) Laceration with intracapsular hematoma (note the stretching of the capsular artery). (*3*) Laceration extending across the renal capsule. (*4*) Internal laceration communicating with the collecting system. (*5*) Renal fracture ("shattered kidney"). (*6*) Pelvic rupture, usually in patients with ureteropelvic obstructing lesions. (*7*) Vascular pedicle injury (thrombosis or rupture). Injuries 3 and 5 generally result in enlargement of the renal contour with extensive hemorrhage into the perirenal spaces. **B.** CT image shows a contusion of the left kidney manifest as an area of low density (*arrow*). **C.** Renal laceration on the left (*solid arrow*) from a stab wound to the left flank. The site of the stab wound is visible posteriorly (*asterisk*). Note the small perirenal hematoma (*arrowhead*). **D.** Massive left renal injury with perinephric hematoma (*H*) and large peripelvic urinoma (*U*). There is extravasated contrast (*arrow*) between the hematoma and the urinoma. **E.** Shattered kidney. There is enlargement of the left renal outline (*arrows*). Even though this is an enhanced scan, no renal function is evident. However, areas of enhancement within the renal capsule represent fragments of renal tissue. **F.** Nonfunctioning right kidney (*arrowheads*) caused by renal vein thrombosis secondary to trauma. The left kidney functions normally on this contrast-enhanced study. **G.** Nonfunctioning left kidney (*arrow*) caused by renal artery thrombosis. The dense streaks in the left kidney are the result of contrast that refluxed through the renal vein.

and adjacent fluid collections (Fig. 9.54). The main strength of US in the evaluation of a renal transplant is its ability to provide rapid detection and quantification of arterial anastomotic stenosis. Additionally, the vascular data obtained during Doppler evaluation of the transplant can be used to detect rejection and identify those patients who should undergo biopsy. US guidance plays a critical role during biopsy by allowing selection of glomeruli-rich cortex and by minimizing vascular complications. US guidance is also used during catheter drainage of postoperative fluid collections. CT, MRI, and nuclear scintigraphy scan are imaging alternatives that can be used to further evaluate an abnormality detected with US.

Vesicoureteral Reflux

Vesicoureteral reflux (VUR) is not infrequently detected in patients (usually children) undergoing evaluation for recurrent urinary tract infection. VUR is most frequently observed during voiding and may be demonstrated by either the VCUG or radionuclide cystogram. The latter study has a lower radiation dose and is the preferred screening examination in children whose siblings have a history of reflux and in patients receiving a follow-up examination. Unrecognized and untreated VUR may result in renal scarring and compromised function.

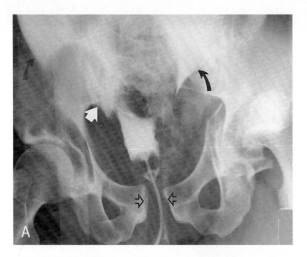

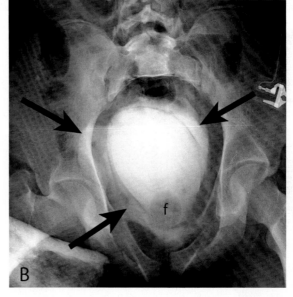

Figure 9.52   Pelvic fractures with bladder rupture.   A. The patient has suffered a severe pelvic injury with dysraphism of the pubic symphysis (*open arrows*) and a comminuted fracture of the left acetabulum with hip dislocation. This cystogram demonstrates extraperitoneal (*white arrow*) as well as intraperitoneal (*curved arrows*) extravasation of contrast from the ruptured bladder. **B.** Another patient with disruption of the pubic symphysis and fractures of the left pubic arches. Contrast is seen outside the bladder (*arrows*). *f* = Foley catheter.

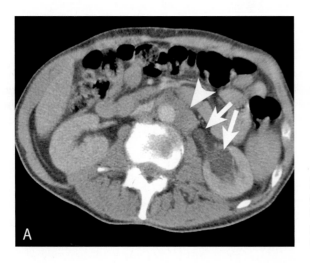

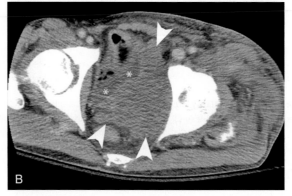

Figure 9.53   Retroperitoneal adenopathy.   A. Contrast-enhanced CT shows retroperitoneal adenopathy (*arrowhead*) and left hydronephrosis and hydroureter (*arrows*). **B.** More inferiorly, a large pelvic mass (*arrowheads*) displaces the bladder (*asterisks*). The mass was due to prostate cancer.

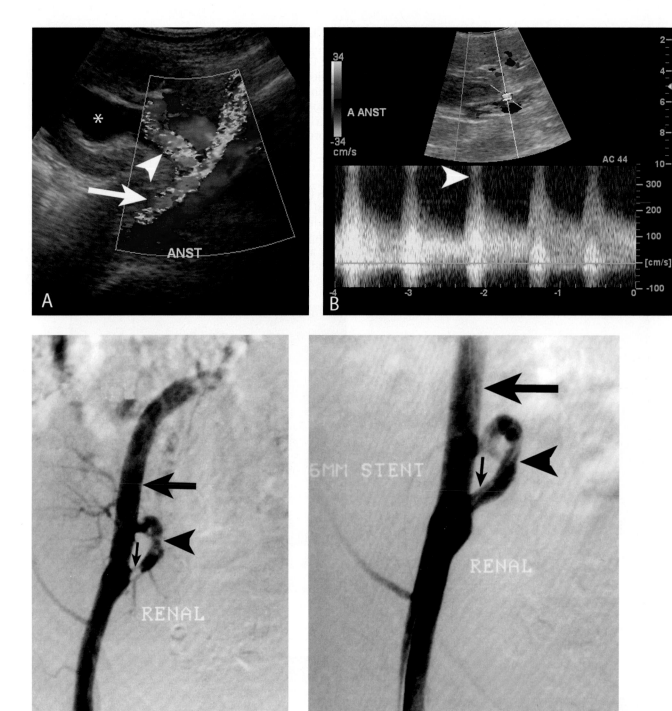

Figure 9.54   Renal artery stenosis in a transplanted kidney.   A. Color Doppler US shows a normal anastomosis between the renal artery *(arrowhead)* and the iliac artery *(arrow)*. The corresponding adjacent venous structures are shown in blue. Note hydronephrosis of the transplanted kidney *(asterisk)*. **B.** Spectral Doppler image shows focally elevated velocity *(arrowhead)* at the arterial anastomosis in another patient, consistent with stenosis. **C.** Digital subtraction angiogram shows stenosis of the anastomosis *(small arrow)* between the renal artery *(arrowhead)* and the iliac artery *(large arrow)*. **D.** After placement of a stent, the lumen *(small arrow)* of the transplanted artery is restored.

Summary and Key Points

▶ The urinary tract can be effectively evaluated by various imaging modalities.

▶ IVU, once the mainstay of uroradiology, has been replaced by US, CT, and MRI in the United States.

▶ The diagnostic accuracy of these modalities is high and increases when different modalities are used in combination.

▶ Pathology of the urinary tract can be due to congenital, infectious, inflammatory, traumatic, vascular, and neoplastic etiologies.

▶ Familiarity with the common pathologic abnormalities affecting the urinary tract, their common imaging findings, and their differential diagnoses is an important component of diagnosis, treatment planning, and patient management.

Suggested Additional Reading

Blickman JG. Pediatric Radiology: The Requisites. 3rd Ed. St. Louis, MO: Mosby-Elsevier, 2009:148–194.

Brant WE, Helms CA. Fundamentals of Diagnostic Radiology. 4th Ed. Philadelphia, PA: Lippincott Williams & Wilkins, 2012:796–837.

Donnelly LF, Jones M, O'Hara S, et al. Diagnostic Imaging: Pediatrics. Philadelphia, PA: WB Saunders, 2006.

Dunnick NR, Sandler CM, Newhouse JH. Textbook of Uroradiology. 5th Ed. Philadelphia, PA: Lippincott Williams & Wilkins, 2012.

Federle MP, Jeffrey RB, Anne V. Diagnostic Imaging: Abdomen. Philadelphia, PA: WB Saunders, 2005.

Heller MT, Tublin ME. Detection and characterization of renal masses by ultrasound: a practical guide. Ultrasound Q 2007;23(4):269–278.

Katz DS, Lane MJ, Sommer FG. Unenhanced helical CT of ureteral stones: incidence of associated urinary tract findings. AJR Am J Roentgenol 1996;166:1319–1322.

Kawashima A, Sandler CM, Corl FM. Imaging of renal trauma: a comprehensive review. Radiographics 2001;21:557–574.

Smith RC, Verga M, McCarthy S, et al. Diagnosis of acute flank pain: value of unenhanced helical CT. AJR Am J Roentgenol 1996;166:97–101.

Tamm EP, Silverman PM, Shuman WP. Evaluation of the patient with flank pain and possible ureteral calculus. Radiology 2003;228:319–329.

Williamson MP, Smith A. Fundamentals of Uroradiology. Philadelphia, PA: WB Saunders, 2000.

Zagoria RJ. Genitourinary Radiology: The Requisites. 2nd Ed. St. Louis, MO: Mosby, 2004.

Ziessman HA, O'Malley JP, Thrall JH. Nuclear Medicine: The Requisites. 3rd Ed. St. Louis, MO: Mosby, 2006.

Zwiebel WJ, Pellerito JS. Introduction to Vascular Ultrasonography. 5th Ed. Philadelphia, PA: WB Saunders, 2005.

chapter 10

Obstetric and Gynecologic Imaging

Paul R. Klepchick   Richard H. Daffner

Diagnostic imaging of the female reproductive tract may be conveniently divided into obstetric and gynecologic imaging. Obstetric imaging relies heavily on diagnostic ultrasound with magnetic resonance imaging (MRI) reserved for detailed evaluation of several specific entities. Gynecologic imaging uses all diagnostic methods available to both the radiologist and the gynecologist. Because of the complexity of the studies performed and their interpretation, this chapter reviews the highlights of obstetric and gynecologic imaging with the goal of discussing indications for various studies and their applications to some common problems.

Technical Considerations

Diagnostic Ultrasound

Diagnostic ultrasound is the primary tool for investigation of the gravid uterus as well as various conditions that may affect the female reproductive tract. Ultrasound is the procedure of choice because there is no ionizing radiation associated with its use to harm either the fetus or ovarian tissue. Furthermore, because of the normal relationships of the uterus and ovaries to the bladder, it is possible to image these organs by surface examination through a distended bladder without degradation of the image by bowel gas. Transvaginal ultrasound provides higher resolution imaging, allowing more accurate diagnosis in most cases.

Computed Tomography and Magnetic Resonance Imaging

Other noninvasive imaging studies performed include computed tomography (CT) and MRI. CT and MR are used primarily in evaluating suspected infections or neoplasms involving the ovaries or uterus. MRI is now used extensively in evaluating specific known or suspected fetal anomalies in the obstetric patient. These studies are employed in much the same way they would be used to evaluate similar abnormalities elsewhere within the abdomen and pelvis.

Hysterosalpingography

Hysterosalpingography is an invasive procedure in which the uterine os is cannulated and water-soluble contrast is injected. It is primarily performed to evaluate patients with infertility in whom congenital uterine abnormalities or tubal occlusion of any origin may exist. Other indications include evaluation of patients with recurrent abortions, to assess the obstruction or patency of the fallopian tubes after ligation, and occasionally before artificial insemination to determine if there are any structural abnormalities present.

Anatomic Considerations

The anatomic aspects of the female reproductive tract are important because of the relationships of the uterus and ovaries to the bladder, rectum, and peritoneum. The uterus lies immediately posterior to and just above the urinary bladder and anterior to the rectum. It is completely extraperitoneal and is surrounded by peritoneal folds that extend between the uterus and the bladder and between the uterus and the colon (*rectouterine pouch of Douglas*). Although variations in uterine shape and position do occur, in most patients, the relationships are as just described and as shown in Figure 10.1. There are three parts to the uterus: the cervix that projects into the vagina; the body, its main portion; and the fundus, or the rounded end. The fallopian tubes begin laterally below the level of the fundus. They are attached to the uterus by the broad ligament. The distal ends of these tubes lie close to the ovary with some of its fingerlike processes (*fimbria*) actually in contact with the gland. Normal ovaries are paired, almond-sized structures attached by the ovarian ligament to the uterus as well as to the broad ligament. They are completely shielded from the bladder anteriorly by the broad ligament.

Although the textbook depiction of the position of the ovaries is as just described, the ovaries are quite mobile and are often located lateral to the broad ligament. Figure 10.2 shows these relationships. The uterus, ovaries, and fallopian tubes are sustained by a rich vascular plexus. In addition, numerous lymphatic channels drain the area. These factors account for the intraabdominal spread of pelvic malignancy.

Obstetric Sonography

The evaluation of the gravid uterus is accomplished primarily through the use of ultrasound. *Obstetric sonography is a highly complex examination that needs to be performed by a carefully trained operator and interpreted with a great degree of skill.* Early in the history of obstetric ultrasound, the primary goal was to confirm the presence of an intrauterine pregnancy, determine the location of the placenta, detect multiple gestations, determine the lie of the fetus, or estimate gestational age. Obstetric ultrasound is now also extensively utilized for detecting both congenital and acquired fetal abnormalities and evaluating fetal growth.

> ▶ Obstetric sonography is a highly complex examination that needs to be performed by a highly trained operator and interpreted with a great degree of skill.

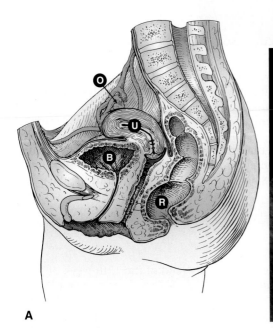

A

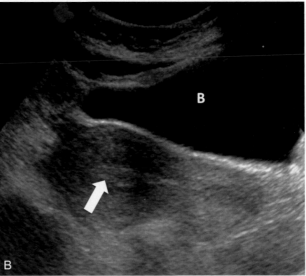

B

Figure 10.1 Normal female pelvic anatomy. A. Midline sagittal drawing showing the ovary (*O*), uterus (*U*), bladder (*B*), and rectum (*R*). **B.** Normal transvaginal longitudinal image of the uterus scanned through the bladder (*B*) shows the endometrium (*arrow*).

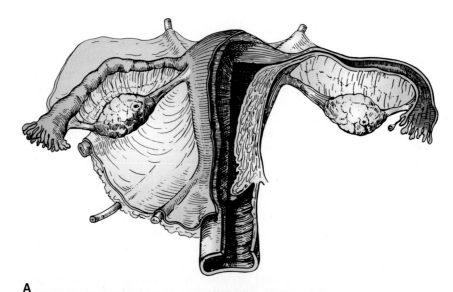

A

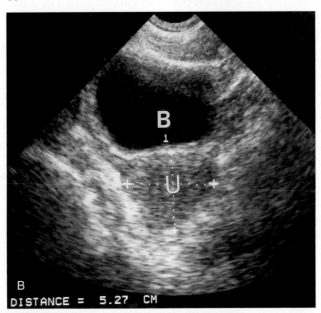

Figure 10.2   Normal coronal anatomy.   A. Cut-away section of the uterus, ovaries, and fallopian tubes. **B.** Axial ultrasound showing the relationship of the uterus (*U*) and the bladder (*B*).

Because ultrasound uses no ionizing radiation, it imposes no adverse biologic effects on either the mother or the fetus. However, this study, like any other, should be performed only when indicated. Table 10.1 lists the indications for obstetric sonography. Note that the indications change with time throughout the pregnancy. The following discussion highlights the normal sonographic changes that may be observed at various intervals during pregnancy. In addition, several common abnormalities are discussed. For a more in-depth treatment of the subject, see the works listed in the "Suggested Additional Reading" section at the end of the chapter.

Normal Pregnancy

First Trimester

The first trimester is the time between conception and the end of the 13th week of gestation. Obstetricians often use the terms *gestational age* and *menstrual age* interchangeably. However, because of variations in ovulation, a 1–2-week discrepancy may occur between the sonographic assessment of menstrual age and the actual gestational age of the fetus. Gestational age typically is determined from the time of conception, and the menstrual age is based on the first day of the last menses. For purposes of discussion, this chapter refers only to gestational age.

Table 10.1 INDICATIONS FOR OBSTETRIC SONOGRAPHY

General Indications
• Confirmation of intrauterine pregnancy
• Estimation of gestational age
• Detection of multiple gestation
• Determination of placental location and texture
• Detection of anatomic and functional abnormalities of the fetus
• Evaluation of other pelvic masses during pregnancy
First Trimester
• Vaginal bleeding
• Suspected threatened, incomplete, or missed abortion
• Distinction between intrauterine and ectopic pregnancy
• Suspected molar pregnancy
• Suspected pregnancy associated with intrauterine contraceptive device
Second Trimester
• Localization and evaluation of placenta
• Polyhydramnios/Oligohydramnios
• Evaluation of fetal growth
Third Trimester
• Possible placenta previa
• Determination of fetal maturity to plan optimal time and mode of delivery
• Determination of fetal presentation
• Biophysical profile for fetal well-being
Other Indications
• Adjunct to amniocentesis
• Maternal abdominal disorders during pregnancy
• Postpartum for suspected retained products of conception

A gestational sac, which may be detected as early as 3 weeks from conception, consists of a round-to-oval area devoid of echoes located within the body or fundus of the uterus (Fig. 10.3). This sonolucency represents the choriodecidual fluid that surrounds the developing embryo. The *embryonic period* occurs between the third and eighth weeks of gestational age. Embryonic development cannot usually be delineated in its early stages. During this period, all major body organs begin forming. Further growth and differentiation occur in the *fetal period*. The exact transition time between embryonic and fetal periods is arbitrary.

 ▶ The exact transition time between embryonic and fetal periods is arbitrary.

Once a fetus is detected, the gestational age may be estimated by measuring the crown-to-rump (long-axis) length of the fetus. This is the most accurate means of determining gestational age, accurate to within 1 week (Fig. 10.4). The following normal structures can also be detected at the times indicated: fetal heart, 6 to 7 weeks; arm buds, 8 weeks; leg buds, 9 to 10 weeks; choroid plexus of the brain, 12 to 16 weeks. Other structures that can be detected during the first trimester include the umbilical stalk and the yolk sac.

Figure 10.3   Early gestational sac.   Transvaginal sagittal image shows the "double decidual sign" of early intrauterine pregnancy. The gestational sac (*S*) is seen between the decidua basalis (*DB*) and the decidua capsularis (*DC*). A thin dark line separates the decidua capsularis from the decidua parietalis (*DP*).

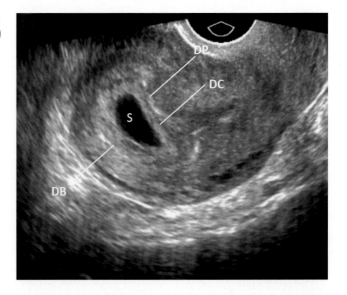

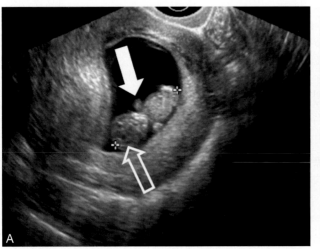

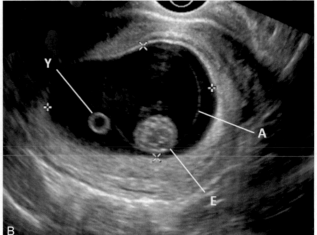

Figure 10.4   Normal first trimester.   A. Embryo at 8 weeks 2 days. The head (*open arrow*) and arm buds (*closed arrow*) are clearly visible at this gestational age. The calipers (+) measure head to rump length. **B.** Transverse view through the gestational sac showing the embryo (*E*), yolk sac (*Y*), and amnionic membrane (*A*).

▶ The gestational age of a fetus may be estimated by measuring the crown-to-rump (long-axis) length.

Measurement of the nuchal translucency thickness has been shown to be efficacious in determining the risks of aneuploidy, especially in trisomy 21. A nuchal translucency thickness of >3 mm is considered abnormal when scans are performed on fetuses between 11 and 14 weeks gestational age. The risk of aneuploidy is based on a combination of nuchal thickness, maternal age, serum free β-hCG, and serum pregnancy associated plasma protein A (PAPP-A) (Fig. 10.5).

Second Trimester

The second trimester of pregnancy is the interval between the 14th and 26th gestational weeks. A more detailed evaluation of the fetus, uterus, and placenta is possible because of their enlargement during this time. It is in the second trimester that amniotic fluid

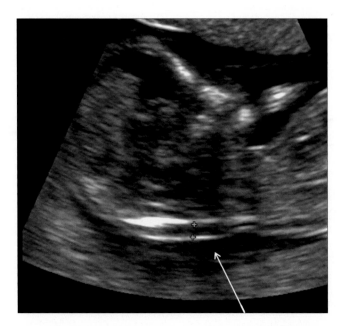

Figure 10.5   Nuchal translucency measurement.   Magnified image of the fetal head, neck, and upper thorax shows calipers (+) placed on the inner borders of the widest aspect of the anechoic nuchal space perpendicular to the long axis of the fetus. The amnion (*arrow*) is seen posteriorly.

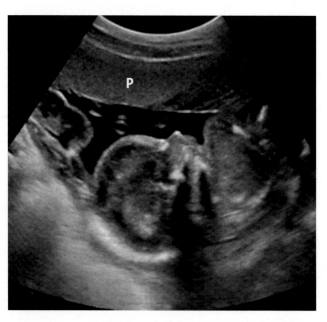

Figure 10.6   Normal second trimester fetus showing an anterior placenta (P).   Facial features are clearly visible.

may be detected surrounding the fetus. As a rule, the volume of amniotic fluid should equal the volume of the fetus. The location and size of the placenta can also be determined (Fig. 10.6). The fetal organs also enlarge and are easily detectable on sonography. It is thus possible to determine the gross morphology and function of the heart by real-time examination. Second trimester sonography, typically referred to as "fetal anatomic survey," is generally performed between 18 and 22 weeks. It is a systematic review of fetal anatomy during which certain structures should be demonstrated based on guidelines described by professional organizations (Table 10.2). In the second trimester, gestational age is established by measuring the biparietal diameter, head circumference, abdominal circumference, and femur length. Comparing a composite of these numbers against standardized tables allows calculation of gestational age to within 1 to 2 weeks during the second trimester. Between 90% and 100% of mothers in North America have one or more sonographic examinations in the antenatal period. The majority of these examinations are done as a "screening examination" to look for fetal abnormalities.

> Gestational age in the second trimester is established by measuring the biparietal diameter, head circumference, abdominal circumference, and femur length.

Third Trimester

The third trimester of pregnancy falls between the 27th week of pregnancy up to the time of delivery (usually at 38 to 40 weeks). During this time, there is continued enlargement of the uterus and fetus, as well as changes within the placenta. Third trimester sonography is primarily used to for follow-up of abnormalities detected earlier in gestation, evaluating growth, and establishing fetal well-being with biophysical profile scoring.

Magnetic Resonance Imaging during Pregnancy

Fetal MRI is gaining widespread use, particularly for confirmation of inconclusive sonographic findings and for evaluation of sonographically occult diagnoses. Neurologic indications well suited to evaluation include ventriculomegaly, agenesis of the corpus callosum, posterior fossa abnormalities, and abnormalities of cortical development.

Table 10.2 FETAL ANATOMIC SURVEY

Fetal Presentation and Lie
Fetal Environment
• Amniotic fluid
• Three vessel cord
• Placental position, placental cord insertion
Skull and Intracranial Structures
• Biparietal diameter, head circumference, head shape, cavum septum pellucidum, thalami
• Lateral ventricles (normal <10 mm)
• Cerebellum, cisternal magnum (normal <10 mm), nuchal skin fold (normal <6 mm)
• Facial structures (chin, lips, orbits, upper palate)
Spine
• Normal
• Dysraphism (spina bifida)
Heart (4-chamber view, right ventricular outflow tract, left ventricular outflow tract)
• Normal
• Anomalies
Abdomen
• Abdominal circumference
• Stomach
• Umbilical cord insertion
• Kidneys (normal renal pelvis <5 mm)
• Bladder
Extremities
• Measure femur
• Movement, shape, and position
• Open hands
• Anomalies

Non-neurologic indications include congenital diaphragmatic hernia (Fig. 10.7), lung abnormalities (pulmonary sequestration, airway obstruction, and congenital cystic adenomatoid malformation), and evaluation of fetal genitourinary (GU) and gastrointestinal (GI) anomalies.

Pathologic Considerations

Obstetric Abnormalities

The vast array of abnormalities that occurs during pregnancy is beyond the scope of this text. Some of the more common abnormalities encountered in daily practice are covered below.

Vaginal bleeding during the first trimester is often referred to as *threatened abortion*. There are no specific sonographic findings in this condition. However, retention of products of conception is referred to as *incomplete abortion*. Retained fetal parts or an endometrial mass are highly specific for incomplete abortion (Fig. 10.8). Endometrial thickening, complex fluid and Doppler blood flow are less specific. Absence of these findings has been shown to have a negative predictive value for retained products of conception of up to 100%.

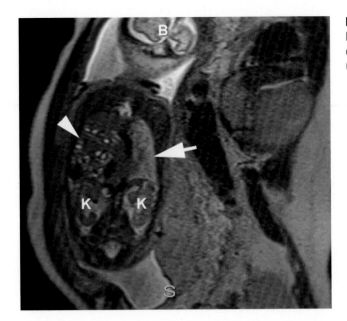

Figure 10.7   Congenital diaphragmatic hernia.   Coronal T2-weighted HASTE image of the fetus shows the normal hyperintense lung (*arrow*). The opposite hemithorax is filled with loops of bowel (*arrowhead*). Note the kidneys (*K*) and brain (*B*).

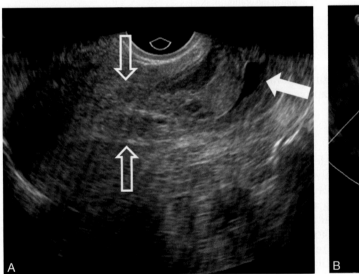

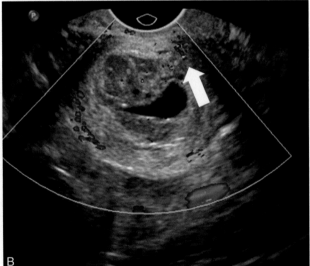

Figure 10.8   Appearance of the uterus after incomplete abortion.   **A.** Sagittal transvaginal scan shows heterogeneous thickening of the endometrium (*between open arrows*) with anechoic fluid in the cervix (*closed arrow*) **B.** Coronal scan at the level of the cervix shows color Doppler flow in the heterogeneous retained products of conception (*closed arrow*).

> ▶ Absence of retained fetal parts or an endometrial mass has been shown to have a negative predictive value for incomplete abortion of close to 100%.

Placenta Previa

Placenta previa is a condition in which a placenta is located either partially or completely across the cervical os (Fig. 10.9). This condition may result in maternal or fetal death from massive hemorrhage at the time of birth. The detection of placenta previa by the middle of the third trimester is necessary so that the fetus can be delivered by cesarean section before the onset of labor.

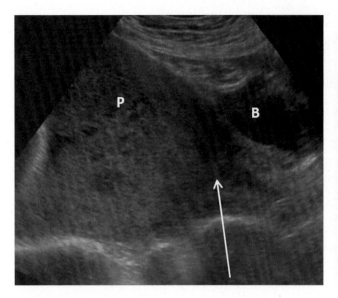

Figure 10.9   Placenta previa.   Transabdominal view of the lower uterine segment showing the placenta (*P*) completely covering the internal cervical os (*arrow*). The bladder is partially seen anteriorly (*B*).

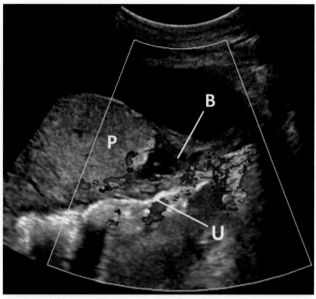

Figure 10.10   Abruptio placentae.   Transabdominal Doppler scan shows heterogeneous blood (*B*) between the caudal tip of the placenta (*P*) and the wall of the uterus (*U*).

Abruptio Placentae

Abruptio placentae is the premature separation of the placenta from the wall of the uterus. This may be detected by sonography as a sonolucent area between the uterine wall and the placental shadows (Fig. 10.10).

Fetal Anomalies

Various fetal anomalies may be detected during the later stages of pregnancy. These include fetal hydrocephalus, anencephaly, spina bifida (Fig. 10.11), and hydranencephaly. Urinary abnormalities such as urinary obstruction detected by oligohydramnios, and multicystic or polycystic kidney disease can also be demonstrated. Abnormalities of the GI tract that are detectable include duodenal atresia, omphalocele (Fig. 10.12), and fetal ascites. Cardiac abnormalities are difficult to detect because of the cardiac motion. However, careful demonstration of the normal relationships of the atria and ventricles and the cardiac outflow tract is useful in excluding many anomalies. Finally, forms of dwarfism such as achondroplasia may be detected. Fractures of the fetal skeleton in utero may be the result of underlying osteogenesis imperfecta.

Ectopic Pregnancy

Ectopic pregnancy occurs when implantation occurs outside the uterine cavity. In most patients with this condition, the products of conception implant in a fallopian tube. Usually, there is tubal scarring as the result of previous pelvic inflammatory disease. Ectopic pregnancy is readily detectable by ultrasound (Fig. 10.13). Failure to demonstrate an intrauterine gestational sac in a patient with a positive serum β-hCG and pelvic pain should be considered suspicious for ectopic pregnancy, even if an ectopic pregnancy is not visualized. In these patients, serial monitoring of serum β-hCG should be performed. Follow-up ultrasound is often necessary. Please refer to our online supplement about ectopic pregnancies for more information.

▶ In most ectopic pregnancies the products of conception implant in a fallopian tube.
▶ Failure to demonstrate an intrauterine gestational sac in a patient with a positive serum β-hCG and pelvic pain should suggest ectopic pregnancy.

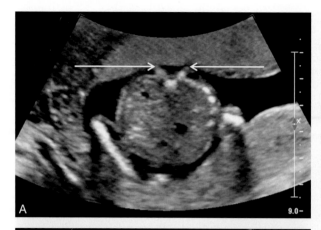

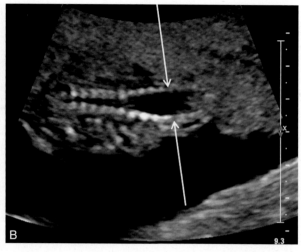

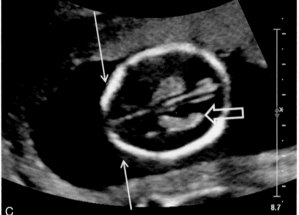

Figure 10.11 Neural tube defect. A. Axial scan through the lower fetal abdomen shows outward splaying of the posterior elements of the spine (*arrows*) **B.** Coronal scan of the fetal lumbosacral spine shows fusiform widening of the spinal canal (*between arrows*). **C.** Flattening of the frontal bones causes a concavity (*thin arrows*) known as the "lemon sign." The choroid plexus (*open arrow*) only partially fills the lateral ventricle.

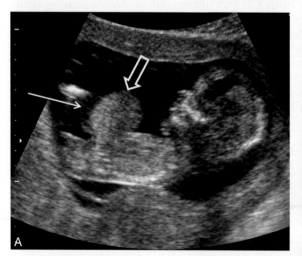

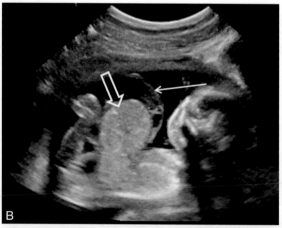

Figure 10.12 Giant omphalocele. A. Sagittal scan of a 13-week 3-day fetus shows the liver (*open arrow*) herniated into the omphalocele sac (*thin arrow*). **B.** Sagittal view in the second trimester again shows the liver (*open arrow*) extending into the sac (*thin arrow*). **C.** Transverse color Doppler image of the umbilical arteries (*small arrows*) at the base of the sac. Note the liver (*large arrow*) within the sac is greater in circumference than the lower abdominal circumference.

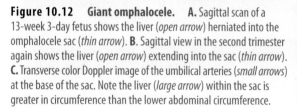

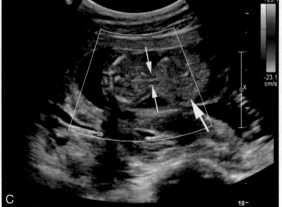

Figure 10.13   Ectopic Pregnancy.
Thick-walled gestational sac (*solid large arrow*) abutting the ovary (*open arrow*). A small embryonic pole (*thin arrow*) is present within the gestational sac.

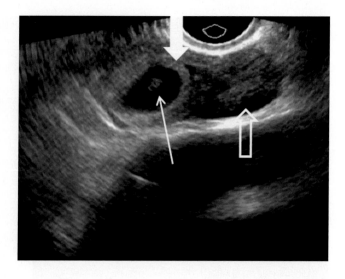

Gynecologic Abnormalities

Evaluation of abnormalities involving a woman's reproductive tract has benefitted greatly by the developments in body imaging. The modalities primarily used are ultrasound, CT, MRI, and hysterosalpingography.

As previously mentioned, ultrasound is noninvasive, uses no ionizing radiation, can be performed rapidly, and is relatively inexpensive. Thus, it is one of the initial studies to be performed in evaluation of abnormalities of the female pelvis. Real-time imaging is a distinct advantage over CT and MRI, allowing patient interaction and opportunity for the examiner to directly focus the examination on an abnormality to improve diagnostic accuracy.

MRI has distinct advantages over both CT and ultrasound in demonstrating tissue qualities; it is particularly useful in evaluating pelvic neoplasms. Hysterosalpingography is the best radiologic technique for delineating the morphology of the uterine lumen as well as the patency of the fallopian tubes in evaluating patients with infertility problems (Figs. 10.14 and 10.15). Thus, the gynecologic imager has many procedures available to diagnose abnormalities.

Pathologic conditions that occur within the female reproductive organs fall into four categories: congenital, physiologic, inflammatory, and neoplastic.

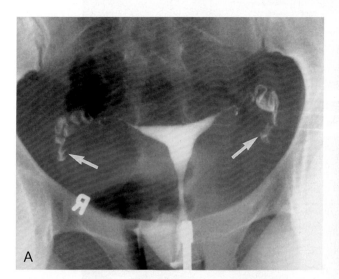

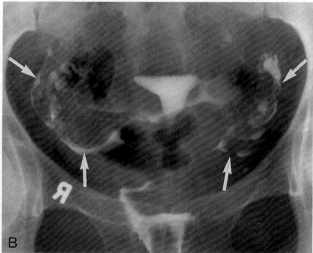

Figure 10.14   Normal hysterosalpingogram.   A. After injection of contrast through the uterine os, there is spillage from both fallopian tubes (*arrows*). **B.** Delayed image shows intraperitoneal contrast outlining loops of bowel (*arrows*).

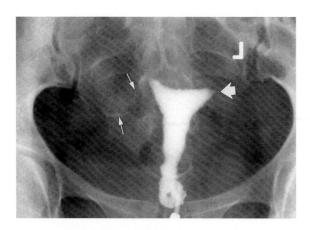

Figure 10.15 Abnormal hysterosalpingogram. The left fallopian tube is occluded near its origin (*large arrow*). In addition, there is irregularity and scarring of the right fallopian tube (*small arrows*).

Congenital Abnormalities

Congenital abnormalities occur primarily in the uterus. Approximately 0.5% of women have congenital anomalies. These may be incidental findings of no clinical significance. However, others, such as bicornuate uterus, may result in pregnancy disorders. Congenital uterine abnormalities are often associated with renal agenesis. For this reason, it is important to image the kidneys when a uterine abnormality is encountered.

Physiologic Abnormalities

Physiologic abnormalities include cystic diseases of the ovary and endometriosis. Because of normal physiologic functions, the vast majority of ovarian cysts as large as 5 cm are simply physiologic—that is, transient and changing, depending on the phase of the menstrual cycle. However, a normal physiologic cyst that fails to regress or enlarges because of a hormonal imbalance or hemorrhage may form a functional or retention cyst. Ovarian cysts are the most common pelvic masses encountered in young women (Fig. 10.16).

 ▶ Ovarian cysts are the most common pelvic masses in a young woman.

Endometriosis

Endometriosis is caused by the presence of endometrial tissue in extrauterine sites. The most common location for endometriosis is within the pelvic cavity. From an imaging standpoint,

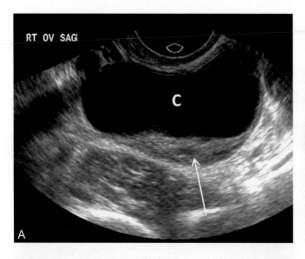
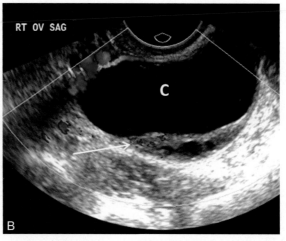

Figure 10.16 Simple ovarian cyst. A. Sagittal transvaginal image of the ovary shows an anechoic thin-walled ovarian cyst (*C*) arising from the surface of the ovary (*arrow*). **B.** Color Doppler image at the same level shows flow (*arrow*) in the ovary but not in the mass.

endometriosis produces cystic masses of various sizes anywhere within the pelvis (Fig. 10.17). These may implant on the colon and produce extraluminal compression.

Pelvic Inflammatory Disease

Pelvic inflammatory disease is the result of an ascending infection from the vagina to the endometrium, the fallopian tubes, and ultimately the pelvic peritoneum. In most instances, the causal organism is gonococcal. Inflammatory collections in the pelvis may be detected on either CT or ultrasound without difficulty. Occasionally, a tuboovarian abscess will be formed (Fig. 10.18).

Neoplasms

Neoplasms of a woman's reproductive organs include both benign and malignant tumors. Common benign tumors include serous cystadenoma (Fig. 10.19), mucinous cystadenoma, mature cystic teratoma (Figs. 10.20 and 10.21), and fibroid tumors (Fig. 10.22). Mature cystic teratomas (dermoids) often contain fat, calcifications, and occasionally dental elements, all of which are easily demonstrable by CT (see Fig. 10.21). Fibroids are extremely common and occur in up to 40% of women over the age of 35 years. They are often found as incidental calcifications on abdominal radiographs (see Fig. 10.22).

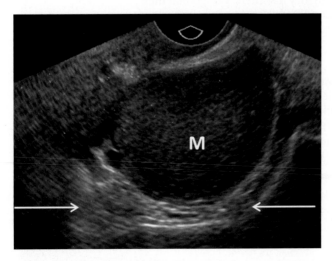

Figure 10.17   Endometrioma. Transvaginal ultrasound shows a hypoechoic mass (*M*) with low level internal echoes pathologically proven to be an endometrioma. Note enhanced through transmission compatible with cystic nature, manifested as increased echogenicity (*between arrows*) behind this mass.

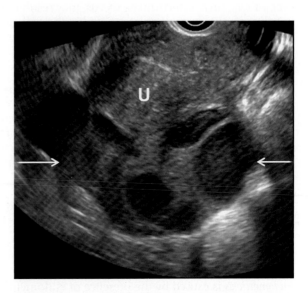

Figure 10.18   Tuboovarian abscess. Transvaginal scan shows a complex heterogeneous mass (*between arrows*) posterior to the uterus (*U*). The ovary and fallopian tube cannot be seen as separate structures.

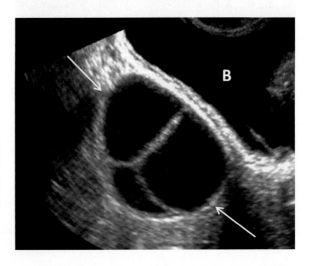

Figure 10.19   Benign ovarian cystadenoma. Transvaginal ultrasound shows a cystic mass (*between arrows*) with thick internal septations in the ovary. The full bladder (*B*) is seen anteriorly.

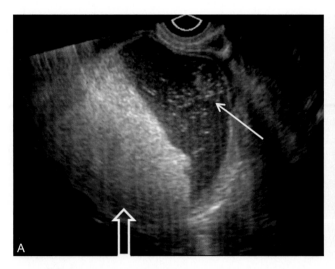

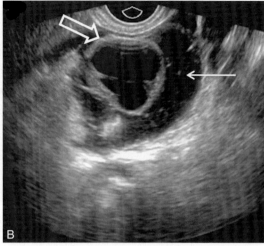

Figure 10.20 Ovarian mature cystic teratoma (dermoid). A. Transvaginal ultrasound shows a heterogeneous mass with internal tiny echogenic dots (*thin arrow*) compatible with hair follicles; this is known as "dermoid mesh." The echogenic shadowing component is known as a "dermoid plug" (*open arrow*). **B.** Different patient with a complex cystic adnexal mass with punctate dots (*thin arrow*) and a thick-walled component (*open arrow*).

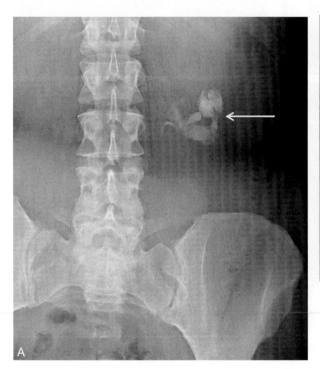

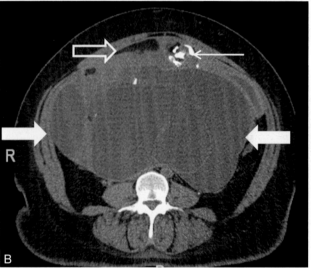

Figure 10.21 Ovarian mature cystic teratoma. A. Abdominal radiograph shows a calcified mass in the left hemiabdomen (*arrow*). **B.** CT scan of the abdomen shows a classic ovarian mature cystic teratoma as a large heterogenous pelvic mass containing calcifications (*thin arrow*), fluid components (*closed arrows*), and a fat-fluid level (*open arrow*).

In some instances they are responsible for dysfunctional uterine hemorrhage and may require hysterectomy or myomectomy. Uterine artery embolization and MRI-guided ultrasound ablation are gaining use as less invasive means of treating fibroids.

Malignant neoplasms are unfortunately common. *Endometrial carcinoma* is the most common invasive gynecologic malignancy. *Ovarian carcinoma* is the second most common gynecologic malignant tumor. It is responsible for 50% of the deaths from gynecologic malignancy and is the fifth most frequent cause of cancer death in women (after lung, breast, colon, and pancreatic cancers). *Cervical carcinoma* is the third most common. Regular Pap tests and the introduction of human papillomavirus (HPV) vaccination has decreased both the incidence of cervical cancer and associated mortality. Malignancies of the vagina, vulva, and fallopian tube are much less common. Multimodality imaging is used in detecting, staging, and follow-up of all these neoplasms (Figs. 10.23 to 10.25). Of particular importance in

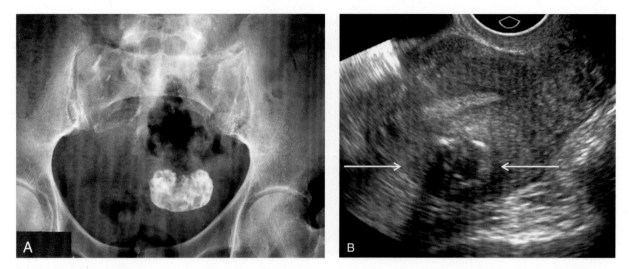

Figure 10.22   Uterine fibroids.   A. Pelvic radiograph shows a calcified mass just to the left of midline. Calcifications in fibroids often look like popcorn. **B.** Transvaginal ultrasound shows an echogenic mass in the posterior uterine wall with internal shadowing from the calcifications (*arrows*).

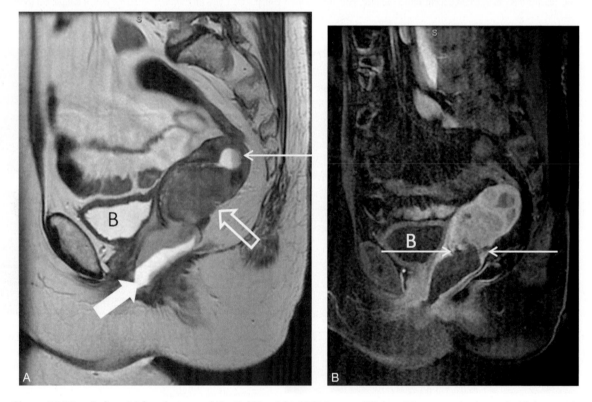

Figure 10.23   Endometrial carcinoma.   A. Sagittal T2-weighted MRI shows a mildly hyperintense mass (*open arrow*) with transmural invasion of the posterior lower uterine segment (*asterisk*). Retained fluid is present in the fundus (*thin arrow*). Hyperintense fluid in the vagina (*closed arrow*) is gel placed before examination to help facilitate evaluation of disease extent. **B.** Sagittal fat suppressed contrast-enhanced T1-weighted MRI is useful in evaluating extent of disease. In this case, the mass extends into the cervical stroma (*between arrows*). Note the bladder (**B**) is hyperintense on the T2 image.

the evaluation of patients with these diseases is the detection of the presence or absence of localized spread through invasion of contiguous tissues. The presence or absence of extension beyond the affected organ will determine the exact staging of the neoplasm according to the standards set by the International Federation of Gynecology and Obstetrics.

> ▶ Endometrial carcinoma is the most common invasive gynecologic malignancy.
> ▶ Ovarian carcinoma is the second most common invasive gynecologic malignancy.
> ▶ Cervical carcinoma is the third most common invasive gynecologic malignancy.

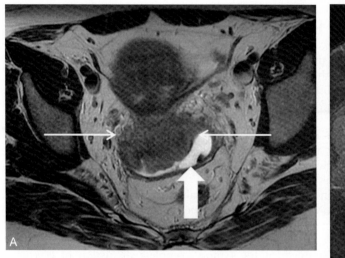
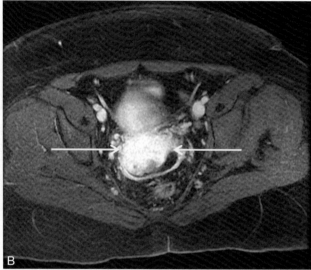

Figure 10.24   Cervical carcinoma.   A. T2-weighted MRI shows a heterogeneously hypointense mass (*thin arrows*) replacing the fibrous cervical stroma protruding into the vagina (filled with ultrasound gel *closed arrow*). **B.** Axial fat suppressed contrast-enhanced T1-weighted MRI shows a homogeneously enhancing cervical mass (*arrows*).

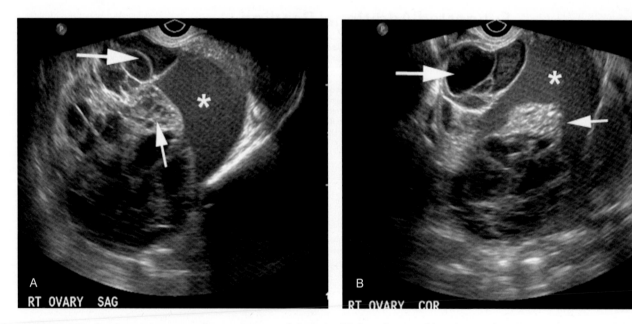

Figure 10.25   Ovarian mucinous cystadenocarcinoma.   A. Sagittal and **B.** Coronal images of the right ovary show a heterogeneous mixed solid (*small arrow*) and cystic mass. The cystic components contain areas of increased (*asterisk*) and decreased (*large arrow*) echogenicity, a common finding in mucinous neoplasms.

Summary and Key Points

▶ This chapter has dealt with the evaluation of the female reproductive tract primarily by sonography. Because of the complexity in the performance and interpretation of obstetrical sonography, the discussion has been limited to basic concepts. See the more-definitive texts listed at the end of this chapter for in-depth discussion of the sophisticated aspects of this subject.

▶ Common obstetric entities include normal pregnancy, placenta previa, abruptio placentae, ectopic pregnancy, and fetal anomalies.

▶ The evaluation of gynecologic abnormalities uses a multimodality imaging approach, although sonography remains the primary tool.

▶ Gynecologic abnormalities include congenital anomalies, physiologic problems, such as cystic disease of the ovaries and endometriosis; pelvic inflammatory disease; and tumors. The evaluation of these abnormalities is performed in the same manner as that of other organ systems.

▶ Please refer to our online supplement for a more complete discussion of ectopic pregnancies with some interactive cases.

Suggested Additional Reading

Benacerraf BR. Ultrasound of Fetal Syndromes. 2nd Ed. Philadelphia, PA: Churchill Livingstone, 2008.
Bowerman RA. Atlas of Normal Fetal Ultrasonographic Anatomy. 2nd Ed. St. Louis, MO: Mosby-Year Book, 1991.
Brant WE, Helms CA. Fundamentals of Diagnostic Radiology. 4th Ed. Philadelphia, PA: Lippincott Williams & Wilkins, 2012:838–857.
Callen, PW. Ultrasonography in Obstetrics and Gynecology. 5th Ed. Philadelphia, PA: Saunders-Elsevier, 2008.
Fleischer AC, Kepple DM. Transvaginal Sonography: A Clinical Atlas. Philadelphia, PA: JB Lippincott, 1991.
Karasick S, Karasick D. Atlas of Hysterosalpingography. Springfield, IL: Charles C. Thomas, 1987.
Rumack CM, Wilson SR, Charboneau JW, Levine D. Diagnostic Ultrasound. 4th Ed. St. Louis, MO: Mosby-Elsevier, 2011.
Woodward PJ, Kennedy AM, Sohaey R, et al. Diagnostic Imaging: Obstetrics. Philadelphia, PA: WB Saunders, 2005.

chapter 11

Musculoskeletal Imaging

Richard H. Daffner

Imaging examinations of the musculoskeletal system are, after chest radiographs, the second most common studies you will encounter. In this age of specialized—computed tomography (CT) and magnetic resonance (MR)—imaging, radiographic analysis of the skeleton still provides considerable information about the overall health of the patient. In addition to obvious abnormalities of the bones and joints themselves, skeletal radiographs may provide clues to the presence of occult systemic inflammatory, metabolic, or neoplastic diseases.

This chapter primarily outlines an approach useful in the interpretation of skeletal radiographs. In addition, the important musculoskeletal applications of other imaging studies are highlighted. A key principle to remember is that, as in the gastrointestinal tract, *lesions in the skeleton appear similar to one another no matter where they are located*. The incidence may vary with the location, but the basic appearance is the same.

▶ Lesions in the skeleton appear similar to one another no matter where they are located.

Technical Considerations

Imaging of the musculoskeletal system encompasses the entire spectrum of diagnostic radiology. Radiography is still the cornerstone for diagnosis, and thus radiographs must be obtained before ordering more sophisticated imaging studies. Radiographs provide the "road map" for further investigation and diagnosis. Overall, radiographs have an intermediate sensitivity but a high specificity for diagnosing bone abnormalities. Many bone lesions have characteristic radiographic appearances that allow confident and accurate pathologic diagnosis, particularly when the findings are interpreted in light of clinical and/or laboratory data (Fig. 11.1). Other lesions have an indeterminate appearance that requires additional imaging or perhaps a biopsy for diagnosis (Fig. 11.2). The basic appearances and management of musculoskeletal radiographic findings can be divided into four categories:

1. Benign, asymptomatic—"leave me alone"
2. Benign, symptomatic—elective excision
3. Malignant ("I think")—biopsy needed
4. Indeterminate—biopsy needed

Fortunately, developments in imaging technology have made the decision process easier. Using CT and MRI, it is possible to increase the confidence levels to put more lesions in categories 1 and 3.

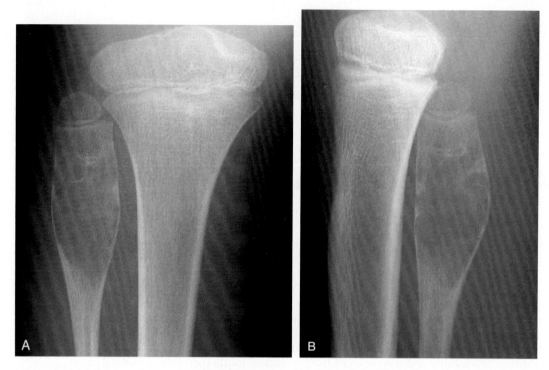

Figure 11.1   Aneurysmal bone cyst of the proximal fibula.   Frontal **(A)** and lateral **(B)** radiographs demonstrate an expanded lesion of the diametaphyseal area of the fibula. The lesion is trabeculated and does not cross the physis. In this skeletally immature patient, the most likely diagnosis is an aneurysmal bone cyst. This lesion is radiologically characteristic enough to allow a confident diagnosis.

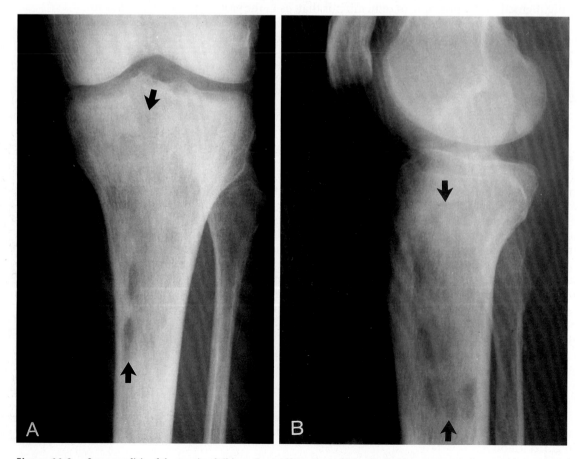

Figure 11.2   Osteomyelitis of the proximal tibia.   Frontal **(A)** and lateral **(B)** radiographs demonstrate a destructive lesion in the diametaphyseal region of the proximal tibia (*arrows*). There is nothing characteristic about this lesion to allow confident diagnosis without a biopsy.

DECISION TREE BASED ON APPEARANCE

▶ Benign, asymptomatic—"leave me alone"
▶ Benign, symptomatic—elective excision
▶ Malignant ("I think")—biopsy needed
▶ Indeterminate—biopsy needed

Computed Tomography

CT is used extensively for evaluating musculoskeletal abnormalities. In addition to providing diagnostic information about bones and soft tissues in another plane, it is a mainstay for safe and accurate biopsy procedures (Fig. 11.3) as well as for CT-guided intervention (Fig. 11.4). CT is used to evaluate suspected tumors (Fig. 11.5); fractures, particularly of the vertebral column (Fig. 11.6); and infections (Fig. 11.7). Another use for CT is to augment arthrograms when MRI cannot be performed. Multiplanar tomographic and three-dimensional reconstructions of CT examinations have been found useful by referring surgeons (Fig. 11.8).

Magnetic Resonance Imaging

MRI of the musculoskeletal system is the second most common use of this technique (after neuroimaging). MRI has revolutionized musculoskeletal radiology because of its abilities to portray detailed images of soft tissues as well as bone in any plane (sagittal, coronal, axial [transverse], and unlimited oblique). It is invaluable in its ability to investigate internal joint derangements, its primary use (Fig. 11.9). MRI has eliminated most conventional arthrography. Indeed, MR arthrography is now the procedure of choice for the definitive diagnosis of many internal joint derangements, especially of the shoulder (Fig. 11.10), because of its ability to leave little doubt as to the nature of the abnormality. It can also aid in the diagnosis of primary (Fig. 11.11) and metastatic tumors (Fig. 11.12), infections (Fig. 11.13), trauma (Fig. 11.14), avascular necrosis (Fig. 11.15), and tendon ruptures (Fig. 11.16).

Ultrasound

Ultrasound is being used more frequently to diagnose soft tissue lesions of the limbs such as cysts (Fig. 11.17), loose bodies (Fig. 11.18), and ligament and tendon ruptures (Fig. 11.19). Throughout Europe and in many US centers, it is also used for assessing

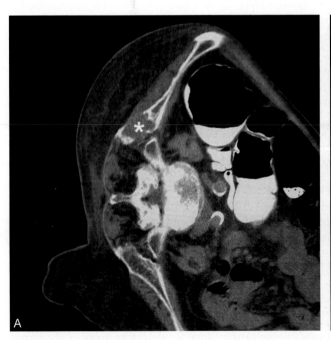
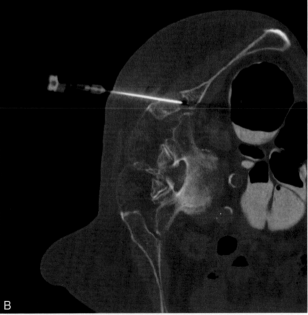

Figure 11.3   CT-guided biopsy.   A. CT image shows a destructive lesion in the right iliac bone (*asterisk*). **B.** CT image shows biopsy needle in the center of the lesion. Diagnosis: metastatic lung carcinoma.

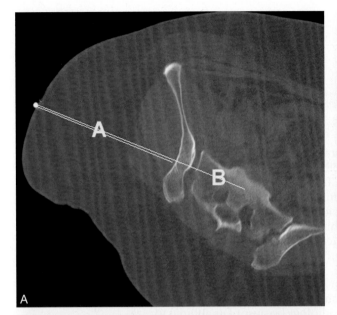

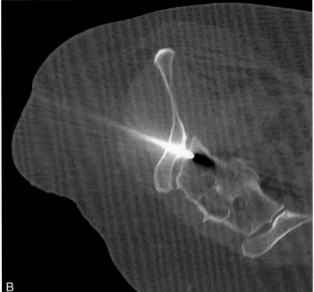

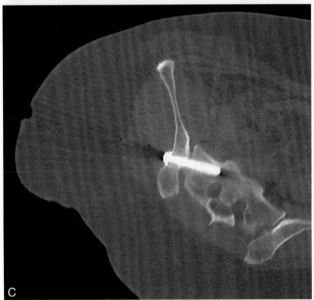

Figure 11.4   CT-guided screw placement.   A. CT image shows proposed trajectory of the screw insertion. *A*, distance from skin to bone; *B*, distance from skin to desired position in the sacrum. **B.** CT image shows screw being placed. **C.** CT image shows final position of screw.

tears of the rotator cuff of the shoulder (Fig. 11.20). However, the greater accuracy of MRI as well as its ease of performance has resulted in poor acceptance of musculoskeletal ultrasound in the United States. Part of this relates to the orthopaedic surgeons' lack of understanding of ultrasonic images. Ultrasound is an excellent choice for diagnosing congenital hip dysplasia in the infant whose femoral head epiphyses have not yet ossified (Fig. 11.21). Ultrasound shows the unossified cartilaginous femoral head and the acetabulum without the danger of irradiation of the pelvis and gonads. Despite the availability and the efficacy of ultrasound, pediatricians still order pelvic radiographs when they suspect congenital hip dysplasia in their patients. Ultrasound is also useful for locating nonopaque foreign bodies in soft tissues.

Nuclear Imaging

Nuclear imaging studies of the skeletal system include the radioisotope bone scan and indium scan. The bone scan is a valuable and useful tool for detecting areas of abnormal metabolic activity within bone. The introduction of technetium 99m–labeled phosphorus compounds (methylene diphosphonate) brought a new dimension of safety and accuracy to nuclear imaging. The phosphorus contained within the isotope is exchanged in areas

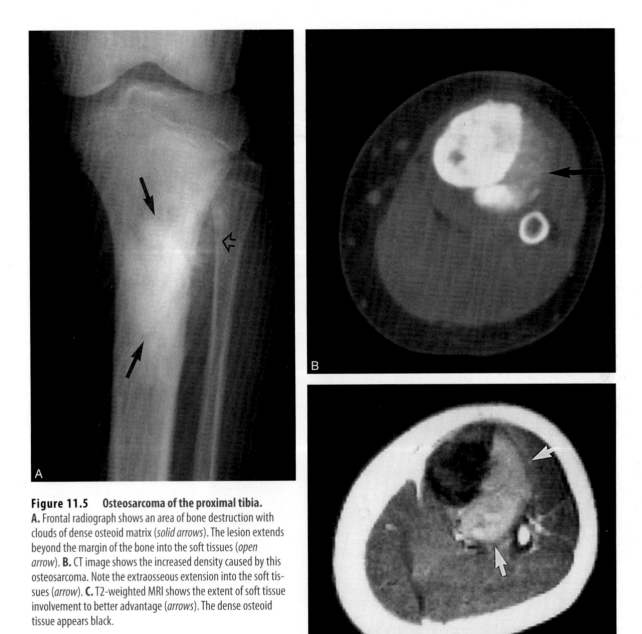

Figure 11.5   Osteosarcoma of the proximal tibia.
A. Frontal radiograph shows an area of bone destruction with clouds of dense osteoid matrix (*solid arrows*). The lesion extends beyond the margin of the bone into the soft tissues (*open arrow*). **B.** CT image shows the increased density caused by this osteosarcoma. Note the extraosseous extension into the soft tissues (*arrow*). **C.** T2-weighted MRI shows the extent of soft tissue involvement to better advantage (*arrows*). The dense osteoid tissue appears black.

of rapid bone turnover (metabolism): destructive lesions such as osteomyelitis, tumors, arthritis, and areas of growing bone. Although the scan itself is not specific for a particular disease, it indicates an area of bony abnormality to which radiography, CT, or MRI may be directed. The bone scan is often positive before radiographs show any abnormality in a particular bone. It should be used as the primary screening examination for detecting metastases (Fig. 11.22) and fractures (Fig. 11.23), and in cases of suspected child abuse (Fig. 11.24). A notable exception, when the bone scan is not useful in diffuse bone disease, is in cases of multiple myeloma. Little or no abnormal uptake of the isotope occurs in that disorder.

Bone Scan

The typical *bone scan* is performed in three phases. First is the *vascular phase,* which consists of serial images performed at 2- to 5-second intervals to follow the flow of the isotope through the vascular system. This phase can indicate areas of increased or

Text continues on page 363

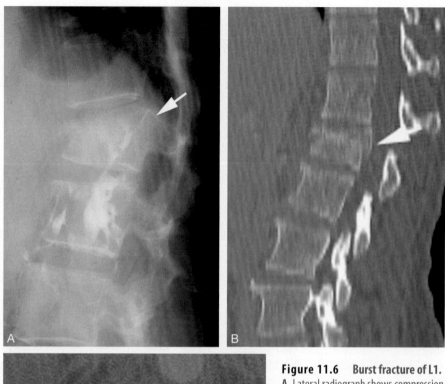

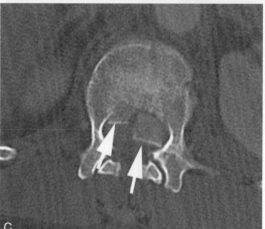

Figure 11.6   Burst fracture of L1.
A. Lateral radiograph shows compression of the body of L1 and retropulsion of fragments from posterior vertebral body line into the vertebral canal (*arrow*).
B. Sagittal reconstructed CT image shows the displaced fragment (*arrow*) narrowing the vertebral canal. **C.** Axial image shows two bone fragments displaced into the vertebral canal (*arrows*).

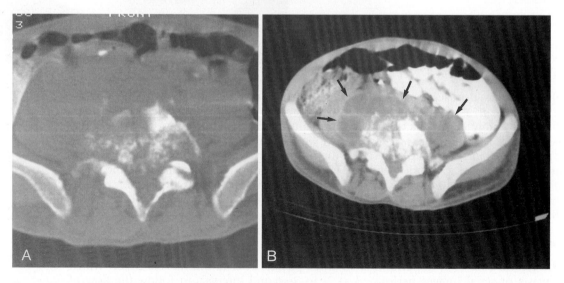

Figure 11.7   Vertebral tuberculous osteomyelitis and paraspinous abscess.   A. CT image near the lumbosacral junction shows a destructive process of L5 and a paraspinal soft tissue mass in front of the vertebrae. **B.** CT image slightly lower made at soft tissue windows after intravenous contrast enhancement shows the large multilocular abscess in the soft tissues (*arrows*). The rim of the abscess is enhanced.

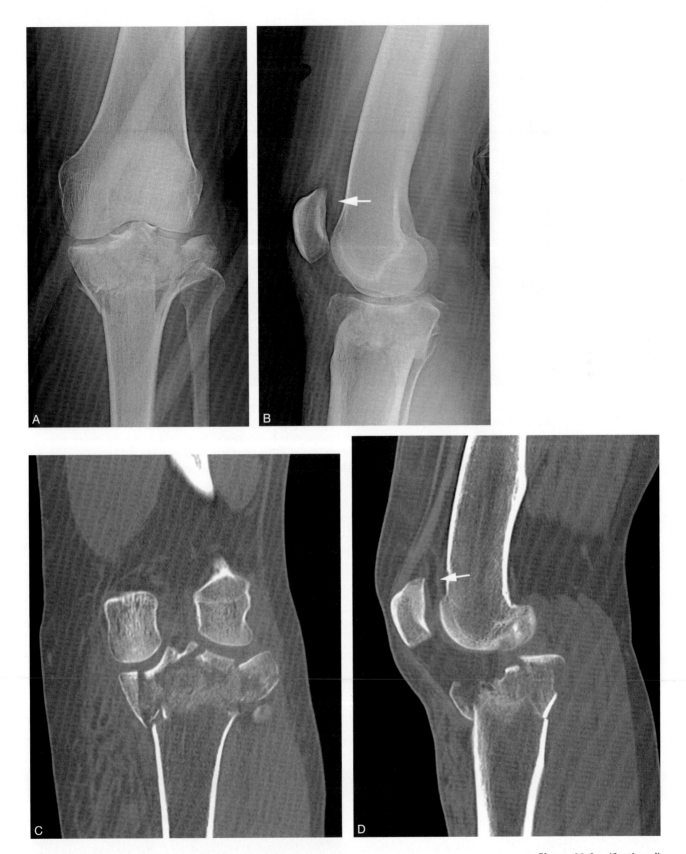

Figure 11.8 (Continued)

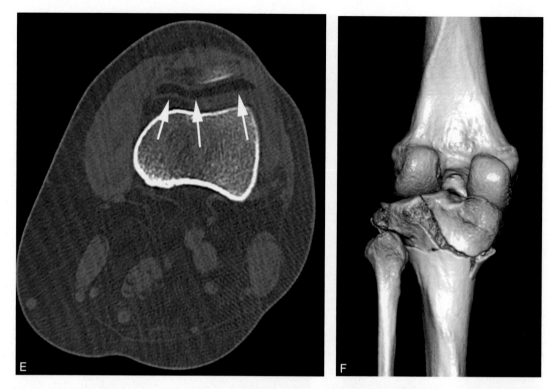

Figure 11.8   Comminuted tibial plateau fracture   A. Frontal and **B.** Lateral radiographs show comminuted fractures through the lateral tibial plateau and proximal tibia. Note the lipohemarthrosis (*arrow*) in the suprapatellar bursa on the lateral view. **C.** Coronal and **D.** Sagittal tomographic reconstructed CT images show the full extent of this severe injury. Note the lipohemarthrosis in **D** (*arrow*). **E.** Axial CT image shows the lipohemarthrosis (*arrows*). **F.** Three-dimensional (3D) reconstructed CT image viewed from behind shows the severe comminution. 3D reconstructions provide a macro view for the surgeon.

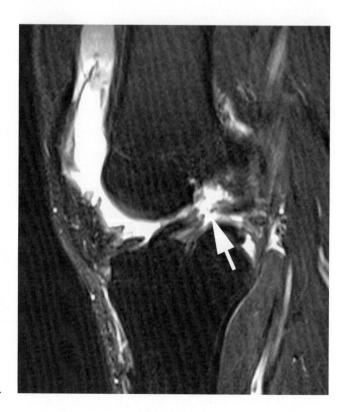

Figure 11.9   Anterior cruciate ligament tear.   Sagittal inversion recovery image shows the torn ligament (*arrow*) and a large joint effusion.

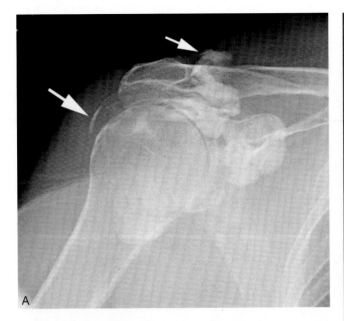

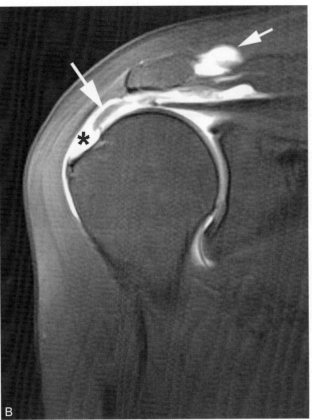

Figure 11.10 Rotator cuff tear. A. Arthrogram shows extravasation of contrast into the subdeltoid bursa (*large arrow*) as well as "geyser sign" (*small arrow*). **B.** MR arthrogram image shows contrast in the subdeltoid/subacromial bursa (*asterisk*) as well as the torn end of the supraspinatus tendon (*large arrow*). Note the "geyser sign" (*small arrow*).

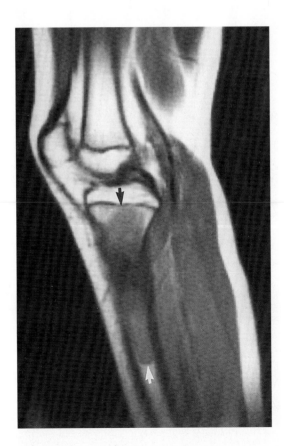

Figure 11.11 Osteosarcoma of the tibia. (This is the same patient as in Fig. 11.5.) Sagittal T1-weighted MRI shows an extensive area of marrow replacement in the proximal tibia (*arrows*). Cortical breakthrough is suggested in the darkest area near the middle.

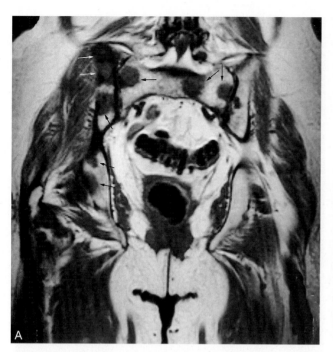

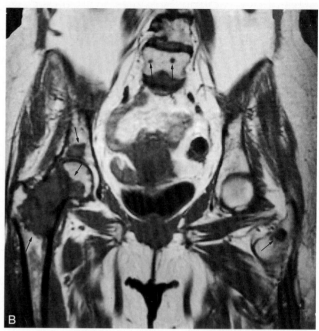

Figure 11.12   Bony metastases.   A and **B.** Coronal T1-weighted MRI demonstrates multiple areas of low signal (*arrows*) involving the iliac bones, sacrum, both proximal femurs, and the lumbar vertebrae.

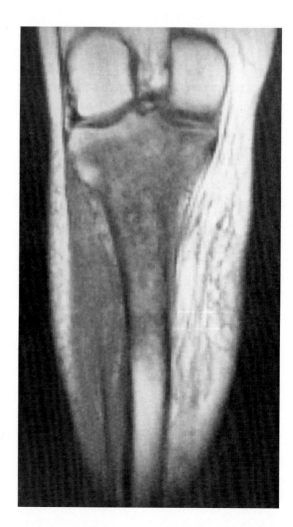

Figure 11.13   Osteomyelitis of the proximal tibia. (This is the same patient as in Fig. 11.2.) Coronal T1-weighted MRI demonstrates an extensive area of low signal within the marrow space of the tibia. The process extends up to the joint line but has not yet crossed it. The actual extent of marrow involvement is greater than the degree of bony destruction seen on the radiograph.

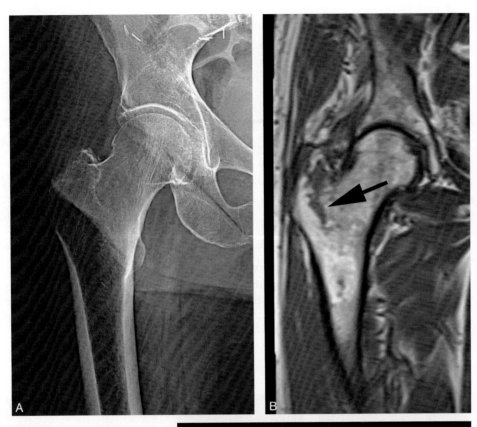

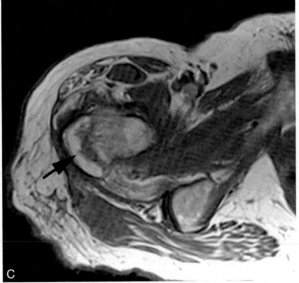

Figure 11.14   Occult hip fracture diagnosed by MRI.   A. Radiograph of the hip is not satisfactory for diagnosing a hip fracture in this elderly patient. **B.** T1-weighted coronal and **C.** Axial MRI shows a vertical line of low signal (*arrows*) representing an intertrochanteric fracture.

decreased blood flow. Second is the *blood-pool phase*, which consists of static images to determine areas of hyperemia, such as would occur in osteomyelitis. Third is the *delayed phase*, which consists of static images of the skeleton obtained 2 to 3 hours after injection to determine areas of increased tracer uptake or areas of decreased uptake (photopenia). On rare occasions, when vertebral collapse from osteoporosis or metastases is suspected, a fourth phase is obtained at 24 hours to compare the ratio of residual isotope in abnormal vertebrae versus normal vertebrae.

Indium Scan

As mentioned previously, the *technetium scan* is often nonspecific. One area where a more specific isotope scan may be used is in suspected osteomyelitis. These studies use

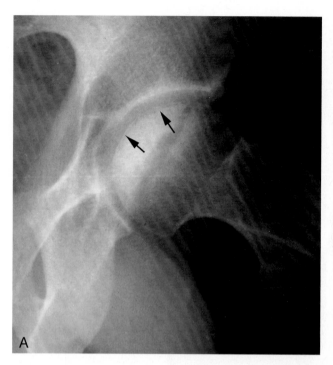

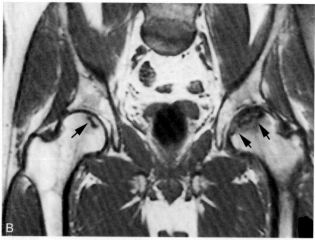

Figure 11.15   Avascular necrosis of the left femoral head.
A. Frogleg lateral radiograph of the left hip demonstrates increased density to the femoral head and subchondral lucency (*arrows*). **B.** T1-weighted image of the pelvis shows low signal within both femoral heads (*arrows*). Radiographs of the right hip were normal.

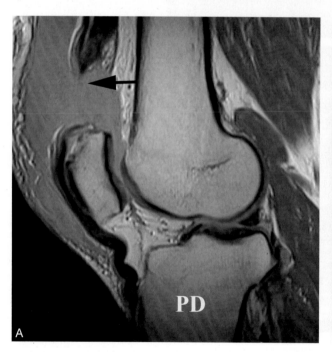

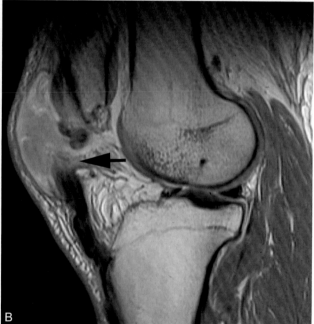

Figure 11.16   Quadriceps (A) and patellar tendon (B) tears (*arrows*) in two different patients demonstrated on gradient echo sagittal MRI.

indium 111–labeled white cells to identify areas of inflammatory activity (Fig. 11.25). This is particularly useful in a patient who may have an infection around a metallic implant (plate, screw, rod, or prosthesis), because the metal often produces artifacts in MRI.

Arthrography

Arthrography is the study of joints using contrast material that is injected into the joint space. Two varieties are performed. In *conventional arthrography,* iodinated contrast is injected without or with air into the shoulder to detect tears of the rotator cuff (Fig. 11.26) or into

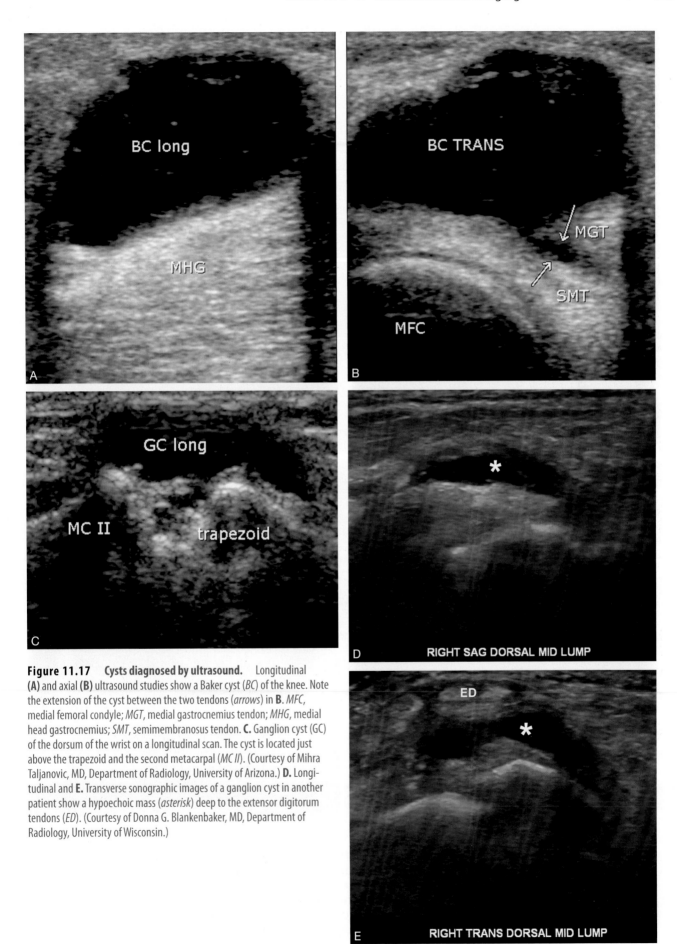

Figure 11.17 Cysts diagnosed by ultrasound. Longitudinal **(A)** and axial **(B)** ultrasound studies show a Baker cyst (*BC*) of the knee. Note the extension of the cyst between the two tendons (*arrows*) in **B**. *MFC*, medial femoral condyle; *MGT*, medial gastrocnemius tendon; *MHG*, medial head gastrocnemius; *SMT*, semimembranosus tendon. **C.** Ganglion cyst (GC) of the dorsum of the wrist on a longitudinal scan. The cyst is located just above the trapezoid and the second metacarpal (*MC II*). (Courtesy of Mihra Taljanovic, MD, Department of Radiology, University of Arizona.) **D.** Longitudinal and **E.** Transverse sonographic images of a ganglion cyst in another patient show a hypoechoic mass (*asterisk*) deep to the extensor digitorum tendons (*ED*). (Courtesy of Donna G. Blankenbaker, MD, Department of Radiology, University of Wisconsin.)

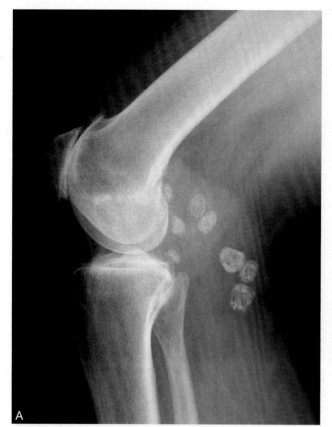

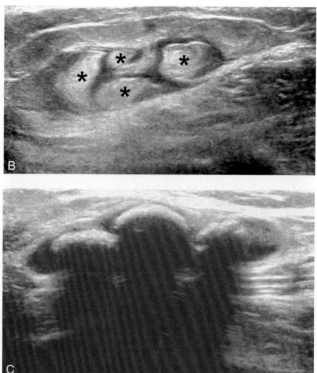

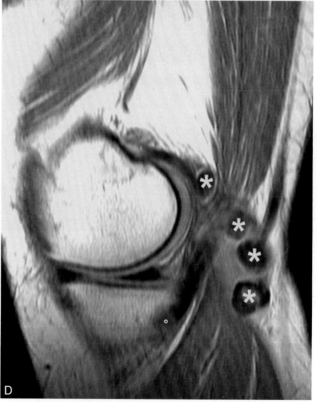

Figure 11.18   Synovial osteochondromatosis.   A. Lateral radiograph shows multiple loose bodies in the popliteal fossa. **B.** Longitudinal ultrasound exam shows multiple bodies (*asterisk*) within a cyst. **C.** Axial ultrasound exam shows shadowing from the loose bodies. This is similar to the picture seen with gallstones. **D.** Sagittal proton density MRI shows the loose bodies (*asterisks*) to be within a Baker cyst.

the wrist for ligamentous tears (Fig. 11.27). This type of study is also used in evaluating patients with painful joint implants (Fig. 11.28). Although conventional arthrography has largely been replaced by MRI, it still is used for patients who are unable to go into the magnet. The second type of arthrography is the *MR arthrogram.* In this procedure, dilute paramagnetic agents are injected into the joint before MR examination (see Fig. 11.10). MR arthrography has the advantage over unenhanced MRI in that it clearly identifies tears

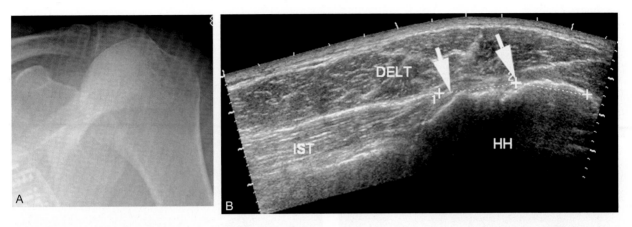

Figure 11.19   Supraspinatus tendon rupture (rotator cuff tear).   A. Radiograph shows elevation of the humeral head and impingement on the acromion. These findings are strongly suggestive of rotator cuff tear. **B.** Oblique coronal ultrasound shows a complete tear of the supraspinatus tendon and demonstrates the free ends of the torn tendon (*arrows*). *DELT*, deltoid; *HH*, humeral head; *IST*, infraspinatus. (Courtesy Mihra Taljanovic, MD, Department of Radiology, University of Arizona.)

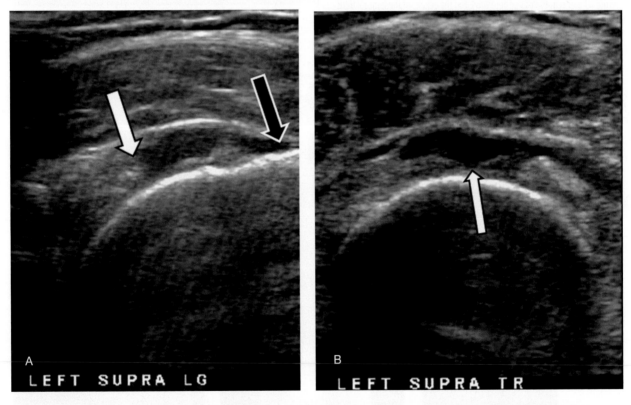

Figure 11.20   Full thickness supraspinatus tendon tear.   A. Longitudinal sonographic image shows fluid signal filling the tear gap between arrows. The torn tendon end (*white arrow*) should attach onto the greater tuberosity footprint (*black arrow*). **B.** Transverse image also depicts the tear (*arrow*). Rotator cuff tears should be confirmed on both longitudinal and transverse images. (Courtesy of Donna G. Blankenbaker, MD, Department of Radiology, University of Wisconsin.)

of cartilage, tendons, and ligaments that may or may not have been demonstrated on the conventional study (Fig. 11.29).

Percutaneous Bone Biopsy

Percutaneous bone biopsy is a procedure that diagnostic radiologists perform using any imaging modality that will show the lesion; however, CT is the method of choice (see Fig. 11.3). In addition to obtaining tissue for pathologic diagnosis, CT-guided excision

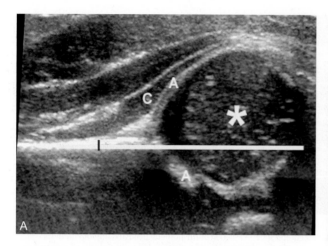

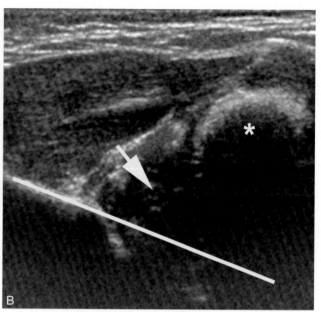

Figure 11.21   Congenital hip dysplasia.   A. Ultrasound examination shows lateral subluxation of femoral head (*asterisk*) with application of pressure. Normally, an extension of a line drawn along the ischium (*I*) should pass through the center of the femoral head. **B.** Dislocation of femoral head. With pressure, the femoral head echoes disappear (*arrow*) and the echoes of the femoral neck now can be seen (*asterisk*). *A*, acetabulum; *C*, cartilaginous portion of acetabular roof. (Courtesy of Leonard E. Swischuk, MD, University of Texas at Galveston.)

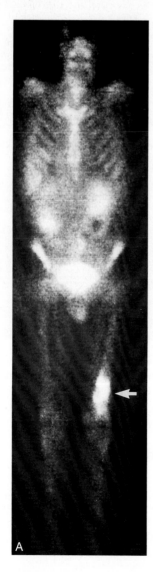

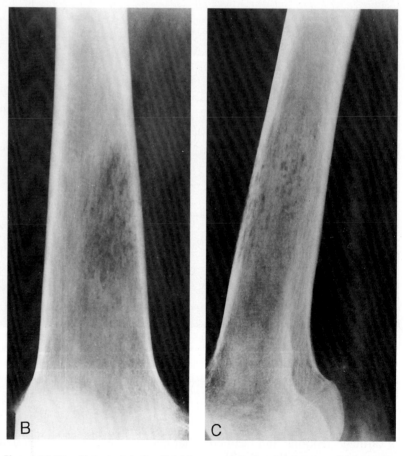

Figure 11.22   Metastasis to the distal femur.   A. Radionuclide bone scan shows extensive areas of increased tracer activity in the sternum, ribs, iliac bones, and distal left femur (*arrow*). Frontal (**B**) and lateral (**C**) radiographs of the distal left femur show moth-eaten to permeative bony destruction.

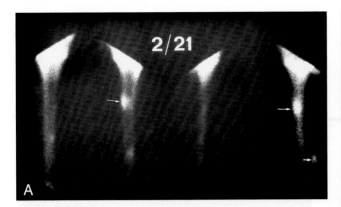

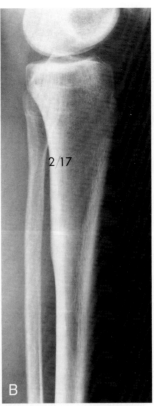

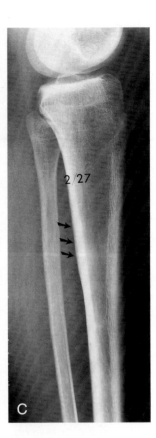

Figure 11.23 Stress fracture of the tibia in a runner.
A. Radionuclide bone scan shows an area of tracer uptake in the proximal tibia (*long arrows*). A second area is present in the distal fibula (*short arrow*). **B.** Lateral radiograph made 4 days earlier is normal. **C.** Lateral radiograph made 10 days after the first shows periosteal new bone formation in the posterior tibia (*arrows*).

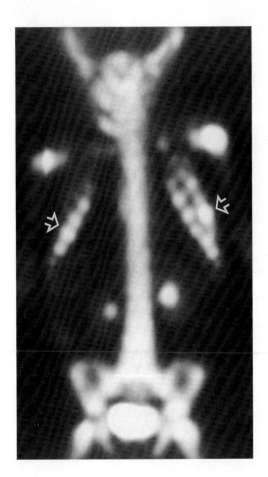

Figure 11.24 Child abuse. Radionuclide bone scan demonstrates multiple areas of tracer activity in the ribs (*arrows*), a finding considered pathognomonic for child abuse.

of osteoid osteomas is replacing conventional surgical excision because of its greater accuracy in localization, lower morbidity, and lower cost. Furthermore, CT-guided injections of steroids, alcohol, or methyl methacrylate into bone tumors or tumorlike lesions is commonplace at large medical centers. A variation on this procedure is the ablation of osteoid osteomas by a radiofrequency probe placed under CT guidance (Fig. 11.30). Another variation of this procedure is CT-guided screw placement for sacroiliac instability (see Fig. 11.4) or for acetabular fractures.

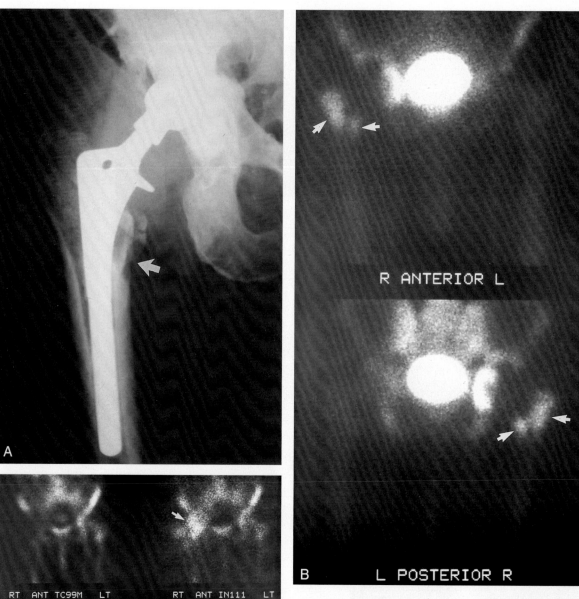

Figure 11.25   Infection at site of hip implant.   A. Radiograph shows a lucency in the vicinity of the lesser trochanter (*arrow*) in a patient with a painful implant. **B.** Conventional bone scan shows increased tracer activity in both trochanters (*arrows*). This could represent postoperative change or evidence of loosening or infection. The main portion of the femoral head is photopenic because of the metal in the implant. **C.** Concomitant technetium 99m bone marrow scan (left) and indium 111 white blood cell scan (right) show the marrow area of the right hip to be photopenic while there is increased white cell concentration on the indium study (*arrows*). This is considered pathognomonic for infection.

Angiography

Angiography is used infrequently to evaluate patients with suspected bone tumors because MRI has largely superseded it for this purpose. However, in these patients, angiography may be performed to localize tumor vessels for either embolization or chemotherapy infusion. Angiography is also used to evaluate blood vessels in severe skeletal trauma where vascular injury is suspected (Fig. 11.31).

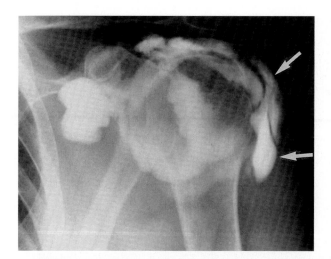

Figure 11.26   Shoulder arthrogram demonstrating a complete rotator cuff tear.   Contrast injected into the glenohumeral joint has extravasated into the subacromial/subdeltoid bursa (*arrows*). An intact rotator cuff prevents this from occurring.

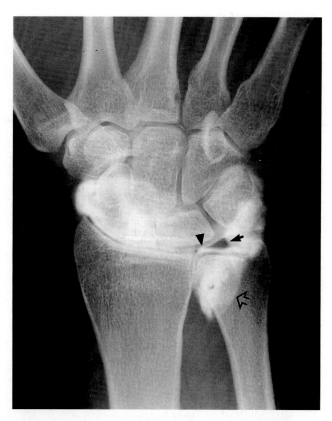

Figure 11.27   Triangular fibrocartilage tear.   Wrist arthrogram demonstrates extravasation of contrast into the distal radioulnar joint space (*open arrow*). Note the tear (*arrowhead*) in the triangular fibrocartilage (*short arrow*) at its point of origin from the distal radius.

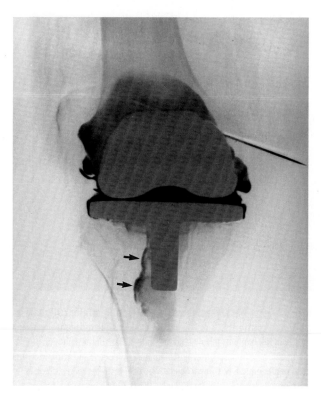

Figure 11.28   Loose total knee implant.   Subtraction radiograph following intraarticular injection of contrast shows the contrast tracking between bone and cement at the site of implantation of the tibial component (*arrows*).

Bone Mineral Density Imaging

Concern for patients with osteoporosis and its subsequent morbidity and mortality has led to the development of several methods of assessing bone mineral density using imaging studies: dual x-ray absorptiometry (DXA), CT densitometry, and a sonogram device for scanning of the calcaneus. Each of these methods has advantages and drawbacks in terms of sensitivity and accuracy. However, at present, DXA scanning is the procedure of choice (Fig. 11.32). This procedure uses a database of normal bone density for comparison and provides an objective assessment of a patient's bone mineral density. This is helpful in initial diagnosis and reevaluation after therapy is initiated. If you have a patient for whom you are considering performing a bone densitometry study, you should consult your radiologist.

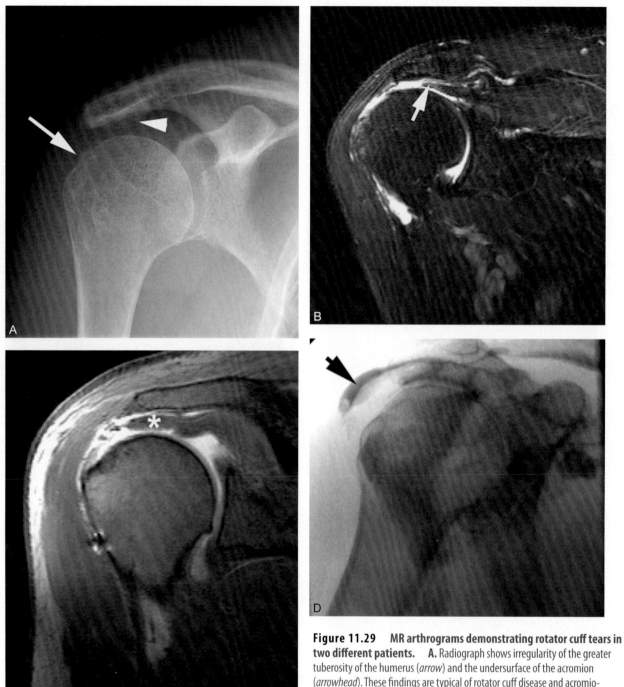

Figure 11.29   MR arthrograms demonstrating rotator cuff tears in two different patients.   A. Radiograph shows irregularity of the greater tuberosity of the humerus (*arrow*) and the undersurface of the acromion (*arrowhead*). These findings are typical of rotator cuff disease and acromiohumeral impingement. **B.** Coronal oblique MRI demonstrates extravasation of contrast into the subdeltoid bursa through a tear in the supraspinatus tendon that is retracted (*arrow*). **C.** Coronal oblique MRI in another patient demonstrates shredding and atrophy of the supraspinatus tendon (*asterisk*) with extravasation of contrast into the subdeltoid bursa. **D.** Fluoroscopic spot film taken at the time of injection shows extravasated contrast (*arrow*) in the subdeltoid bursa.

Anatomic Considerations

We will not review the anatomy of each of the 206 bones in the skeleton or of the important ligaments and muscles you will encounter on musculoskeletal imaging studies. For that purpose, consult an anatomy textbook. However, you should remember that because you are dealing with three-dimensional structures in the skeleton, many bony projections

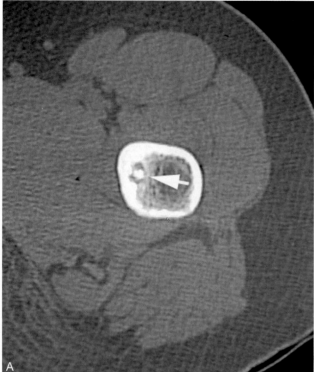

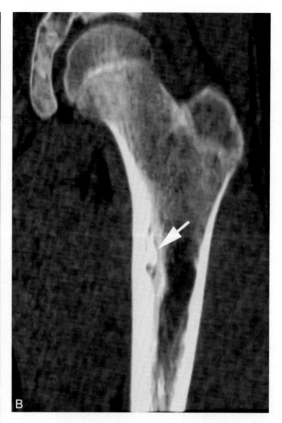

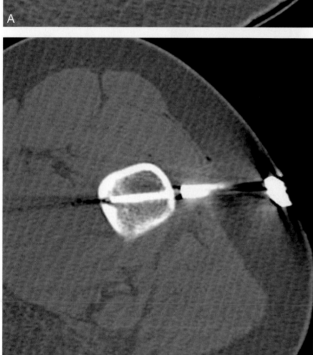

Figure 11.30   CT-guided radiofrequency ablation of an osteoid osteoma.   Axial (**A**) and coronal (**B**) reconstructed CT images of the proximal femur shows the osteoid osteoma (*arrows*). **C.** Axial shows the radiofrequency probe placed into the tumor.

on radiographs may overlap and produce "strange" images with which you are not familiar. The best way to avoid this confusion is to have a thorough knowledge of the anatomy of the bone being studied. For difficult cases CT has been proven effective in resolving the issues.

Bones are grouped into five types based on their shapes:

- ○ *Long bones,* which have two ends and a shaft (femur, humerus, and, interestingly, phalanges, which are miniature long bones)
- ○ *Short bones,* which are typically six sided (carpals and tarsals)

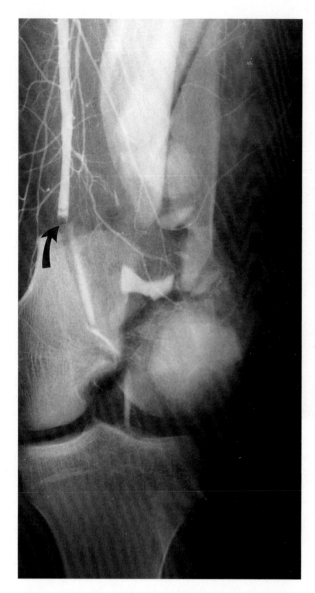

Figure 11.31   Transected femoral artery (*arrow*) in a patient with a severely comminuted intercondylar fracture of the distal femur.

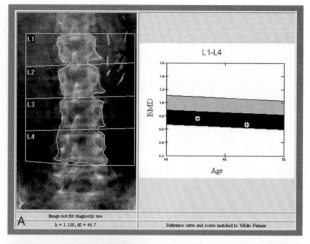

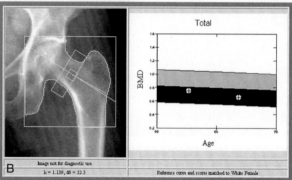

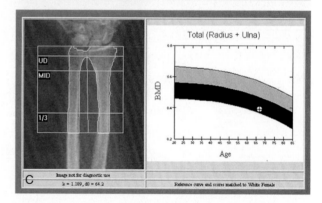

Figure 11.32   Dual x-ray absorptiometry (DEXA) bone densitometry scans.   A. Lumbar scan. **B.** Right hip scan. **C.** Right wrist scan. The images show the areas studied at each level. The data from each measurement reflect the bone mineral density (BMD). A graphic printout for each level shows the patient's average density (+) is below the mean for her age. A complete scan has charts of all the measurements.

○ *Flat bones* (calvaria, ribs, os coxae, and sternum)
○ *Irregular bones,* which have many sides (vertebrae)
○ *Sesamoid bones,* which lack periosteum and develop in tendons (the largest is the patella)

Furthermore, there are two architectural types of bone: *compact* (dense) and *cancellous* (spongy). The distribution of these types of bones depends on the stress to which each bone is subjected.

There are three locations within a long bone: the *epiphysis,* or growth center; the *metaphysis,* an area that lies just beneath the *physis,* or growth plate; and the *diaphysis,* or shaft. Accessory growth centers called *apophyses* serve as anchoring points for tendons. Examples of apophyses are the greater and lesser tuberosities of the proximal humerus, the distal medial epicondyle of the humerus, and the greater and lesser trochanters of the proximal femur. Bone growth occurs at the physis. The blood supply to the metaphysis is the most prominent, which explains the frequent occurrence of infections and tumors at that location. Apophyses and flat bones such as the os coxae have *metaphyseal equivalent* areas. As will be discussed later, these locations are of considerable importance in predicting the nature of some bone lesions.

Pathologic Considerations

The analysis of bone and joint lesions can be as simple as the ABCS:

- ○ Anatomic appearance and alignment abnormalities
- ○ Bony mineralization and texture abnormalities
- ○ Cartilage (joint space) abnormalities
- ○ Soft tissue abnormalities

Each of these is discussed in detail later in the chapter. Using this analytical approach, however, you will find how adept you will be at recognizing and diagnosing many bone and joint lesions.

"ABCS" OF MUSCULOSKELETAL ABNORMALITIES

- ▶ Anatomic and alignment abnormalities
- ▶ Bony mineralization and texture abnormalities
- ▶ Cartilage (joint space) abnormalities
- ▶ Soft tissue abnormalities

There are six basic pathologic categories of skeletal disease: *congenital, inflammatory, metabolic, neoplastic, traumatic,* and *vascular.* A seventh category, *miscellaneous* or *other,* might be added to encompass diseases that do not fall strictly into one of the first six.

The logical approach to musculoskeletal radiology begins by defining the *distribution* of a lesion and by applying a number of factors called *predictor variables* that can further narrow the diagnostic choices.

Distribution

The distribution of a bone or joint lesion provides important clues to the etiology of that lesion. Lesions may be *monostotic* or *monoarticular*—confined to one bone or joint; *polyostotic* or *polyarticular*—located in many bones or joints; or *diffuse*—involving virtually every bone or joint. Applying this distribution pattern to the six pathologic categories produces the scheme shown in Table 11.1. As the table shows, only two disease categories may occur diffusely: metabolic and neoplastic. Metabolic disease by definition is a diffuse disease; however, occasionally monostotic or polyostotic forms occur. Examples of these lesions are shown in Table 11.2.

Table 11.1 DISTRIBUTION OF BONE DISEASE BY PATHOLOGIC CATEGORY

Category	Monostotic/Articular	Polyostotic/Articular	Diffuse
Congenital	X	X	
Inflammatory	X	X	
Neoplastic	X	X	X
Metabolic	(X)	(X)	X
Traumatic	X	X	
Vascular	X	X	

Table 11.2 EXAMPLES OF DISTRIBUTION: PATHOLOGIC RELATIONSHIPS

Category	Monostotic/Articular	Polyostotic/Articular	Diffuse
Congenital	Cervical rib	Cleidocranial dysplasia	
Inflammatory	Osteomyelitis, gout	Gout, rheumatoid arthritis	
Neoplastic	Any bone tumor	Myeloma	Metastasis
Metabolic	(Paget disease)	(Paget disease, fibrous dysplasia)	hyperparathyroidism, osteopetrosis
Traumatic	Single fracture	Multiple fractures, battered child	
Vascular	Perthes disease	Perthes disease, sickle cell	Sickle cell

Predictor Variables

Eleven predictor variables may be applied to the radiographic appearance of any bone or joint lesion to help you make a correct diagnosis:

- Behavior of the lesion
- Bone or joint involved
- Location within bone or joint
- Age, gender, and race
- Margin of lesion
- Shape of lesion
- Joint space involvement
- Bony reaction
- Matrix production
- Soft tissue changes
- History of trauma or surgery

Although many of these variables apply to the diagnosis of bone tumors you should be aware that primary bone tumors, exclusive of myeloma, are rare lesions. You should also recognize that, in many instances, you may not be able to make a specific diagnosis even after applying all these factors. Radiologists should be satisfied that they have done their best when they have been able to categorize a difficult lesion as either *aggressive* or *nonaggressive* and have thus decided whether the lesion needs to undergo biopsy. Table 11.3 summarizes these predictor variables.

Behavior of the Lesion

Bone lesions may be primarily *osteolytic* (*osteoclastic* or *bone destroying*) or *osteoblastic* (*bone forming, reactive,* or *reparative*); occasionally, you will see a mixture of the two. Lytic lesions are usually the result of increased osteoclastic activity. The pathologic entity (infection or tumor) stimulates the multinucleated osteoclasts or giant cells to literally make room for it. This explains the presence of giant cells in the pathology of many bone lesions. There are three forms of osteolytic bone destruction: geographic, moth-eaten, and permeative. A *geographic* appearance implies that large areas of bone have been destroyed and are easily visible with the unaided eye (Fig. 11.33). While geographic destruction suggests a less aggressive lesion, we must look at other predictor variables (discussed below) to make that determination. A *moth-eaten* appearance is one in which there are many discrete, small holes throughout the bone, similar to a piece of clothing ruined by moth larvae (Fig. 11.34). A moth-eaten appearance suggests a more aggressive lesion. A *permeative* pattern is one in which there is fine bony destruction (Fig. 11.35). Pathologically, this represents a lesion diffusely infiltrating bone through the Haversian system. In many instances, a magnifying lens is required to see the bone destruction. Permeative destruction implies a very aggressive process, such as the round cell tumors of bone (Ewing tumor, malignant lymphoma, myeloma), or osteomyelitis.

Table 11.3 PREDICTOR VARIABLES FOR BONE AND JOINT LESIONS

Behavior of the lesion
• Osteolytic
• Osteoblastic
• Mixed
Bone or joint involved
Location within a bone or joint
• Epiphysis (or apophysis)
• Metaphysis (or equivalent)
• Diaphysis
• Articular (cartilage)
• Para-articular ("bare areas")
Age, gender, and race of patient
Margin of lesion
• Sharply defined
• Poorly defined
Shape of lesion
• Longer than wide
• Wider than long
• Cortical breakthrough
• No breakthrough
Joint space involvement
Bony reaction
• Sclerosis
Buttressing
• Periosteal
• Solid
• Laminated ("onionskin")
• Spiculated, sunburst, "hair on end" Codman triangle
Matrix production
• Osteoid
• Chondroid
• Mixed
• None
Soft tissue changes
History of trauma or surgery

Bone or Joint Involved

Some diseases have a predilection for certain bones or joints. Figure 11.36 illustrates the preferred locations of many common bone and joint lesions. Note, for example, that chondrosarcomas (Fig. 11.37) favor the pelvis, whereas enchondromas (Fig. 11.38) favor the phalanges and metacarpals; Paget disease commonly affects the pelvis, skull, spine, and tibia but spares the fibula (Fig. 11.39); gout favors the joints of the hands and feet (Fig. 11.40) as does rheumatoid arthritis (Fig. 11.41); and hyperparathyroidism commonly affects the skull, distal clavicles, and the hands and feet (Fig. 11.42). It is important to remember, however, that any lesion may be found in an unusual site (for example, a chondrosarcoma of the skull base). When that occurs, the lesion usually has all the characteristics of the entity at a more typical location. When confronted by a lesion in what may seem an unusual site, mentally transfer that lesion to the knee, one of the most common locations for benign and malignant processes, and the identity may become more apparent.

Text continues on page 382

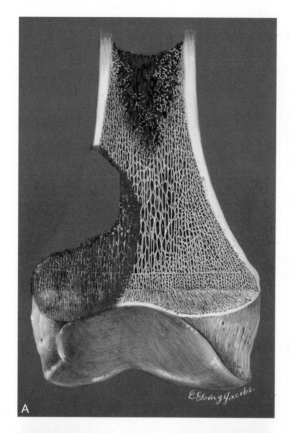

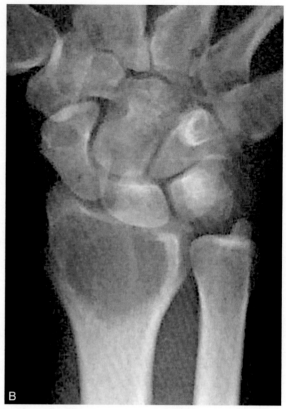

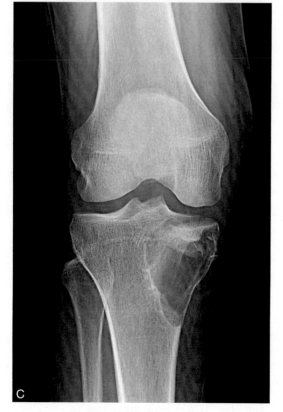

Figure 11.33   Geographic bone destruction.   A. Drawing showing a large destructive lesion that is easily seen with the unaided eye. **B.** Giant cell tumor of the distal radius with poorly defined borders. **C.** Giant cell tumor of the proximal medial tibia with well-defined borders.

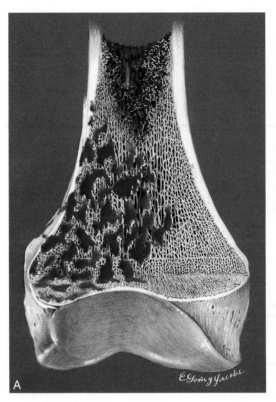

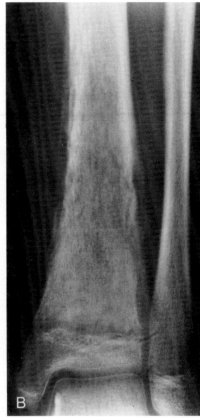

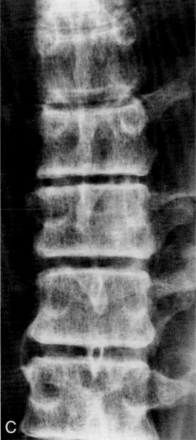

Figure 11.34   Moth-eaten bone destruction.   A. Drawing showing typical appearance of moth-eaten destruction. In most instances, this may be seen with the unaided eye. **B.** Osteomyelitis of the distal tibia, an example of moth-eaten bony destruction.

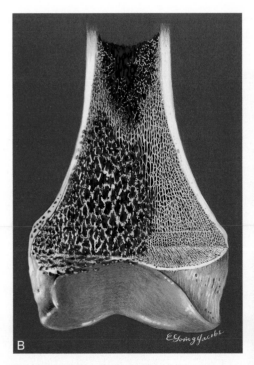

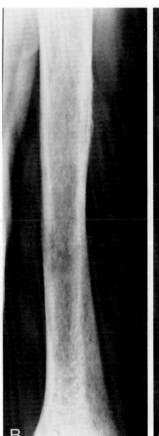

Figure 11.35   Permeative or infiltrative bone destruction.
A. Drawing showing the pathologic process infiltrating the Haversian system. Magnification may be required to see the lesion. **B.** Permeative bony destruction in a patient with metastatic breast carcinoma involving the entire humerus. Note the severe soft tissue wasting, an indication of cachexia in this patient. **C.** Permeative destruction of the vertebrae in a patient with multiple myeloma. At first glance, this appears like osteoporosis. On closer inspection, there is actual bone destruction.

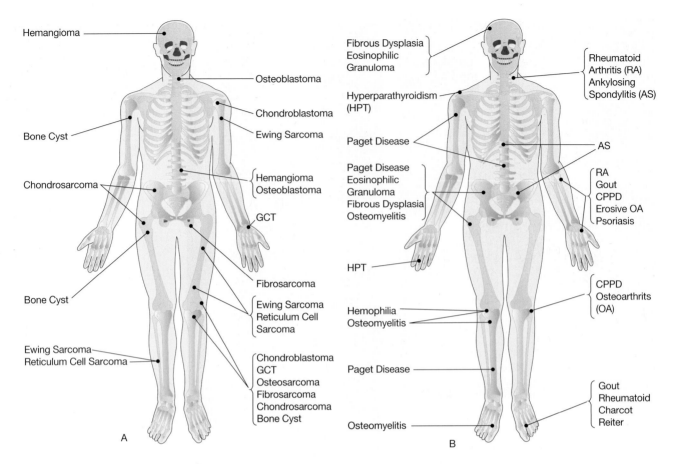

Figure 11.36   **Preferred locations for bone lesions.**   **A.** Neoplastic conditions. **B.** Nonneoplastic conditions. *AS,* ankylosing spondylitis; *CPPD,* calcium pyrophosphate deposition disease; *GCT,* giant cell tumor; *HPT,* hyperparathyroidism; *OA,* osteoarthritis; *RA,* rheumatoid arthritis.

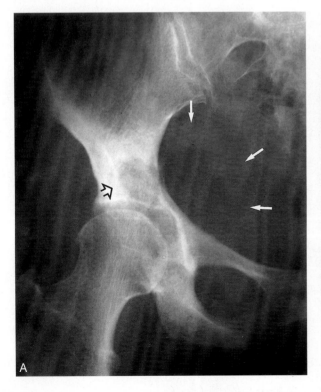

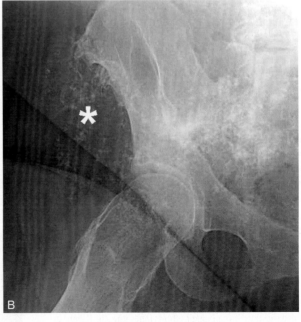

Figure 11.37   **Chondrosarcoma of the pelvis in two patients.**
A. There is a large lytic lesion just above the acetabulum (*open arrow*). An associated soft tissue mass with flocculent calcification extends into the pelvis (*closed arrows*). **B.** Oblique view in another patient shows the popcornlike chondroid matrix (*asterisk*). Chondrosarcomas tend to be large when located in the pelvis.

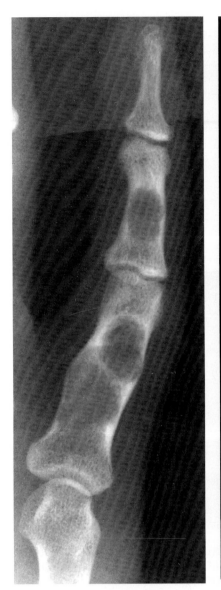

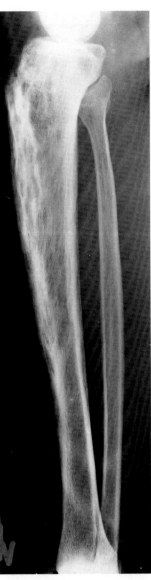

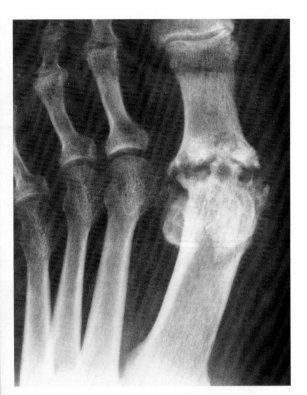

Figure 11.40 Gout. The metatarsophalangeal joint of the great toe is severely involved in this patient with long-standing gout.

Figure 11.38 Enchondromas of the proximal and middle phalanges.

Figure 11.39 Paget disease of the tibia. Note that the fibula is spared.

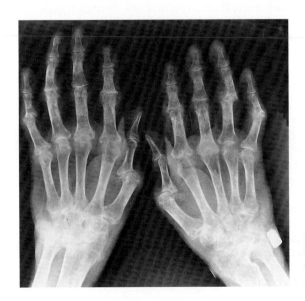

Figure 11.41 Rheumatoid arthritis of the hands and wrists. Note the involvement of the wrist joints, the metacarpophalangeal joints, and interphalangeal joints.

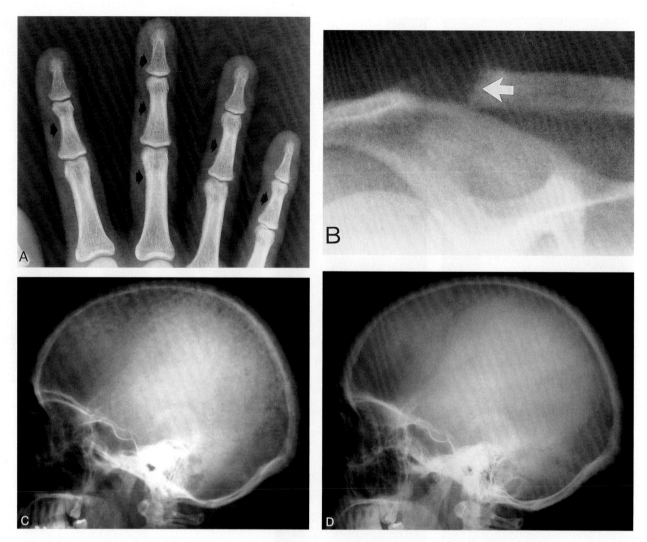

Figure 11.42   Hyperparathyroidism.   A. Detail view of the hands shows subperiosteal resorption in the phalanges (*arrows*). **B.** Detail views of distal clavicle shows subchondral resorption (*arrow*). **C.** Skull radiograph shows the typical "salt and pepper" appearance caused by the osteoporosis. **D.** Skull radiograph of same patient 6 months after removal of the patient's parathyroid adenoma. The bones have returned to normal.

 ▶ When confronted by a lesion in what may seem an unusual site, mentally transfer that lesion to the knee.

Location within Bone or Joint

The location of a lesion within a bone or joint also provides important clues to its identity. Many lesions have a predilection for the epiphysis, metaphysis, or diaphysis. The common locations of bone tumors are shown in Figure 11.43. Similarly, nonneoplastic lesions also have a predilection for favored areas of bones or joints; for example, osteoarthritis prefers the weight-bearing surfaces of the large joints (Fig. 11.44), whereas rheumatoid arthritis affects the entire surface of the same joint (Fig. 11.45). Osteomyelitis favors the diam-etaphyseal region where red marrow is prevalent. Similarly, Langerhans cell histiocytosis (histiocytosis X, eosinophilic granuloma) is found in areas rich in red marrow.

The various arthritides favor not only joints but also sites within and around a joint. Each synovial joint consists of three parts: a cartilage-bearing surface, an area devoid of cartilage called the "bare" or paraarticular area, and a joint capsule. Both the areas with and without cartilage are contained within the joint capsule (Fig. 11.46). Diseases such as rheumatoid arthritis and osteoarthritis primarily involve the cartilage areas (Fig. 11.47), while gout, psoriatic arthritis, and reactive arthritis affect the bare (paraarticular) areas (Fig. 11.48).

Locus within bone

Round cell lessions } Ewing tumor
Malignant lymphoma
Myeloma

Chondrosarcoma
osteosarooma

Non-assifying fibroma

Chondromyxoid fibroma

Bone cyst
fibrosarcoma

Giant cell tumor

Osteolytic osteosarcoma

Chondrosancoma
ostecearcoma

Chondroblasloma

Figure 11.43   Common locations of bone tumors. Chondroblastoma favors the epiphysis in the skeletally immature patient. Round cell lesions favor the diaphysis. The majority of other lesions favor the metaphysis. Giant cell tumors will extend to the joint surface in a skeletally mature patient.

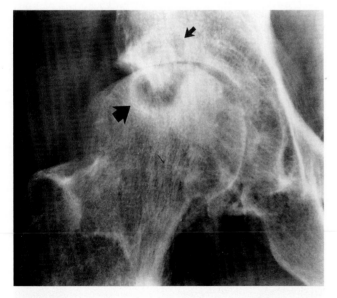

Figure 11.44   Osteoarthritis of the hip. The hip joint is narrowed, particularly superiorly. Large degenerative synovial cysts (geodes) are present in both the femoral head (*fat arrow*) and acetabulum (*small arrow*). Note the osteophyte formation in both the acetabulum and femoral head.

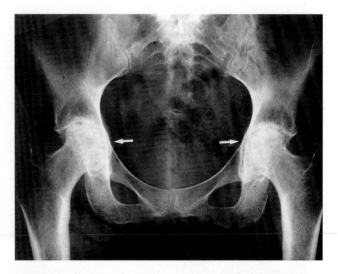

Figure 11.45   Rheumatoid arthritis of the hips. There is medial migration of both femoral heads (acetabular protrusion, *arrows*). Note that the entire joint is involved in rheumatoid arthritis. Compare with Figure 11.44.

Age, Gender, and Race of the Patient

The diagnosis of bone diseases also depends on the patient's age. A 10-year-old child with a permeative lesion of the shaft of a long bone is likely to have Ewing tumor (Fig. 11.49). A lesion of similar appearance in a much older patient should suggest malignant lymphoma (reticulum cell sarcoma) of bone. The clinician can often predict the type of a

Figure 11.46   Drawings illustrating joint surfaces.   A. The two areas within the joint capsule are the cartilage area (*open arrows*) and the "bare" (paraarticular) areas (*solid arrows*). **B.** Rheumatoid arthritis and osteoarthritis primarily affect the cartilage areas. Psoriatic arthritis, gout, and reactive arthritis affect the bare areas. In the late stages of all arthropathies, all areas of the joint are involved.

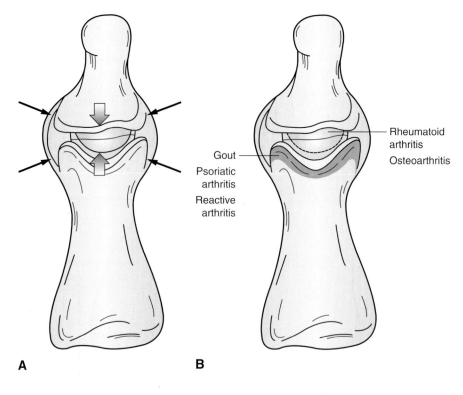

A

B

Gout

Psoriatic arthritis

Reactive arthritis

Rheumatoid arthritis

Osteoarthritis

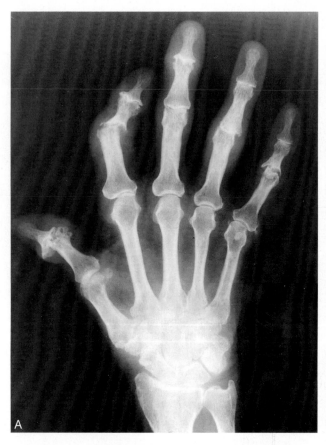

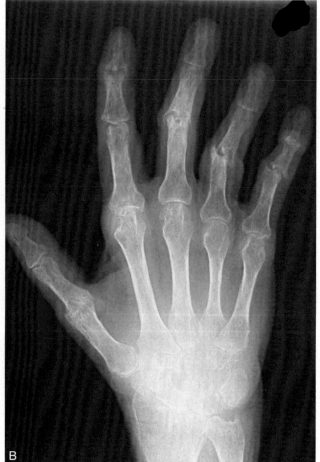

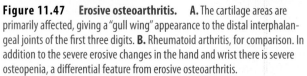

Figure 11.47   Erosive osteoarthritis.   A. The cartilage areas are primarily affected, giving a "gull wing" appearance to the distal interphalangeal joints of the first three digits. **B.** Rheumatoid arthritis, for comparison. In addition to the severe erosive changes in the hand and wrist there is severe osteopenia, a differential feature from erosive osteoarthritis.

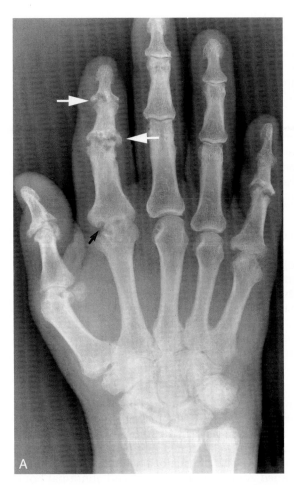

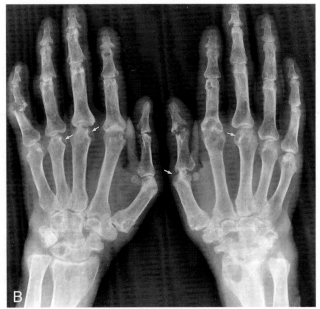

Figure 11.48   Involvement of the "bare" (paraarticular) areas.
A. Psoriatic arthropathy (advanced). The disease affects the bare areas initially, as shown in the second metacarpophalangeal joint (*small arrow*). Note the new bone formation at the bases of the middle and distal phalanges of the second digit (*large arrows*), giving a "mouse ear" configuration. In addition there is the "single ray phenomenon," in which all the joints of the first, second, and fifth digits are involved. **B.** Gout showing involvement of the paraarticular areas of multiple distal metacarpals (*arrows*).

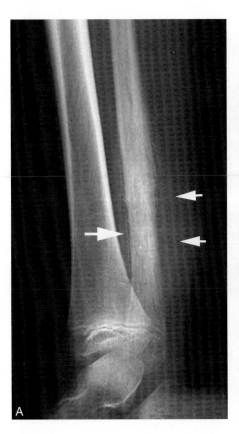

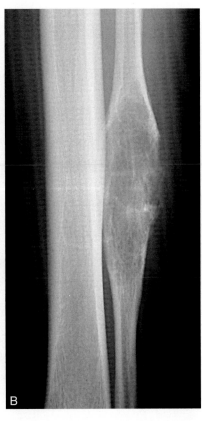

Figure 11.49   Round cell tumors of the fibula.   A. A permeative lesion is present in the diametaphyseal region. Note the interrupted laminated and "hair-on-end" periosteal reaction (*arrows*). This lesion may easily be confused with an osteosarcoma. The open physes in the tibia and fibula indicates the patient is of an age that would favor Ewing tumor. **B.** Lymphoma of bone in the mid diaphysis of the fibula. This lesion is poorly defined, has broken out of the bone indicating that it is aggressive. Biopsy is needed to make the diagnosis.

malignant bone tumor on the basis of the patient's age. For example, the most common type of tumor in patients under 1 year of age is neuroblastoma; in the first decade, Ewing tumor of tubular bone; ages 10 to 30 years, osteosarcoma and Ewing tumor of flat bones; between ages 30 and 40 years, most of the malignant sarcomas; and over age 40 years, metastatic carcinoma, along with multiple myeloma and chondrosarcoma.

BONE TUMORS AND AGE
- <1 year   Neuroblastoma
- 1–10 years   Ewing tubular bones
- 11–30 years   Ewing flat bones, osteosarcoma
- 30–40 years   Osteosarcoma, chondrosarcoma, fibrosarcoma
- >40 years   Myeloma, metastases, chondrosarcoma

Similarly, nonneoplastic lesions also occur more commonly in certain age groups. For example, Paget disease is almost never seen in patients younger than age 40 years. Infantile cortical hyperostosis (Caffey disease) does not occur in patients over age 1 year.

Many lesions also have a gender distribution. Paget disease and psoriatic arthritis are found more commonly in males. Rheumatoid arthritis, fibrous dysplasia, and congenital hip dysplasia are more common in females.

In addition to gender predominance, there is a racial predominance in some diseases, such as sickle cell disease (African descent), thalassemia (Mediterranean descent), and Gaucher disease (Ashkenazic Jewish descent).

Margin of Lesion

The border between normal and abnormal bone is called the *transition zone*. Careful attention to this area yields a wealth of information regarding the biologic behavior of bone lesions. In general, an abrupt transition zone that appears as a dense area of sclerosis between a lesion and normal bone or as a thin, well-defined line between normal and abnormal bone (Fig. 11.50) indicates a nonaggressive or usually a benign process. On the other hand, a broad or wide, poorly defined zone between normal and abnormal bone indicates a more aggressive lesion (Fig. 11.51). The differences in the growth rate of these

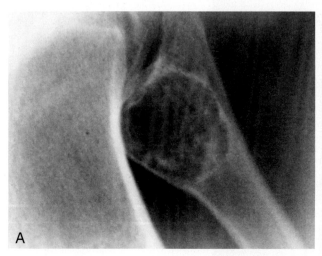

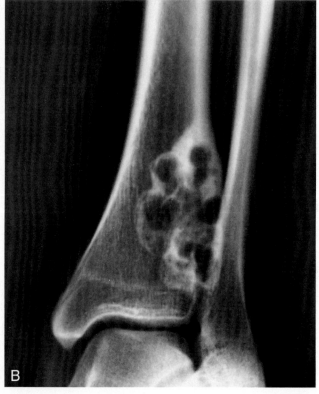

Figure 11.50   Benign lesions demonstrating a sharp transition zone. A. Enchondroma of the head of the fibula. Note the flocculent chondroid matrix within the lesion. **B.** Benign fibrous cortical defect (fibroxanthoma). A sclerotic border around this bubbly benign lesion clearly defines the transition between normal and abnormal bone. If asymptomatic, both of these lesions should be left alone.

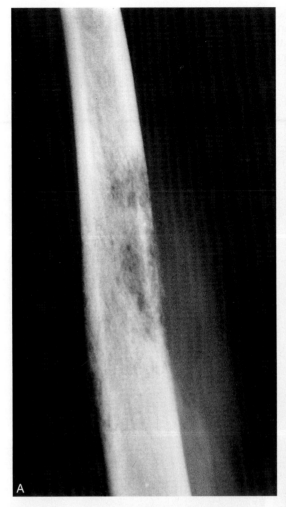

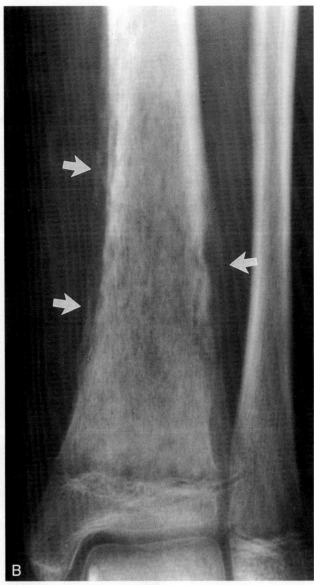

Figure 11.51 **Aggressive lesions demonstrating poor transition zone.** **A.** Metastatic lung carcinoma. **B.** Osteomyelitis. It is impossible to tell where normal bone is. Note the periosteal reaction (*arrows*). Each of these lesions requires a biopsy to make a diagnosis.

lesions account for the differences in their appearance. Slow-growing, benign lesions such as a fibroxanthoma of bone (see Fig. 11.50B) or a focus of tuberculosis progress at a rate slow enough to allow the bone to react in an attempt to contain them. An aggressive lesion, such as a malignant tumor or osteomyelitis, progresses at a rapid rate, and the bone is unable to respond adequately. Furthermore, a sclerotic margin that is thick with fuzzy borders should suggest an inflammatory lesion such as sclerosing osteomyelitis or tuberculosis.

▶ An abrupt transition zone indicates a nonaggressive or usually a benign process.
▶ A broad or wide, poorly defined zone between normal and abnormal bone indicates a more aggressive lesion.
▶ A lesion with a thick sclerotic margin with fuzzy borders suggests an inflammatory etiology.

Shape of Lesion

The shape of a lesion also indicates its growth rate in the same way that the margin does. A lesion that is longer than it is wide—that is, oriented with the shaft of the bone—is likely to be a nonaggressive benign process. In this situation, the lesion is growing with the bone and not faster than the bone. On the other hand, a lesion that is wider than the bone, has broken out of the bone, and has extended into the soft tissues is a more aggressive type of lesion (Fig. 11.52). MRI is particularly useful for assessing the extraosseous extent of bone lesions.

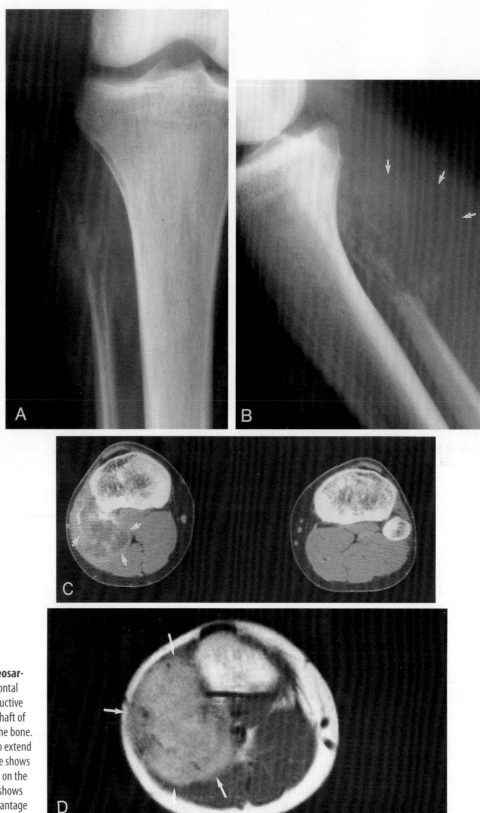

Figure 11.52   Telangiectatic osteosarcoma of the proximal fibula.   A. Frontal radiograph shows a poorly defined destructive lesion involving the head and proximal shaft of the fibula. The lesion has broken out of the bone. **B.** Lateral radiograph shows the lesion to extend into the soft tissues (*arrows*). **C.** CT image shows the lesion extending into the soft tissues on the right side (*arrows*). **D.** T2-weighted MRI shows the soft tissue involvement to better advantage (*arrows*).

▶ A lesion that is longer than it is wide is likely to be a nonaggressive benign process.
▶ A lesion that is wider than the bone, has broken out of the bone, and extends into the soft tissues is an aggressive process.

Joint Space Involved or Crossed

If a lesion involves or crosses a joint space, it most likely has an inflammatory origin. This is generally the case, no matter how aggressive or malignant the process may appear (Fig. 11.53). Infections will extend across a joint space, but tumors will not. Preservation of the vertebral end plates in a patient with a collapsed or destroyed vertebral body generally rules out infection as the cause of that collapse (Fig. 11.54). Tumors that have a predilection for the ends of bones, such as chondroblastoma and giant cell tumor (Fig. 11.55), will extend to the joint but will not cross it. Furthermore, even the most malignant bone tumors respect the joint cartilage or the physes (Fig. 11.56). On the other hand, abnormalities found on both sides of a joint that has *intact cortical margins* should suggest a polyostotic disorder rather than an arthropathy or infection.

▶ Preserved vertebral end plates in a patient with a collapsed or destroyed vertebral body generally rules out an infection as the cause. Abnormalities found on both sides of a joint that has intact cortical margins should suggest a polyostotic disorder rather than an arthropathy or infection.

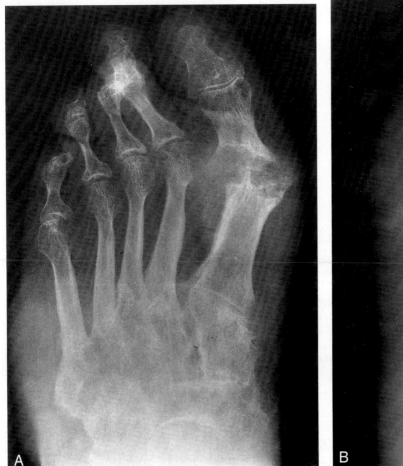
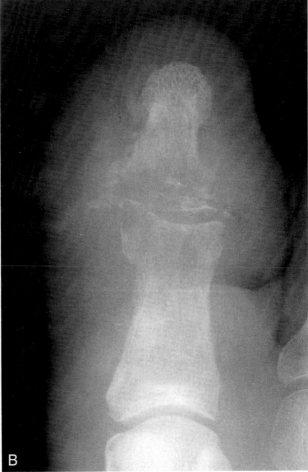

Figure 11.53   Joint space involvement.   A. Tophaceous gout. **B.** Osteomyelitis and joint space infection in a diabetic patient. These extensive destructive lesions involve both sides of the joint. This signifies that the process is either an arthropathy or an infection.

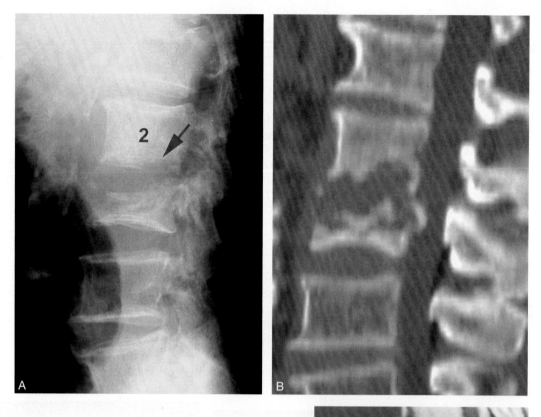

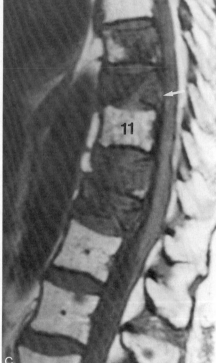

Figure 11.54   Importance of disc space involvement.
A. Vertebral osteomyelitis and disc space infection at L2-L3. There is bony destruction with partial collapse of L3. Note the involvement of L2 as well (*arrow*). **B.** Sagittal reconstructed CT image shows that both vertebrae are involved with most of the destruction centered on the disc space. **C.** T1-weighted sagittal CT image in a patient with diffuse metastatic disease. Although multiple vertebrae are involved the disc margins are spared. Note the involvement of the vertebral canal at T10 (*arrow*).

Bony Reaction

Bony responses to insult include periosteal reaction, sclerosis, and buttressing. *Periosteal reaction* is of four varieties: solid, laminated or onionskin, spiculated ("sunburst" or "hair on end"), or Codman triangle. *Solid* (uninterrupted, organized, or wavy) periosteal reaction (greater than 2 mm) indicates a benign process. It most often occurs in osteo-myelitis (Fig. 11.57) and fracture healing. A *laminated* (layered) or *onionskin* type of

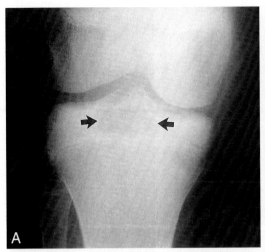

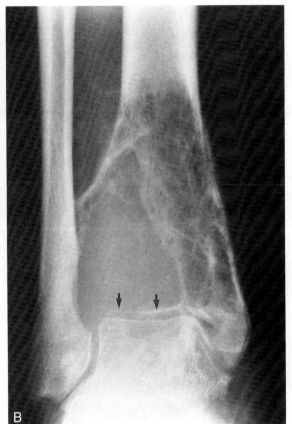

Figure 11.55 Epiphyseal tumors. A. Chondroblastoma (*arrows*) of the proximal tibia. The lesion has not crossed the physis. **B.** Giant cell tumor of the distal tibia. This large bubbly lesion extends down to the joint line (*arrows*) but has not crossed it. As a rule, tumors respect joint surfaces and physes.

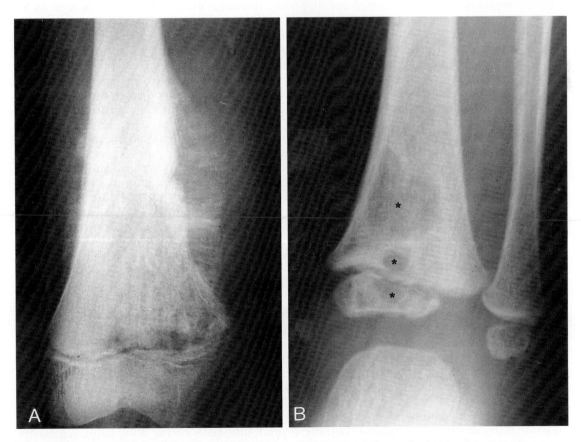

Figure 11.56 Relationship of lesions to the physis. A. Osteosarcoma extends down to the physis but does not cross it.
B. Tuberculous osteomyelitis has produced cystic lesions (*asterisks*) on both sides of the physis. The ankle joint is still not crossed.

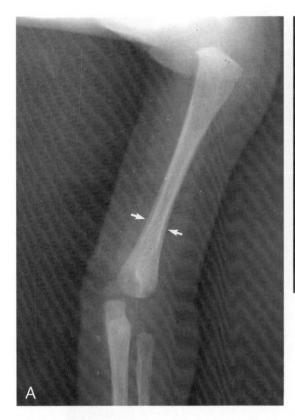

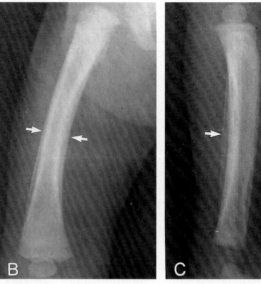

Figure 11.57   Solid periosteal reaction (*arrows*) in a patient with congenital syphilis.   A. Humerus. **B.** Femur. **C.** Tibia, lateral view.

periosteal reaction indicates *repetitive injury* to bone. This was previously thought to be pathognomonic of Ewing tumor or malignant lymphoma of bone. However, this type of reaction also occurs in any type of repetitive injury to bone, such as in child abuse. Once again, the nature of the laminated periosteal reaction may be determined by its thickness. In Ewing tumor, the periosteal reaction is thin, irregular, and disorganized (Fig. 11.58), whereas in a benign process such as osteomyelitis or repetitive trauma, such as child abuse (Fig. 11.59), the reaction is considerably thicker and often wavy. A *spiculated,* "*sunburst,*" or "*hair-on-end*" appearance is almost always associated with a malignant bone lesion (Fig. 11.60), most often an osteosarcoma. Occasionally, this type of periosteal pattern occurs in Ewing tumors and in metastatic squamous cell tumors. This form of periosteal reaction is the result of the neoplastic process breaking through a layer of periosteal new bone, followed by new periosteal response and subsequent breakthrough. The *Codman triangle* represents triangular ossification of a piece of periosteum that has been elevated (see Figs. 11.58A and 11.60B). In the past, this finding was also thought to be pathognomonic of tumor. However, it occurs in many benign conditions, including subperiosteal hemorrhage of any cause, such as postoperatively, in scurvy, and in child abuse.

 ▶ Laminated periosteal reaction indicates repetitive injury to bone.

Sclerosis is an attempt by the bone to wall off a diseased area. It generally indicates a benign process (Fig. 11.61). *Buttressing* is an attempt by the bone to reestablish architectural integrity; the term is derived from the flying buttresses of Gothic architecture (Fig. 11.62). The most common example of this is the *osteophyte* of degenerative arthritis (see Fig. 11.62B,C) or the *syndesmophyte* of inflammatory arthritis (Fig. 11.63). An osteophyte represents ossification along the corners of a joint. As a rule, it first grows horizontally before turning vertically. A syndesmophyte, on the other hand, represents ossification of Sharpey fibers in the disc. It is always oriented vertically. In ankylosing spondylitis, syndesmophytes are thin, delicate, and symmetric. In diffuse idiopathic

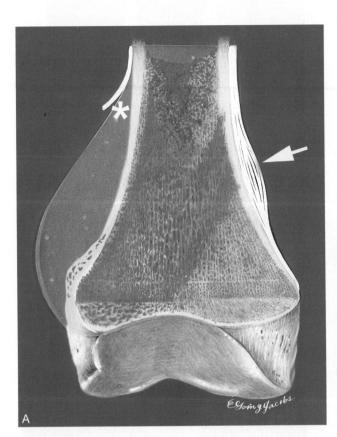

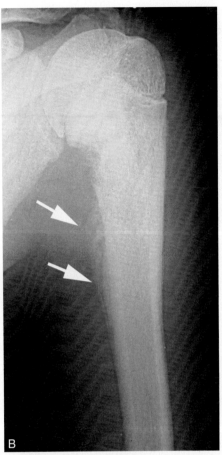

Figure 11.58 Laminated periosteal reaction. **A.** Drawing showing laminations (*solid arrow*). A Codman triangle is illustrated on the opposite side (*asterisk*). **B.** Irregular interrupted laminated periosteal reaction (*arrows*) in a patient with Ewing tumor.

skeletal hyperostosis (DISH), they are thicker, coarser, and usually symmetric. In other inflammatory arthropathies, such as psoriatic arthritis, reactive arthritis, or the spondyloarthropathy of inflammatory bowel disease, they are thick and asymmetric.

The *enthesophyte* is a variant of osteophytes and syndesmophytes. *Entheses* are the tendinous or ligamentous attachment points on bones. Some diseases, such as psoriatic arthropathy, produce ossification of entheses (Fig. 11.64).

Matrix Production

Matrix is a substance produced by certain bone tumors. It may be *chondroid* (cartilaginous), *osteoid* (bony), or mixed. Chondroid matrix appears as fine, stippled calcification; as rings, or Cs and Os; or as multiple popcornlike calcifications. Matrix frequently occurs in bulky masses of tumor within the soft tissues (Fig. 11.65). Osteoid matrix, on the other hand, is dense, usually of the same radiographic density as bone. It occurs most often in osteosarcoma (Fig. 11.66) but also may be seen in the benign ossifying condition called myositis ossificans (Fig. 11.67), in which soft tissue ossification results from injury and hemorrhage. Tumor matrix may be differentiated from the calcification of myositis ossificans or bone infarction by observing its distribution. As a rule, calcified tumor matrix is concentrated in the *center* of the lesion (Fig. 11.68A), whereas calcification of other sources (myositis ossificans or bone infarct) occurs initially in the *periphery* and then spreads centrally (Fig. 11.68B). CT may be required to identify and characterize matrix (Fig. 11.69).

 Calcified tumor matrix is concentrated in the center of the lesion, whereas calcification due to other causes occurs initially in the periphery and then spreads centrally.

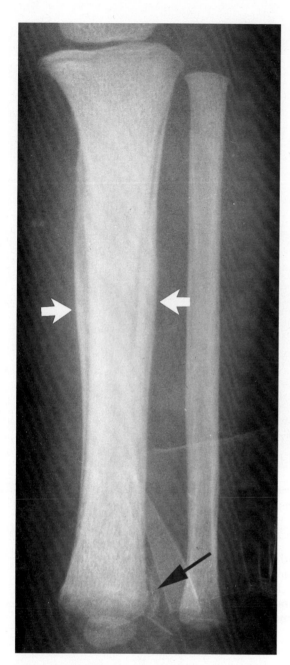

Figure 11.59   Laminated but solid periosteal reaction (*white arrows*) in an abused child.   Note the metaphyseal corner fracture in the distal tibia (*black arrow*).

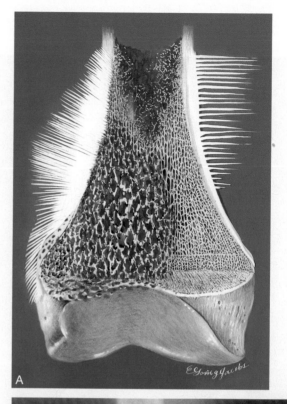

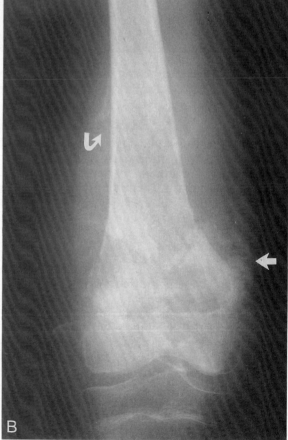

Figure 11.60   Spiculated periosteal reaction.   A. Drawing showing variations on spiculated periosteal reaction. **B.** Osteosarcoma demonstrating spiculated periosteal reaction (*straight arrow*). Note the Codman triangle (*curved arrow*).

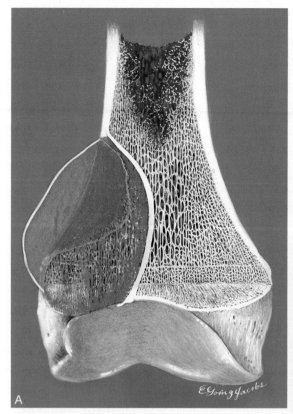

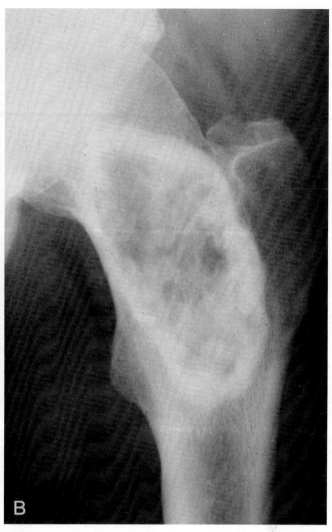

Figure 11.61   Reactive sclerosis.   A. Drawing showing sclerotic rim around a geographic lesion. **B.** Sclerosis around a focus of fibrous dysplasia of the proximal femur.

Soft Tissue Changes

By analyzing the soft tissues, you may obtain important clues regarding an underlying injury, disease process, or a specific bone lesion. For example, diffuse muscle wasting suggests a patient with paralysis, primary muscle disease, or severe inanition caused by disseminated carcinomatosis or AIDS. The presence of soft tissue swelling may be indicative of a mass (Fig. 11.70), hemorrhage, inflammation, or edema. The loss or displacement of fat lines normally found in the soft tissues is another indication of adjacent abnormality. For example, displacement or obliteration of the pronator quadratus fat line in the wrist (Fig. 11.71) usually indicates a fracture of the wrist. Elevation or displacement of the fat pads of the elbow indicates fluid within the joint capsule, usually the result of trauma (Fig. 11.72), but sometimes is found in inflammatory conditions such as rheumatoid arthritis. The presence of a *lipohemarthrosis* or fat-fluid level in the suprapatellar space on a horizontal beam lateral radiograph of the knee is indicative of a fracture communicating with the joint (Fig. 11.73). Lipohemarthroses are also commonly found on CT examinations of fractures (Fig. 11.74).

Calcifications within the soft tissues may be the result of old trauma or connective tissue disorders. Occasionally, old parasitic disease will manifest with soft tissue calcifications.

Gas in the tissues indicates trauma, recent surgery or injection, infection, or gas gangrene. Other soft tissue findings include the presence of foreign bodies, abdominal aortic aneurysm, or renal calculi in patients being evaluated for back pain.

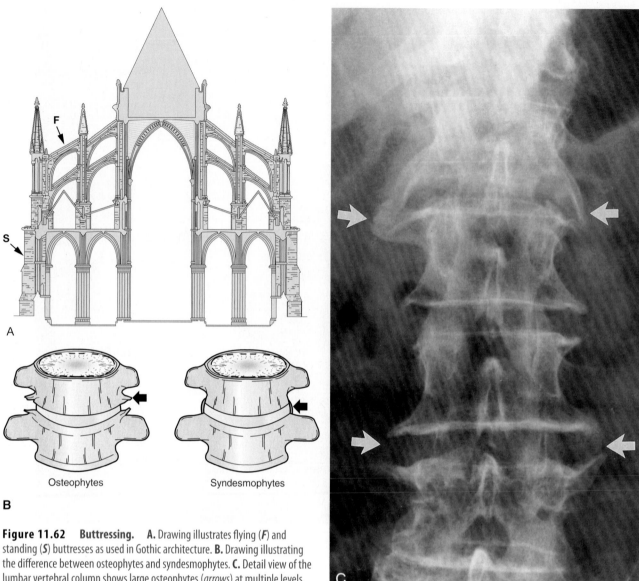

Osteophytes   Syndesmophytes

B

Figure 11.62   Buttressing.   A. Drawing illustrates flying (**F**) and standing (**S**) buttresses as used in Gothic architecture. **B.** Drawing illustrating the difference between osteophytes and syndesmophytes. **C.** Detail view of the lumbar vertebral column shows large osteophytes (*arrows*) at multiple levels.

History of Trauma or Surgery

Because trauma is the most common bone "disease" you will encounter, it is very important to elicit a history of trauma whenever possible. A stress fracture (Fig. 11.75) may be misdiagnosed as a malignant bone tumor unless a specific history of trauma (pain with an unusual activity, condition worsening with that activity, and relief achieved by rest) is obtained. Occasionally, however, a history of trauma will be deliberately withheld, as in the case of child abuse or of a child or adult who, prior to injury, was doing something prohibited or illegal.

Similarly, it is important to know whether the patient has had surgery or a recent injection on a particular bone or joint. Healing surgical sites, particularly those used for bone graft donation (Fig. 11.76), may have ominous radiographic appearances if encountered within a few months of the procedure. It is therefore imperative to know about any previous operations.

It is also important to know whether a patient has undergone radiation therapy to an area of bony abnormality. Radiation may produce bizarre findings of mixed lucency and bony sclerosis (Fig. 11.77). Some bone sarcomas are the result of previous radiation (Fig. 11.78). In addition, radiation of bones makes them more susceptible to the insufficiency type of stress fracture, particularly in the pelvis and sacrum (Fig. 11.79).

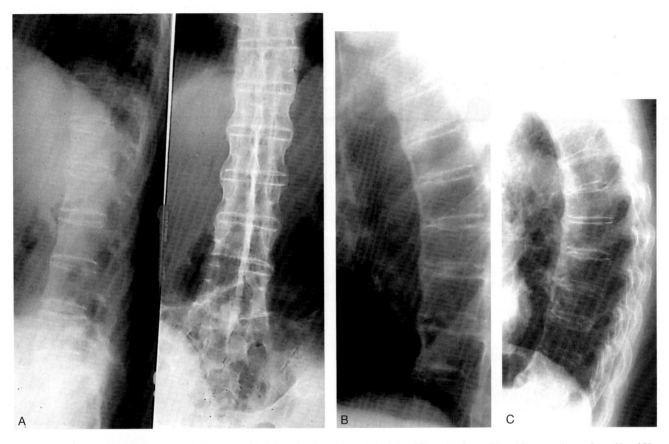

Figure 11.63   Syndesmophytes in ankylosing spondylitis and diffuse idiopathic skeletal hyperostosis.   Thin, delicate syndesmophytes **(A** and **B)** extend across the intervertebral discs in these two patients with ankylosing spondylitis. **C.** In a patient with diffuse idiopathic skeletal hyperostosis (DISH), the flowing syndesmophytes are coarser and primarily anterior.

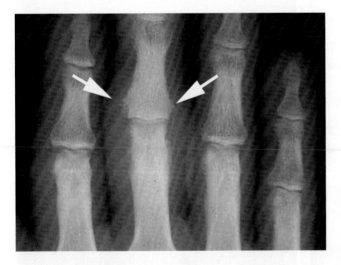

Figure 11.64   Enthesophytes in psoriatic arthropathy.   Irregular new bone formation (*arrows*) is seen along the proximal portions of the middle phalanx. Similar changes are in the proximal phalanx.

Additional Observations

Abnormalities of Bony Anatomy and Alignment

Deformities in bone generally indicate a congenital abnormality (Fig. 11.80). However, they may also occur as a result of poorly treated trauma (Fig. 11.81). Two types of malalignment may occur in joints: subluxations and dislocations. *Subluxation* is a partial loss of continuity between articulating surfaces; *dislocation* is the complete loss of continuity

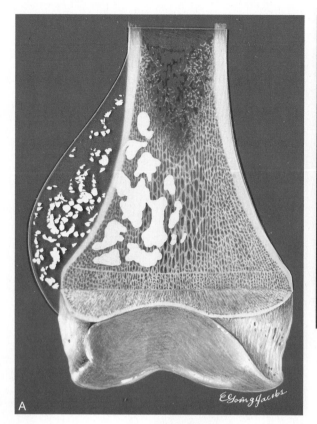

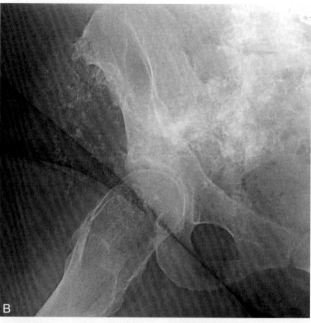

Figure 11.65   Matrix formation.   A. Drawing showing lumpy and flocculent types of matrix. **B.** Chondroid matrix in a patient with chondrosarcoma. Note the flocculent calcifications within the soft tissues adjacent to the iliac bone.

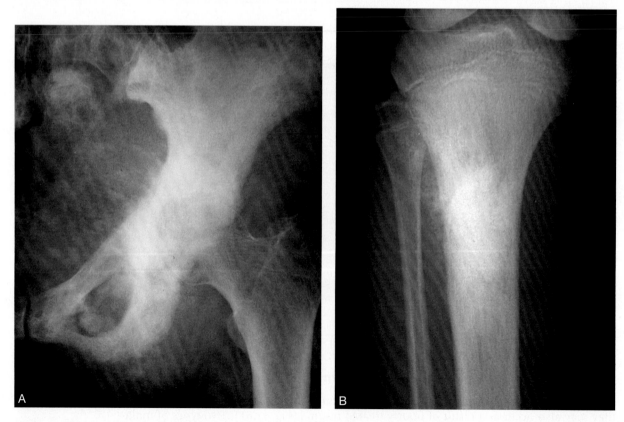

Figure 11.66   Osteosarcoma demonstrating osteoid matrix.   A. Pelvis. **B.** Tibia. Note how dense the lesions are because of the osteoid matrix formation.

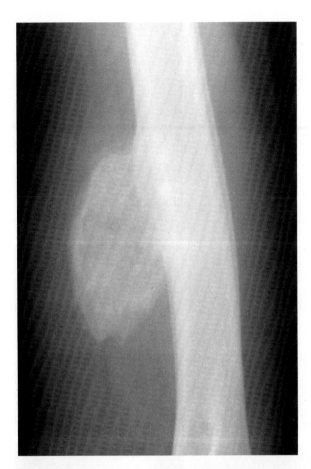

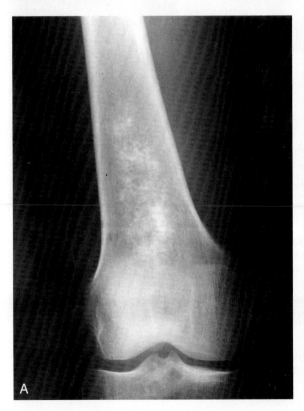

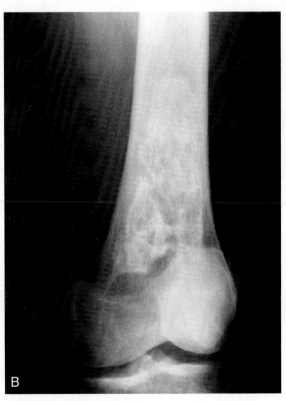

Figure 11.67 Myositis ossificans of the humerus. The lesion is well defined, with uniform ossification that is slightly denser in the periphery. Note the laminated but solid periosteal reaction.

Figure 11.68 Difference between matrix and heterotopic calcification. A. Enchondroma of the distal femur demonstrates flocculent matrix resembling rings, or *C*s and *O*s. It is concentrated in the *center* of the lesion. **B.** Heterotopic calcification in a bone infarct. The calcification is mainly in the *periphery* of the lesion and has a wavy or serpentine appearance.

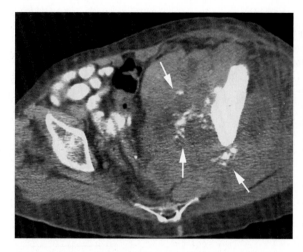

Figure 11.69   Osteosarcoma.   This is the same patient as in Figure 11.66**A**. CT image shows the osteoid matrix (*arrows*). Note how much denser the left acetabulum is compared to the right. Note also the large soft tissue mass.

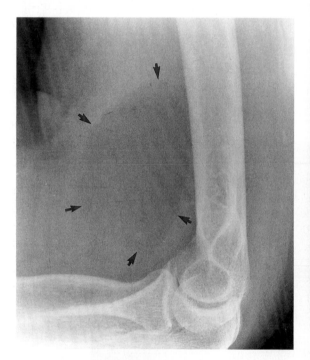

Figure 11.70   Lipoma of the antecubital fossa (*arrows*).   The lucency within this large mass indicates that a major component is fat.

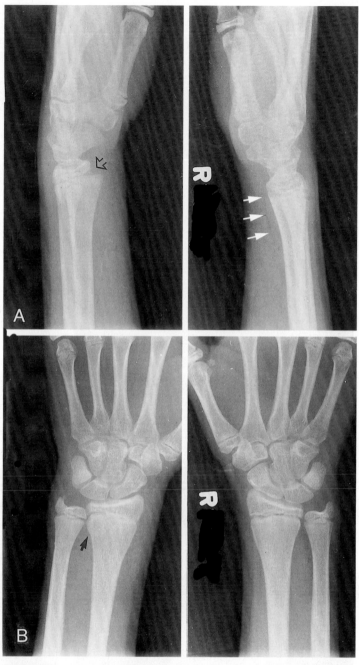

Figure 11.71   Soft tissue changes in a patient with a Salter-Harris-Ogden type 2 fracture of the distal radius.   **A.** Lateral views show the normal pronator quadratus fat stripe (*white arrows*) on the right. Note the obliteration of this line and overall soft tissue swelling on the left. There is widening of the physis on the left (*open arrow*). **B.** Frontal views show buckling of the ulnar cortex of the distal radius on the left (*black arrow*). Note the differences in soft tissue compared with the right. The changes on the frontal views are even more subtle than those on the lateral views.

at that joint space. These are illustrated in Figure 11.82. Shoulder, hip, and finger dislocations are the most commonly encountered. Artificial joints occasionally dislocate (Fig. 11.83).

 ▸ Subluxation is a partial loss of continuity between articulating surfaces; dislocation is complete loss of continuity at the joint.

Figure 11.72 Elbow fat pad.
A. Lateral radiograph shows elevation of the anterior (*large arrow*) and posterior (*curved arrow*) in a patient with a subtle fracture of the distal humerus. **B.** Lateral radiograph of the opposite side shows the normal position and appearance of the anterior fat pad (*arrow*). The posterior fat pad is never visible under normal circumstances.

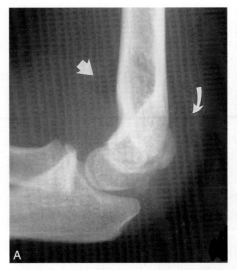
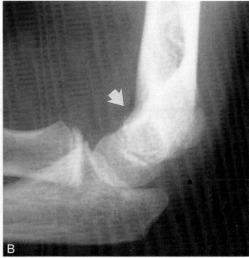

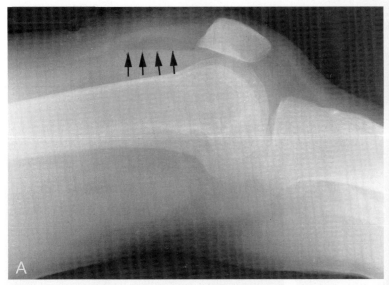
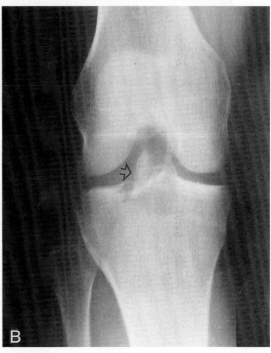
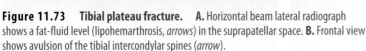

Figure 11.73 Tibial plateau fracture. **A.** Horizontal beam lateral radiograph shows a fat-fluid level (lipohemarthrosis, *arrows*) in the suprapatellar space. **B.** Frontal view shows avulsion of the tibial intercondylar spines (*arrow*).

Abnormalities of Bony Mineralization and Texture

The degree of mineralization of a bone is directly related to the patient's age, the physiologic state, and the amount of activity or stress being placed on that bone. Furthermore, the *texture* of the trabeculae (thin, delicate, coarsened, smudged) may tell you something about the patient's metabolic state. It is important to differentiate the terms osteopenia and osteoporosis. *Osteopenia* is a term used to define a decrease in mineralization of bones as demonstrated on radiographs. *Osteoporosis* is a term that defines a specific pathologic state in which there is diminution of bone substance. It may be determined by either bone densitometry or by biopsy and mineral analysis.

Osteoporosis commonly occurs in elderly patients and in postmenopausal women. However, an acute form of osteoporosis may occur after a limb is immobilized. Diminished mineralization is also a common manifestation of inactivity as well as of certain diseases such as renal osteodystrophy, rheumatoid arthritis (Fig. 11.84), and scurvy.

Renal osteodystrophy is a complex of several metabolic conditions with four prominent radiographic manifestations: osteopenia, coarsening of bony trabeculae, osteomalacia,

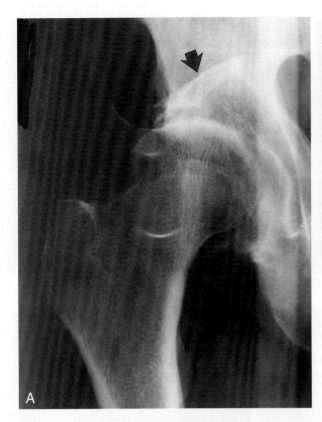

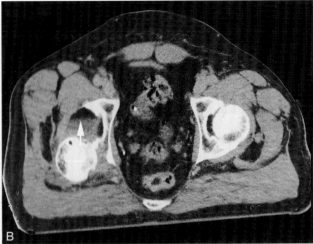

Figure 11.74   Femoral head dislocation and acetabular fracture.
A. Detail frontal view shows superior displacement of the femoral head in association with a fracture of the acetabulum (*arrow*). **B.** CT image using soft tissue windowing shows the right femoral head to be displaced posteriorly. There is a lipohemarthrosis within the hip joint capsule (*arrow*).

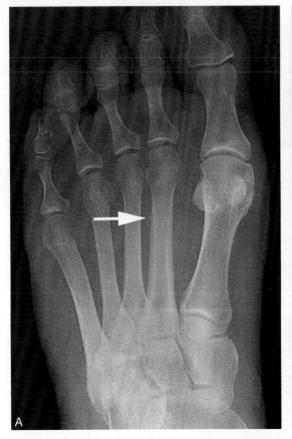

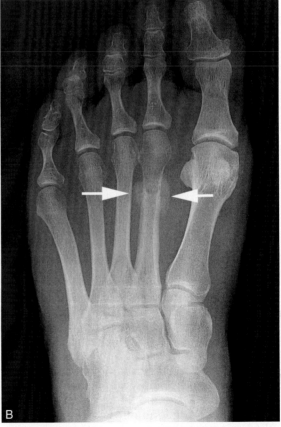

Figure 11.75   Stress fracture of the second metatarsal.   A. Frontal radiograph made 1 week after onset of symptoms shows a break in the cortex and irregular periosteal reaction along the midshaft of the second metatarsal (*arrow*). The underlying bone appears moth eaten. **B.** Three weeks after onset of symptoms, more healing has occurred. Note the periosteal reaction across the fracture site (*arrows*).

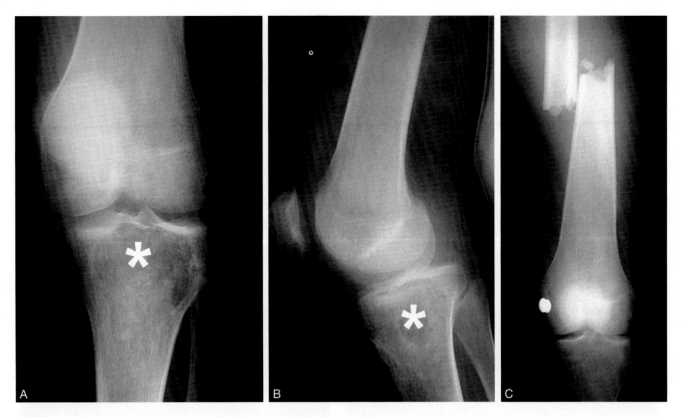

Figure 11.76   Bone graft donor site.   Frontal **(A)** and lateral **(B)** radiographs show a large, lucent lesion in the proximal tibia (*asterisks*). Giant cell tumor or chondrosarcoma might be suspected unless given the history that 3 months before, the patient underwent surgical plating and bone grafting for multiple long bone fractures. The proximal tibia was the site for the donor bone. **C.** Radiographs of the region at the time of the original injury show a femoral fracture. The proximal tibia is normal.

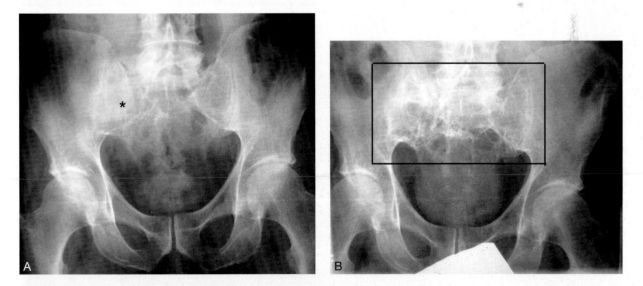

Figure 11.77   Radiation changes in the pelvis in a patient who was treated for multiple myeloma.   A. Pelvic radiograph shows a bubbly destructive lesion on the right side of the sacrum (*asterisk*). Compare with the left. **B.** Pelvic radiograph 1 year later shows sclerosis in the sacrum. Note that the abnormal bone is confined to the area subtended by the radiation portal (*rectangle*).

and hyperparathyroidism. It is most often encountered in patients with chronic renal failure. The radiographic picture may feature one of the components more prominently than others or simply be a combination of all four. Features of osteomalacia include osteopenia, *smudged and indistinct trabeculae,* resorption about the physes in

Figure 11.78   Radiation-induced chondrosarcoma.   Shoulder radiograph shows flocculent tumor matrix. The patient had been irradiated for breast carcinoma.

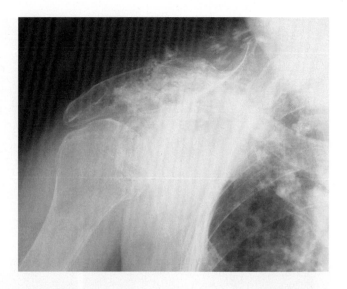

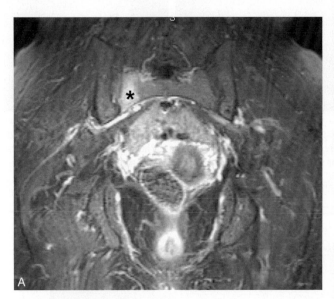

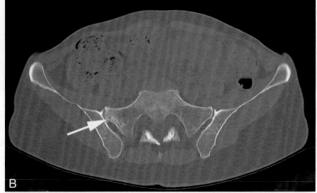

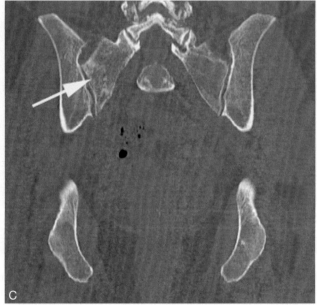

Figure 11.79   Insufficiency stress fracture of the sacrum.
A. Coronal short T1 inversion recovery MRI shows a linear area of increased signal in the body of the sacrum on the right (*asterisk*). A radionuclide bone scan (not shown) had increased tracer activity in this area. **B.** Axial CT image shows a linear area of sclerosis in the same area of the sacrum (*arrow*). **C.** Coronal reconstructed CT image shows the same finding (*arrow*). Radiographs (not shown) were normal.

the skeletally immature (Fig. 11.85), and a curious appearance in the vertebral column of alternating horizontal bands of osteoporosis centrally with osteosclerosis along the vertebral end plate termed "*rugger jersey spine*" (Fig. 11.86) because it resembles the horizontal stripes of a rugby jersey. Hyperparathyroidism, on the other hand, produces

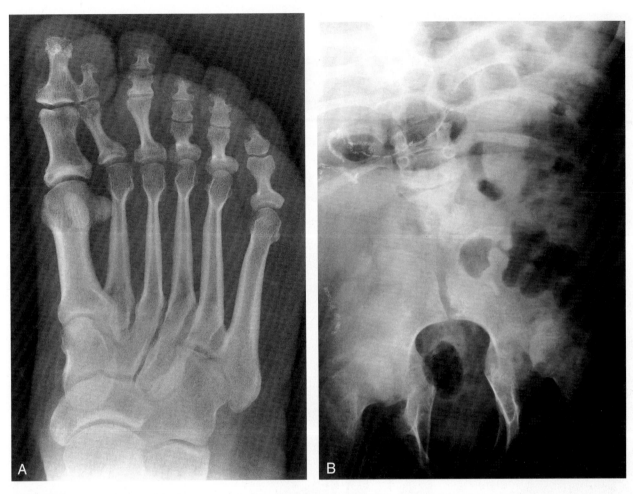

Figure 11.80   Congenital deformities.   A. Polydactyly in a patient with six toes. **B.** Sacral agenesis in a patient with caudal regression syndrome.

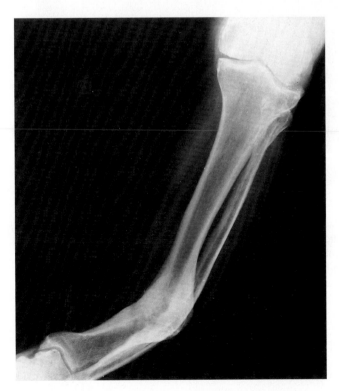

Figure 11.81   Deformity of the distal tibia and fibula secondary to poorly managed fractures.

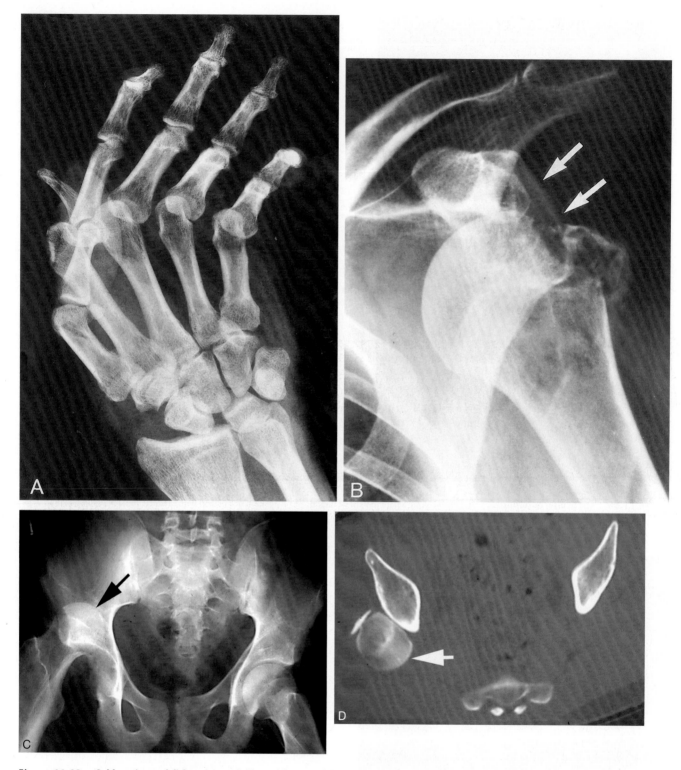

Figure 11.82   Subluxation and dislocation.   A. Ulnar subluxation of the carpus and metacarpophalangeal joint subluxations in a patient with systemic lupus erythematosus. **B.** Anterior inferior humeral dislocation. There is complete loss of continuity between the joint surfaces. Also evident are a naked glenoid (*arrows*) and a fracture of the humeral head (Hill-Sachs deformity). **C.** Hip dislocation. Pelvic radiograph shows superior displacement of the right femoral head (*arrow*). **D.** CT image shows the dislocated femoral head to be posterior as well as superior (*arrow*). A small sliver of bone from the acetabulum sits just lateral to the femoral head.

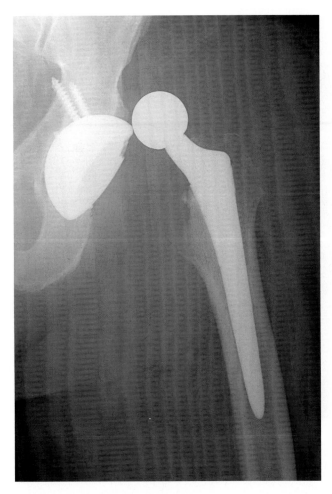

Figure 11.83   Dislocated total hip implant.   The femoral component is dislocated superiorly and posteriorly.

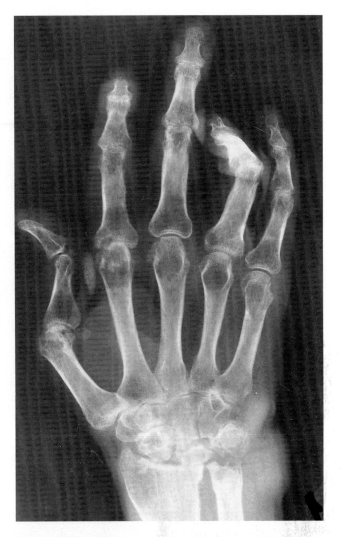

Figure 11.84   Advanced rheumatoid arthritis.   This disease primarily involves the wrist joint, the metacarpophalangeal joints, and the proximal interphalangeal joints. Note the erosive changes in these locations, as well as diffuse osteopenia.

osteopenia, resorption of the tufts of the distal phalanges, subperiosteal resorption along the radial borders of phalanges, and resorption about symphyseal joints such as the acromioclavicular joint (see Fig. 11.42B), the sacroiliac joints, and the pubic symphysis (Fig. 11.87). In addition there is resorption along *entheses* (tendinous insertion points) and a curious mixed pattern of osteopenia and fluffy sclerosis in the skull called *salt and pepper skull* (see Fig. 11.42C).

It is sometimes difficult to differentiate osteoporosis from permeative bone destruction on either radiographs or CT. In these situations, MRI can help make the differentiation. Osteoporosis produces a study that shows fatty replacement of marrow that is of high signal on T1-weighted images. Infiltrative disorders generally produce low signal in the marrow spaces on T1-weighted studies (Fig. 11.88). Furthermore, osteoporotic vertebral fractures, if recent, usually have more of a *linear* distribution of abnormal signal (Fig. 11.89) than does that associated with infiltration. In some instances, biopsy may be necessary to establish the proper diagnosis.

Patients with osteoporosis (of any origin) are subject to *insufficiency* stress fractures. These fractures result from the effect of normal muscle activity on bone that is deficient in mineral. In contradistinction, *fatigue* stress fractures result from excessive muscular activity on bones of normal mineralization. The typical patient with an insufficiency stress fracture is an elderly woman who has engaged in some low-impact activity, such

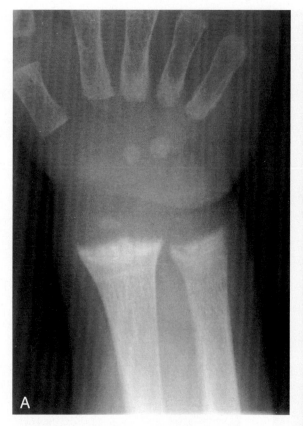

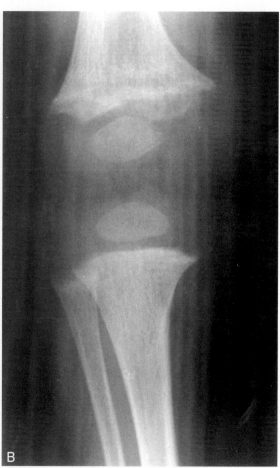

Figure 11.85   Rickets in a child.   A. Wrist radiograph shows irregular frayed metaphyses and coarsened trabeculae. **B.** Knee radiograph shows similar findings.

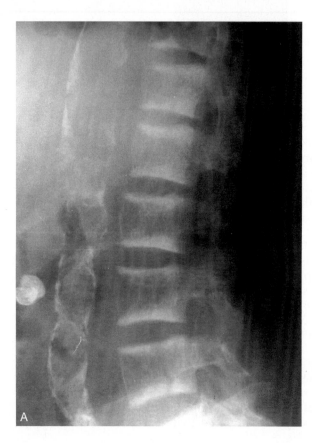

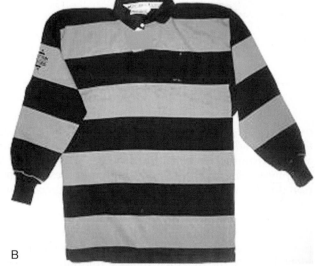

Figure 11.86   "Rugger jersey spine" in a patient with chronic renal failure and osteomalacia.   A. Note the striped appearance from the alternating areas of osteosclerosis along the disc plates with central osteoporosis. The relatively lucent disc spaces also contribute to the striped appearance. **B.** Rugby jersey.

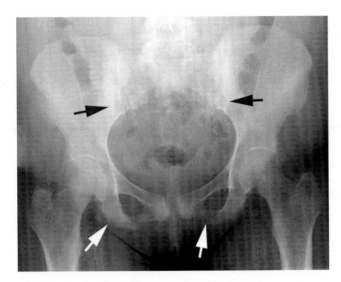

Figure 11.87 Bony resorption in hyperparathyroidism. Pelvic radiograph shows subchondral resorption along the sacroiliac joints (*black arrows*) and subperiosteal resorption of the ischial tuberosities (*white arrows*).

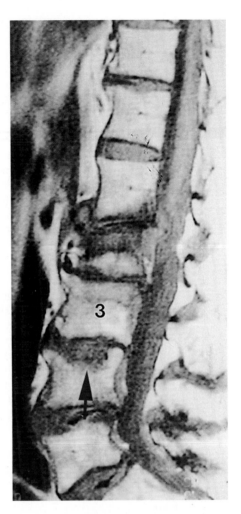

Figure 11.89 Osteoporotic collapse of L2. A T1-weighted image shows collapse of the body of L2. There is low signal in a *linear* distribution, typical of nonpathologic collapse. Note the central Schmorl node of L4 (*arrow*). Compare with Figure 11.88.

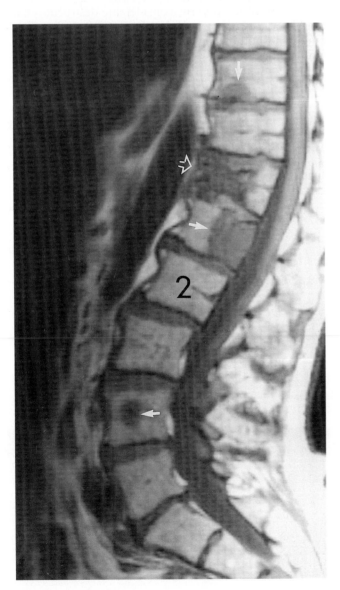

Figure 11.88 Metastases (*solid arrows*) and pathologic collapse (*open arrow*) of T12 as demonstrated on a T1-weighted MRI. The abnormal signal in the collapsed vertebra extends throughout the vertebra, typical of metastases. Compare with Figure 11.89.

as walking through a mall, with sudden onset of sacral, groin, or lower limb pain (see Fig. 11.79). Typically, the pain is worse with activity and is relieved by rest. In many instances, the patient's clinical picture may be clouded by a history of previous malignancy and radiation therapy.

For an excellent in-depth discussion of bone mineral physiology and pathology, consult Resnick's *Diagnosis of Bone and Joint Disorders*.

Joint Space Abnormalities

The width of the joint space and the appearance of the distal ends of articulating bones are important in the diagnosis of arthritis. The distribution, location, and erosive patterns produced by the various arthritides allow considerable accuracy in radiologic diagnosis, particularly when correlated with clinical and laboratory findings. You should familiarize yourself with the changes in the five most common types of arthritis you will encounter: rheumatoid, degenerative, gout, calcium pyrophosphate deposition, and neuropathic. The salient features of these diseases are summarized here.

Rheumatoid Arthritis

The radiographic findings of rheumatoid arthritis depend on the stage of the disease. Early findings include fusiform pericapsular swelling, joint effusion, and subtle demineralization of the subarticular bone. As the disease progresses, marginal erosions occur, usually associated with narrowing of the joint space (Fig. 11.90). The degree of osteopenia has also progressed. In the late form of the disease, considerable destruction has taken place about the joints, and subluxations occur. In the end stage, ankylosis occurs (Fig. 11.91). Ankylosis is the common end point of all severe joint disorders, regardless of the cause. Rheumatoid arthritis affects the cervical vertebral column in at least 50% of patients with the disease; most of these patients have no cervical symptoms. This is an

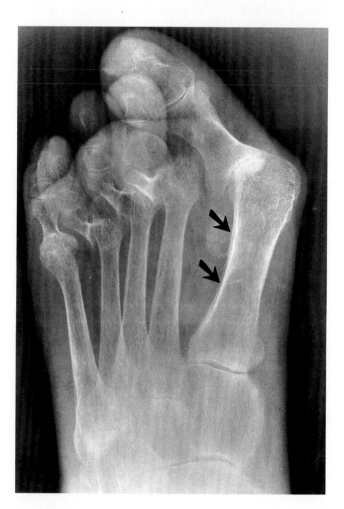

Figure 11.90   Rheumatoid arthritis of the foot with lateral subluxations of the metatarsophalangeal joints.   There are erosive changes in the second through fifth metatarsophalangeal joints. There is periosteal reaction (*arrows*) along the shaft of the first metacarpal.

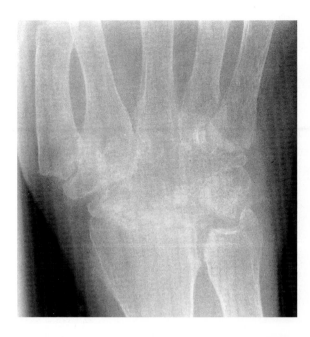

Figure 11.91   End-stage rheumatoid arthritis with bony ankylosis in the wrist.   Normal anatomic margins of the carpal bones cannot be identified. Note the severe osteopenia.

important fact to know because the most serious complication of cervical rheumatoid arthritis is atlantoaxial subluxation (Fig. 11.92) or cranioverterbral settling (Fig. 11.93). In the large joints, such as the hips and knees, joint space loss is severe but without the extensive proliferative changes that occur with osteoarthritis. MRI is being used more frequently to confirm synovial proliferation in the earliest stage of the disease (Fig. 11.94). This allows rheumatologists to begin using the new powerful disease-modifying antirheumatic drugs (DMARDs) before there are recognizable radiographic signs of erosion. In some centers, ultrasound is also used for this purpose.

▸ Ankylosis is the common end point of all severe joint disorders.
▸ Rheumatoid arthritis affects the cervical spine in at least 50% of patients, most of whom have no cervical symptoms.

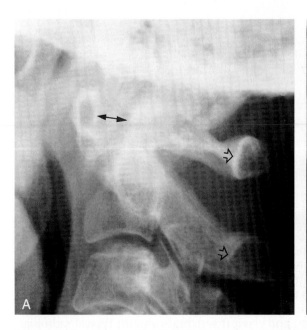
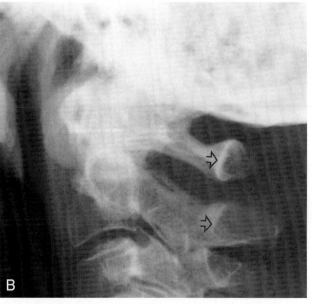

Figure 11.92   Atlantoaxial subluxation in a patient with rheumatoid arthritis.   A. Lateral radiograph in flexion shows anterior subluxation of C1 on C2. Note the widening of the predental space (*double arrow*) and malalignment of the spinolaminar lines of C1 and C2 (*open arrows*). **B.** Lateral radiograph in extension shows the subluxation to have reduced nearly completely. The spinolaminar line (*open arrows*) is still not anatomically aligned.

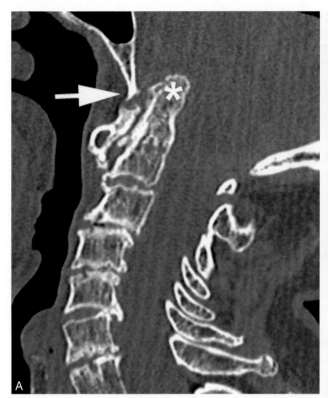

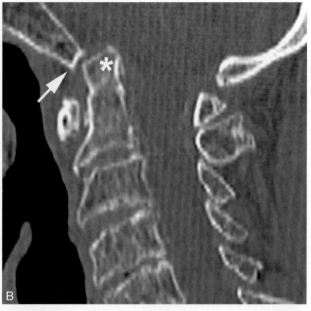

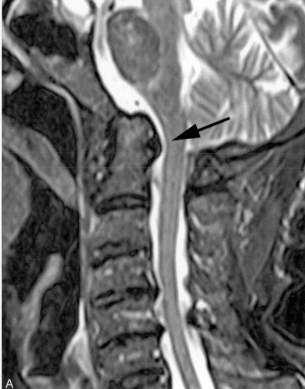

Figure 11.93   Craniovertebral settling in rheumatoid arthritis.
A and **B.** Sagittal reconstructed CT images in two different patients show the tip of the dens (*asterisks*) protruding through the foramen magnum. The dens should normally be 12 mm below the basion (*arrows*). **C.** Sagittal STIR MRI shows impingement of the dens on the medulla (*arrow*).

Juvenile Rheumatoid Arthritis

Juvenile rheumatoid arthritis (JRA) is one of the chronic polyarthritides of childhood that is similar in pathology to its adult counterpart. However, the involvement of growing bones produces clinical and radiologic features that are uniquely different. Unlike the adult form of the disease, which primarily affects the smaller joints, the clinical and radiologic manifestations of JRA are found early on in larger joints (knee, ankle, shoulder) as well as in the smaller joints of the hands, wrists, and cervical vertebral column. Typical radiologic changes include soft tissue swelling, overgrowth and squaring of the epiphyses because of hyperemia, and early ankylosis. Erosive changes that are the hallmark of the adult disease are seldom found in JRA. Figure 11.95 shows typical features of JRA.

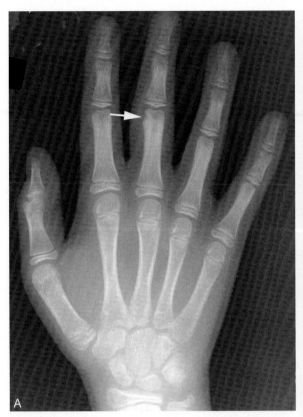

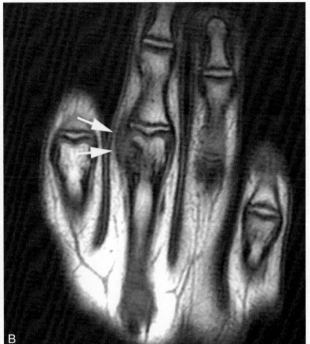

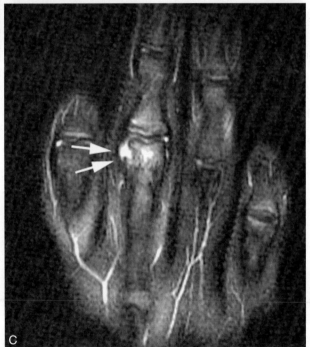

Figure 11.94   Utility of MRI in early juvenile rheumatoid arthritis.   A. Radiograph shows fusiform soft tissue swelling and localized osteopenia around the proximal interphalangeal joints of the second and third digits. There is a small cyst (*arrow*) in the distal end of the proximal phalanx of the second digit on the radial side. **B.** T1-weighted and **C.** T2-weighted coronal images show the cyst as well as synovial thickening (*arrows*) and bone edema.

Degenerative Arthritis (Osteoarthritis)

Osteoarthritis may be primary or secondary. The primary form results from the aging process and the "wear and tear" that process inflicts on joints. The secondary form is the result of any injury or disease that disrupts articular cartilage or interferes with the normal motion of the affected joint(s). There are three salient features of degenerative arthritis: narrowed joint spaces, subarticular reactive sclerosis, and spur formation (Fig. 11.96). Mineralization generally remains normal. In severe forms, subarticular cysts or *geodes* occur. There may also be chondrocalcinosis, particularly in the knees. A particularly aggressive form of this disease that affects middle-aged and elderly women is known as *erosive osteoarthritis.* It primarily affects the distal interphalangeal joints of the hands (see Fig. 11.47A).

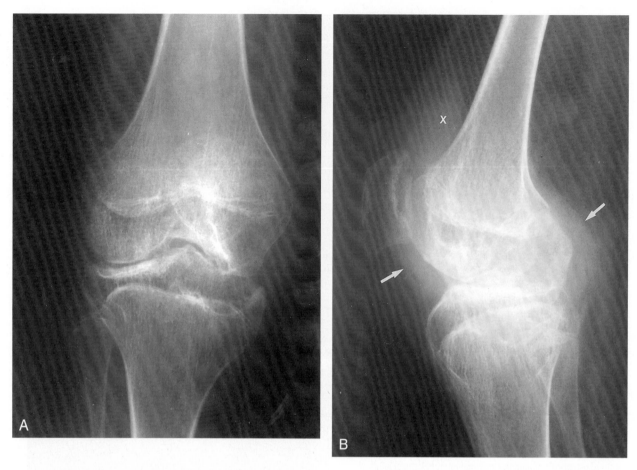

Figure 11.95   Juvenile rheumatoid arthritis of the knee.   A. Frontal view shows hypertrophy of the epiphyses and joint space narrowing. **B.** Lateral view shows epiphyseal hypertrophy with erosions along the joint surface. There is a suprapatellar effusion (*X*) and evidence of synovial hypertrophy anteriorly and posteriorly (*arrows*).

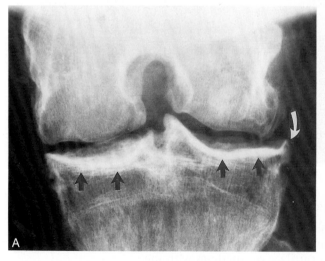

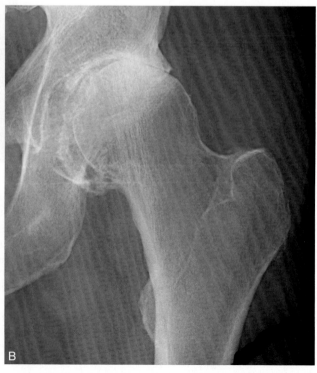

Figure 11.96   Osteoarthritis.   A. Knee. There is subchondral sclerosis (*straight arrows*) and a large marginal osteophyte (*curved arrow*) laterally. **B.** Hip. There is marked joint space narrowing superiorly as well as osteophyte formation.

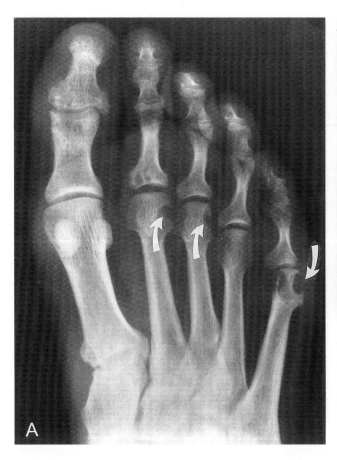

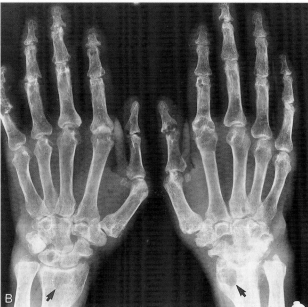

Figure 11.97   Gout.   A. Detail view of a foot shows paraarticular punched-out lesions in the distal metatarsals (*arrows*). Other joints are involved as well. **B.** Involvement of the hands and wrists in the same patient shows multiple lesions. Note the asymmetry, predominantly paraarticular involvement, and overall preservation of mineralization around the joints. There are intraosseous tophi in the distal radii (*arrows*).

Gout

Gout arises from abnormal urate metabolism. In the early stages of this disease, soft tissue swelling is the only radiographic finding. Indeed, the disease must be present for 5 to 7 years before erosive changes and large punched-out lesions are seen. These erosions may be articular or paraarticular (more common) and result from *tophus* formation; often they have overhanging edges (Fig. 11.97) and have the appearance of a rat bite. The erosions are more common in the "bare" (paraarticular) areas. The degree of mineralization is usually normal except in an acute attack.

Calcium Pyrophosphate Deposition Disease (CPPD)

Calcium pyrophosphate deposition disease (CPPD), a common disorder, often termed *pseudogout,* is another of the crystalline arthropathies. The clinical picture of this disease is identical to that of an acute gouty attack. However, aspiration of the affected joint(s) reveals pyrophosphate crystals instead of urate crystals. CPPD, unlike gout, responds to treatment with nonsteroidal antiinflammatory drugs. Radiographically, the hallmark of CPPD is chondrocalcinosis of both hyaline and fibrocartilage and the paucity of large osteophytes. The knee and the wrist are the two joints most commonly involved (Fig. 11.98).

Neuropathic Osteoarthropathy (Charcot Joint)

This disorder is the result of denervation of joints caused by preexisting diseases such as diabetes mellitus, syringomyelia, or, in the past, neurosyphilis (tabes dorsalis). In the United States, diabetes is the most common etiology. Denervation of the joints allows the microfractures that occur in everyone as the result of daily "wear and tear" on the bones to go undetected by the patient. Continued activity on those compromised bones and joints results in propagation of the fractures. Ultimately, the affected part disintegrates into a "bag of bones." The main radiographic features of neuropathic disease are severe fragmentation, dislocation, and reactive changes (Fig. 11.99). The appearance has been described by skeletal radiologist Frieda Feldman as "osteoarthritis with a vengeance."

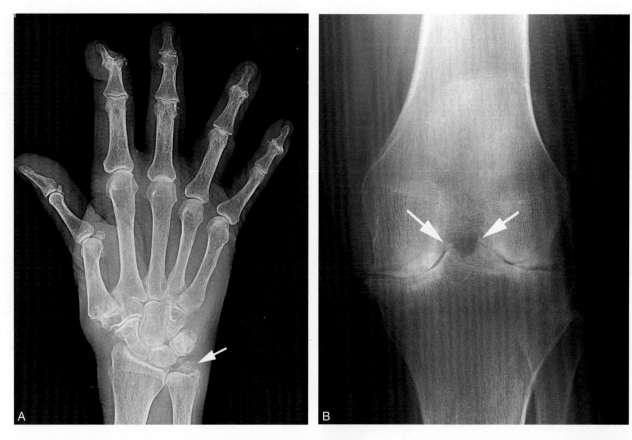

Figure 11.98   Calcium pyrophosphate deposition disease (CPPD, pseudogout).   A. Radiograph of the hand and wrist show narrowing of virtually all of the joints. The radiocarpal and metacarpophalangeal joints are most severely involved. Note the chondrocalcinosis of the triangular fibrocartilage (*arrow*). **B.** Radiograph of the knee shows symmetric narrowing of the joint space without osteophyte formation. There is faint chondrocalcinosis (*arrows*).

Often the appearance will suggest previous surgical resection with straight margins (pseudoamputation sign) (Fig. 11.100). The foot is the most common location in diabetics and the shoulder is the most common location in patients with syringomyelia. Vertebral neuropathic joints are not uncommon. Neuropathic changes in the hips and knees used to be common in patients with tertiary syphilis. Today, diabetes accounts for these unusual findings. Charcot joints from neurosyphilis are now a medical curiosity and radiographic examples of them are found only in teaching files.

Trauma

As previously mentioned, skeletal trauma is the most common bone disorder. *A fracture is really a soft tissue injury in which a bone is broken.* In most instances, the bone, left to itself, will heal. However, in dealing with fractures, you must be concerned with associated soft tissue injuries. For example, a fracture of the skull itself may be trivial. However, if there is damage to the underlying meningeal vessels or brain, the injury is significant. Similarly, vertebral fractures are often associated with neurologic deficit from damage to the spinal cord. Therefore, in evaluating a patient who has sustained skeletal trauma, it is important to also assess the status of the adjacent soft tissue structures. *In patients who have suffered severe multisystem trauma, the goal of imaging should be to diagnose those abnormalities that are most likely to be life threatening, such as cranial, thoracic, visceral, or vascular injuries.* Often radiographic assessment of the skeleton will have a lower priority.

▶ A fracture is a soft tissue injury in which a bone is broken.
▶ The goal of imaging of victims of severe trauma should be to diagnose those abnormalities that are most likely to be life threatening.

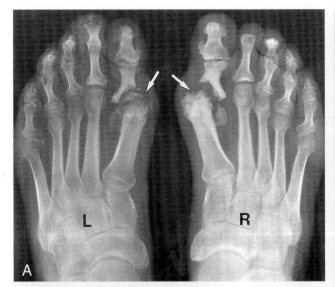

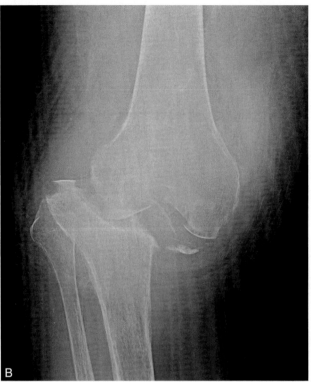

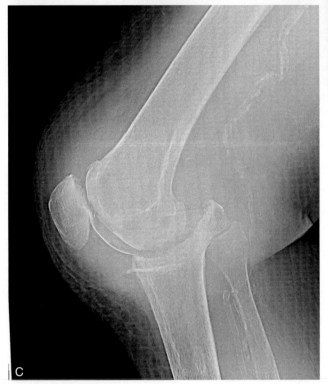

Figure 11.99   Neuropathic (Charcot) joints in two diabetic patients.   A. Radiographs of both feet show bilateral neuropathic joints at the first metatarsophalangeal joints (*arrows*). On the left there is periarticular osteopenia, indicating superimposed infection. Frontal (**B**) and lateral (**C**) knee radiographs of another patient show disintegration of the knee joint with considerable bony debris ("bag of bones") and a large joint effusion. In the past, involvement of this joint was usually caused by neurosyphilis.

In trauma patients, views other than those considered routine may be necessary to demonstrate suspected fractures. Furthermore, *comparison views* with the opposite, uninjured limb may be necessary, particularly in evaluating possible epiphyseal injuries in children (Fig. 11.101). I recommend selective use of comparison views—that is, only in special circumstances and never routinely (with the exception of the pediatric elbow, where there are six growth centers). Occasionally, stress views to test ligamentous stability and arteriography to investigate the possibility of vascular injury may be necessary.

The *descriptive terminology* of fractures is important; the referring clinician, orthopaedic surgeon, and radiologist must all speak the same language. Fractures are described by location within the bone (head, neck, shaft, etc.); type (spiral, comminuted, oblique, green-stick); and position of the fragments (degrees of angulation, displacement, overriding, distraction; Fig. 11.102). Figure 11.103 shows several common types of fractures and their descriptive terminology. For a further discussion of terminology, refer to *The Handbook of Fractures*, by Egol et al.

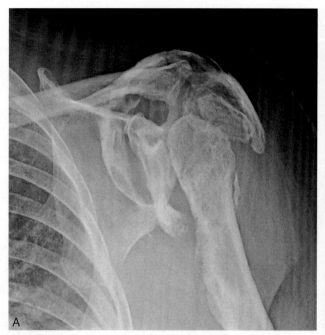

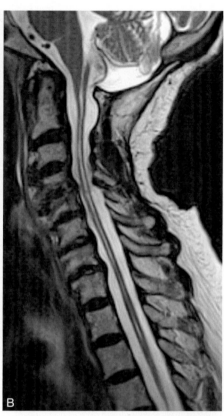

Figure 11.100   Neuropathic (Charcot) joint disease of the shoulder in a patient with syringomyelia.   A. Frontal radiograph shows fragmentation of the articular surfaces of the humeral head and the glenoid. In addition, there is a large amount of bony debris ("bag of bones") and heterotopic ossification. **B.** Sagittal T2-weighted MRI shows increased signal in the central portion of the atrophic spinal cord as a result of syringomyelia.

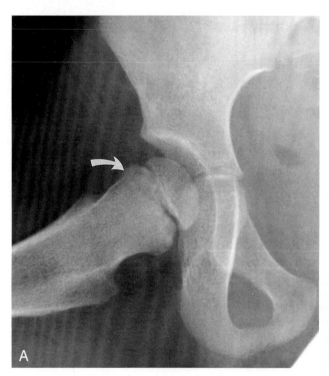

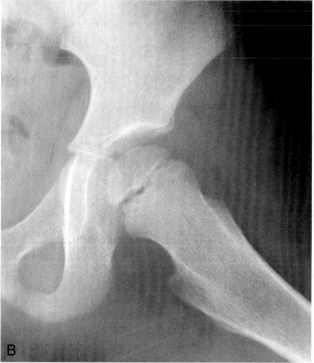

Figure 11.101   (Continued)

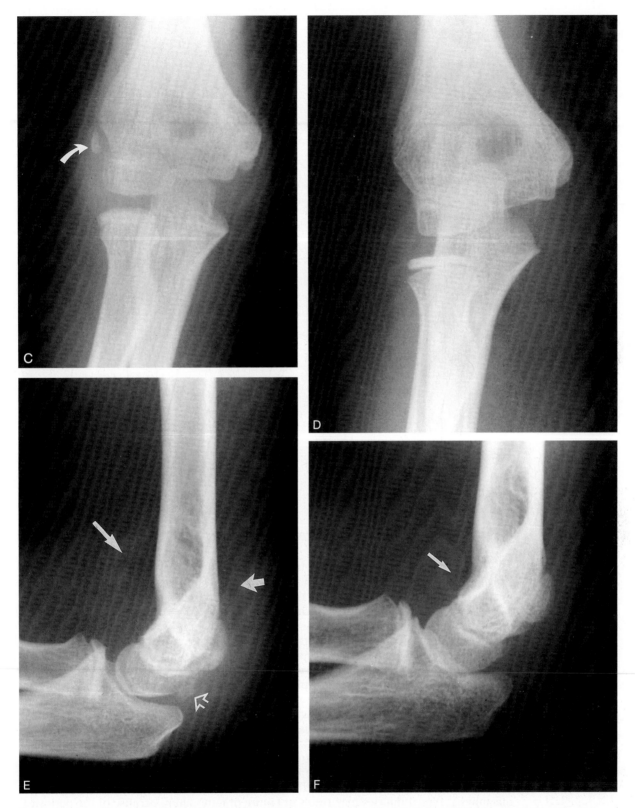

Figure 11.101   Use of comparison views in trauma.   A. Frogleg lateral view of the right hip in a child demonstrates buckling of the metaphyseal cortex (*arrow*). **B.** Comparison view of the left side is normal. **C.** Frontal view of the right elbow of a child shows soft tissue swelling laterally and a bone fragment (*arrow*). Is this a fracture or the apophysis of the lateral epicondyle? **D.** Comparison view of the opposite side shows no additional ossicles and no soft tissue swelling. **E.** Lateral radiograph of the symptomatic side in the same patient shows elevation of the anterior (*thin arrow*) and posterior (*fat arrow*) fat pads in addition to the avulsed bone fragment (*open arrow*). **F.** Comparison view of the opposite side shows a normal anterior fat pad (*arrow*) and no avulsed bone fragment. The lateral epicondylar apophysis usually ossifies around age 12; this patient is considerably younger.

Figure 11.102   Schematic drawing of fracture terminology. *AP,* anterior-posterior; *Lat,* lateral.

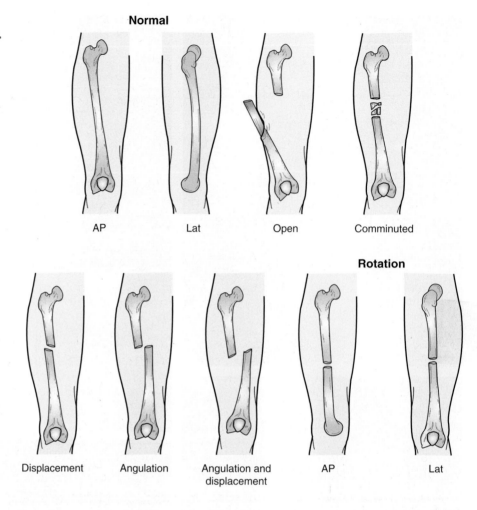

Normal

AP   Lat   Open   Comminuted

Rotation

Displacement   Angulation   Angulation and   AP   Lat
displacement

Special Pediatric Considerations

Salter-Type Fractures

Fractures in children occur in two distinct patterns, depending on whether the injury is near the physis or the shaft. Injuries about the physis are described according to the *Salter-Harris-Ogden (S-H-O)* classification, which is based on the degree of involvement of the epiphysis, physis, or metaphysis. The type 1 injury is a pure epiphysiolysis. The type 2 injury, the most common, involves the epiphysis and a small metaphyseal fragment. The type 3 injury is a vertical fracture of the epiphysis with epiphysiolysis of the fracture fragment. Type 4 is a vertical epiphyseal fracture with metaphyseal involvement. Type 5, the rarest, is uniform compression of the physeal plate. Type 6 is a compression of part of the physeal plate with lysis of the other part. Type 7 is an osteochondral fracture of the epiphysis. Type 8 injuries affect the metaphyseal growth and remodeling areas. Type 9 injuries are those of periosteal portions of the diaphysis. Figure 11.104 illustrates the S-H-O classification. Types 1 and 2 are said to produce little or no growth disturbance; types 3 through 6 have a higher potential for growth disturbance, and type 7 has no potential for disturbance but can produce joint problems from the intraarticular loose fragments. Type 8 injuries may result in epiphysiolysis caused by ischemia from disruption of the blood supply in the metaphysis. Type 9 injuries may result in failure of remodeling because of the periosteal injury. Colloquially, these injuries are usually called Salter-type fractures.

Slipped Capital Femoral Epiphysis

Slipped capital femoral epiphysis (SCFE) is an S-H-O type 1 injury that occurs most frequently in boys in their early teens. In many instances, the child is overweight. At least half of the patients report some history of trauma. Hip pain and limp are the most common presenting symptoms; however, up to one-fourth of patients may present with knee

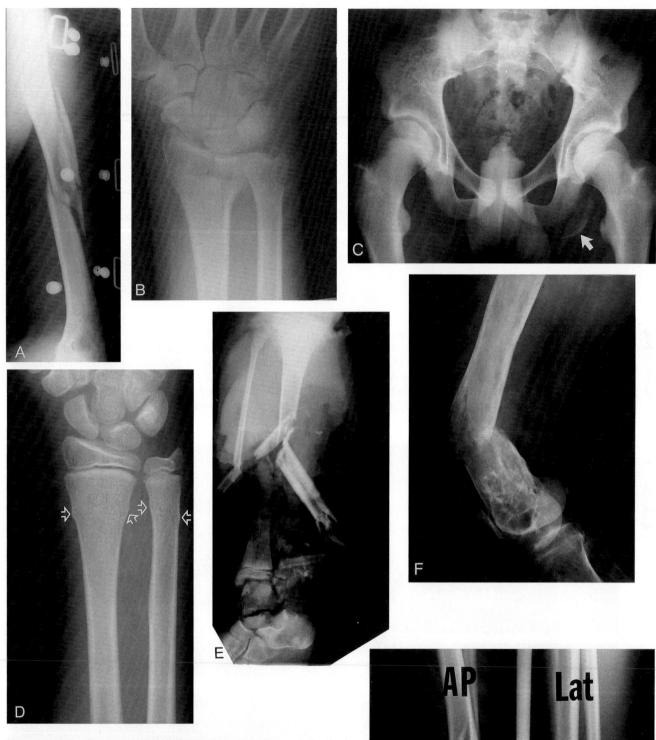

Figure 11.103 Fractures and their descriptive terminology. **A.** Spiral comminuted fracture of the midshaft of the humerus. **B.** Comminuted, intraarticular compression fracture of the distal radius. There is also a fracture of the ulnar styloid. **C.** Avulsion fracture (*arrow*) of the ischial apophysis. **D.** Green-stick (torus) fractures of the distal radius and ulna (*arrows*). The torus fracture presents as a bulge along the surface of the otherwise smooth bone. **E.** Comminuted open fractures of the distal tibia and fibula. **F.** Pathologic fracture of the distal femur in a patient with a malignant bone tumor. Note the bone destruction around the fracture. **G.** Fracture dislocation of the ankle. There are fractures of the distal fibula and posterior lip of the tibia (*arrow*). The foot is dislocated *and* rotated laterally. Note the orientation markers on the radiographs. *AP*, anterior-posterior; *Lat*, lateral.

Figure 11.104   Salter-Harris-Ogden classification of growth region injuries. See text for description.

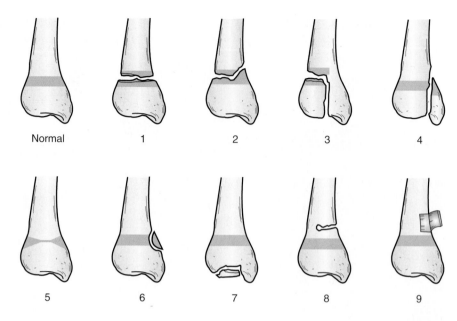

Normal   1   2   3   4

5   6   7   8   9

pain. In some instances the slip may be bilateral. The radiographic manifestations are often subtle on an anterior-posterior projection. A line drawn along the lateral border of the femoral neck should normally intersect the femoral capital epiphysis with approximately 20% of the diameter of the head lying lateral to this line. With SCFE, too much or too little of the femoral head will lie lateral to this line (Fig. 11.105). Frogleg lateral views often show the slippage better than the frontal views (see Fig. 11.105B). Complications of

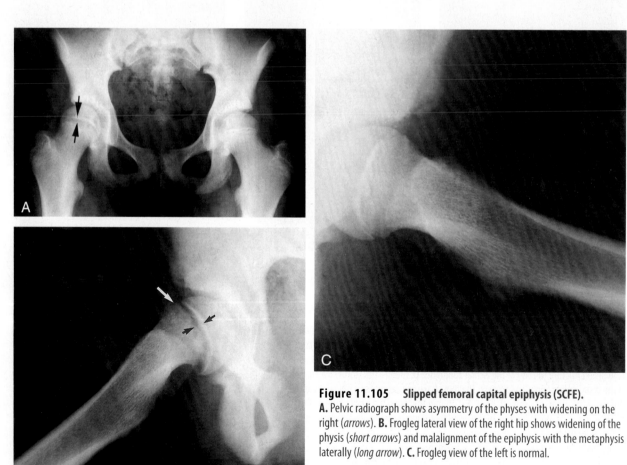

Figure 11.105   Slipped femoral capital epiphysis (SCFE).
A. Pelvic radiograph shows asymmetry of the physes with widening on the right (*arrows*). **B.** Frogleg lateral view of the right hip shows widening of the physis (*short arrows*) and malalignment of the epiphysis with the metaphysis laterally (*long arrow*). **C.** Frogleg view of the left is normal.

this injury include avascular necrosis and chondrolysis. The former condition may result from damage to the blood supply to the femoral head at the time of injury or as a result of surgical pinning to treat the disorder.

Fractures of Bone Shafts

Fractures of the shafts of bones may be either complete or of the green-stick variety. Three types of green-stick fractures are recognized: *classic green-stick* (fracture on one side of the bone, bent on the other); *torus,* resembling the base of a Greek column (buckling of cortex on both sides of the bone); and *"lead pipe"* (one side buckled, one side cracked). Of these, the torus variety (see Fig. 11.103D) is the most common.

Stress Fractures

Fatigue Fractures

Stress fractures, as previously mentioned, are the result of increased muscle activity on normal bone (*fatigue fracture*) or of normal muscle activity on bone with compromised mineral content (*insufficiency fracture*). In the typical fatigue fracture, the activity is new or in excess of the structural tolerance of the patient's bone(s). The activity is usually vigorous and repetitive. The typical history in a patient with a stress fracture (any type) is of pain with activity that is relieved by rest and made worse by resuming the activity. Tumors and infections typically produce pain at rest as well as with activity. *Stress fractures are common injuries that occur at predictable sites with specific activities.* For example, running typically produces fractures of the proximal posterior medial tibia (Fig. 11.106) or of the distal fibula (Fig. 11.107). Other common sites include the metatarsal shafts in military

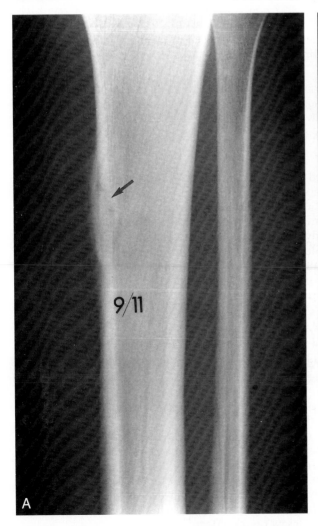

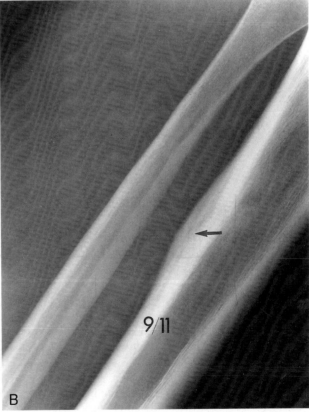

Figure 11.106   Tibial stress fracture in a runner.   A. Detail view of a frontal radiograph of the tibia shows the fracture along the medial cortex (*arrow*). Laminated periosteal reaction indicates the patient continued to run despite the pain. **B.** Lateral view shows the fracture involves the posterior cortex (*arrow*). This is the typical site for a stress fracture caused by running.

Figure 11.107   **Stress fracture** (*arrow*) of the distal fibula in runner.

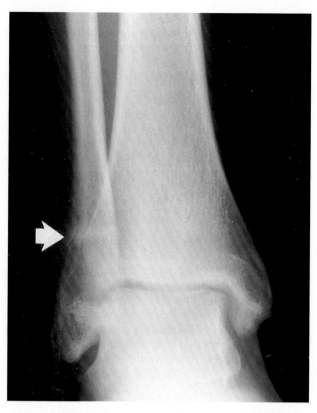

recruits ("march fractures"), calcaneus in people engaged in jumping activities, and pars interarticularis of the lumbar vertebrae in gymnasts.

 ▶ Stress fractures typically produce pain with activity that is relieved by rest and made worse by resuming the activity. Tumors and infections typically produce pain at rest as well as with activity.

Insufficiency Fractures

Insufficiency fractures were discussed under abnormalities of bone mineralization. Common locations for this type of stress fracture are the sacrum, pubic arches, and femoral necks. The initial radiographs of a patient with a stress fracture may be normal; the patient should be treated symptomatically and return for a repeat radiographic examination in 7 to 10 days. For elderly patients in whom a diagnosis needs to be made immediately, as well as in elite athletes or persons in whom rest will interfere with their jobs, MRI may be performed because it will show the occult abnormalities before the radiographs (Fig. 11.108). If time is not of the essence in making such a diagnosis, a radionuclide bone scan may be performed instead.

Fracture Summary

Although an in-depth description of fractures is beyond the scope of this book, you should follow some of the principles listed here when evaluating patients with skeletal trauma:

○ *Assume a fracture is present if there is pain, swelling, and discoloration over a bony surface in a child, even without a history of trauma.* It is best to treat patients for fractures and bring them back in 7 to 10 days for follow-up radiographs rather than let them leave the emergency department with untreated fractures.
○ Comparison views should be made only when you and your radiologist are uncertain about the presence or absence of a fracture (particularly in small children whose physeal lines could be confused for a fracture).
○ Acute fractures typically have irregular margins that resemble the pieces of a jigsaw puzzle. You can mentally put the pieces together even if they are displaced (Fig. 11.109). Old, ununited fractures or accessory ossicles have smooth, rounded margins and do not have the "jigsaw puzzle effect."

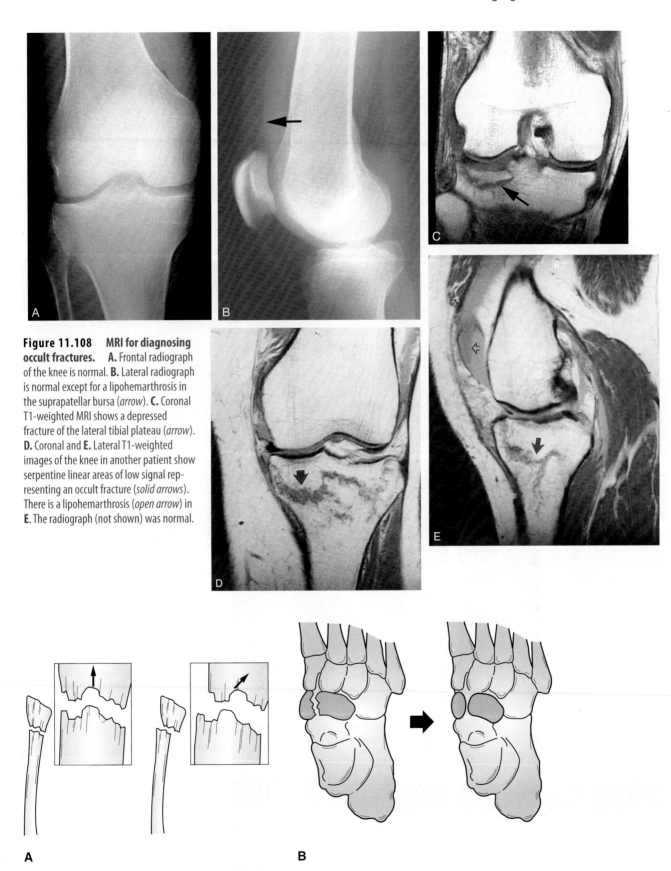

Figure 11.108   MRI for diagnosing occult fractures.   A. Frontal radiograph of the knee is normal. **B.** Lateral radiograph is normal except for a lipohemarthrosis in the suprapatellar bursa (*arrow*). **C.** Coronal T1-weighted MRI shows a depressed fracture of the lateral tibial plateau (*arrow*). **D.** Coronal and **E.** Lateral T1-weighted images of the knee in another patient show serpentine linear areas of low signal representing an occult fracture (*solid arrows*). There is a lipohemarthrosis (*open arrow*) in **E.** The radiograph (not shown) was normal.

A   **B**

Figure 11.109   "Jigsaw puzzle effect" with fractures.   A. The irregular margins of a fracture may be matched perfectly, like the pieces of a jigsaw puzzle, even if there is displacement (indicated by *arrows*). Accessory ossicles or old ununited fractures do not match perfectly. **B.** Drawing showing a fracture of the tarsal navicular bone on the left that went to nonunion. Note the change in configuration of the margins of the ossicles.

○ A CT scan is useful for evaluating fractures of certain joints such as the shoulder, knee (Fig. 11.110), and ankle. It is also the best method of assessing pelvic fractures (Fig. 11.111), in establishing the extent of vertebral fractures, and determining whether or not a fracture extends intraarticularly.

○ MRI is useful in assessing the extent of spinal cord compression in vertebral fractures (Fig. 11.112). It is also helpful in determining whether or not an occult fracture is present, particularly in the elderly (see Fig. 11.108D, E). In these instances, we perform a limited examination consisting of T1-weighted images in two planes only.

▶ A child with pain, swelling, and discoloration over a bony surface should be presumed to have an underlying fracture.

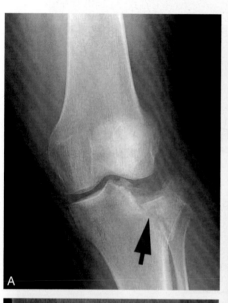

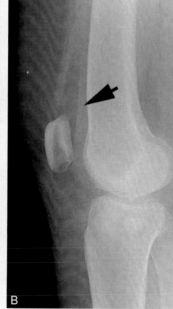

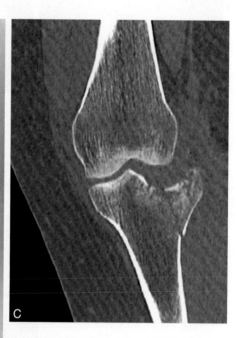

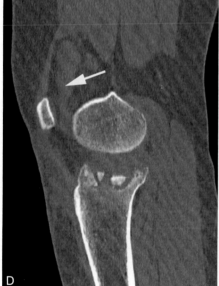

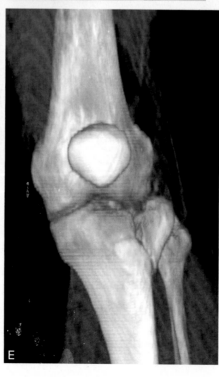

Figure 11.110   Lateral tibial plateau fracture.   A. Frontal radiograph shows a severely comminuted depressed fracture of the lateral tibial plateau (*arrow*). **B.** Lateral radiograph (made with a horizontal beam) shows a lipohemarthrosis in the suprapatellar space (*arrow*). **C.** Coronal reconstructed CT image shows the fracture in detail. **D.** Sagittal reconstructed CT image shows the lipohemarthrosis (*arrow*). **E.** Three-dimensional volumetric reconstructed image shows the fracture from the vantage point that the orthopaedist would see at the time of surgery.

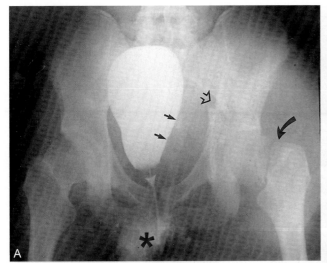

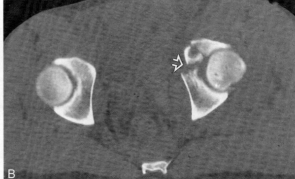

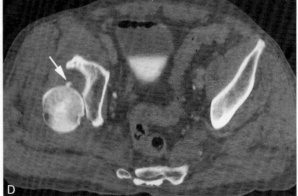

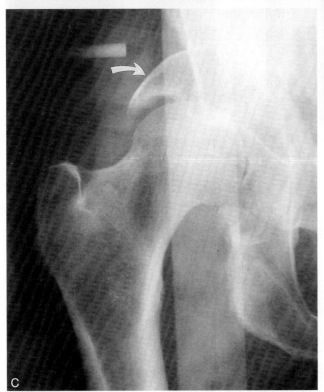

Figure 11.111   Pelvic fractures.   A. Frontal radiograph shows fractures involving the left acetabulum (*open arrow*) and left femoral neck (*curved arrow*). A large pelvic hematoma compresses and displaces the contrast-filled bladder to the right (*small arrows*). There is extravasated contrast (*asterisk*) just below the pubic symphysis as a result of a urethral injury. The floor of the bladder is elevated as another manifestation of this injury. **B.** CT image through the hips shows the severely comminuted acetabular fracture on the left (*arrow*). **C.** Acetabular fracture of the right hip (*arrow*) in another patient with posterior and superior dislocation of the femoral head. **D.** CT image shows the posterior dislocation of the femoral head and an intraarticular bone fragment (*arrow*).

Postoperative Changes

A large number of joint implants and appliances are used in orthopaedics today. You should familiarize yourself with the more common of these and their appearance in the bone (Fig. 11.113). Furthermore, the sites of previous screw holes, osteotomies, or implants may present a variety of bony defects that are easily recognizable if you are familiar with the types of procedures used in orthopaedic surgery (Fig. 11.114). Remember, straight lines and rectangular margins are human made (Fig. 11.115); nature prefers curves and circles.

▶ Straight lines and rectangular margins suggest human intervention; nature prefers curves and circles.

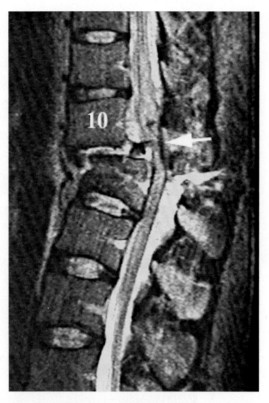

Figure 11.112   Fracture dislocation of T10 on T11.
Sagittal MR T2-weighted image shows the dislocation and resultant cord transection (*arrow*).

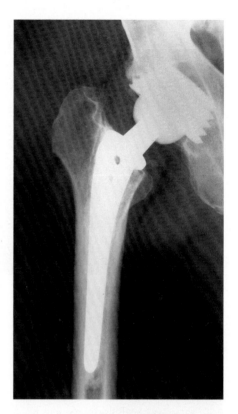

**Figure 11.113   Normal postoperative
appearance of a total hip implant.**

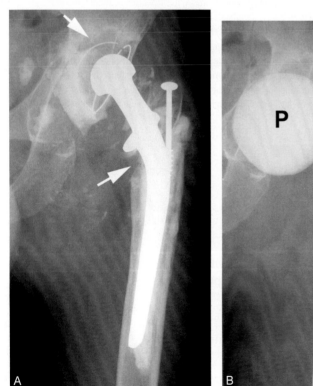

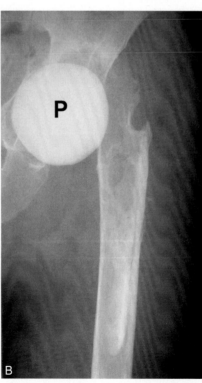

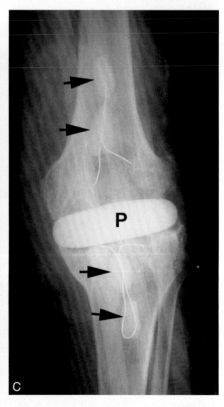

Figure 11.114   Antibiotic cement in place after removal of joint implants.   A. Radiograph shows loosening of a total hip implant. Note the spaces
between the acetabular and the femoral components and their respective bones (*arrows*). **B.** After removal of the device, a large puck (*P*) of antibiotic methyl
methacrylate cement has been inserted as a spacer until a new device is implanted. **C.** Knee radiograph following removal of a total joint implant and insertion of
a puck (*P*) and intramedullary beads (*arrows*) of cement. The beads are connected by wire to make removal easier.

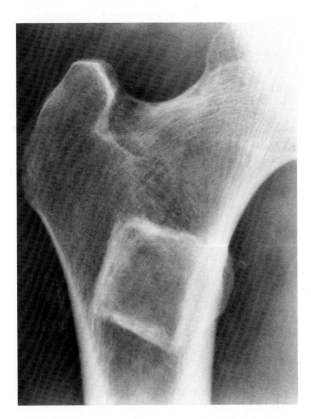

Figure 11.115   Bone biopsy excision site.
The *square*, straight margins of this sclerotic lesion indicate the iatrogenic nature of the lesion. Naturally occurring lesions have rounded margins.

Summary and Key Points

▶ Bone abnormalities are among the most common you will encounter. Of these, fractures and arthritic conditions occur most frequently.

▶ Most bone lesions fall into one of six basic pathologic categories: congenital, inflammatory, metabolic, neoplastic, traumatic, and vascular.

▶ By recognizing patterns of destruction and the use of a series of predictor variables, it is possible to reduce the complexities of skeletal radiology to a workable format.

▶ The application of the mnemonic **ABCS** was introduced to describe the analysis of bone and joint lesions: **A**natomy and alignment abnormalities, **B**ony mineralization and texture abnormalities, **C**artilage (joint space) abnormalities, and **S**oft tissue abnormalities.

▶ A number of common entities were discussed, as were the principles of fracture diagnosis.

Suggested Additional Reading

Brower AC, Flemming DJ. Arthritis in Black and White. 3rd Ed. Philadelphia, PA: Elsevier WB Saunders, 2012.

Chew FS. Skeletal Radiology: The Bare Bones. 3rd Ed. Philadelphia, PA: Lippincott Williams & Wilkins, 2010.

Egol, KA, Koval KJ, Zuckerman JD. Handbook of Fractures. 4th Ed. Philadelphia, PA: Lippincott Williams & Wilkins, 2010 .

Greenspan A. Orthopaedic Imaging: A Practical Approach. 5th Ed. Philadelphia, PA: WB Saunders, 2010.

Helms CA. Fundamentals of Skeletal Radiology. 3rd Ed. Philadelphia, PA: WB Saunders, 2005.

Helms CA, Major NM, Anderson MW, Kaplan P, Dussault R. Musculoskeletal MRI. 2nd Ed. Philadelphia, PA: WB Saunders, 2009.

Kleinman PK. Diagnostic Imaging of Child Abuse. 2nd Ed. St. Louis, MO: Mosby, 1998.

Ogden JA. Skeletal Injury in the Child. 2nd Ed. Philadelphia, PA: WB Saunders, 1990.

Ozonoff MB. Pediatric Orthopedic Radiology. 2nd Ed. Philadelphia, PA: WB Saunders, 1992.

Resnick DL. Diagnosis of Bone and Joint Disorders. 4th Ed. Philadelphia, PA: WB Saunders, 2002.

Resnick DL, Kang HS, Pretterklieber ML. Internal Derangements of Joints. 2nd Ed. Philadelphia, PA: WB Saunders, 2007.

Resnick DL, Kransdorf MJ. Bone and Joint Imaging. 3rd Ed. Philadelphia, PA: WB Saunders, 2005.

Stoller DW. Magnetic Resonance Imaging in Orthopaedics and Sports Medicine. 3rd Ed. Philadelphia, PA: Lippincott Williams & Wilkins, 2006.

Stoller DW, Tirman P, Bredella MA. Diagnostic Imaging: Orthopaedics. Philadelphia, PA: WB Saunders, 2004.

Swischuk LE. Imaging of the Newborn, Infant, and Young Child. 5th Ed. Philadelphia, PA: Lippincott Williams & Wilkins, 2004:747–755.

Van Holsbeeck MT, Introcaso JT. Musculoskeletal Ultrasound. 2nd Ed. St. Louis, MO: Mosby, 2001.

Weissman BNW, Sledge CB. Orthopedic Radiology. 2nd Ed. Philadelphia, PA: WB Saunders, 1999.

chapter 12

Cranial Imaging

Michael F. Goldberg   Richard H. Daffner

Neuroradiology is the subspecialty concerned with radiologic investigation and intervention of the brain and spinal cord. It is this area that has been most dramatically changed by the technical developments in imaging of the past 40 years. Computed tomography (CT), magnetic resonance imaging (MRI), digital subtraction angiography (DSA), and positron emission tomography (PET) scanning have been major breakthroughs in the imaging of the brain and spinal cord. Although abnormalities in other areas of the body may be grossly evident, the changes present on studies of the central nervous system (CNS) are often subtle. The student or house officer who is confronted with a neuroradiologic study is often frustrated and feels insecure. Remember, however, that neuroradiology is founded on the same principles of anatomy, physiology, and pathology as any other diagnostic area. This chapter focuses on cranial imaging; Chapter 13 discusses vertebral and spinal cord imaging.

Neuroradiologic examinations are often complex. For this reason, detailed descriptions of the various entities are beyond the scope of this book. However, the pertinent aspects of each type of study, their indications, and a basic discussion of the main pathologic entities is included to provide you with the foundation you need to select the appropriate studies for your patients.

Technical Considerations

The cranial contents are studied by CT, MRI, angiography, and nuclear imaging. Prior to the development of cross-sectional imaging, cranial evaluations were performed to display the effects of certain intracranial abnormalities on structures that could be opacified. Hence, the main purpose of skull radiographs was to detect enlargement of the sella turcica, intracranial calcifications, and shifts in the calcified pineal gland. Cerebral angiography was a primary tool to detect *neovascularity* (new tumor vessels) and to show displacement and encasement of vessels by intracranial masses. It was also used to show brain compression from extracerebral masses such as subdural and epidural hematomas. *Pneumoencephalography* was performed to outline the cerebral ventricular system and to show the effects of neoplasms and other lesions on those structures. Of these modalities, only angiography has as important a role today, as is discussed later in the chapter.

Although CT and MRI are the prime investigative tools for cranial imaging, there is still a limited role for skull radiography: penetrating injury, destructive lesions, dental abnormalities, metabolic bone disease, congenital anomalies, screening for metallic foreign bodies (prior to MRI evaluation), and postoperative changes. In addition, facial radiographs are still effective for screening for suspected facial fractures; in practice, however, CT has replaced radiography for the detection of calvarial and facial fractures.

Computed Tomography

CT examination of the brain and surrounding tissue is usually performed as the initial study for evaluation of patients with suspected intracranial abnormalities, especially in the emergency department setting. Cranial CT is generally performed without intravenous (IV) contrast since iodinated contrast can mimic the appearance of intracranial hemorrhage. With the greater availability of MRI, the role for a contrast-enhanced head CT has greatly diminished; when a contrast-enhanced CT has been ordered, a discussion with the referring clinician often reveals that the clinical question to be addressed can be better answered by MRI. For patients with contraindications to MRI, the contrast-enhanced CT can serve as an alternative procedure of choice.

 ▶ The greater availability of MRI has diminished the role of contrast-enhanced cranial CT. When such a study is ordered a discussion between the clinician and the radiologist often shows that the clinical question to be addressed could be better answered by MRI.

Computed Tomographic Angiography

Computed tomographic angiography (CTA) has emerged as a key diagnostic test in a variety of clinical settings, largely replacing the role of diagnostic cerebral angiogram (see below). Most commonly, CTA is employed for the acute workup of subarachnoid hemorrhage (SAH) for the detection of aneurysm. In addition, in the setting of acute ischemia, CTA is used to assess for proximal vascular stenosis or occlusion.

Computed Tomography of the Face and Sinuses

CT of the face and sinuses is also performed to evaluate patients with suspected trauma or infection, respectively. Although radiographs of those areas are valuable, CT provides more information, particularly about displacement of bone fragments and the presence of ocular injury in trauma and about possible bone destruction in sinusitis.

Magnetic Resonance Imaging

MRI is one of the greatest technological improvements for evaluating suspected intracranial lesions. It is the primary investigative tool for suspected intracranial abnormalities, such as tumors and multiple sclerosis, because it can display the brain in exquisite detail in axial, coronal, and sagittal planes. Cranial MR is performed using T1- and T2-weighted spin echo sequences as well as various gradient echo and inversion recovery (STIR and FLAIR) sequences. Diffusion-weighted imaging (DWI) is also essential for the evaluation of patients with suspected acute ischemia; DWI also plays a critical role in the characterization of other disease processes, including pyogenic abscesses and highly cellular tumors, such as lymphoma. The scanning parameters of these studies are adjusted to optimize the characteristics of certain intracranial lesions. In addition, MR angiography is now commonly performed either alone, or after IV contrast enhancement, as a noninvasive mechanism for evaluating the carotid, vertebral, and cerebral arteries.

Cerebral Angiography

Cerebral angiography is still used to evaluate vascular lesions such as atherosclerotic occlusive disease, aneurysms, and arteriovenous malformations (AVMs). As mentioned above, CTA is commonly done prior to or in place of conventional cerebral angiography, since CTA is less invasive and involves less ionizing radiation. Interventional vascular procedures (see Chapter 3) are now commonly performed to occlude those abnormalities. DSA allows the neuroradiologist to perform the studies using minimal amounts of contrast media.

Nuclear Imaging

Nuclear imaging of the brain was the only noninvasive cranial procedure before the development of CT and MRI. The latter technologies have largely replaced nuclear medicine for the study of the CNS. However, a role still persists in select clinical settings. Four types of nuclear studies are performed: conventional scintigraphy with blood-barrier agents, cerebral perfusion, cisternography, and PET scanning

Cerebral Perfusion Imaging

Cerebral perfusion imaging with single photon computer emission tomography (SPECT) technology is still used for patients who are being considered for carotid endarterectomies or intracranial vascular aneurysm occlusion. By placing an intraluminal balloon in the diseased carotid artery, subsequent radioisotope injection of technetium 99m–tagged diethylenetriamine pentaacetic acid (DTPA) can provide information about cerebral cortex perfusion on the ipsilateral side. This allows the physician to determine whether sacrificing a carotid artery will compromise cortical perfusion and function.

Another use of cerebral perfusion is in providing visual corroboration of a clinical diagnosis of brain death. By injecting technetium 99m–tagged DTPA and performing immediate flow images in the region of the head and neck, intracranial perfusion is assessed. Absence of arterial flow on early images as well as lack of pooling in the venous system on subsequent "blood pool" images is consistent with brain death.

Indium 111 Radionuclide Cisternography

Indium 111 radionuclide cisternography is used to identify sites of cerebrospinal fluid leakage, to evaluate shunt patency, and to diagnose normal pressure hydrocephalus. Studies for cerebrospinal fluid leakage are usually performed in collaboration with neurosurgeons. Using indium 111–labeled radiotracers, imaging is possible up to 3 days after the initial time of administration, allowing imaging at multiple time points.

Positron Emission Tomography Scanning

PET scanning is used primarily for brain perfusion and metabolism evaluation. The conventional isotope is F 18 fluoro-2-deoxyglucose (F^{18} FDG), which is produced by a cyclotron. By injecting F^{18} FDG and performing multiplanar imaging, information regarding gray and white matter perfusion can be obtained. The drawback to F^{18} FDG PET for brain imaging is the high background glucose metabolism of normal gray matter. Thus, other radiotracers have been developed for PET imaging of the brain, including radiolabeled amino acids, such as methyl-[C^{11}]-L-methionine (MET); radiolabeled cell membrane components, such as methyl-[C^{11}]-choline (CHO); and radiolabeled nucleosides, such as 3-deoxy-3-[F^{18}]-fluoro-L-thymidine (FLT). Clinical applications include differentiating radiation necrosis from residual tumor, localizing seizure foci for planning of surgery, and diagnosing Alzheimer disease.

Anatomic Considerations

Skull radiographs, as previously mentioned, can be used whenever there is a history of penetrating trauma, facial fracture, sinus disease, destructive lesion, or metabolic problem. However, with the increased availability of CT and increased speed of image acquisition, CT has largely replaced radiography for the evaluation of trauma and sinus disease.

Skull anatomy is complex. However, the symmetry of the skull provides, in most instances, a ready "comparison view" of the unaffected side. The standard radiographic views of the skull are the posterior-anterior (PA), lateral, AP half-axial (Towne), and base. Each view is designed to demonstrate particular areas of the skull. The *PA view* shows the frontal bones, frontal and ethmoid sinuses, nasal cavity, superior orbital rims, and mandible (Fig. 12.1). The *lateral view* demonstrates the frontal, parietal, temporal, and occipital bones, the mastoid region, the sella turcica, the roofs of the orbits, and the lateral aspects of the facial bones (Fig. 12.2). The *modified half-axial projection* (Towne, occipital view; Fig. 12.3) shows the occipital bone, the mandibular condyles and temporomandibular (TM) joints, the mastoid and middle ear regions, the foramen magnum, and the zygomatic arches. The *base view* (Fig. 12.4) shows the major basal foramina and the zygomatic arches. This view is not as useful as thin CT sections through the skull base, because the latter examination portrays the anatomy in greater detail (Fig. 12.5). The occipitomental (*Waters*) projection (Fig. 12.6) is used primarily to study the facial bones and sinuses. Dentists and oral surgeons also use a *panoramic* type of tomogram to study the mandible and facial bones (Fig. 12.7). The TM joints are best studied by CT and MRI.

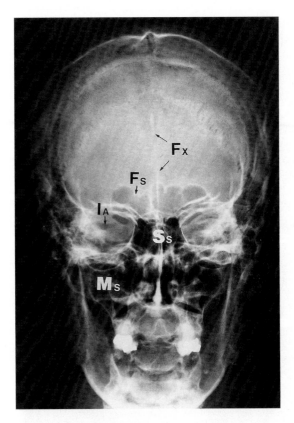

Figure 12.1   PA skull radiograph.   The following structures are visible: falx cerebri (*Fx*), frontal sinus (*Fs*), internal auditory canal (*IA*), sphenoid sinus (*Ss*), and maxillary sinus (*Ms*).

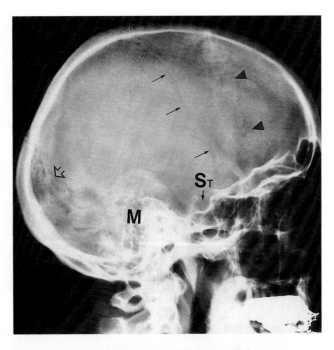

Figure 12.2   Lateral radiograph of the skull.   The following structures are visible: coronal suture (*arrowheads*), occipital suture (*open arrow*), middle meningeal vascular grooves (*straight arrows*), sella turcica (*St*), and mastoid air cells (*M*).

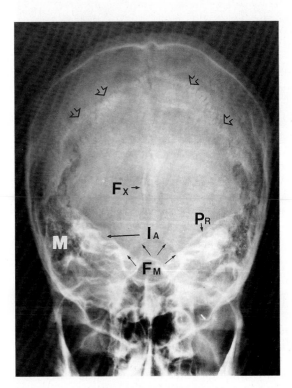

Figure 12.3   Modified half-axial projection (Towne).   The following structures are visible: occipital sutures (*open arrows*), mastoid air cells (*M*), falx cerebri (*Fx*), internal auditory canal (*IA*), petrous ridge (*PR*), and foramen magnum (*FM*).

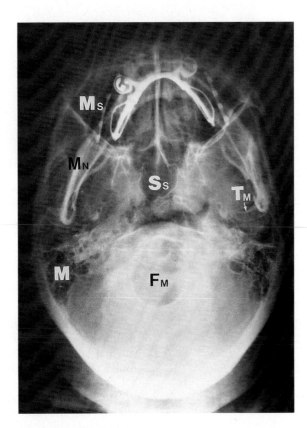

Figure 12.4   Base view.   The following structures are visible: mastoid air cells (*M*), mandible (*MN*), maxillary sinus (*Ms*), sphenoid sinus (*Ss*), foramen magnum (*FM*), and temporomandibular joint (*TM*).

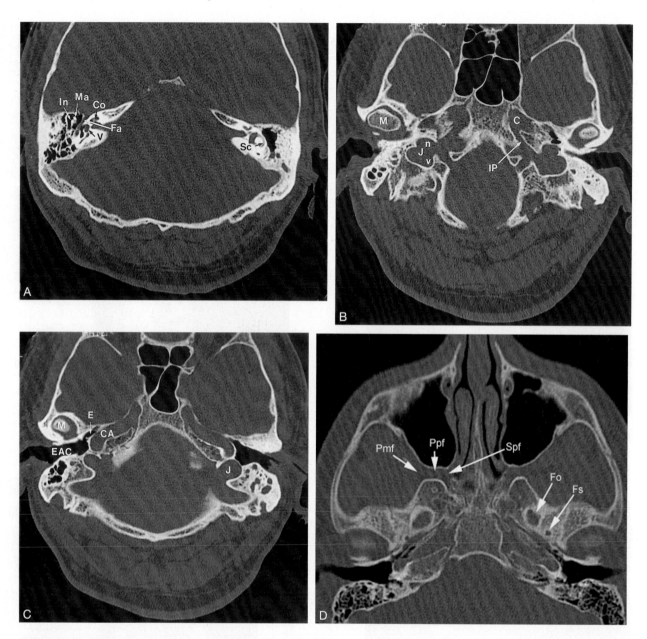

Figure 12.5   Skull base anatomy as demonstrated on high-detail CT.   A. Level of the mastoids. **B.** Level of the mandibular condyles. **C.** Level of the external auditory canals. The following structures are visible: incus (*In*); malleus (*Ma*); cochlea (*Co*); facial nerve canal (*Fa*); vestibule (*V*); semicircular canal (*Sc*); mandibular condyle (*M*); jugular foramen (*J*) with its anterior pars nervosa (*n,* containing cranial nerve IX) and pars vascularis (*v,* containing cranial nerves X and XI); inferior petrosal sinus (*IP*); carotid-cavernous sinus (*C*); carotid artery (*CA*); opening of the eustachian tube (*E*); and external auditory canal (*EAC*). **D.** Level of the maxillary sinuses. The following structures are visible: foramen spinosum (*Fs*); foramen ovale (*Fo*); pterygomaxillary fissure (*Pmf*); pterygopalatine fossa (*Ppf*); and sphenopalatine foramen (*Spf*).

A large variety of normal structures and conditions may cause diagnostic concern. These include prominent vascular grooves (Fig. 12.8), hyperostosis frontalis interna (Fig. 12.9), calcified falx cerebri (Fig. 12.10), and persistent anomalous sutures (Fig. 12.11). When in doubt, review the radiographs with a radiologist.

CT and MRI allow visualization of the brain, its coverings, the extraaxial spaces, the calvarium, and skull base. The advantages of CT include faster scanning times, lower cost, and superior spatial resolution. The primary advantage of MRI is great contrast resolution with greater ability to characterize normal tissue structures as well as disease processes. Figures 12.12 through 12.15 show representative CT images and their MR counterparts of the various normal intracranial structures. Facial CT is now the primary investigative tool for evaluating facial fractures as well as sinus disease. Thin section axial images are

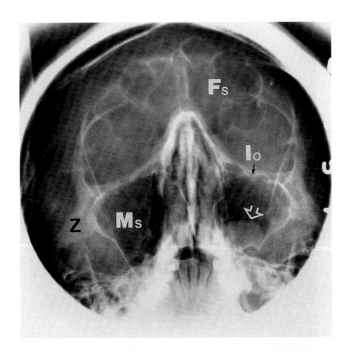

Figure 12.6 Occipitomental (Waters) projection. The following structures are visible: zygomatic arch (*Z*), maxillary sinus (*Ms*), frontal sinus (*Fs*), and inferior orbital rim (*Io* and *small arrow*). A mucous retention cyst (*open arrow*) is in the left maxillary sinus.

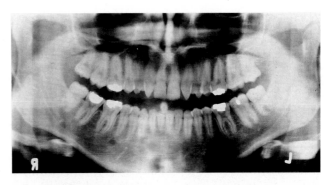

Figure 12.7 Panoramic tomogram of the mandible.

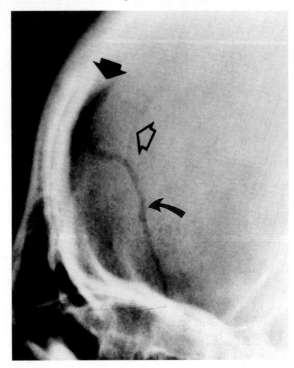

Figure 12.8 Prominent vascular groove (*curved arrow*) that ends in a venous lake (*large black arrow*). Note the branch (*open arrow*).

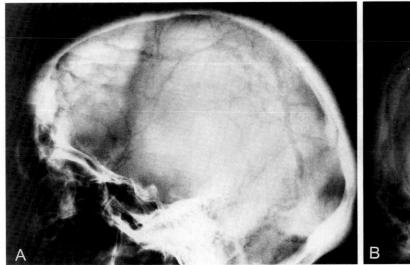

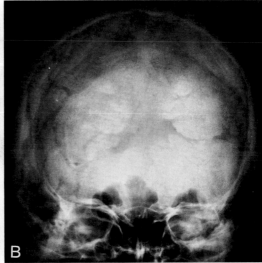

Figure 12.9 Hyperostosis frontalis interna. Lateral (**A**) and frontal (**B**) radiographs show the thickened internal table of the skull. This is a normal variant.

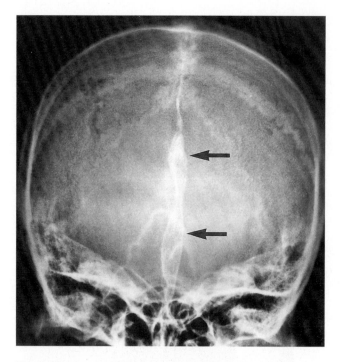

Figure 12.10   Calcified falx cerebri (*arrows*).

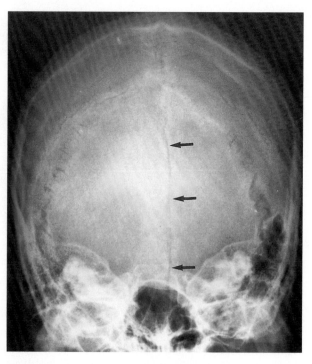

Figure 12.11   Persistent metopic suture (*arrows*).   This could be mistaken for a fracture.

routinely obtained. From the sources images, multiplanar and volume-rendered three-dimensional (3-D) images can be obtained. Figures 12.16 and 12.17 show normal facial anatomy in axial and coronal planes, respectively. Oral, maxillofacial, and plastic surgeons have found three-dimensional volume-rendered reformation of facial images to be extremely useful (Fig. 12.18).

Pathologic Considerations

The most common abnormalities you will encounter in the CNS are trauma, neoplasms, vascular disease, inflammatory disease, infections, and age-related and degenerative changes.

Trauma

Indications for CT examination after trauma include signs and symptoms of neurologic abnormality: loss of consciousness and abnormal neurologic findings on examination. Because the treatment of skull fractures, with two notable exceptions, is directed toward treating the neurologic abnormality, the presence or absence of a fracture itself makes little difference in the management of the patient. You will encounter many patients in whom a skull fracture is present without neurologic findings or sequelae, as well as patients with head injury without fracture where significant neurologic damage has occurred. Remember, as mentioned in Chapter 11, *a fracture is a soft tissue injury in which a bone is broken.*

 ▶ A fracture is a soft tissue injury in which a bone is broken.

Skull Fractures

Two situations in which the *skull fracture* itself is significant are the depressed fracture and the fracture associated with penetration of a bullet or other foreign object. However, in both these instances, associated neurologic abnormalities are usually present and will dictate CT examination before corrective therapy. Brain injury is indicated by brain

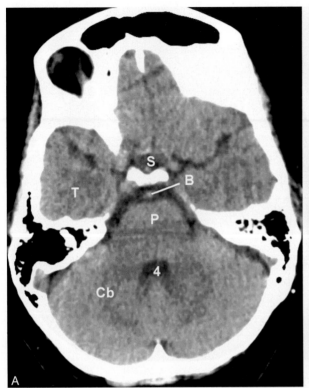

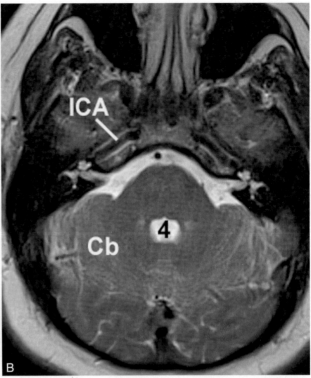

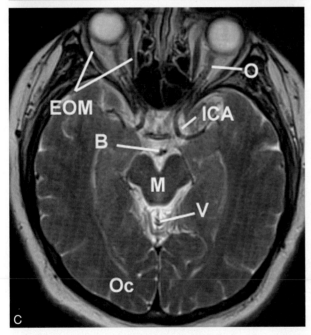

Figure 12.12 **Normal structures of the brain near the skull base.** **A.** CT scan. **B.** Axial T2W MR image. **C.** Axial T2W MR image at the level of the orbits. The following landmarks are visible: cerebellum (*Cb*), fourth ventricle (*4*), pons (*P*), temporal lobe (*T*), basilar artery (*B*), sella turcica (*S*), infundibulum of the pituitary (*I*), internal carotid arteries (*ICA*), occipital lobe (*Oc*), midbrain (*M*), vermis (*V*), optic nerve (*O*), and extraocular muscles (*EOM*).

edema or hemorrhage. On CT, brain edema is manifest as an area of low density, acute hemorrhage as an area of high density. Figures 12.19 to 12.22 illustrate skull fractures and their associated findings. MRI portrays brain edema as areas of low signal intensity on T1-weighted images and increased signal intensity on T2-weighted images. One caveat is that gunshot wounds to the skull that cross the midline are uniformly fatal injuries. In these instances, the most cost-effective study is the AP radiograph of the skull to demonstrate that this has occurred.

 ▶ In patients with a gunshot wound to the head, the AP skull radiograph is the most cost-effective imaging exam. If the bullet has crossed the midline, the wound is fatal.

Text continues on page 443.

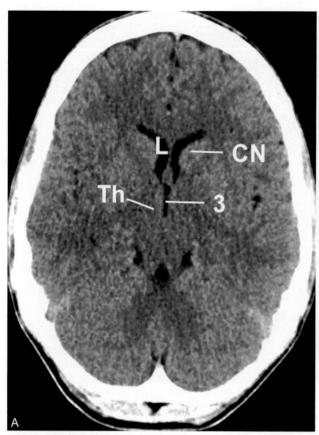

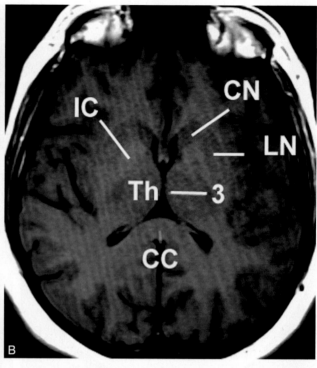

Figure 12.13   Normal cerebral anatomy.   A. CT scan. **B.** Axial T1W MRI. The following structures are visible: head of the caudate nucleus (*CN*), lateral ventricle (*L*), fornix (*F*), thalamus (*Th*), third ventricle (*3*), splenium of the corpus callosum (*CC*), internal capsule (*IC*), and lentiform nucleus (*LN*).

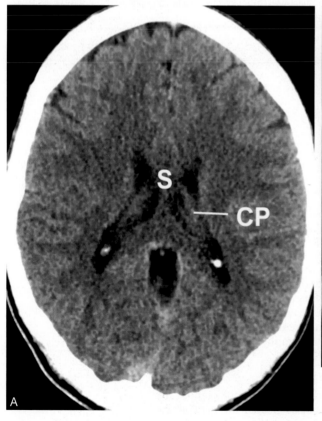

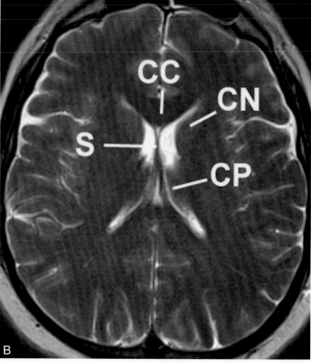

Figure 12.14   Normal cerebral anatomy.   **These views are slightly higher than those in Fig. 12.13. **A. CT scan. **B.** Axial T2W. The following structures are visible: interventricular septum (*S*), choroid plexus (*CP*), genu of the corpus callosum (*CC*), and caudate nucleus (*CN*).

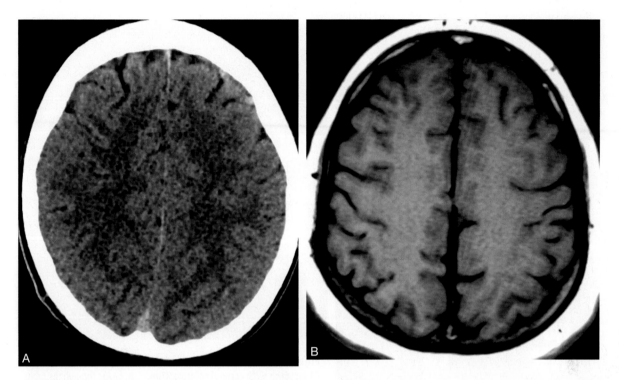

Figure 12.15   High cerebral cortex.   A. CT scan. **B.** Axial T1W MRI.

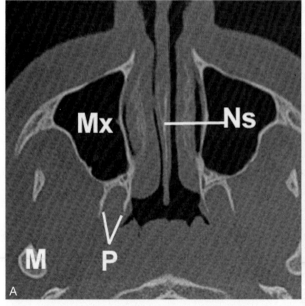

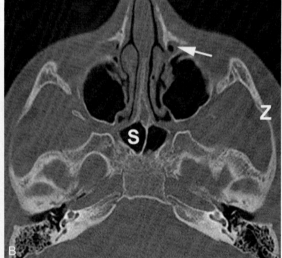

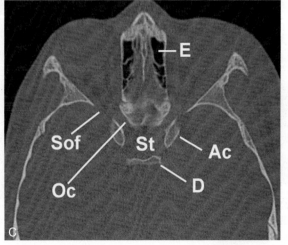

Figure 12.16   Normal facial anatomy as demonstrated by axial CT imaging.   A. Image through the lower maxilla shows the following structures: maxillary sinus (*Mx*), pterygoid plates (*P*), nasal septum (*Ns*), and mandibular condyle (*M*). **B.** Image through mid-maxilla shows the following structures: zygomatic arch (*Z*), sphenoid sinus (*S*), and nasolacrimal duct (*arrow*). **C.** Image through mid-orbits shows the following structures: ethmoid sinus (*E*), sella turcica (*St*), dorsum sellae (*D*), anterior clinoid process (*Ac*), optic canal (*Oc*), and superior orbital fissure (*Sof*). In addition, note the intraocular muscles in each eye.

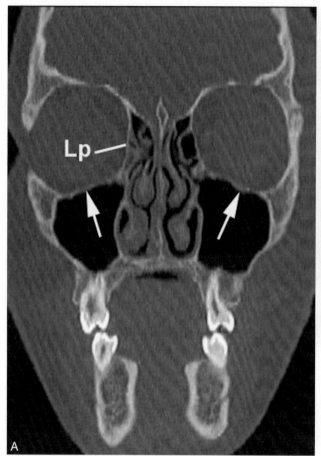

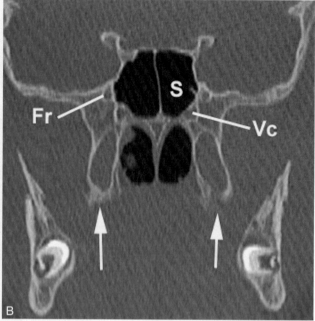

Figure 12.17   Normal facial anatomy as demonstrated by axial CT imaging with coronal reformatting.   A. Image through the orbits shows the orbital floors (*arrows*) and lamina papyracea (*Lp*). Note the intraocular muscles and the optic nerves within the orbits. **B.** Image through the sphenoid sinus shows the pterygoid plates (*arrows*), the sphenoid sinus (*S*), vidian canal (*Vc*), and foramen rotundum (*Fr*).

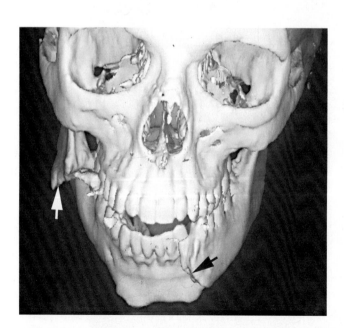

Figure 12.18   Value of three-dimensional CT in a patient with bilateral mandibular fractures (*arrows*).   This is the view that the surgeon would see at the time of surgery.

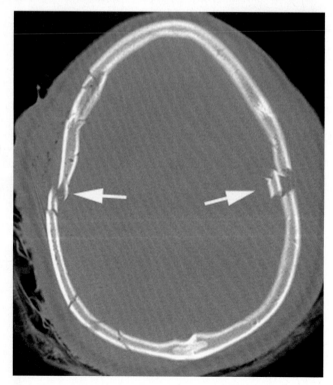

Figure 12.19   Multiple skull fractures, some of which are depressed (*arrows*).

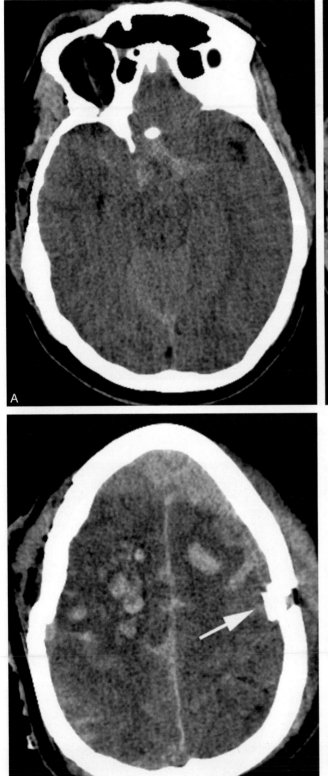

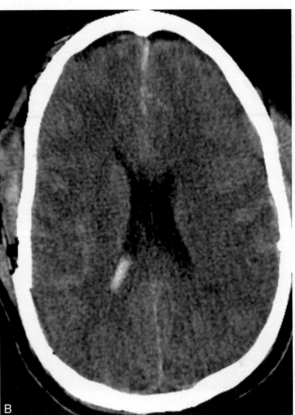

Figure 12.20 Depressed skull fracture with intracerebral hemorrhage. (Same patient as in Fig. 12.19). CT images **(A** and **B)** in a brain algorithm parenchymal and extraaxial hemorrhage (*white areas*). **C.** CT image shows the depressed fragment (*arrow*).

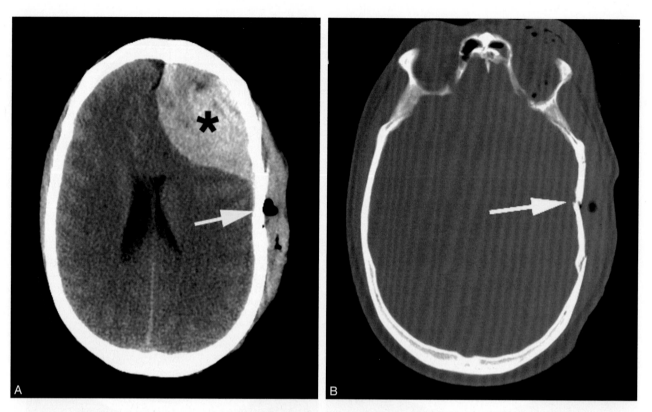

Figure 12.21   Skull fracture in the left temporal region with epidural hematoma.   A. CT image at brain window shows the lentiform epidural hematoma (*asterisk*) in the left frontal region. Note the superficial hematoma and gas in the left temporal region (*arrow*). **B.** CT image slightly lower at bone window shows the depressed fracture (*arrow*). Epidural hematomas are not always located directly over fractures.

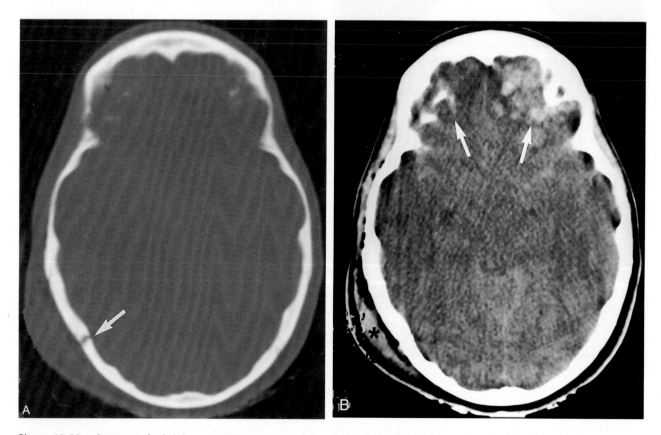

Figure 12.22   Contrecoup brain injury.   A. CT image at bone window shows a fracture in the right posterior parietal bone (*arrow*). **B.** Same image at brain window shows areas of intracerebral hemorrhage in the frontal lobes (*arrows*). Note the scalp hematoma (*asterisk*) in the right occipital area.

Posttraumatic Intracranial Hemorrhage

Posttraumatic intracranial hemorrhage can be intraaxial or extraaxial. Intraaxial or intracerebral hemorrhage in the setting of trauma can be referred to as hemorrhagic contusion. Extraaxial hematomas occur in the subarachnoid, subdural, and epidural spaces. Intracranial hemorrhage, regardless of whether it is intraaxial or extraaxial, presents on CT as areas of increased density in the acute stage. Frequently, intracerebral hemorrhages are associated with bleeding into the ventricles (Fig. 12.23 **A**, **B**). On MRI,

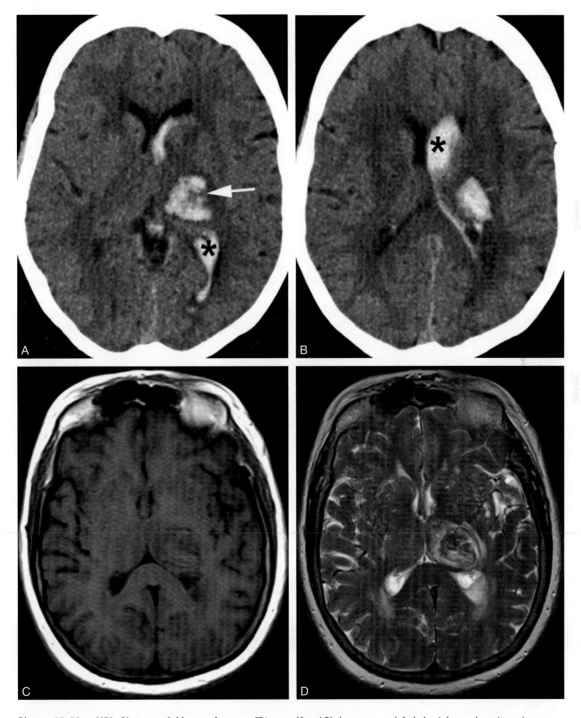

Figure 12.23   MRI of intracranial hemorrhage.   CT images (**A** and **B**) show an acute left thalamic hemorrhage (*arrow*), a classic location for hypertensive hemorrhage; patient presented in hypertensive crisis. Note the intraventricular blood (*asterisk*). MRI was performed approximately 12 hours after onset of left-sided weakness. **C.** T1W MR demonstrates hypointense and isointense signal and **D.** T2W MR demonstrates hypointense and hyperintense signal. Findings reflect a combination of oxyhemoglobin and deoxyhemoglobin, consistent with an acute/subacute hemorrhage.

the signal of the hemorrhage depends on its age and may range from low to high intensity (Fig. 12.23C and D); its characteristics on T1- and T2-weighted sequences can be used to estimate the age of the blood products (Table 12.1).

▶ Intracranial hemorrhage presents on CT as areas of increased density in the acute stage, regardless of its location.

Epidural, Subdural, and Subarachnoid Hematomas

Epidural, subdural, and subarachnoid hematomas all can result from cranial trauma. They are each managed in different ways, and the role of the radiologist is not only to identify the presence of acute intracranial hemorrhage, but also to localize it to the correct intracranial compartment. Fortunately, each type of extraaxial hematoma has unique imaging features.

▶ Subarachnoid, epidural, and subdural hematomas are managed in different ways and the role of the radiologist is to not only identify the presence of the abnormality but also to localize it to the correct intracranial compartment.

Epidural Hematomas

Epidural hematomas are usually the result of skull fractures that involve one of the meningeal arteries. Most commonly, epidural hematomas occur secondary to fractures of the temporal bone with injury to the middle meningeal artery. As blood accumulates between the dura and inner table of the skull, these hematomas characteristically have a *lentiform* or biconvex shape (Figs. 12.24 and 12.25; see Fig. 12.21) and do not cross calvarial sutures; they can, however, cross the midline.

Subdural Hematomas

Subdural hematomas are due to head injury that results in shearing of the bridging meningeal veins that cross the subdural space. They are especially common in elderly patients secondary to cerebral atrophy, which is a risk factor for the shearing injury. In the acute stage, the subdural hematomas conform to the contour of the brain and have a *crescentic* shape (Figs. 12.26 and 12.27). In contrast to epidural hematomas, a subdural hematoma can cross sutures, but will not cross the midline. Subdural hematomas can extend along the falx and tentorium.

▶ Epidural hematomas do not cross calvarial sutures but can cross the midline. Subdural hematomas can cross sutures but will not cross the midline.

Table 12.1 MRI CHARACTERISTICS OF INTRACRANIAL HEMORRHAGE

Phase	Time	T1W	T2W	Hemoglobin
Hyperacute	<6 h	Mild hyperintensity	Hyperintensity with peripheral hypointensity	Central oxyhemoglobin with peripheral deoxyhemoglobin
Acute	>6–72 h	Isointensity and hypointensity	Hypointensity	Deoxyhemoglobin
Early subacute	3–7 d	Hyperintensity	Hypointensity	Intracellular methemoglobin
Late subacute	1 wk–months	Hyperintensity	Hyperintensity	Extracellular methemoglobin
Chronic	2 wk–years	Hypointensity	Hypointensity	Hemosiderin

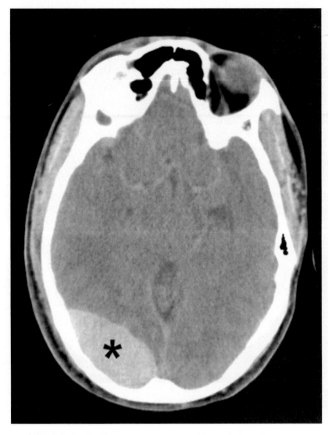

Figure 12.24 Acute epidural hematoma (*asterisk*), CT appearance. Note the typical lentiform or biconvex shape to the hematoma.

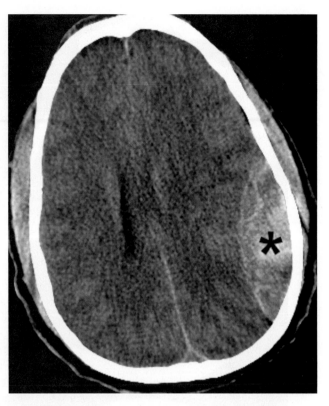

Figure 12.25 Acute epidural hematoma (*asterisk*), MRI appearance. T2-weighted image shows the typical biconvex shape, similar to that seen on a CT image.

Acute subdural hematomas have a high mortality rate because of their ability to exert a significant amount of mass effect, including midline shift and various herniation syndromes. Subfalcine herniation is the most common herniation syndrome and occurs when mass effect results in displacement of the cingulated gyrus under the falx, compression of the ipsilateral ventricle, and possible trapping or dilation of the contralateral ventricle (due to obstruction of the foramen of Monro). There can also be impingement of the ipsilateral anterior cerebral artery against the falx with resultant anterior cerebral artery (ACA) territory infarct.

Uncal or transtentorial herniation is the second most common herniation syndrome and occurs when mass effect results in medial displacement of the medial temporal lobe (uncus) into the incisura. This can be detected by the radiologist by effacement of the ipsilateral suprasellar and quadrigeminal cisterns. In severe cases, the medial temporal lobe can be displaced into the upper cerebellopontine angle with compression of the midbrain. Complications include compression of the posterior cerebral artery (PCA) with resultant PCA territory infarcts, compression of the oculomotor nerve (CN III) with resultant CN III palsy, and midbrain (Duret) hemorrhage. Uncal herniation often requires emergency neurosurgical decompression; if the radiologist detects this finding, an immediate phone call to the referring physician is required.

> ▌ Uncal herniation requires emergency neurosurgical compression and the radiologist is required to call the referring physician immediately.

Subarachnoid Hemorrhage

Traumatic *SAH* is due to injury of the vessels within the subarachnoid space. On CT, acute SAH appears as hyperdensity in the subarachnoid space, (Fig. 12.28) most commonly in the sulci adjacent to other traumatic injuries, including skull fractures, contusions, as

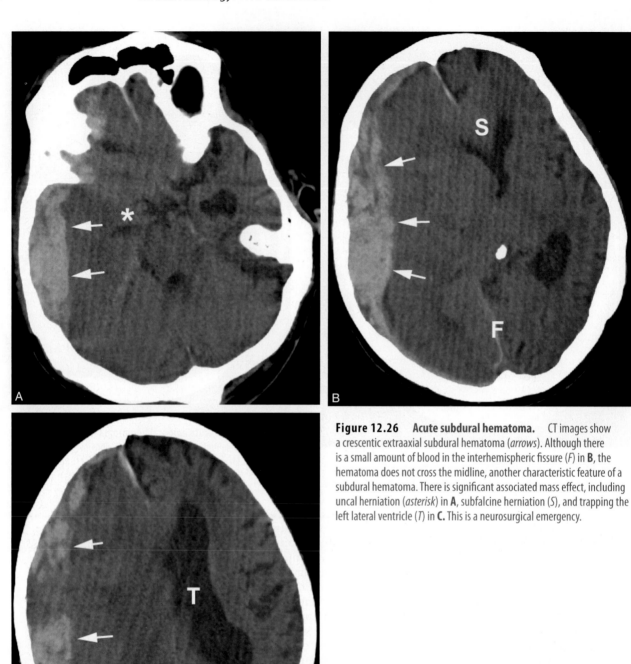

Figure 12.26 **Acute subdural hematoma.** CT images show a crescentic extraaxial subdural hematoma (*arrows*). Although there is a small amount of blood in the interhemispheric fissure (*F*) in **B**, the hematoma does not cross the midline, another characteristic feature of a subdural hematoma. There is significant associated mass effect, including uncal herniation (*asterisk*) in **A**, subfalcine herniation (*S*), and trapping the left lateral ventricle (*T*) in **C.** This is a neurosurgical emergency.

well as subdural and epidural hematomas. Traumatic SAH may also be seen in the basilar cisterns and within the ventricles. This can present a diagnostic dilemma, as aneurysmal SAH can have an identical imaging appearance. Correlation with the patient's history and physical examination is critical in this situation. If there is a suspicion that the SAH may be aneurysmal, rather than traumatic, angiographic imaging (usually CTA) should be performed.

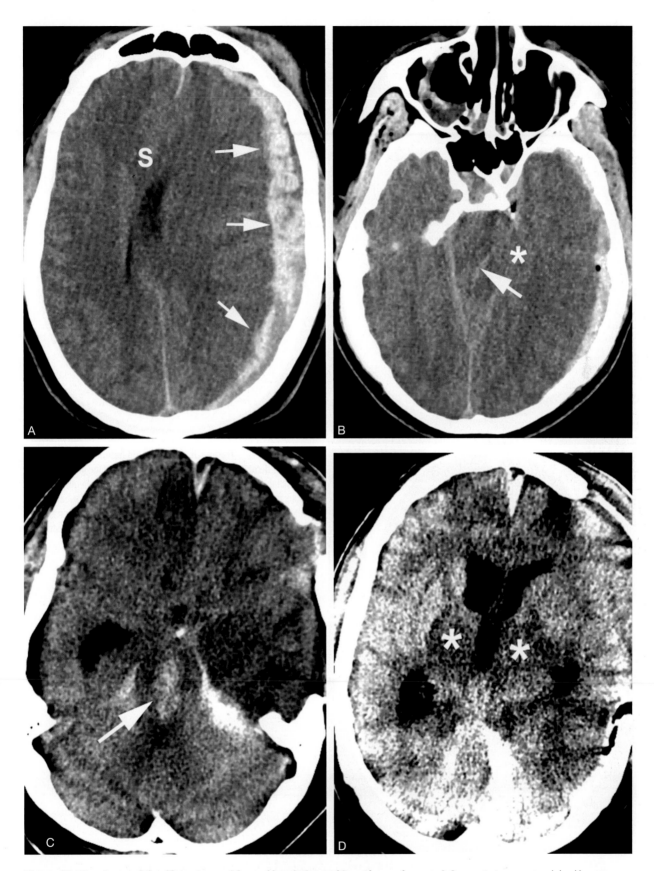

Figure 12.27 Acute subdural hematoma with uncal herniation and Duret hemorrhage. A. Demonstrates an acute subdural hematoma (*arrows*) with subfalcine herniation (*S*). **B.** At the level of the midbrain, there is complete effacement of the left basilar cistern (*asterisk*). Thin, linear hemorrhage within the midbrain is consistent with a Duret hemorrhage (*arrow*). On admission, the patient had a Glasgow Coma Scale (GCS) score of 3. **C.** Repeat CT performed 8 hours later (after decompressive craniectomy) shows expansion of Duret hemorrhage (*arrow*). **D.** Hypodensities within both thalamic areas (*asterisks*) are consistent with acute bilateral PCA territory infarcts, secondary to uncal herniation. Brain death was declared the following day.

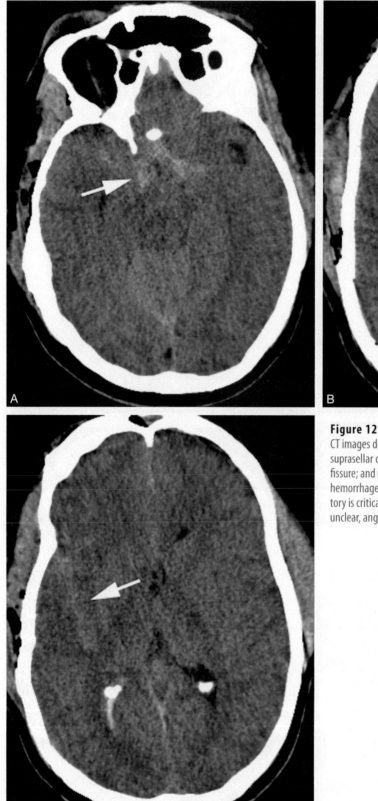

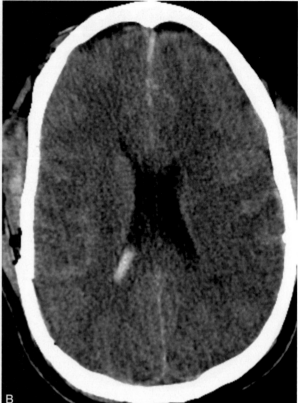

Figure 12.28   Traumatic subarachnoid hemorrhage.
CT images demonstrate acute subarachnoid hemorrhage in the **(A)** suprasellar cistern (*arrow*); **(B)** ventricles, sulci, and interhemispheric fissure; and **(C)** right Sylvian fissure (*arrow*). This pattern of subarachnoid hemorrhage could also be due to a ruptured aneurysm. The clinical history is critical in determining the appropriate management; if history is unclear, angiographic imaging should be performed.

▶ Angiographic imaging (CTA) should be performed whenever there is suspicion that a SAH is aneurysmal rather than traumatic.

Facial Fractures

Facial fractures are common injuries. At our level I trauma center, facial fractures occurred in approximately 15% of the 25,000 trauma patients seen over the past decade. Facial fractures occur in various patterns that produce characteristic radiographic and CT abnormalities reflecting the distinctive type of injury. For example, a direct blow to the eye (usually from a fist) is likely to result in an *orbital blowout fracture* (Fig. 12.29) of either the floor or medial wall. Similarly, a blow to the malar region (from a fist) is most likely to produce a *zygomaticomaxillary complex* (ZMC) fracture, characterized by fractures of the zygomatic arch, the frontozygomatic suture, the anterior inferior orbital rim, and the anterior maxillary wall (Fig. 12.30). This fracture is sometimes erroneously called a *tripod fracture* because it produces a triangular bone fragment. Other more severe forms of facial trauma include various degrees of maxillofacial separation (the *LeFort fractures*; Fig. 12.31); 3-D CT imaging is very useful for complete evaluation of these patients (Fig. 12.32). CT is also extremely useful for postoperative evaluation of patients with facial fractures.

Cervical Vertebral Trauma

An associated abnormality that often occurs in patients with skull or facial trauma is *cervical vertebral trauma*. A direct blow to the skull or face is usually of sufficient force to produce enough stress on the cervical vertebrae in flexion, extension, or lateral flexion to cause a fracture or ligamentous disruption. At our medical center, every patient evaluated for skull or facial trauma is considered "at high risk" for vertebral injury (see Chapter 13) and, therefore, undergoes cervical CT examination at the same time the cranial examination is obtained.

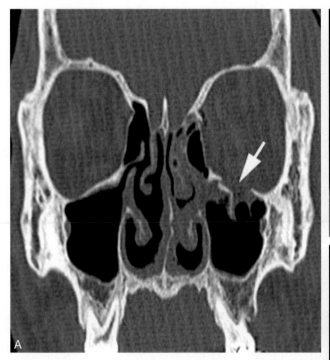

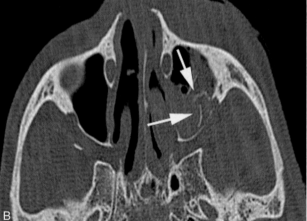

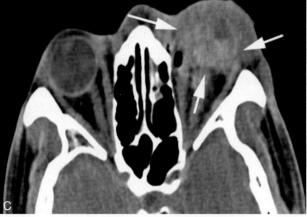

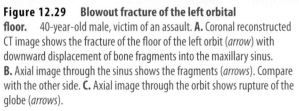

Figure 12.29 Blowout fracture of the left orbital floor. 40-year-old male, victim of an assault. **A.** Coronal reconstructed CT image shows the fracture of the floor of the left orbit (*arrow*) with downward displacement of bone fragments into the maxillary sinus. **B.** Axial image through the sinus shows the fragments (*arrows*). Compare with the other side. **C.** Axial image through the orbit shows rupture of the globe (*arrows*).

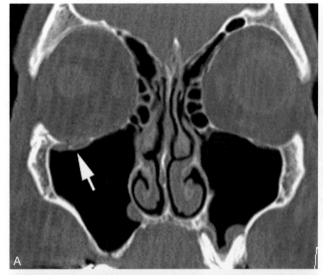

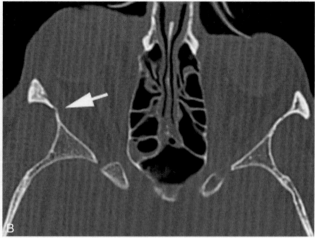

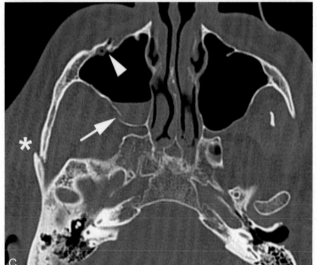

Figure 12.30   Zygomaticomaxillary complex (ZMC) fracture on the right.   A. Coronal reconstructed CT image shows a small fracture of the inferior orbital wall (*arrow*). **B.** Axial CT image shows a fracture (*arrow*) of the lateral orbital wall in the region of the sphenozygomatic suture. **C.** Axial CT image shows fractures of the zygomatic arch (*asterisk*), lateral maxillary wall (*arrow*), and anterior maxillary wall (*arrowhead*).

Neoplasms

Cranial CT and MRI have greatly aided the diagnosis of primary and metastatic brain tumors. Although some of your patients will have these lesions, the actual interpretation of their imaging studies will be performed by neuroradiologists, neurologists, and neurosurgeons. For this reason, the discussion of neoplasms here is brief, concentrating on the imaging appearances.

Intraaxial or Extraaxial

When an intracranial mass is identified, the first step is to determine whether the mass is intraaxial or extraaxial. Proper localization of the mass is critical in the attempt to characterize it. Findings that suggest an extraaxial location include "buckling" of the white (or gray) matter, maintenance of gray-white differentiation, and a "CSF cleft" (Fig. 12.33). Findings that suggest an intraaxial location include expansion of the white matter and blurring of the gray-white differentiation (Fig. 12.34).

> ❯ When an intracranial mass is identified a determination should be made whether it is intraaxial or extraaxial.

Common intraaxial and extraaxial tumors are listed in Table 12.2.

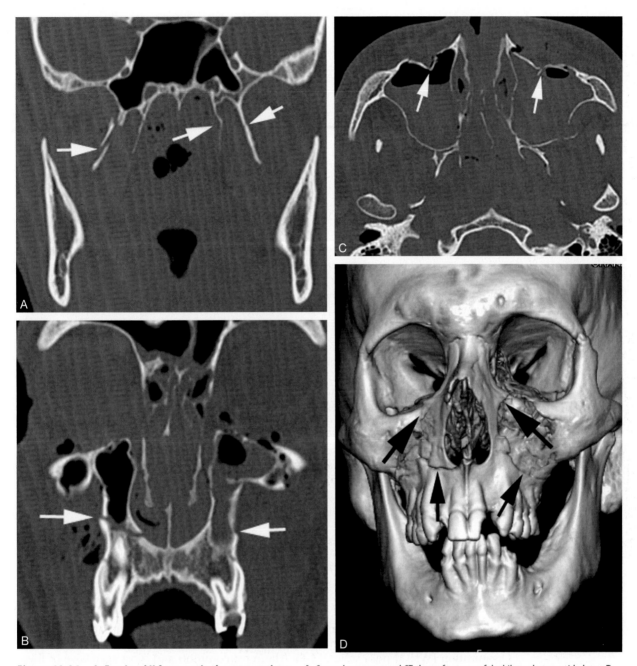

Figure 12.31   LeFort I and II fractures in the same patient.   A. Coronal reconstructed CT shows fractures of the bilateral pterygoid plates. **B.** Coronal reconstructed CT more anteriorly shows the horizontally oriented LeFort I fracture (*arrows*) involving the maxillary alveolar ridge as well as the lateral and medial walls of the maxillary sinus. **C.** Axial CT image shows fractures (*arrows*) of the anterior walls of the maxillary sinuses. **D.** Volume-rendered 3D image shows both LeFort I (*large arrows*) and LeFort II (*small arrows*).

Extraaxial Masses

If a mass is determined to be extraaxial, the differential is limited. The most common extraaxial mass in adults is a meningioma. Its characteristic imaging features include broad dural-based mass; avid, homogenous enhancement; and, less commonly, reactive hyperostosis in the overlying bone (Fig. 12.35). Common locations include cerebral convexity, sphenoid wing, olfactory groove, and the cerebellopontine angle. Depending on its size, a meningioma will exert varying levels of mass effect on the adjacent brain parenchyma. Meningiomas tend to grow at a very slow rate and there is often little, if any, edema within the adjacent brain parenchyma.

The differential diagnosis for extraaxial masses also includes dural metastasis, lymphoma, and hemangiopericytoma. These can often (but not always) be distinguished from a meningioma by their more aggressive features, including *heterogeneous enhancement,*

Figure 12.32   Value of three-dimensional CT for facial fractures.   Volume-rendered 3D image of a patient with a LeFort II injury shows fractures of the orbital floors (*long arrows*) and frontal bone (*open arrows*), as well as fractures of the anterior wall of the maxilla. The right-sided maxillary fracture (*short arrows*) has not separated as has the fracture on the left (*arrowheads*).

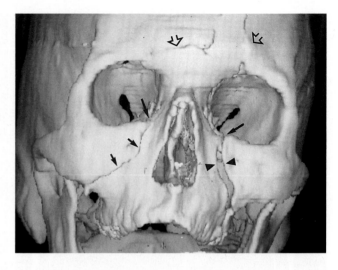

rapid growth, brain and bone invasion, and large amount of edema in the adjacent brain parenchyma.

Intraaxial Masses

There is a more extensive differential diagnosis for intraaxial masses, and more complex image analysis is required to arrive at the right diagnosis (or appropriate differential diagnosis). The components of a tumor that determine its imaging appearance include cellular composition, blood products, calcification, and enhancement. The presence of enhancement is indicative of disruption of the blood-brain barrier. (It should be noted that there are several nonneoplastic intraaxial processes that result in enhancement, including inflammatory and infectious diseases, subacute/chronic infarcts, and radiation necrosis.) More recently, radiologists are using MR spectroscopy, MR perfusion, and PET to characterize a mass's metabolic components, neovascularity, and metabolic activity, respectively, to more definitely characterize an intracranial mass.

▶ Intracranial masses are more definitely characterized regarding their metabolic components, neovascularity, and metabolic activity by using MR spectroscopy, MR perfusion, and PET, respectively.

Gliomas

Approximately half of all primary CNS tumors arise from glial cells and are thus termed *"gliomas."* Of these, the vast majority are astrocytomas, which are graded by the World Health Organization (WHO) on a scale of I–IV. The most common and most aggressive of these tumors is *glioblastoma multiforme* (GBM), classified as WHO IV. It is characteristically located in the supratentorial white matter, demonstrating thick and irregular ring-enhancement with central necrosis and surrounding signal abnormality (a combination of edema and nonenhancing infiltrative tumor) (Fig. 12.36). The differential diagnosis for a ring-enhancing mass includes metastasis and abscess. There are additional, less common etiologies for a ring-enhancing mass which can be remembered by the "MAGIC DR" mnemonic (Table 12.3).

▶ Less common ring-enhancing masses can be remembered using the "MAGIC DR" mnemonic.

Finally it should be mentioned that a number of tumors may contain calcification. These lesions may be remembered with the mnemonic *"Old Elephants Age Gracefully."*
- Oligodendroglioma
- Ependymoma
- Astrocytoma
- Glioblastoma multiforme

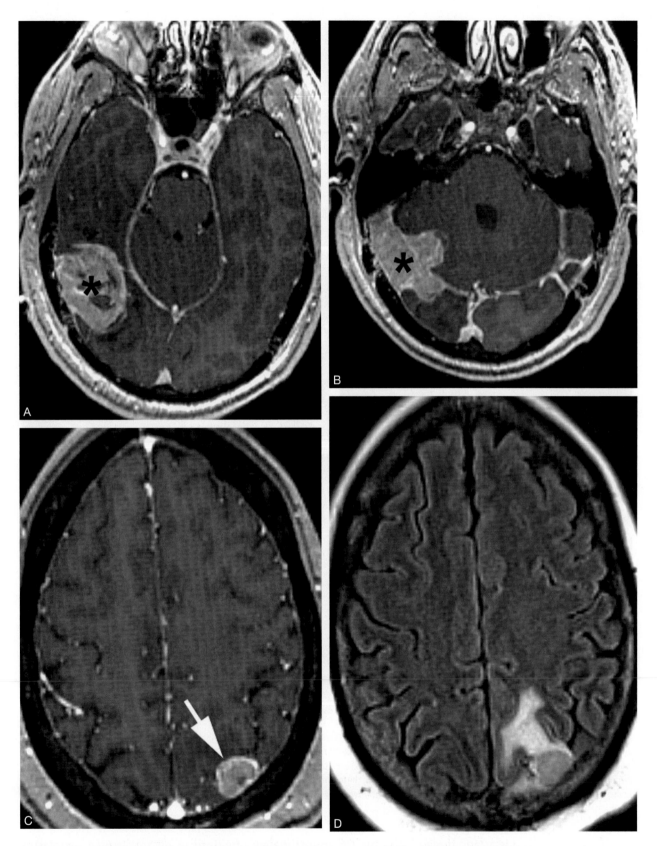

Figure 12.33   Differential for extraaxial mass.   A, B. Hemangiopericytoma. Axial T1W contrast-enhanced images show an extraaxial mass (*asterisk*) extending above **(A)** and below **(B)** the tentorium with invasion of the right transverse sinus. Heterogenous enhancement would be atypical for a meningioma. **C.** Dural metastasis (*arrow*) from breast cancer. Axial T1W weighted image shows an avidly enhancing extraaxial mass. Based solely on this image, it would be difficult to distinguish this from a meningioma. **D.** Axial FLAIR in the same patient shows surrounding edema, suggestive of more rapid growth than would be expected for a meningioma.

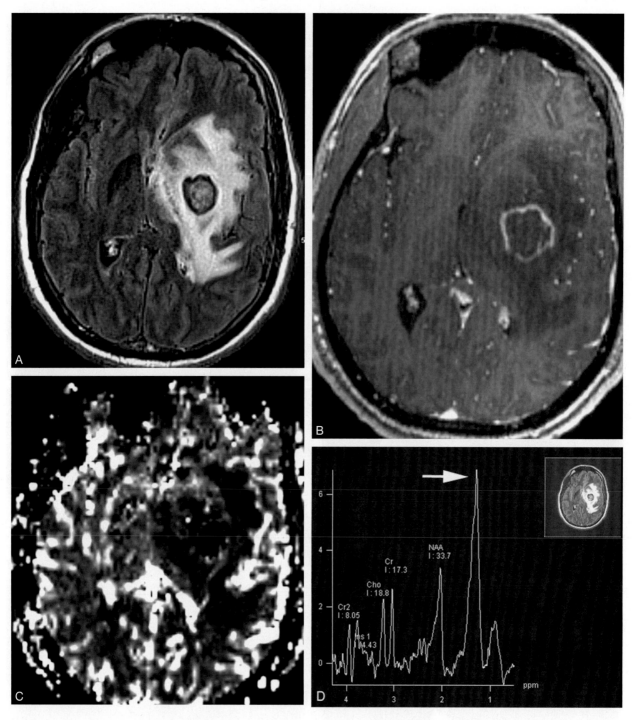

Figure 12.34 **Advanced imaging in characterization of an intraaxial mass.** **A.** Axial FLAIR MRI shows left basal ganglia mass with a large amount of surrounding edema. **B.** Axial T1W contrast-enhanced image shows ring-enhancement of the mass. **C.** Perfusion-weighted image shows no evidence of increased cerebral blood volume. **D.** MR spectroscopy shows a relative low choline peak (*Cho*) and an increased lipid/lactate peak (*arrow*). Although the differential is quite broad based on features of **A** and **B**, the information provided in **C** and **D** strongly suggest that this ring-enhancing mass is nonneoplastic and likely an abscess. Further workup of this patient revealed he was HIV positive, and the lesion resolved with anti-toxoplasmosis therapy.

Metastatic Disease

Metastatic disease accounts for approximately one-third of all intracranial neoplasms in adults. When the radiologist encounters numerous enhancing intraaxial masses, the diagnosis of metastatic disease is often straightforward (Fig. 12.37). However, 30% of all intracranial metastases are solitary. Although not definitive, metastases are generally associated with more surrounding edema (relative to the tumor's size) than a primary tumor. MR spectroscopy can also play a role in differentiating primary versus metastatic tumor.

Table 12.2 COMMON INTRAAXIAL AND EXTRAAXIAL BRAIN TUMORS

Intraaxial Tumors
Gliomas (most are astrocytomas or oligodendrogliomas)
Lymphoma
Metastasis
Non-glial and mixed glial tumors (e.g., ganglioglioma, DNET)

Extraaxial Tumors
Meningioma
Dural metastasis
Lymphoma
Hemangiopericytoma

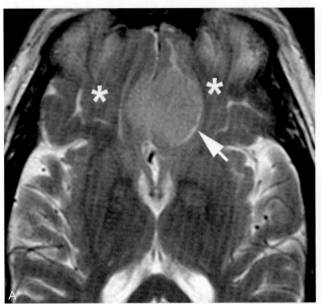

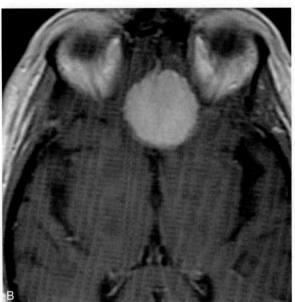

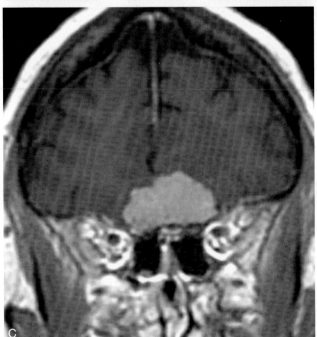

Figure 12.35   Meningioma of the planum sphenoidale.
A. Axial T2W image shows mass of the anterior cranial fossa. Extraaxial location is suggested by CSF cleft (*arrow*) and "buckling" of surrounding cortex (*asterisk*). Axial **(B)** and coronal **(C)** T1W contrast-enhanced images show homogenous, avid enhancement of this mass, consistent with meningioma.

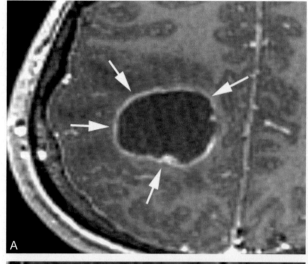

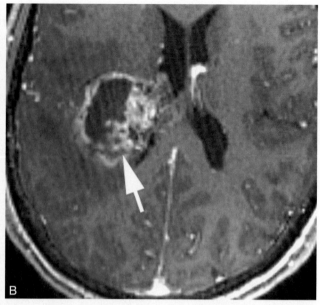

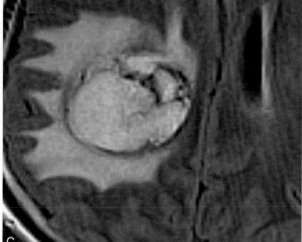

Figure 12.36   Glioblastoma multiforme.   A and **B.** Axial T1W contrast-enhanced images show a ring-enhancing mass *(arrows)* in **A.** Eccentric nodularity *(arrow)* in **B** is suggestive of GBM. **C.** Axial FLAIR shows large amount of increased signal surrounding the mass, representing a combination of edema and infiltrative, nonenhancing tumor.

Table 12.3 "MAGIC DR" MNEMONIC FOR RING-ENHANCING MASSES

Metastases
Abscess
Glioblastoma multiforme
Infarct (subacute/chronic)
Contusion/hematoma (resolving)
Demyelinating disease
Radiation necrosis

Other less common intracranial tumors include low-grade astrocytomas (WHO I), such as a subependymal giant cell astrocytoma (Fig. 12.38), gliomatosis cerebri (WHO II) (Fig. 12.39), and oligodendroglioma (Fig. 12.40). Oligodendrogliomas are often calcified, and the radiologist should be aware of other tumors that can calcify (see Table 12.2).

Computed Tomography Guidance

Neurosurgeons now use stereotactic biopsy of brain tumors using CT guidance to pinpoint the exact location. In order to perform this examination, a stereotactic template is clamped to the patient's skull prior to the study, and location coordinates are obtained through measurements from the relationships of the tumor to the template.

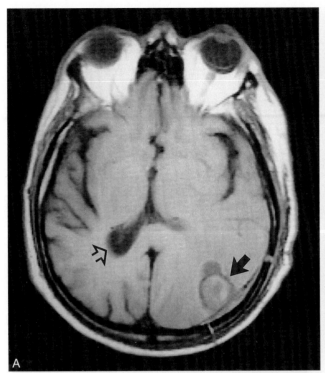

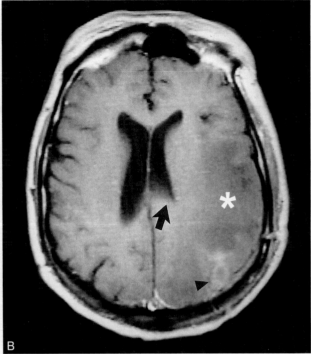

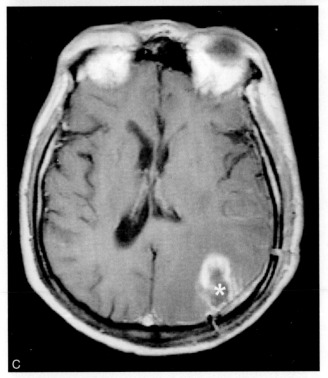

Figure 12.37   Metastases.   A. T1W MRI shows that the metastatic lesion (*solid arrow*) in the left occipital lobe has compressed the posterior horn of the left lateral ventricle. Compare with the normal right ventricle (*open arrow*). **B.** Higher section shows brain edema as an area of lower signal (*asterisk*) than the normal brain. Note the loss of convolutional markings on the left, ventricular compression (*arrow*), as well as the tumor itself (*arrowhead*). **C.** Following intravenous contrast enhancement with gadolinium, the tumor is much more prominent. The unenhanced portion of the tumor (*asterisk*) represents necrosis.

Intraoperative Ultrasound

Neurosurgeons also use intraoperative ultrasound to locate brain tumors. The ultrasound transducer is placed directly on the dura or brain surface to provide both location and depth information to the surgeon.

Vascular Disease

Vascular-related abnormalities are a common cause of CNS disease. This group of disorders includes infarction secondary to atherosclerotic or embolic occlusion (Fig. 12.41),

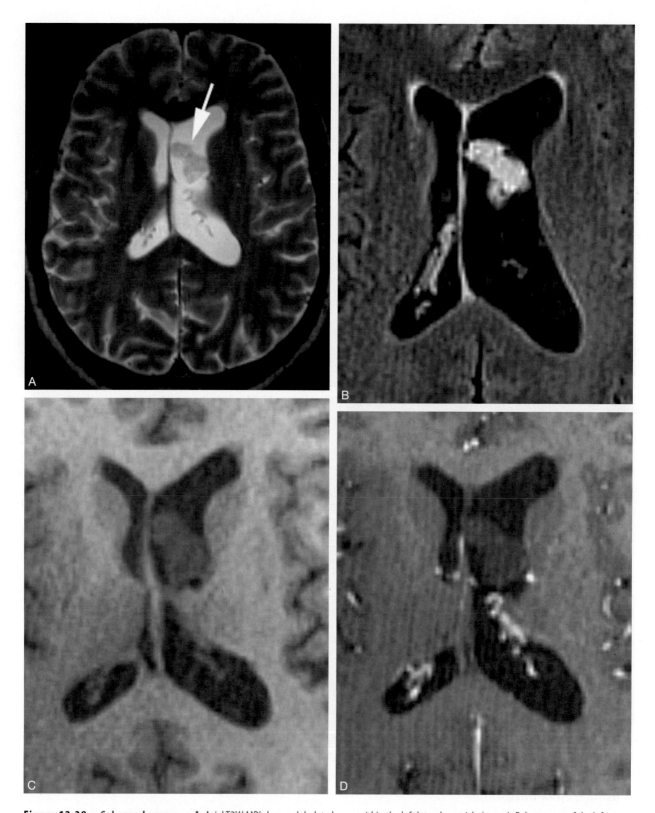

Figure 12.38   Subependymoma.   A. Axial T2W MRI shows a lobulated mass within the left lateral ventricle (*arrow*). Enlargement of the left lateral ventricle may be due to partial obstruction of the foramen of Monro. **B.** Mass appears more conspicuous on the FLAIR image. **C.** Unenhanced T1W shows the mass to be isointense to gray matter. **D.** T1W contrast-enhanced image shows no enhancement.

vascular malformations (Fig. 12.42), and aneurysms (Figs. 12.43 and 12.44). All these may be readily diagnosed by CT and/or MR examinations. Furthermore, examination of the carotid arteries in the neck by Doppler ultrasound (Fig. 12.45) is used to evaluate patients with suspected ischemic cerebral problems.

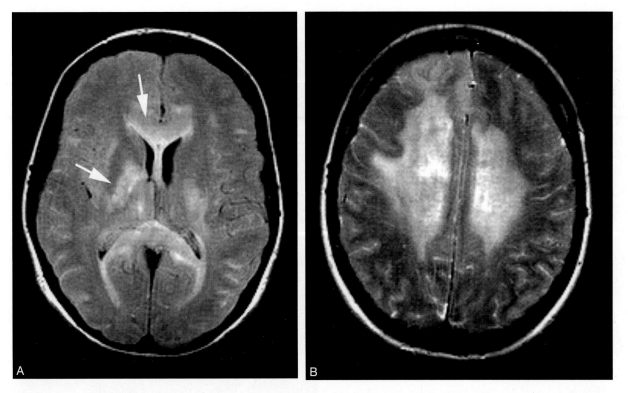

Figure 12.39 Gliomatosis cerebri. A. Axial FLAIR image shows abnormal signal hyperintensity within the right basal ganglia, right thalamus, and corpus callosum (*arrows*). Note the mild expansion of the genu and splenium of the corpus callosum. **B**. Axial T2 weighted image shows abnormal signal hyperintensity within the bilateral centrum semiovale and right frontal cortex. Note the gyral expansion of the right frontal lobe. Findings are consistent with an infiltrative process, and biopsy demonstrated gliomatosis cerebri.

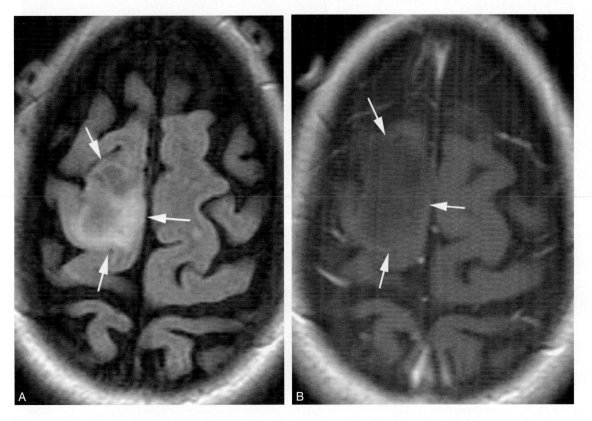

Figure 12.40 Oligodendroglioma. A. FLAIR MRI shows a heterogenous mass involving both subcortical white matter and cortex (*arrows*). **B.** T1W contrast-enhanced image showed no enhancement (*arrows*).

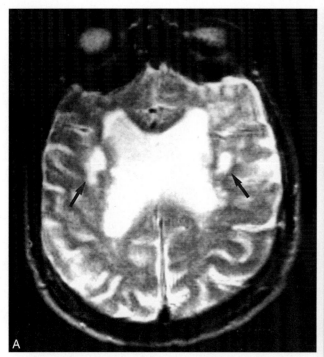

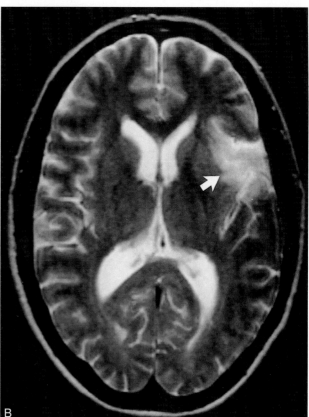

Figure 12.41   Brain infarcts.   A. T2-weighted MRI shows bilateral areas of high signal (*arrows*). Note the ventricular dilation in this elderly patient. **B.** T2-weighted image in another patient shows a large area of high signal in the left parietal region (*arrow*).

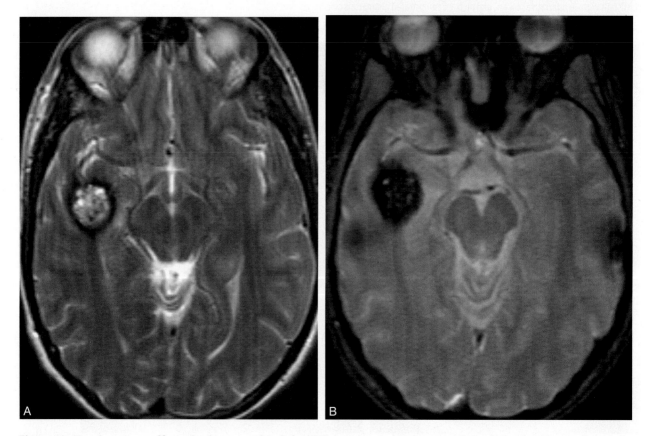

Figure 12.42   Cavernous malformation (cavernoma).   A. Axial T2W shows a mass within heterogenous signal internal within a complete rim on low signal. This appearance has been referred to as the "popcorn ball," typical of this vascular malformation. **B.** Axial T2* gradient-recalled echo (GRE) image shows marked susceptibility artifact or "blooming."

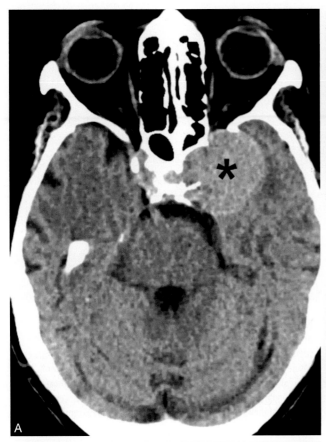

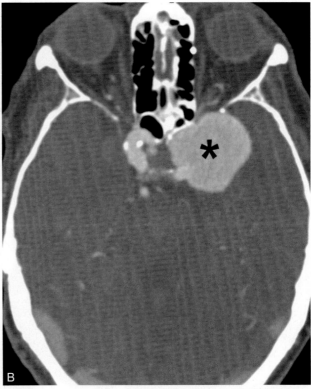

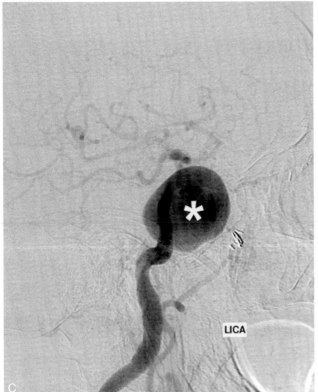

Figure 12.43 Saccular aneurysm. A. Unenhanced CT image shows a round, dense, well-circumscribed mass (*asterisk*) arising from the left cavernous sinus. Patient presented with headaches and diplopia from left CN III, IV, and VI palsies. Differential diagnosis was aneurysm and meningioma. **B.** CTA shows a large aneurysm (*asterisk*) arising from the cavernous portion of the left ICA. Compression of the cranial nerves within the cavernous sinus explains the diplopia. **C.** Lateral projection from cerebral angiogram confirms the diagnosis (*asterisk*).

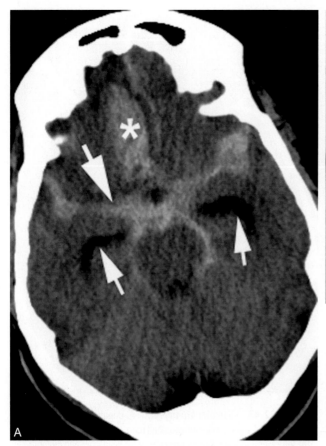

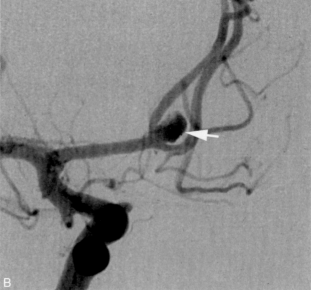

Figure 12.44   Aneurysm of the anterior communicating artery.   A. Axial CT shows acute subarachnoid hemorrhage within the suprasellar cistern (*large arrow*) within extension into the interhemispheric fissure and inferior right frontal lobe (*asterisk*). Note dilated temporal horns of the lateral ventricles (*small arrows*) consistent with hydrocephalus secondary to intraventricular hemorrhage (not shown). **B.** Cerebral angiogram shows the aneurysm arising from the anterior communicating artery (*arrow*).

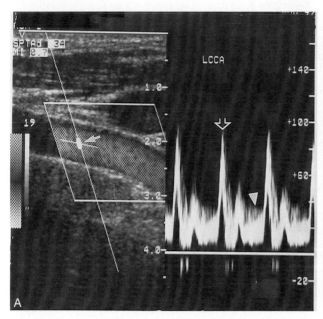

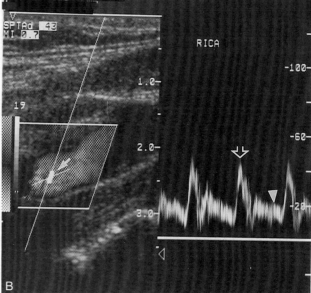

Figure 12.45   Carotid Doppler ultrasound examination.   A. Normal left common carotid artery (LCCA). The gray-scale image of a portion of the LCCA shows the vessel to be widely patent. The vessel walls are smooth, without visible atheromatous plaques. The rectangle within the vessel lumen (*small arrow*) is the Doppler sample site from which the flow characteristics and velocities generate the Doppler waveform tracing shown to the right of the gray-scale image. There is a normal peak systolic flow velocity of approximately 90 cm/sec (*open arrow*); (normal <125 cm/sec) as well as antegrade blood flow velocity of 40 cm/sec at the end of diastole (*arrowhead*). **B.** Significant stenosis in the right internal carotid artery (RICA). The gray-scale image of a portion of a *RICA* shows gross vessel wall irregularity with significant stenosis near the Doppler sample site (*small arrow*). The peak systolic flow velocity is only 45 cm/sec (*open arrow*). The antegrade blood flow velocity at the end of diastole is 20 cm/sec (*arrowhead*). Compare with the flow velocities in **A.**

Stroke

Imaging of stroke is of particular importance, since this condition affects approximately 800,000 patients each year in the United States, and is the leading cause of disability and third leading cause of death. Stroke is a nonspecific clinical term referring to the acute onset of a neurologic deficit from either an ischemic or hemorrhagic insult. Ischemia accounts for approximately 87% of all strokes and can be due to large vessel embolic or thrombotic disease, cardioembolism, or small vessel occlusion.

Imaging plays an important role in both diagnosis and treatment of acute stroke, particularly since IV tissue plasminogen activator (TPA) has been approved for the treatment of acute ischemic stroke. With the increasing use of pharmacologic and mechanical thrombolysis, CT or MR perfusion imaging is used to identify not only the region of infarcted tissue, but also the penumbra, the tissue surrounding the ischemic core that is hypoperfused but still viable.

> ▶ With the increasing use of pharmacologic and mechanical thrombolysis, CT or MR perfusion imaging is used to identify not only regions of infarcted brain tissue but also the penumbra, the tissue surrounding the ischemic core that is hypoperfused but still viable.

Computed Tomography Scanning

CT is now critical for the evaluation of patients with suspected ischemic infarcts. First, CT will detect whether there are any contraindications to using TPA, such as intracranial hemorrhage and presence of large infarct. Findings of acute infarct on CT include loss of gray-white differentiation, sulcal effacement, and the "dense MCA sign" (Fig. 12.46). It should be noted that CT is insensitive for ischemic infarcts less than 4 hours old. MRI with diffusion-weighted imaging can be employed for its excellent sensitivity in depicting hyperacute and acute ischemia (see Fig. 12.46**D**).

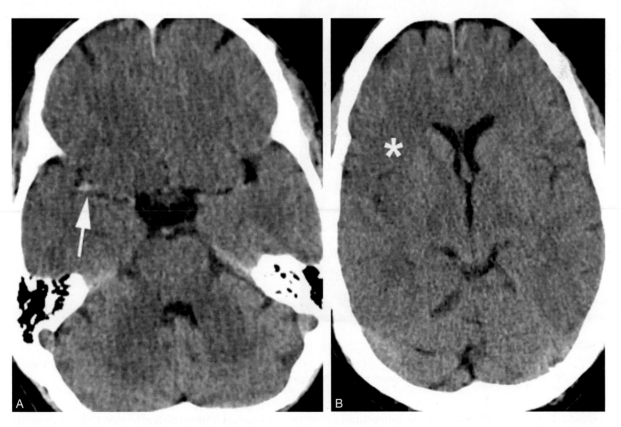

Figure 12.46   **(Continued)**

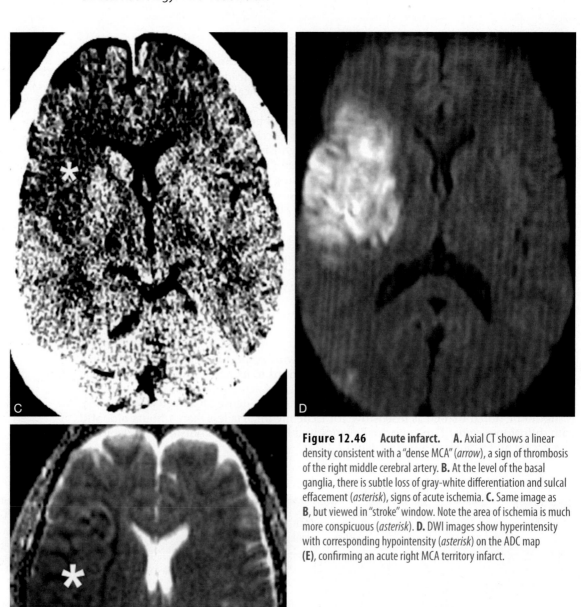

Figure 12.46   Acute infarct.   A. Axial CT shows a linear density consistent with a "dense MCA" (*arrow*), a sign of thrombosis of the right middle cerebral artery. **B.** At the level of the basal ganglia, there is subtle loss of gray-white differentiation and sulcal effacement (*asterisk*), signs of acute ischemia. **C.** Same image as **B**, but viewed in "stroke" window. Note the area of ischemia is much more conspicuous (*asterisk*). **D.** DWI images show hyperintensity with corresponding hypointensity (*asterisk*) on the ADC map **(E)**, confirming an acute right MCA territory infarct.

 CT findings of an acute brain infarct are loss of gray-white differentiation, sulcal effacement, and the "dense MCA sign."

There is a broad differential for acute intracranial hemorrhage. However, depending on the patient's age, clinical presentation, and location of hemorrhage vascular malformations, such as AVM (Fig. 12.47), and aneurysm should also be considered. These lesions

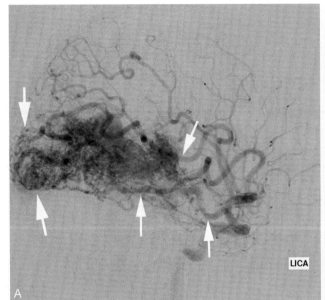

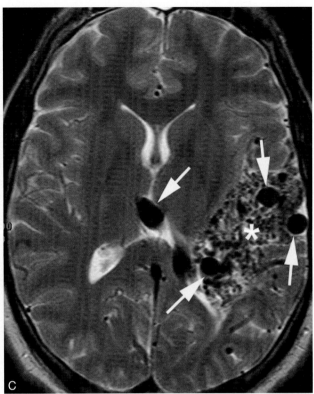

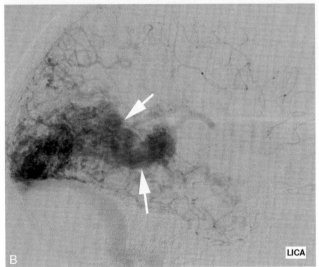

Figure 12.47 Arteriovenous malformation. Lateral projection from a selective left ICA catheterization shows three components of an AVM. **A.** Enlarged feeding arteries (*small arrows*) and the nidus (*large arrows*). **B.** Early opacification of enlarged draining veins (*arrow*). **C.** Axial T2W shows "bag of worms" appearance of left temporal lobe AVM in a patient presenting with seizures. Note the numerous flow voids of the nidus (*asterisk*) and draining veins (*arrows*).

have imaging characteristics identical to their counterparts found in other parts of the body. While we generally think of intracranial hemorrhages occurring in older patients, premature infants are also prone to these entities. Transcranial ultrasound of the newborn skull can detect these hemorrhages and identify ventricular changes that indicate developing hydrocephalus (Fig. 12.48).

Ruptured Intracranial Aneurysms

Ruptured intracranial aneurysms often present with SAH in a characteristic pattern that can help distinguish it from the above-described traumatic SAH. Specifically, the majority of blood from a ruptured aneurysm is generally found in the basilar cisterns, in close proximity to the circle of Willis, where most intracranial aneurysms occur (Fig. 12.49). Traumatic and other causes of nontraumatic SAH tend to have less pronounced involvement of the basilar cisterns. Regardless of the pattern, the finding of SAH will often lead to angiographic imaging to determine the source of blood.

Arteriovenous Malformation

AVMs have a characteristic appearance on T2W MRI, demonstrating a cluster of serpiginous flow voids that has been termed a "bag of worms" or "honey comb" appearance (see Figs. 12.42 and 12.47). The definitive diagnosis is made with catheter angiography.

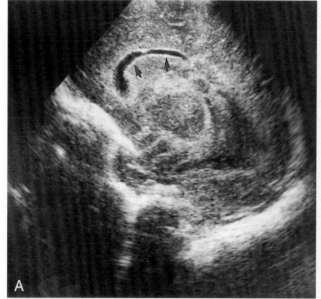

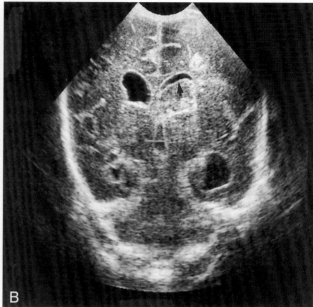

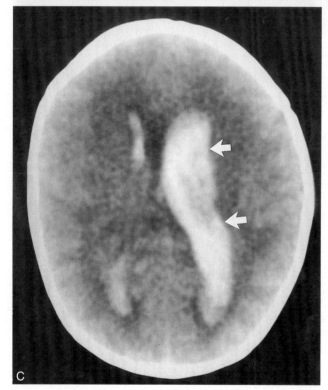

Figure 12.48   Intracranial hemorrhage in a premature newborn.   A. Sagittal transcranial ultrasound image demonstrates a mass within the lateral ventricle (*arrows*). **B.** Coronal image shows the clot within the left lateral ventricle (*arrow*). Compare with the opposite side. **C.** CT image shows blood in both lateral ventricles, forming a ventricular cast (*arrows*) on the left.

Many of these vascular lesions can be treated using the interventional techniques described in Chapter 3.

Cerebral Autosomal Dominant Arteriopathy with Subcortical Infarcts and Leukoencephalopathy

Two less common vascular diseases are worth mentioning due to their distinctive imaging features. *Cerebral autosomal dominant arteriopathy with subcortical infarcts and leukoencephalopathy* (CADASIL) is a hereditary disease of small vessels that leads to ischemic strokes at a young age (30–50 years of age). Periventricular and subcortical white matter lesions are almost always present, but are nonspecific. Lesions involving the anterior temporal lobes, insula, and external capsule are more specific for CADASIL (Fig. 12.50). The diagnosis can be confirmed with genetic testing.

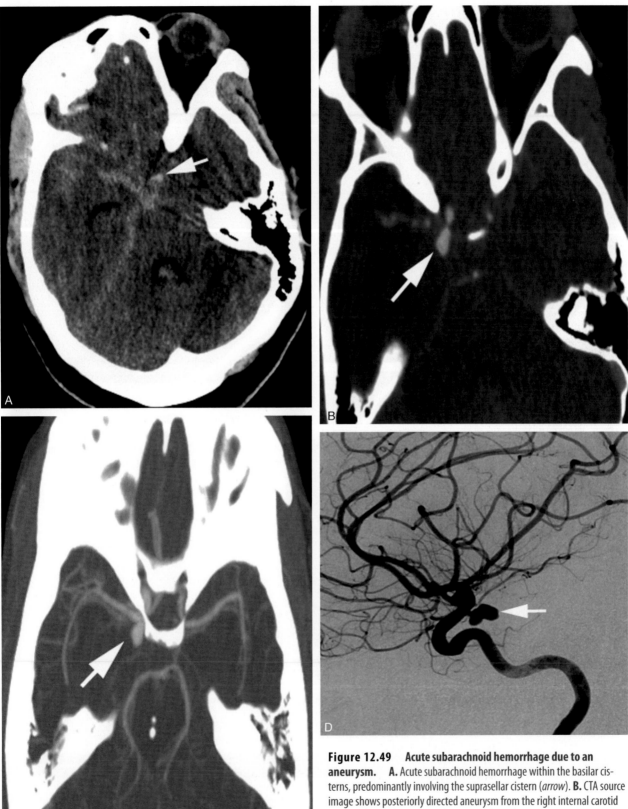

Figure 12.49   Acute subarachnoid hemorrhage due to an aneurysm.   A. Acute subarachnoid hemorrhage within the basilar cisterns, predominantly involving the suprasellar cistern (*arrow*). **B.** CTA source image shows posteriorly directed aneurysm from the right internal carotid artery (RICA) at the expected location of the right posterior communicating artery (*arrow*). **C.** Maximum-intensity projection (MIP) and **D.** Lateral projection of a selective catheterization of the RICA confirm this finding (*arrow*). It was subsequently treated with endovascular coiling.

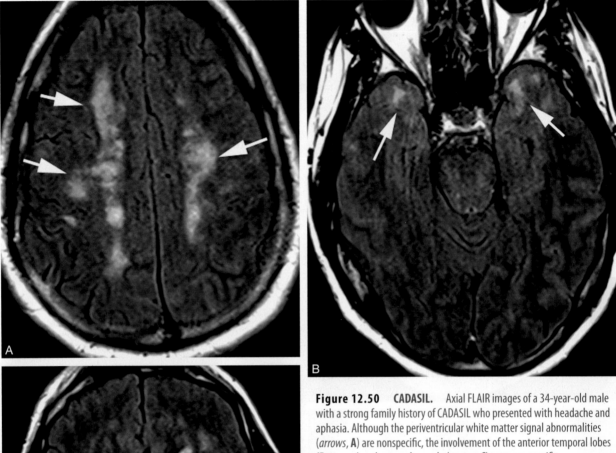

Figure 12.50   CADASIL.   Axial FLAIR images of a 34-year-old male with a strong family history of CADASIL who presented with headache and aphasia. Although the periventricular white matter signal abnormalities (*arrows*, **A**) are nonspecific, the involvement of the anterior temporal lobes (**B**, *arrows*) and external capsule (*arrows*, **C**) are more specific.

Moyamoya

Moyamoya is a disease characterized by early onset of transient ischemic attacks (TIA) and strokes secondary to the progressive stenosis of the intracranial internal carotid arteries and circle of Willis vessels. Moyamoya "disease" is idiopathic, whereas "Moyamoya" occurs secondary to other diseases, including sickle cell disease and neurofibromatosis 1 (NF-1). On MRI and MRA, narrowed flow voids and reduced flow-related enhancement, respectively, of the affected vessels will be seen. Leptomeningeal enhancement from lenticulostriate collateral vessels will also be seen. These tiny collateral vessels appear as a "puff of smoke" (translation of "moyamoya" in Japanese) on angiography (Fig. 12.51).

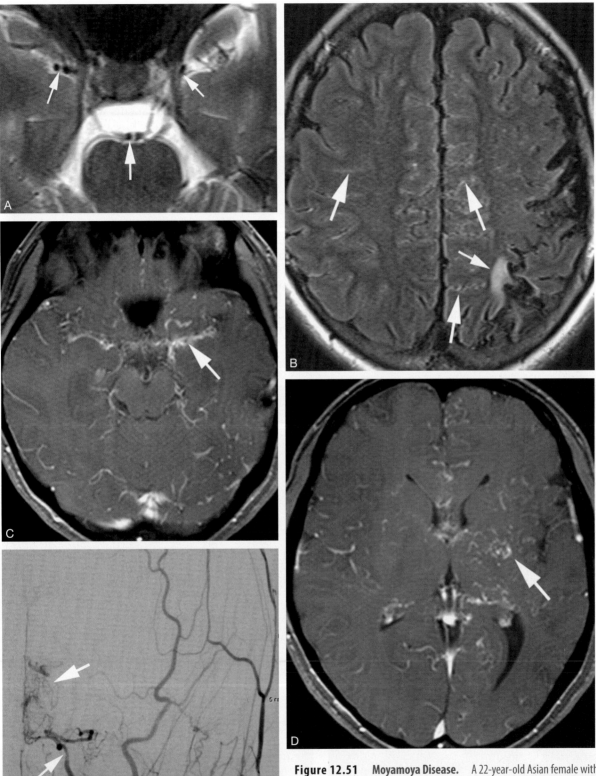

Figure 12.51   Moyamoya Disease.   A 22-year-old Asian female with right-sided hemiplegia presenting with TIAs. **A.** Axial T2W image at the level of the sella show abnormal narrowing of the bilateral internal carotid arteries (ICAs) (*small arrows*). Note the basilar artery in this patient is larger than the ICA (*large arrow*). **B.** Axial FLAIR shows abnormal signal hyperintensity in the sulci secondary to engorged pial vessels and arachnoid thickening (*long arrows*). Note the old left parietal lobe infarct (*small arrow*). **C** and **D.** Axial T1W contrast-enhanced images show abnormal leptomeningeal enhancement and lenticulostriate collaterals (*arrows*) respectively. **E.** Frontal projection of a left common carotid catheterization confirmed narrowing of the left ICA (*small arrow*) and prominence of lenticulostriate collaterals ("puff of smoke") (*large arrow*).

Historically, nuclear imaging had a role in evaluating patients with suspected cerebro-vascular problems. However, CTA and MRI have relegated nuclear studies to making the diagnosis of brain death (Fig. 12.52).

Multiple Sclerosis

Multiple sclerosis (MS) is a demyelinating disease that predominantly affects young females. MRI is the primary imaging method for evaluating patients with suspected MS. MRI clearly demonstrates the plaques that form within the white matter of the brain (Fig. 12.53). Classically, these plaques are hyperintense lesions on T2W in the periven-tricular white matter, perpendicularly oriented to the ventricles. These periventricular extensions are referred to as *"Dawson's fingers."* Enhancing lesions are often found in the midst of active demyelination. MRI is used to assess progression of the disease and complications of treatment.

Infections

A brain abscess often presents as a mass. The clinical history is not always one of acute onset of neurologic symptoms. Nearly every patient has an established focus of infection elsewhere in the body. The typical appearance of a pyogenic abscess is a ring-enhancing mass. As mentioned above, there is a broad differential for a ring-enhancing mass. Features that are suggestive of an abscess include (1) a hypointense rim on T2W imaging; (2) a large amount of surrounding edema; and (3) a smooth, enhancing rim, thinnest on

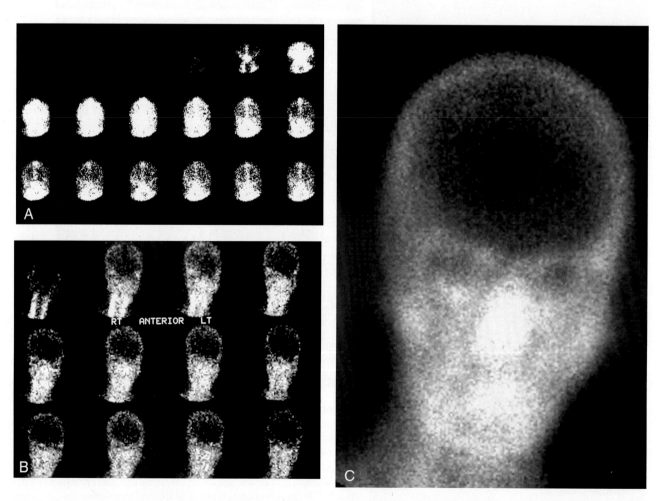

Figure 12.52   Brain death.   A. Normal patient. Radionuclide isotope flow study shows normal blood flow to the brain. **B.** In brain death, there is no circu-lation to the brain. Isotope is seen in the carotid vessels and the face. Compare to **A. C.** Delayed image shows no intracerebral isotope and concentration of isotope in the nasal cavity ("hot nose sign"). This pattern is considered pathognomonic for brain death.

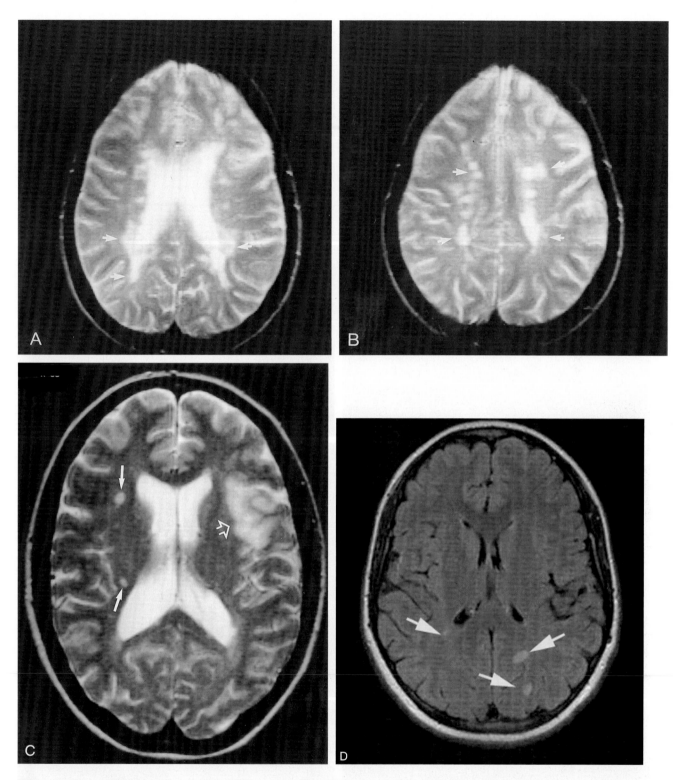

Figure 12.53   Multiple sclerosis.   A and **B.** Contiguous T2-weighted MRI shows areas of ventricular plaques of high signal (*arrows*). **C.** T2-weighted image in another patient shows small periventricular plaques (*solid arrows*) as well as an area of left parietal infarction (*open arrow*). **D.** T1-weighted image in another patient shows plaques in the white matter (*arrows*).

the side closest to the ventricle (Fig. 12.54). Based solely on T1 and T2 weighted imaging, however, distinction of an abscess from other ring-enhancing masses can be difficult. Fortunately, the presence of restricted diffusion is highly sensitive and specific in the diagnosis of pyogenic abscess. MR spectroscopy can also be used to help confirm a diagnosis (see Fig. 12.54E).

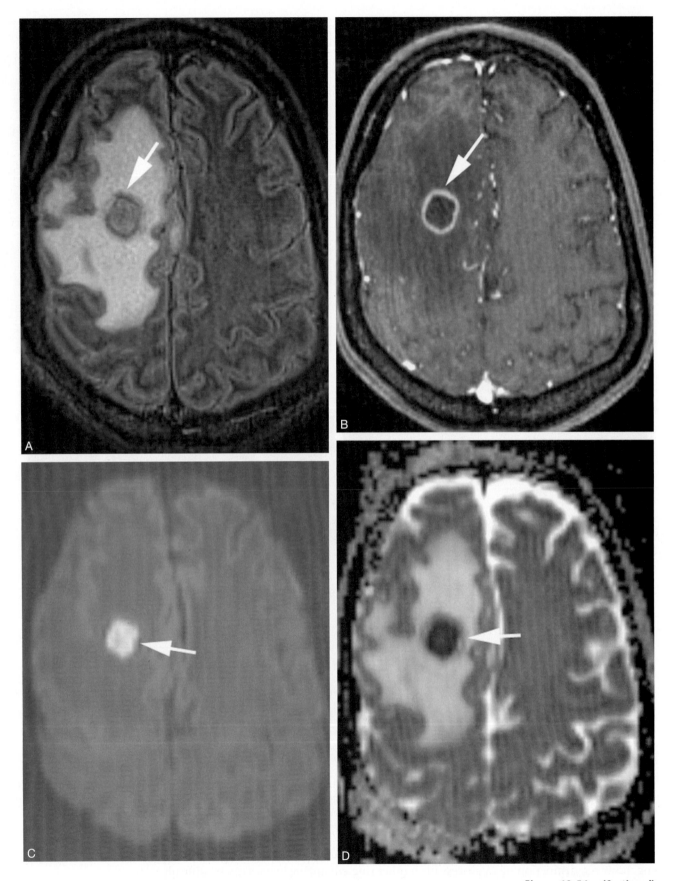

Figure 12.54   (Continued)

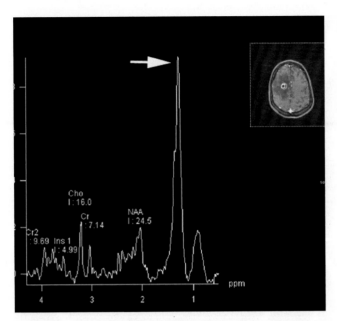

Figure 12.54   Pyogenic abscess.   A. Axial FLAIR images show around mass with low signal-intensity rim and a large amount of surrounding edema (*arrow*). **B.** Axial T1W contrast-enhanced shows a ring-enhancing mass (*arrow*). **C.** Axial DWI shows signal hyperintensity (*arrow*). **D.** Low signal on ADC map confirms restricted diffusion (*arrow*). **E.** MR spectroscopy shows elevated lipid/lactate peak (*arrow*). Combination of conventional and advanced imaging confirms pyogenic abscess.

▶ Distinction of a brain abscess from other ring-enhancing masses solely on T1 and T2 weighted imaging is difficult. The presence of restricted diffusion is highly sensitive and specific for diagnosing pyogenic abscess.

Encephalitis

Encephalitis caused by the type 1 herpes simplex virus typically affects the limbic system (medial temporal and inferior frontal cortex). While CT imaging often reveals no abnormality, MRI usually demonstrates characteristic findings, including cortical/subcortical hyperintensity on T2W, cortical expansion, patchy enhancement, and restricted diffusion (Fig. 12.55). Bilateral involvement is common. Although the presence of restricted diffusion may cause one to think of acute ischemia, the affected areas of the brain rarely conform to a typical vascular territory. Early diagnosis is important because of the importance of early antiviral therapy.

Human Immunodeficiency Virus Infections

As many as two-thirds of patients with human immunodeficiency virus (HIV) infection commonly develop neurologic symptoms. In most instances, these symptoms are from vascular insults, direct HIV neurotoxicity, or opportunistic infections. Toxoplasmosis is the most common opportunistic organism to involve HIV patients. The typical toxoplasma lesion is that of one or more enhancing masses throughout the brain (Fig. 12.56). Primary CNS lymphoma (PCNSL) can have an identical appearance on MRI. Thallium 201 SPECT can be employed if the diagnosis is in doubt, as PCNSL will show increased activity. If the diagnosis continues to be unclear, one can treat empirically for toxoplasmosis and assess for improvement.

Progressive multifocal leukoencephalopathy (PML) can be seen in the setting of severely immunocompromised AIDS patients. The classic MR appearance is scattered subcortical white matter lesions without mass effect or enhancement (Fig. 12.57).

Intracranial Parasitic Infections

Intracranial parasitic infections are relatively rare in the United States. They are endemic in the developing world, including Latin America, India, and Africa. Parts of the United States, particularly the Southwest, are seeing an increasing frequency of this type of infection. Neurocysticercosis (Fig. 12.58) is the most common intracranial parasitic infection. The infection has four different stages with associated characteristic imaging features: (1) Vesicular: cystic lesion which is isointense compared to cerebrospinal fluid (CSF); (2)

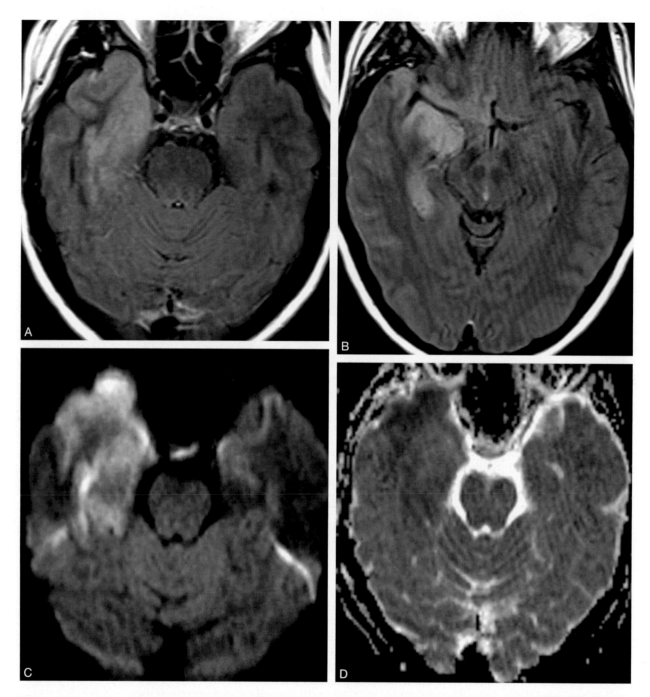

Figure 12.55   Herpes Encephalitis.   A 40-year-old female presenting with seizures. Axial FLAIR images **(A and B)** show cortical and subcortical hyperintensity with gyral expansion of the right temporal lobe, including the hippocampus. Axial DWI **(C)** and ADC map **(D)** show restricted diffusion. Although an infarct could be a consideration, the region of abnormal signal involves both MCA and PCA vascular territories, which would be atypical. Thus, herpes encephalitis was favored.

Colloidal vesicular: the cyst contents become more turbid and are hyperintense compared to CSF on FLAIR; (3) Granular nodular: Cyst shrinkage with thickening of the cyst wall; and (4) Nodular calcified: Focal calcification.

Creutzfeldt-Jakob Disease (CJD) classically presents with rapidly progressive dementia. It is caused by a prion, an infectious protein without nucleic acids (DNA or RNA). On imaging, the diagnosis can be suggested when one sees T2 hyperintensity and restricted diffusion in the basal ganglia, thalamus, and cortex (Fig. 12.59).

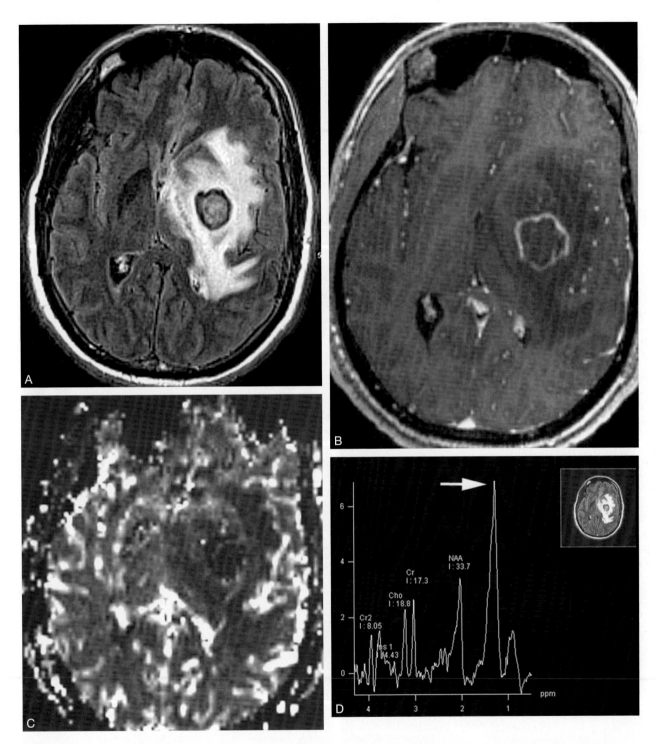

Figure 12.56   Toxoplasmosis abscess.   A. Axial FLAIR MRI shows left basal ganglia mass with a large amount of surrounding edema. **B.** Axial T1W contrast-enhanced image shows a ring-enhancing mass. **C.** Perfusion-weighted image shows no evidence of increased cerebral blood volume. **D.** MR spectroscopy shows a relative low choline peak (*Cho*) and an increased lipid/lactate peak (*arrow*). Although the differential is quite broad based on features of **A** and **B**, the information provided in **C** and **D** strongly suggest that this ring-enhancing mass is nonneoplastic and likely an abscess. Further workup of this patient revealed he was HIV positive, and the lesion resolved with anti-toxoplasmosis therapy.

Cerebral Atrophy and Hydrocephalus

Cerebral Atrophy

Cerebral atrophy occurs from many causes, including infarction, previous trauma, and aging. The typical CT and MR appearance of this disorder is deepening of the sulci and widening of the ventricles (Fig. 12.60). A certain amount of cerebral atrophy is part of the

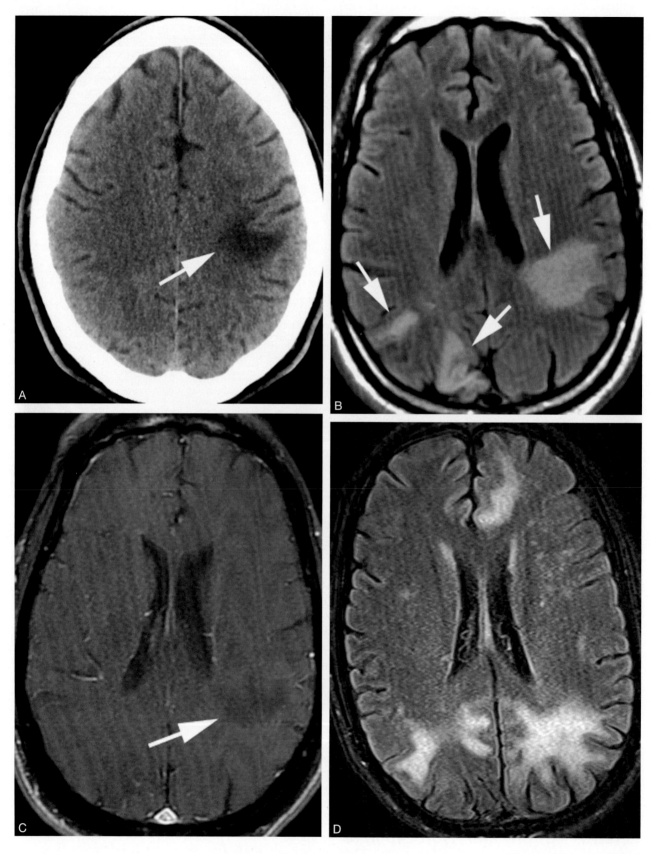

Figure 12.57   (Continued)

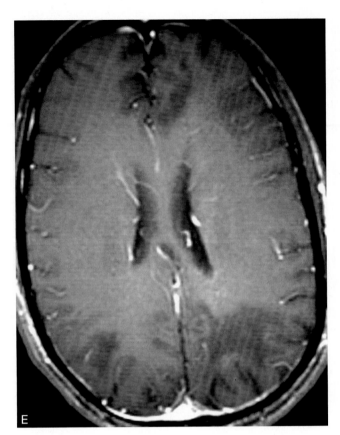

Figure 12.57 **Progressive multifocal leukoencephalopathy.**
A. Axial CT shows a low attenuation of the subcortical white matter (*arrow*).
B. Axial FLAIR shows multiple hyperintense lesions (*arrows*) of the periventricular and subcortical white matter. Note scalloped appearance, extension to gray matter, and lack of mass effect. **C.** Axial T1W unenhanced image shows no pathologic enhancement (*arrow*). **D.** FLAIR and **E.** Axial T1 contrast-enhanced images show similar findings in a different patient.

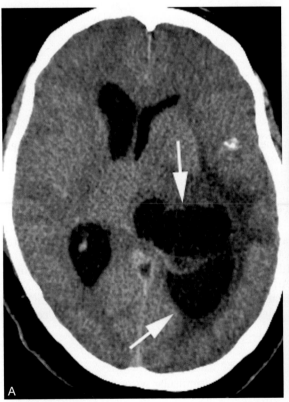

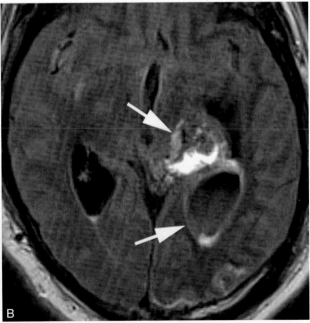

Figure 12.58 **(Continued)**

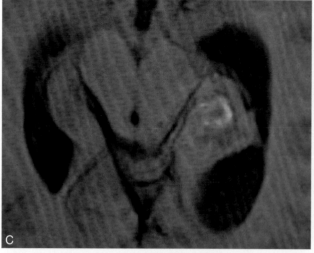

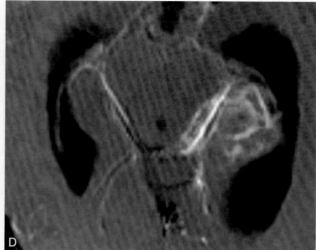

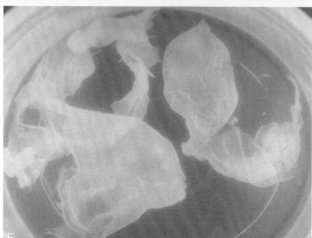

Figure 12.58   Neurocysticercosis.   Axial CT **(A)** and axial FLAIR **(B)** show complex cystic mass (*arrows*) likely centered with the left ambient cistern. Intraventricular extension is present. Chronic, calcified infection is seen more anteriorly. Unenhanced **(C)** and enhanced **(D)** axial T1-W shows heterogenous enhancement. **E.** Gross surgical specimen reveals translucent cyst wall.

normal aging process. Patients with Alzheimer disease also demonstrate these findings. PET scanning is particularly helpful in confirming the diagnosis (Fig. 12.61).

Hydrocephalus

Massive dilation of the ventricular system produces *hydrocephalus*. This dilation compresses other brain structures and impairs function: hence the necessity for early diagnosis and shunting. Hydrocephalus may be congenital or acquired. Congenital hydrocephalus is usually the result of a syndrome that includes brain abnormalities such as the Chiari II malformation and spina bifida. These conditions may be identified in the prenatal period through obstetric ultrasound (see Fig. 10.10A). On CT or MRI, hydrocephalus appears as massive dilation of the ventricular system (Fig. 12.62). If there is proportional ventricular and sulcal enlargement, one should think of cerebral atrophy.

 ▶ Hydrocephalus appears as dilation of the ventricular system out of proportion to the sulci on CT and MRI.

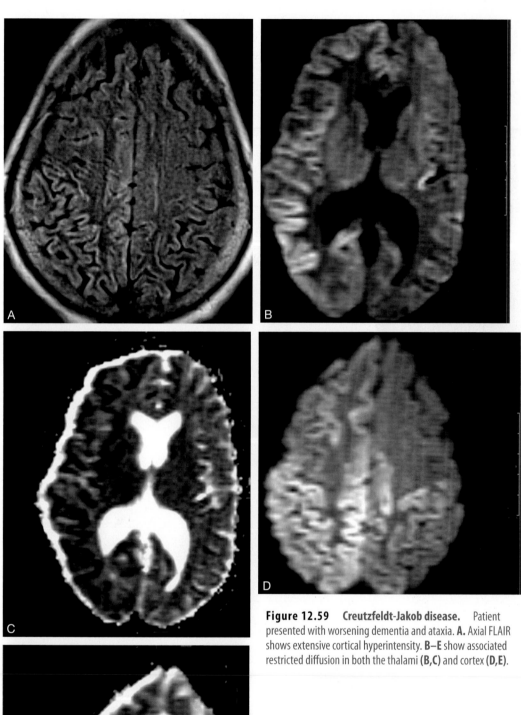

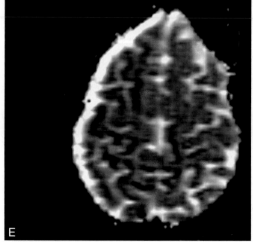

Figure 12.59 **Creutzfeldt-Jakob disease.** Patient presented with worsening dementia and ataxia. **A.** Axial FLAIR shows extensive cortical hyperintensity. **B–E** show associated restricted diffusion in both the thalami (**B,C**) and cortex (**D,E**).

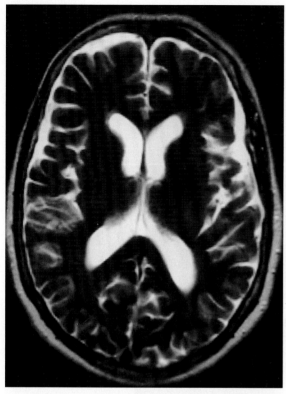

Figure 12.60   Cerebral atrophy. Inversion recovery MRI shows enlargement of the ventricles and deepening of the intracerebral sulci.

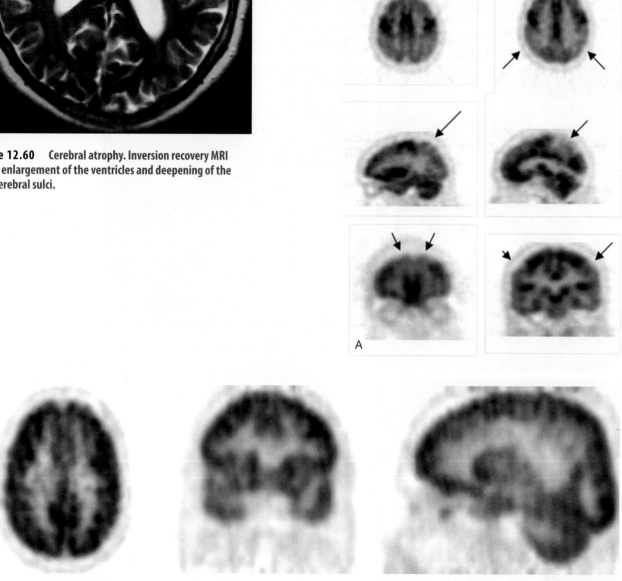

Figure 12.61   PET scan of patient with Alzheimer disease compared with that of a normal patient.   A. Focal decrease in perfusion with F[18] FDG of parietotemporal as well as frontal and posterior cingulate cortex (*arrows*), with preservation of cortical perfusion in motor cortex and temporal lobes, is characteristic for the diagnosis of Alzheimer disease. **B.** Symmetric cortical perfusion in a normal patient.

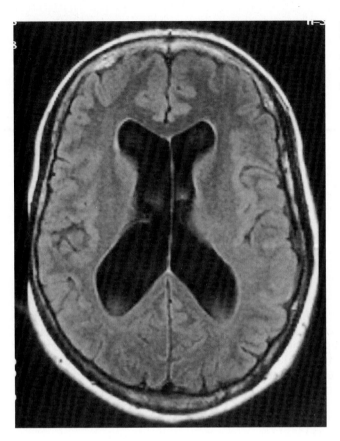

Figure 12.62   Hydrocephalus.
T1-weighted MRI shows massive dilation of the lateral ventricles with blunting of their apices. The cortex is shallow and the sulci are effaced.

Summary and Key Points

▶ This chapter emphasizes the impact that cranial CT, MRI, and PET scanning have had on neuroradiology.

▶ Six pathologic entities—trauma, tumor, vascular disease, multiple sclerosis, infections, and cerebral atrophy and hydrocephalus—were discussed briefly.

▶ Most of these studies will be interpreted by a neuroradiologist, neurologist, or neurosurgeon.

Suggested Additional Reading

Brant WE, Helms CA, eds. Fundamentals of Diagnostic Radiology. 4th Ed. Philadelphia, PA: Lippincott Williams & Wilkins, 2012:42–240.
Daffner RH. Imaging of facial trauma. Curr Prob Diag Radiol 1997;26:159–184.
Goldberg MF, Chawla S, Melhem E. PET and MR imaging of brain tumors. PET Clin 2008;3:293–315.
Harnsberger HR, Glastonbury CM, Michel MA, Koch BL. Diagnostic Imaging: Head and Neck. 2nd Ed. Salt Lake City, UT: Amirsys Inc, 2012.
Osborne AG, Salzman KL, Barkovich AJ. Diagnostic Imaging: Brain. 2nd Ed. Salt Lake City, UT: Amirsys Inc, 2012.
Som PM, Curtin HD, eds. Head and Neck Imaging. 5th Ed. St. Louis, MO: Mosby-Elsevier 2011.
Yousem DM, Zimmerman RO, Grossman RI. Neuroradiology: The Requisites. 3rd Ed. St. Louis, MO: Mosby-Elsevier, 2010.

chapter 13

Spine Imaging

Michael F. Goldberg   Richard H. Daffner

The vertebral column (spine) is an integral part of two anatomic systems. The vertebrae themselves are an important skeletal link between the cranium, upper limbs, and lower limbs. The spinal cord, including its meninges, vascular supply, and peripheral nerves, is part of the nervous system. Disease or injury to one part of this complex often affects both components. This chapter discusses using various imaging techniques to evaluate the vertebral column and its contents.

Technical Considerations

Four types of imaging examinations are used to evaluate the vertebral column and its contents: radiography, computed tomography (CT), magnetic resonance imaging (MRI), and myelography. Image-guided interventional procedures performed on the spine include biopsy and aspiration, discography, nerve block, and vertebroplasty.

Radiography

Radiography is still important for the diagnosis of diseases affecting the vertebral column. The only exception to this is suspected trauma, where CT has replaced radiography for screening. Radiographs should be obtained before any special examination because often abnormalities not only will be apparent on them but also may have findings characteristic enough to allow for diagnoses. Furthermore, the radiograph serves as a road map to aid in interpreting a CT or MR study by allowing confident identification of levels. The standard examination of the cervical vertebral column consists of lateral, frontal (anterior-posterior [AP]) views of the lower column and occipitoatlantoaxial region ("open mouth"), and oblique views. Flexion and extension views may be obtained if necessary. In the thoracic and lumbar regions, standard frontal and lateral radiographs are obtained. We also obtain a "swimmer view" of the cervicothoracic junction.

> ▶ Despite the widespread use of CT, radiography is still important for diagnosing spinal disorders.

A review of the normal radiographic anatomy of the cervical region shows similarities that may be applied throughout the vertebral column (Fig. 13.1). On the lateral view, the anterior and posterior aspects of the vertebral bodies are aligned. The *spinolaminar line,* a dense white line that represents the junction of the laminae to form the spinous process, also is normally aligned. The facet or *apophyseal* joints overlap in an orderly fashion (*imbrication*). The distances between spinous processes and between the laminae are uniform and should not vary by more than 2 mm. The disc and joint spaces are also uniform. The prevertebral soft tissues are normal. A ringlike density over the central portion of the

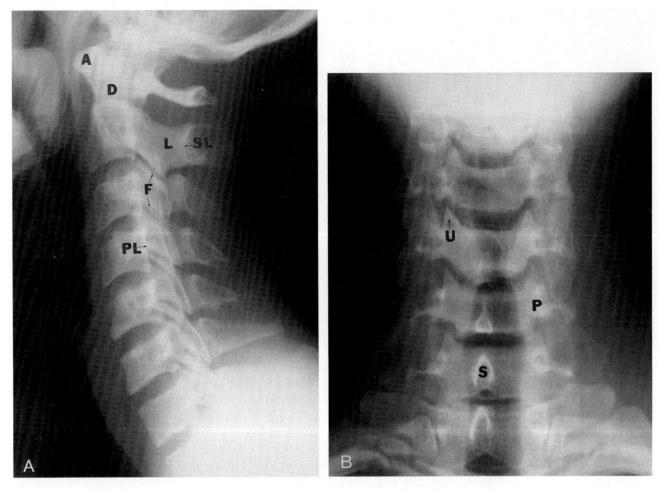

Figure 13.1 Normal cervical radiographs. A. Lateral view. Note the normal alignment of the anterior and posterior portions of the vertebral bodies. The posterior vertebral body line (*PL*) is solid. The spinolaminar line (*SL*) is also aligned. The facet joints (*F*) are uniform and symmetric. The spaces between the laminae (*L*) are uniform with the exception of C2–C3, a normal variant. Note the position of the dens (*D*) and its relation to the anterior arch of the atlas (*A*). The width of the body of C2 does not exceed that of C3. Note the ringlike structure immediately below the dens. This structure is actually a composite of normal images. Disruption of this "ring" is an important finding in trauma. **B.** Frontal view. Note the alignment of the spinous processes (*S*), the pedicles (*P*), and the uncinate processes (*U*).

body of C2 is an important radiologic landmark. This so-called Harris ring is actually a confluence of radiographic shadows from the superior articular facet of C2 superiorly, the posterior vertebral body line posteriorly, the transverse foramen inferiorly, and the anterior vertebral body anteriorly. This "ring" is often disrupted in fractures through the body of C2.

The frontal view shows normal alignment of the lateral margins of the vertebrae. The pedicles are normally aligned, and the distance between them does not vary more than 2 mm from level to level. The interlaminar (interspinous) spaces are uniform, and the distance between them should also not vary by more than 2 mm from level to level. The uncinate processes are small, pointed projections along the posterolateral margins of the cervical vertebrae only.

Computed Tomography

CT is one of the most frequently used examinations for evaluating the vertebral column and its contents. CT scans are more sensitive for finding fractures than are radiographs and do so with considerable time savings. CT is particularly advantageous for areas that do not lend themselves well to diagnosis, such as the craniovertebral and the cervicothoracic junctions, the articular pillars, and the upper thoracic column. In addition to providing transverse images of the vertebrae and showing the surrounding soft tissues, a CT scan provides a further dimension to evaluation of vertebral disease and injury (Fig. 13.2). Sagittal, coronal, and, on occasion, three-dimensional reconstructions should be obtained as well as the axial

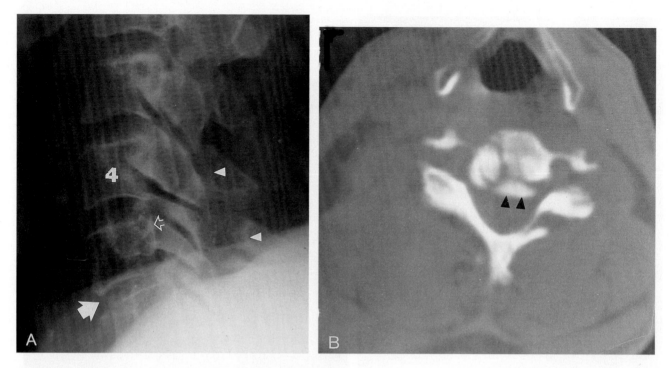

Figure 13.2   C5 burst fracture.   A. Lateral radiograph shows anterolisthesis of C5 on C6 (*large arrow*). There is bowing of the posterior vertebral body line (*open arrow*) and disruption of the spinolaminar line (*arrowheads*). The fact that the spinolaminar line of C5 is not forward indicates that there are bilateral laminar fractures at that level. **B.** CT image shows fractures of the body of C5 with retropulsion of a bone fragment into the vertebral canal (*arrowheads*).

images (Fig. 13.3). Although inferior to MRI, CT can also be used to evaluate herniated intervertebral discs (Fig. 13.4). In this regard, it may be combined with MRI to enhance a diagnosis. CT is also used in various infectious and neoplastic disorders to show not only the extent of destruction but also the spread of the lesion into the soft tissues (Fig. 13.5).

> ▶ CT is one of the most frequently used examinations for evaluating the vertebral column and its contents.

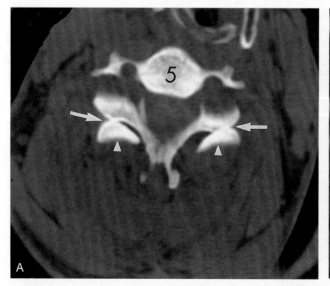

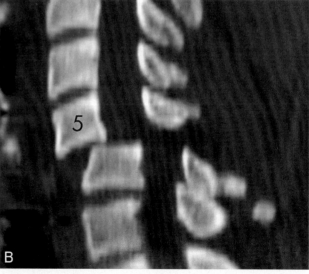

Figure 13.3   (Continued)

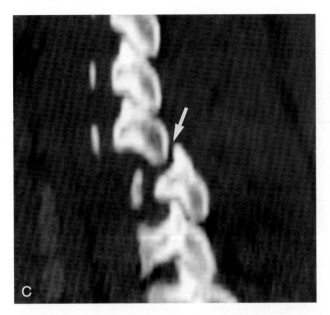

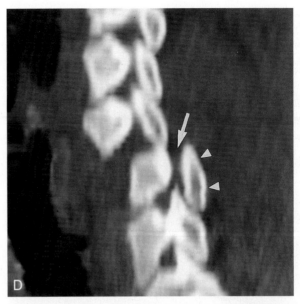

Figure 13.3 **Multiplanar CT reconstruction in a patient with a C5 dislocation on C6.** **A.** Axial CT image shows bilateral jumped and locked facets at C5–C6 (*arrows*). Note the "naked" facets of C6 (*arrowheads*). **B.** Midline sagittal reconstruction shows the degree of dislocation. Left **(C)** and right **(D)** parasagittal reconstructions of the facets show the locked facets (*arrows*). In **D**, a fracture of the articular pillar has resulted in a separate fragment (*arrowheads*).

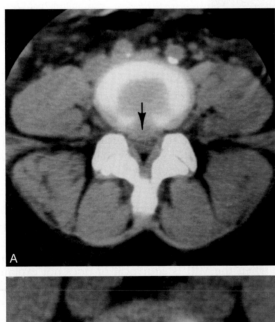

Figure 13.4 Herniated nucleus pulposus.
A. CT image shows a soft tissue density (*arrow*) encroaching the thecal sac. **B.** Myelogram shows extradural compression of the contrast-filled thecal sac (*arrows*) in the same patient. **C.** CT myelogram in a different patient shows herniated disc material compressing the contrast-filled thecal sac (*arrow*).

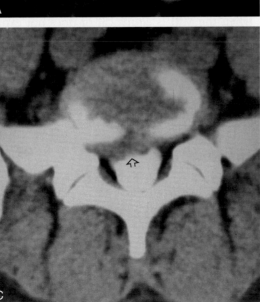

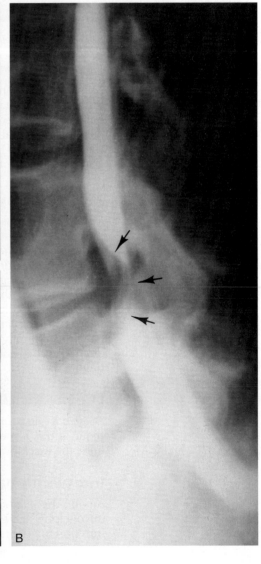

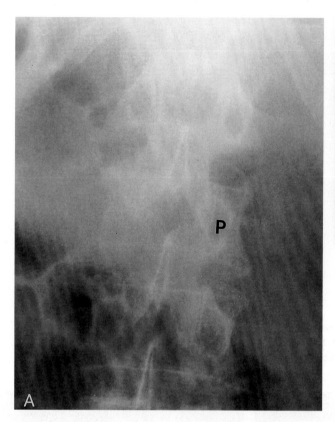

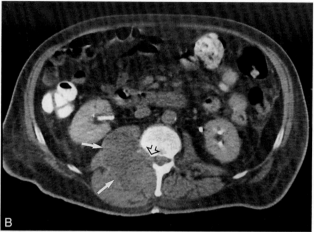

Figure 13.5   Metastatic carcinoma with cord compression.
A. Frontal radiograph shows destruction of the pedicle and body of L2 on the right. Note the normal pedicle (*P*) on the left. **B.** CT image through the same area shows a large paraspinal mass (*solid arrows*). Note the destroyed pedicle on the right (*open arrow*).

Magnetic Resonance Imaging

MRI is used for vertebral abnormalities almost as much as for cranial abnormalities. There are several advantages of MRI over CT, including an improved ability to visualize the spinal cord and other contents of the spinal canal. Thus, it is useful for demonstrating herniated intervertebral discs (Fig. 13.6), infections (Fig. 13.7), tumors (Fig. 13.8), as well as trauma (Fig. 13.9). In addition, MRI can show marrow abnormalities, such as infection, trauma, and tumor, which may be occult on CT (Fig. 13.10).

Myelography

Myelography was used more extensively before the development of MRI for evaluating compressive lesions involving the spinal cord. It is used now when there is a contraindication to MRI, such as the presence of a cardiac pacemaker. Myelography may also be requested by a spine surgeon when the MRI is equivocal or does not explain the patient's signs/symptoms. Myelography is performed by introducing water-soluble, low-osmolar contrast media into the subarachnoid space, most commonly at the level of the mid-lumbar spine. Radiographs are then made after the patient is placed in the appropriate position to allow the contrast to fill the area of interest. Following the radiographic portion of the exam, the patient is typically sent for a CT examination (Fig. 13.11; see Fig. 13.4C). It is used most often to evaluate herniated nucleus pulposus (see Fig. 13.4B). Myelography is also used in trauma patients to evaluate for suspected nerve root avulsions (Fig. 13.12).

Diagnostic Ultrasound

Diagnostic ultrasound is used intraoperatively to evaluate spinal cord lesions. This technique allows a special ultrasound transducer to be placed directly on the dura to determine the exact location of a spinal cord tumor.

Interventional Procedures

Among the *interventional procedures* performed on the spine are biopsy and aspiration, discography, nerve blocks, and vertebroplasty. A *biopsy and aspiration* of a suspected area of infection is performed under CT guidance. It is, in all respects, identical to a biopsy and

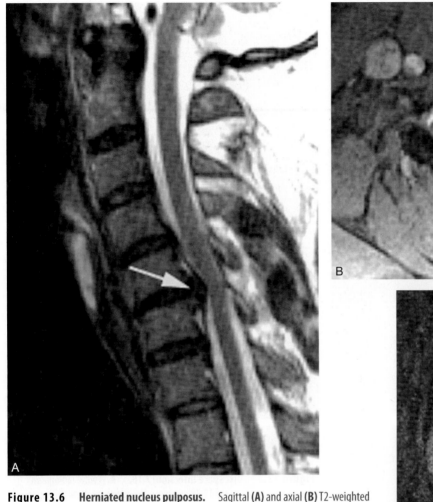

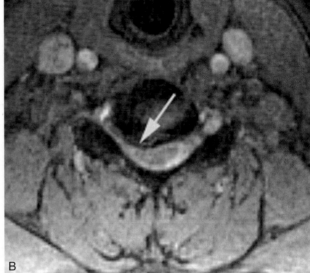

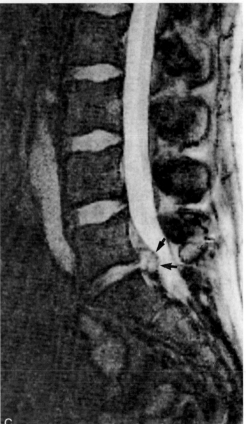

Figure 13.6   Herniated nucleus pulposus.   Sagittal **(A)** and axial **(B)** T2-weighted images show a herniated cervical disc (*arrows*). **C.** Sagittal gradient echo MRI in another patient shows the herniated nuclear material (*arrows*) impinging on the thecal sac in the lumbar region.

aspiration performed anywhere else on the skeleton. The only caveat is that there must be a safe path for the needle to traverse.

Discography

Discography is occasionally used for symptomatic patients who have several levels of disc abnormality on MR studies. Asymptomatic disc herniations are common in patients over age 40 years. Discography is used to determine which abnormal disc is causing the patient's symptoms. Under fluoroscopic or CT guidance, a needle is placed into the nucleus pulposus, and contrast is injected not only to outline the margins of the nucleus and show herniation but also to reproduce the patient's symptoms.

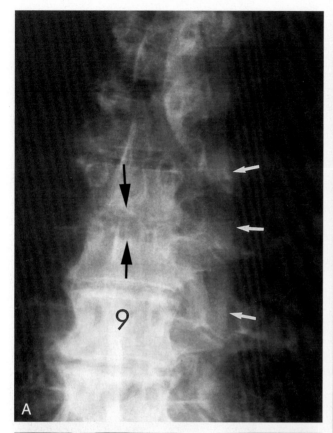

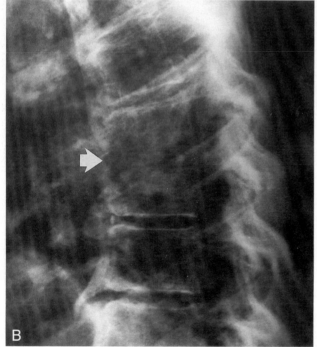

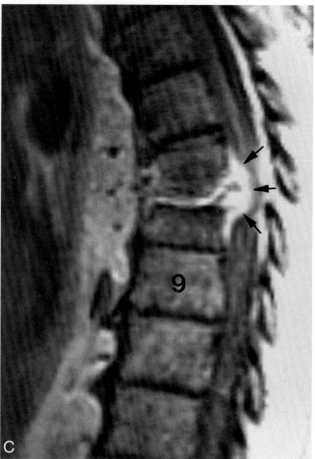

Figure 13.7   Disc space infection T7-T8.   A. Frontal radiograph shows erosions along the T7-T8 disc space (*black arrows*). Note the increased width of the prevertebral soft tissues (*white arrows*). **B.** Lateral radiograph shows the destroyed disc space (*arrow*). Compare to the discs above and below. **C.** Gradient echo MRI shows an epidural abscess (*arrows*) compressing the thecal sac at T7-T8.

Nerve Blocks

Nerve blocks are performed under fluoroscopic or CT guidance to relieve pain from impingements of osteophytes or disc herniations (Fig. 13.13). The injections are a mixture of a long-acting local anesthetic and steroid. Similarly, epidural blocks can also be performed.

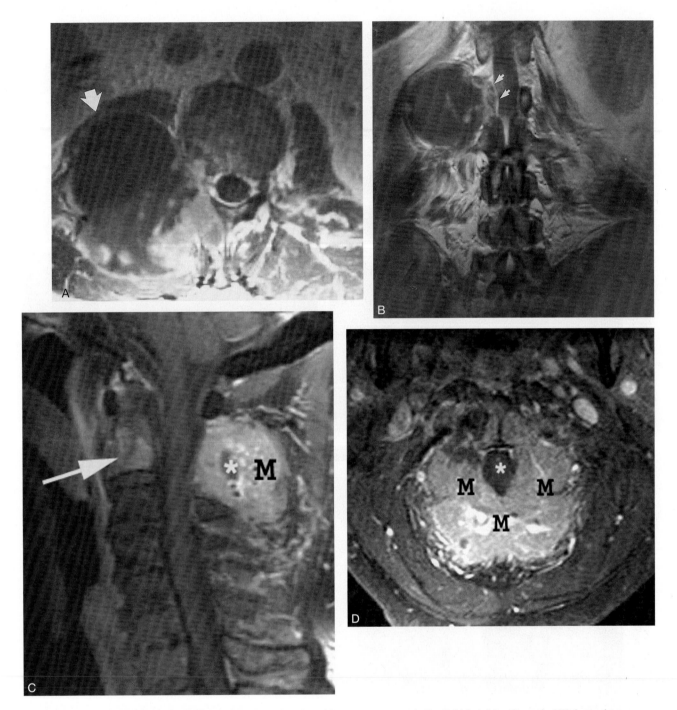

Figure 13.8 **Metastatic tumor invading vertebral canal.** (**A** and **B** are same patient as in Fig. 13.5.) **A.** Axial gradient echo MRI shows a large paraspinal mass (*arrow*). **B.** Coronal image shows compression of the epidural space (*arrows*) by the large mass. **C.** Contrast-enhanced T1-weighted sagittal image in another patient with metastatic renal carcinoma. Note the involvement of the body of C2 by tumor (*arrow*) as well as replacement of the C2 posterior elements by a tumor mass (*M*). There is a central zone of necrosis (*asterisk*) in this mass. **D.** Axial image of same patient as in **C** shows the spinal cord (*asterisk*) compressed by the surrounding mass (*M*), which has virtually replaced C2.

Vertebroplasty and Kyphoplasty

Vertebroplasty and *kyphoplasty* are interventional procedures in which methylmethacrylate is injected into vertebral bodies to relieve pain, reestablish the anatomic height of vertebrae, or treat bone destruction caused by a tumor. These procedures are performed primarily by neurosurgeons and orthopaedic spine surgeons as well as by interventional neuroradiologists.

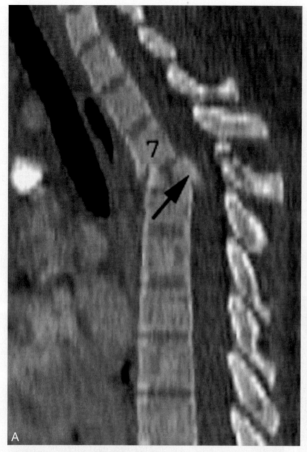

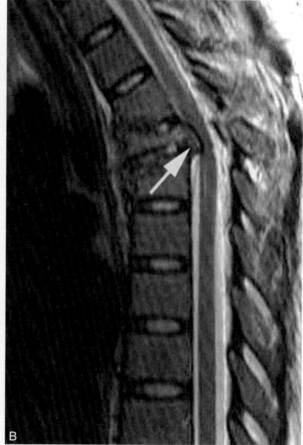

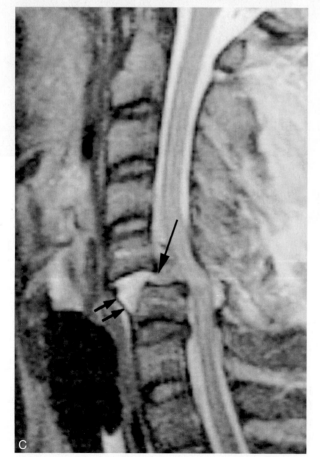

Figure 13.9   Utility of MRI in vertebral trauma.   A. Sagittal reconstructed CT image shows a burst fracture of T1 with retropulsion of a bone fragment into the vertebral canal (*arrow*). **B.** T2-weighted sagittal MRI shows the cord compression (*arrow*). **C.** Sagittal proton density image of the patient shown in Figure 13.3 demonstrates dislocation of C5 on C6, rupture of the posterior longitudinal ligament (*long arrow*), and stripping of the anterior longitudinal ligament (*short arrows*) from C6. In addition, note the signal change in the swollen spinal cord at the injury site.

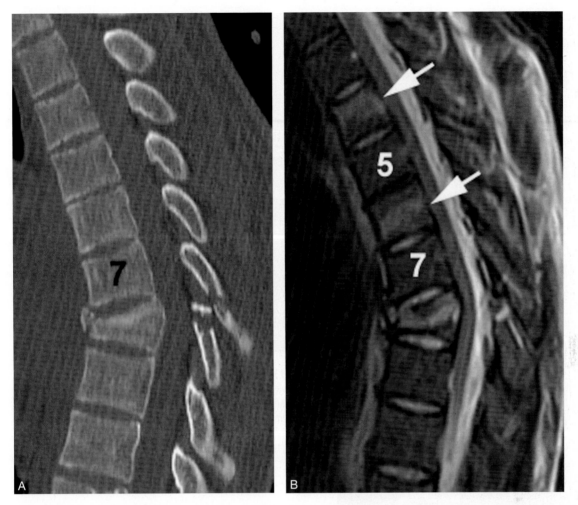

Figure 13.10   Occult vertebral body fractures.   Motorcycle accident. **A.** Sagittal-reformatted CT image of the thoracic spine demonstrates a Chance fracture of T8. No other fractures were identified. **B.** Sagittal STIR MR performed 1 day later confirms presence of acute fracture at T8. Signal hyperintensity within T4 and T6 (*arrows*) is consistent with edema from acute fractures that were not demonstrated on the CT.

Anatomic Considerations

The vertebral column is a collection of 33 irregular bones extending from the base of the skull through the entire length of the neck and trunk. Because of the attached muscles, ligaments, and intervertebral discs, this column is a strong flexible support for the body that also protects the spinal cord. The upper 24 presacral vertebrae remain separate throughout life. The remaining five sacral and four coccygeal segments are fused and thus called the fixed vertebrae.

There are certain common characteristics of all the moveable presacral vertebrae. With the exception of the atlas (C1) and the axis (C2), all these "typical" vertebrae include an anterior *body* that serves a weight-bearing function and a *vertebral arch* located posterior to the body that acts as a protective shell for the spinal cord, meninges, peripheral nerves, and blood vessels (Fig. 13.14). The vertebral arch comprises two *pedicles* and two *laminae*. The pedicles join the arch to the vertebral body; the laminae join the pedicles to form the posterior wall of the *spinal canal*, which encloses the spinal cord. Seven projections or processes are attached to the vertebral arch: two *transverse processes*, one *spinous process*, and four *articular processes*. The transverse processes and spinous process serve as the attachment points for muscles and ligaments. In the cervical region, the transverse processes point downward: in the thoracic region, they point upward. This difference allows for accurate distinctions between the cervical and thoracic vertebrae on a frontal radiograph. The articular processes determine the direction and degree of motion permitted by the

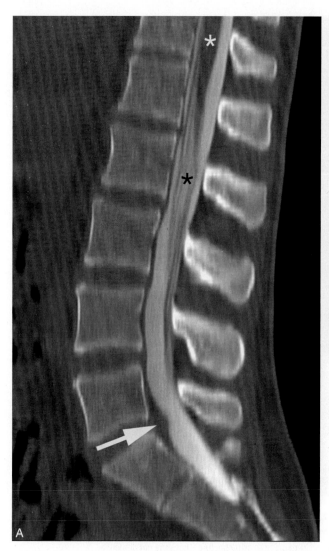

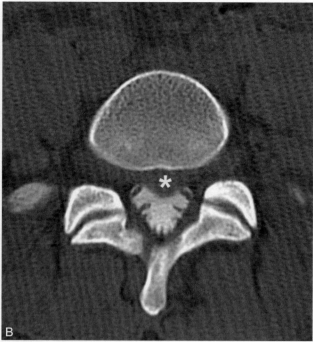

Figure 13.11   Herniated intervertebral disc.   A. Sagittal reconstructed view of a CT myelogram shows a herniated disc compressing the contrast-filled thecal sac (*arrow*). Note the spinal cord (*white asterisk*) ending at the filum terminale (*black asterisk*). **B.** Axial CT image shows the central herniated disc (*asterisk*) compressing the thecal sac. The filling defects in the periphery represent branches of the filum terminale.

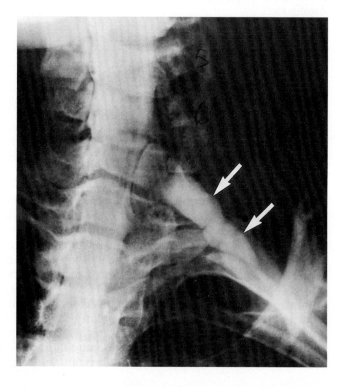

Figure 13.12   Nerve root avulsion after trauma.   Myelogram shows extravasation of contrast along the root sheath (*arrows*).

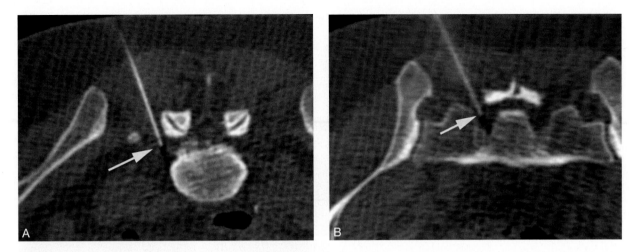

Figure 13.13   CT-guided nerve blocks.   A. L5 root. **B.** S1 root. Arrows show the needle placements adjacent to the neural foramina.

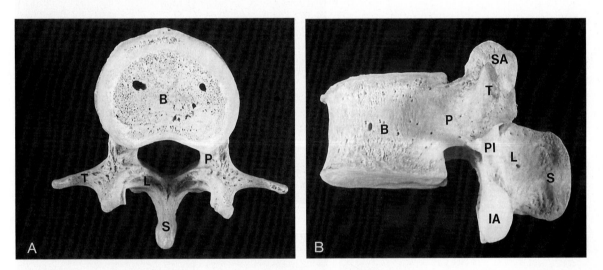

Figure 13.14   "Typical" vertebra (L2).   A. Top view. The following structures are visible: *B,* vertebral body; *P,* pedicle; *S,* spinous process; *L,* lamina; *T,* transverse process. **B.** Side view. The following additional structures are visible: *SA,* superior articular facet; *IA,* inferior articular facet; *PI,* pars interarticularis. All vertebrae, with the exception of C1, have these structures.

particular segment of the vertebral column. The cervical articular processes are joined to form the *articular pillars.*

▶ In the cervical region, the transverse processes point *downward*; in the thoracic and lumbar regions, they point *upward*.

The posterior vertebral body line is an important radiographic structure to recognize on all lateral radiographs and sagittal CT reconstructed images. In the cervical and upper thoracic regions, it is a single, uninterrupted vertical line along the posterior margin of the vertebral body (see Fig. 13.1). In the lower thoracic and lumbar regions, this line is interrupted centrally by the nutrient vessels (Fig. 13.15). At C2, the posterior vertebral body line continues with the dens. *Any displacement, rotation, angulation, bowing, or absence of this line is abnormal* (Fig. 13.16).

▶ Any displacement, rotation, angulation, bowing, or absence of the posterior vertebral body line is abnormal.

Figure 13.15   Normal lateral view of lumbar vertebra.   The posterior vertebral body line (*arrows*) is interrupted centrally by a nutrient vessel.

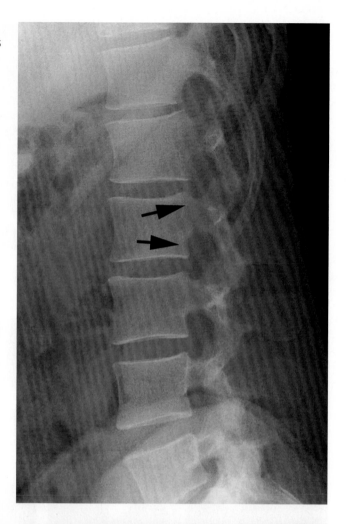

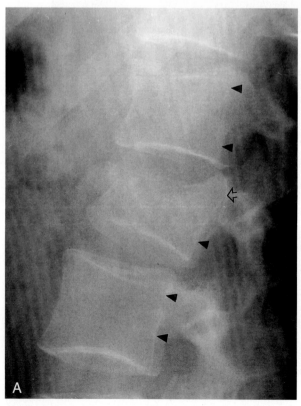

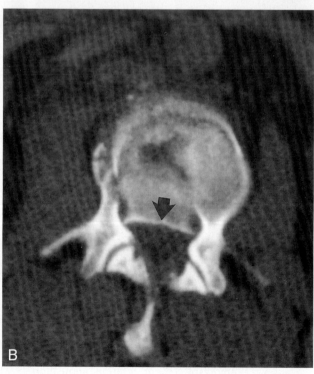

Figure 13.16   (Continued)

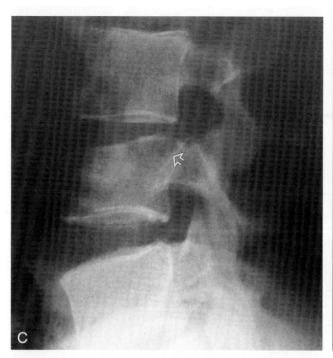
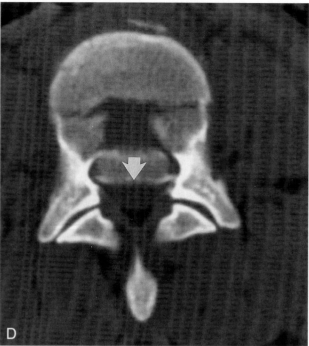

Figure 13.16 **Posterior vertebral body line (PVL) disruption in two patients with burst fractures.** **A.** Lateral radiograph shows posterior bowing of the upper PVL at L2 (*open arrow*). The normal PVL of the neighboring vertebrae are straight (*arrowheads*). **B.** CT image shows a large fragment of the PVL displaced posteriorly into the vertebral canal (*arrow*). **C.** Lateral radiograph in another patient shows posterior angulation of the upper portion of the PVL of L4 (*arrow*). Compare with the neighboring vertebrae. **D.** CT image shows a large fragment of the PVL displaced posteriorly into the vertebral canal (*arrow*). Any displacement, rotation, angulation, bowing, or absence of a portion of or all of the PVL is abnormal.

Vertebrae

Differences in the structure of the vertebrae occur at each level. All cervical vertebrae have, as distinguishing features, *transverse foramina* in each transverse process. The transverse foramina house and protect the V2 or foraminal segments of both vertebral arteries; a fracture from C1 through C6 involving this fracture should prompt an angiographic evaluation of vertebral artery injury.

The atlas, C1, has no body. The axis, C2, on the other hand, has a toothlike projection from the upper portion of its body—the *dens* or *odontoid process*. C3 through C7 also have uncinate processes along the posterolateral margin of the upper surface of the vertebral body that develop during adolescence and provide additional stabilization. Degenerative changes along the articulations (*Luschka joints*) that these uncinate processes form with the vertebrae above, termed *uncovertebral hypertrophy*, are a common cause of neck pain in older individuals.

The *thoracic vertebrae* all have one or more paired facets to accept the ribs. The upper thoracic vertebrae more closely resemble cervical vertebrae (but without transverse foramina), and the lower thoracic vertebrae more closely resemble lumbar vertebrae. The spinous processes of the thoracic vertebrae point downward.

Lumbar vertebrae lack both the transverse foramina and costal facets. Their spinous processes are large and rectangular. Their main function is support. The area between the facets is called the *pars interarticularis,* or simply the *pars.* This area is composed of bone that is thinner than the remainder of the vertebra and is subject to shearing and torsional stresses. For this reason, fractures called pars interarticularis defects (or *spondylolyses*) are not uncommon (Fig. 13.17).

Vertebral Joints

The vertebrae are separated and articulated by a series of joints and supporting ligaments. There are basically two types of joints: slightly movable *symphyseal* joints (the intervertebral discs), and freely movable *synovial* (facet or apophyseal) joints. Motion in these joints is of a gliding nature. The intervertebral disc comprises a laminated outer portion called

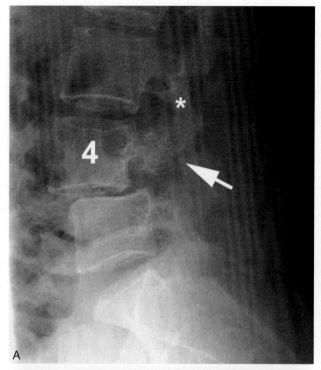

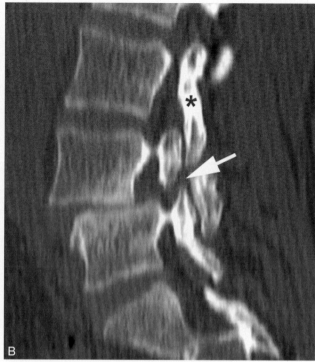

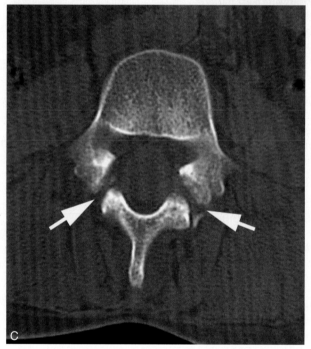

Figure 13.17   Bilateral pars interarticularis defects of L4.
A. Lateral radiograph shows complete interruption of the pars at L4 (*arrow*) with resultant anterolisthesis. Compare with L3 (*asterisk*) and Figure 13.14**B**. **B.** Sagittal CT reconstructed image shows the defect (*arrow*). Note the normal pars at L3 (*asterisk*). **C.** Axial CT image shows the bilateral pars defects (*arrows*).

the *annulus fibrosis* and a jellylike inner portion called the *nucleus pulposus*. The nucleus pulposus is eccentrically located with the shorter distance toward the spinal canal. Therefore, herniation of this material into the spinal canal is more common than herniation anteriorly. The supporting ligaments (Fig. 13.18) serve to stabilize the vertebral column and restrict motion.

Vertebral Motion

Motion permitted in the cervical region is flexion, extension, and rotation. Most rotation occurs with lateral flexion. At C1 and C2, the maximum allowable range in flexion and extension is 20° and 40° of rotation, respectively. The remainder of the cervical column

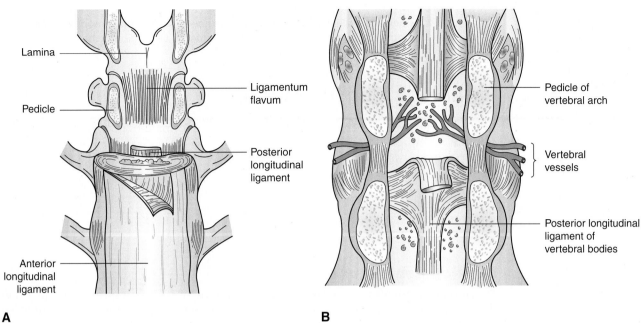

Figure 13.18   Normal vertebral ligaments.   A. As viewed from the front. **B.** As viewed from behind. **C.** Sagittal view of the craniovertebral junction.

has a maximum allowable range of flexion and extension of up to 20°. The thoracic region is relatively restricted by the attached ribs. A minimal amount (at 5°) of flexion occurs in the upper thoracic vertebrae. However, at the thoracolumbar junction (T11–L2), a greater degree of flexion and minimal extension is allowed (12°). In the lumbar region, flexion and extension, to a lesser degree than that in the cervical region, are also allowed. A minor degree of rotation is also permitted predominantly at the thoracolumbar junction. The reason for the allowable motion relates to the orientation of the facet joints at each level. In the cervical region, the joints are oriented at 45°: in the thoracic, at 60°. However, at the thoracolumbar junction, the facets are oriented at 90° to each other. This arrangement greatly restricts motion and accounts for the high incidence of injuries to these levels. The greater degree of allowable motion in the cervical region accounts for the incidence of injuries in that region. As one ages, the craniovertebral junction becomes the most mobile segment, accounting for the higher incidence of injuries to this region in the elderly.

> ▶ As one ages, the craniovertebral junction becomes the most mobile segment, accounting for the higher incidence of injuries to this region in the elderly.

Pathologic Considerations

In your practice, you will encounter six categories of abnormalities involving the vertebral column:

○ Developmental
○ Degenerative and arthritic
○ Traumatic
○ Neoplastic
○ Infectious
○ Postoperative

Developmental Abnormalities

Developmental abnormalities are not uncommon, occurring in an estimated 1 in 1,000 live births. These anomalies may range from nothing more serious than an unfused spinous process (*spina bifida occulta;* Fig. 13.19A) to a severe form of spinal dysraphism, usually with multiple associated abnormalities (Fig. 13.19B). Other anomalies include hemivertebrae, congenital fusions, both of which often result in scoliosis, and cervical ribs. Among the plethora of associated findings are neurologic abnormalities such as hydrocephalus and urinary tract problems. Because of advancements in medical, surgical, and rehabilitation therapy, patients with severe spinal abnormalities can survive into adulthood and lead productive lives.

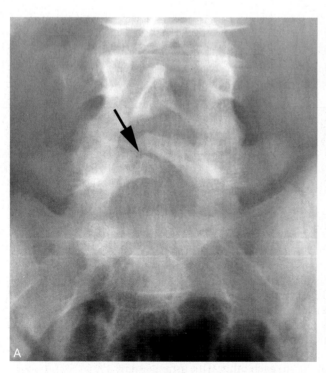

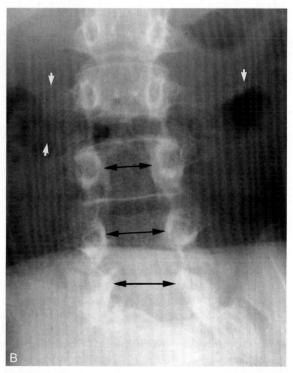

Figure 13.19   Vertebral dysraphism.   A. Spina bifida occulta. There is failure of fusion of the laminae of L5, producing a cleft (*arrow*). This is a normal variant with no associated neurologic or clinical findings. **B.** Severe spina bifida. There is wide dysraphism with congenital absence of the laminae of L3, L4, and L5 (*double arrows*). This anomaly is usually associated with a myriad of neurologic abnormalities including hydrocephalus. Note the ventriculoperitoneal shunt catheter (*small arrows*).

More common are segmentation anomalies occurring in the lumbar region and producing either *lumbarization* of S1 or *sacralization* of L5 (Fig. 13.20). This terminology can be a source of confusion and some have recommended the use of the term *transitional lumbosacral vertebra*. If surgery or radiation therapy is to be performed, it is important for the correct level to be identified. Therefore, it is imperative that radiographs be obtained to accompany all vertebral CT and MR studies.

Degenerative and Arthritic Abnormalities

Vertebral degenerative disease (*spondylosis*) is one of the most common entities that you will encounter. The extent of those degenerative changes range from mild disc space narrowing and osteophyte formation (Fig. 13.21) to severe *spondylosis deformans*, in which there is disc space narrowing, facet joint narrowing, and spur formation (Fig. 13.22). Combined, these changes can encroach on either the intervertebral foramina or the spinal canal to produce stenosis and compression of those structures. Impingement on the spinal cord or peripheral nerves is best evaluated by MRI (Fig. 13.23).

Herniations

Degeneration of the intervertebral disc frequently results in either a disc bulge or herniation of the semisolid nucleus pulposus into the spinal canal. The nomenclature used to

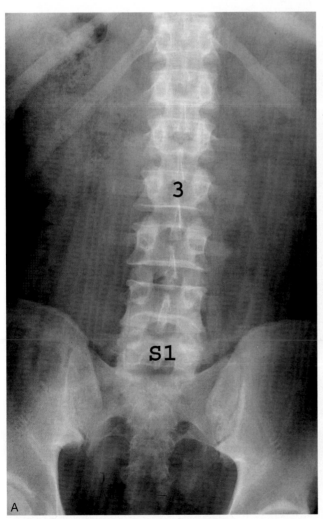

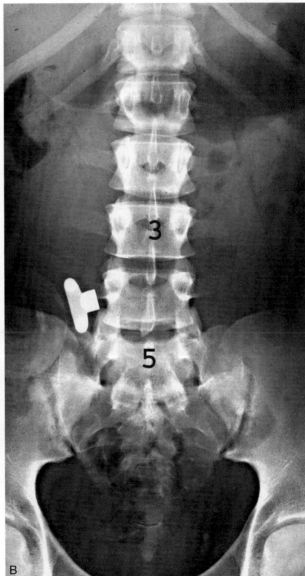

Figure 13.20   Segmentation anomalies of the lumbar spine.
A. Lumbarization of S1. **B.** Sacralization of L5. The transverse processes of L3 are usually the longest. Furthermore, a line drawn horizontally across the iliac crests should pass through or very close to the L4 disc space.

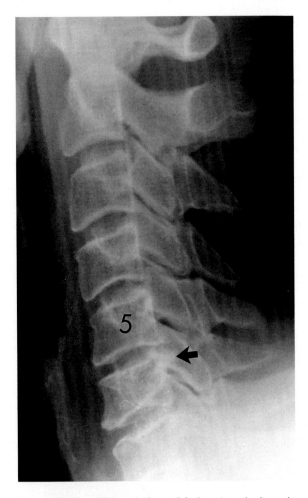

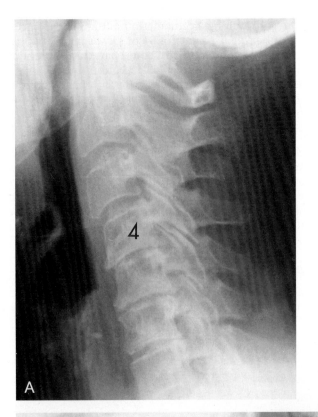

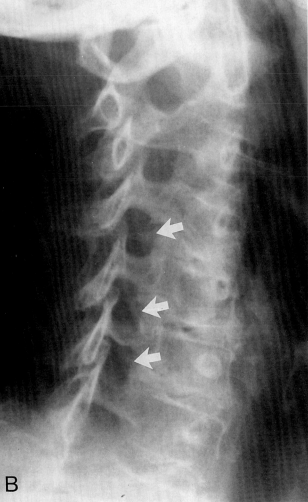

Figure 13.21   Mild cervical spondylosis.   Lateral radiograph shows narrowing of the C5 disc space. Posterior spurs (*arrow*) impinge on the vertebral canal.

Figure 13.22   Severe cervical spondylosis.   A. Lateral radiograph shows narrowing of all the disc spaces below C4. Spurs encroach the vertebral canal at each disc level. Note the sclerosis of the facet joints. **B.** Oblique view shows spurs encroaching the neural foramina at multiple levels (*arrows*).

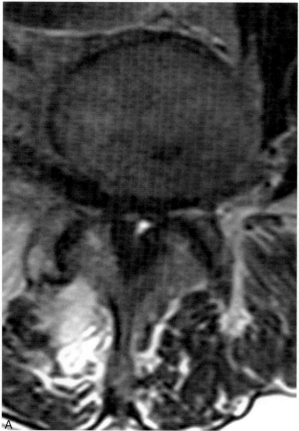
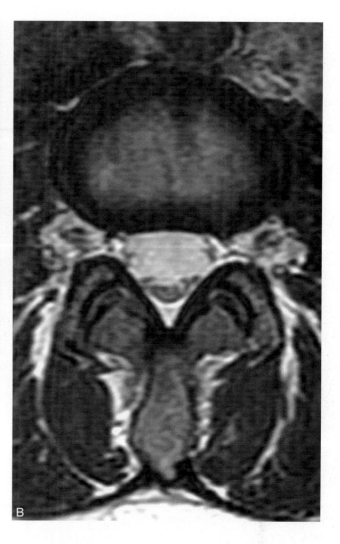

Figure 13.23 **Spondylotic changes.** Axial T2-weighted images of the lumbar spine. **A.** A combination of facet hypertrophy, ligamentum flavum hypertrophy, and disc bulge all contribute to severe spinal canal stenosis. **B.** Normal appearance of the ligamentum flavum and facets in a different patient. For comparison purposes, note the patency of the spinal canal without disc bulge/herniation.

describe disc pathology is a source of much confusion for radiologists, trainees, patients, and referring physicians. For some, this has been a source of concern, as confusion over nomenclature could lead to misdiagnosis and either overtreatment or undertreatment. For this reason, in 2003, a consensus document was created by several spine surgical and radiologic professional societies. A disc *herniation* has been defined as displacement of disc material from its normal location in *association with disruption of the annulus fibrosus*. Since evaluation of the annulus can often be inconclusive, a *herniation* is defined as displacement of disc beyond the ring apophyses involving *greater than 50%* of the circumference of the disc. A disc *bulge* is a displacement that involves *less than 50% of the circumference of the disc*. Thus, a herniation is not a bulge and vice versa. A herniation can be further characterized as either a *protrusion* or *extrusion*, depending on the herniation's morphology (Figs. 13.24 and 13.25).

If the herniated disc material moves superior or inferior to the level of the herniation, it is described as having *migrated* (Fig. 13.26). If the disc herniation is no longer contiguous with the parent disc, it is described as *sequestered*. Additional detail on nomenclature of lumbar disc pathology is beyond the scope of this text; for further detail, consultation with the consensus document listed in the Suggested Additional Reading section is recommended.

Herniated intervertebral discs in the lumbar region are found very commonly as incidental findings in asymptomatic patients. However, once a patient becomes symptomatic, MRI is extremely accurate in locating the extent of degenerative disc disease. Specifically, MRI can often determine whether displaced disc material, in conjunction with other degenerative changes, is compressing nerve roots within the spinal canal or neural foramen (Fig. 13.27).

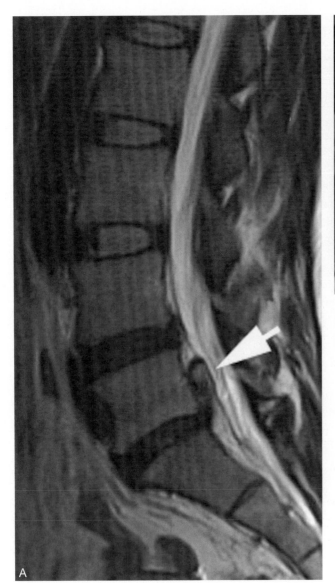

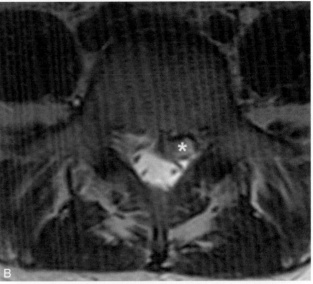

Figure 13.24   Disc extrusion. A. Sagittal T2-weighted MRI of the lumbar spine. Note the herniated disc material at L5-S1 with superior migration (*arrow*). The relative narrow base compared to the overall extent of the herniation is consistent with an extrusion. **B.** Axial T2-weighted image demonstrates the extrusion to be in a left paracentral location (*asterisk*) with mass effect on the exiting left L5 nerve root.

Schmorl Node

A common variation of disc herniation is the *Schmorl node.* This condition results from herniation of disc material *into* the vertebral body, producing a "die-punch" deformity (Fig. 13.28). Some Schmorl nodes may be quite large. Anterior herniations may produce a corner fracture of the vertebral body—the so-called *limbus deformity* (Fig. 13.29). Both of these lesions are associated with narrowing of the affected disc space.

Scheuermann Disease

Scheuermann disease is a posttraumatic osteochondrosis of the ring apophysis of the lower thoracic vertebrae in teenage boys and girls. It produces irregularity, Schmorl nodes, and fragmentation of the disc plate (Fig. 13.30). In severe cases there is a wedge deformity of the vertebral body, which can result in significant kyphosis. Typically, the involved disc spaces are narrow.

Arthritis

Arthritis commonly involves the vertebral column. It is estimated that as many as 50% of patients with rheumatoid arthritis have cervical involvement. The diseases known as the *seronegative spondyloarthropathies* test negative for the HLA B-27 antigen and

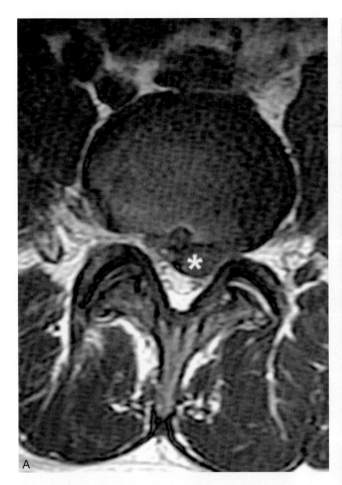

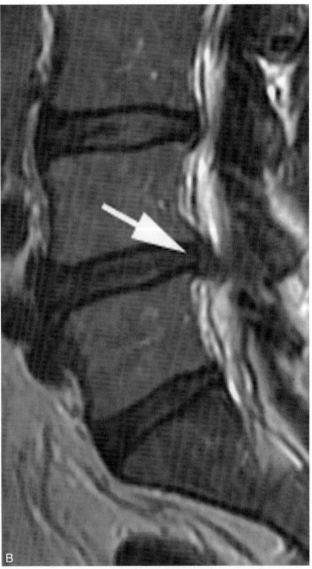

Figure 13.25 **Disc protrusion.** **A.** Axial T2-weighted image shows left paracentral disc herniation at L4-L5 (*asterisk*). Its relative broad base is consistent with a *protrusion*. There is a compression of the traversing left L5 nerve root, which cannot be visualized on this image. **B.** Left parasagittal T2-weighted image shows protrusion (*arrow*) with compression of the left L5 nerve root.

cause peripheral and vertebral arthritic changes. These disorders include ankylosing spondylitis (Fig. 13.31), psoriatic arthropathy, reactive arthritis, and the arthropathy of inflammatory bowel disease. These conditions are characterized by involvement of the sacroiliac joints and the formation of *syndesmophytes* rather than osteophytes (Fig. 13.32). Syndesmophytes represent ossification of the annulus fibrosis and are oriented vertically; osteophytes represent ossification of Sharpey fibers at the margin of the disc and are oriented horizontally at their points of origin. Syndesmophytes are most commonly encountered in a condition known as *diffuse idiopathic skeletal hyperostosis or more commonly DISH* (Fig. 13.33). This disorder, when severe can result in a rigid spine, similar to ankylosing spondylitis. Furthermore, ossification of the posterior longitudinal ligament may produce spinal stenosis. Diseases that produce syndesmophytes may be differentiated by the characteristics of those ossifications. In ankylosing spondylitis the syndesmophytes are thin, delicate, and symmetric. In DISH they are coarse and usually symmetric. In the other HLA B-27 spondyloarthropathies they are coarse and asymmetric.

> ❯ Syndesmophytes represent ossification of the annulus fibrosis and are oriented vertically; osteophytes represent ossification of Sharpey fibers at the margin of the disc and are oriented horizontally at their points of origin.

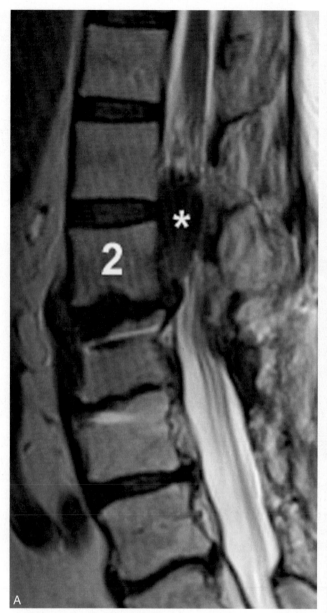

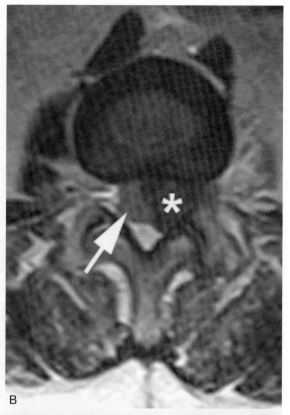

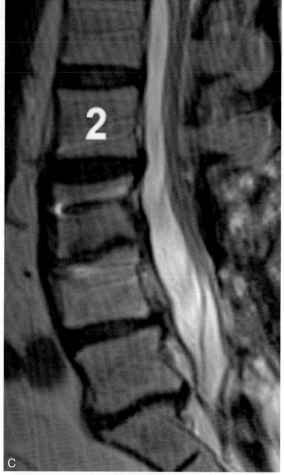

Figure 13.26   Migrated disc extrusion.   A. Sagittal T2-weighted MRI shows a large disc extrusion at L2-L3 with extensive superior migration (*asterisk*). **B.** Axial T2-weighted image demonstrates the low-signal extrusion (*asterisk*) displacing the cauda equina (*arrow*) to the right and compressing the left-sided nerve roots. **C.** Sagittal T2-weighted images performed 1.5 years prior show normal appearance of the L2-L3 disc.

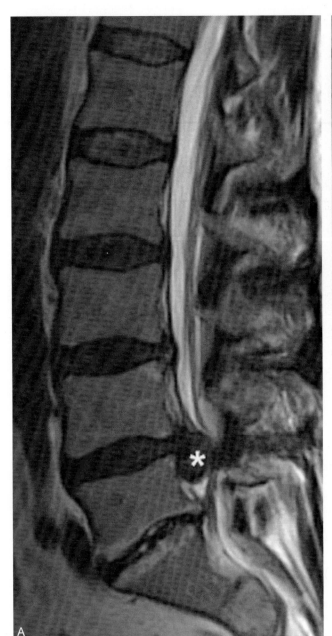

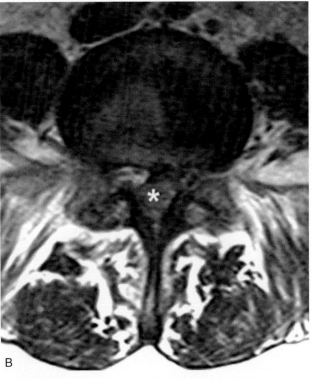

Figure 13.27   Disc Extrusion.   Patient with 3 days of severe bilateral lower extremity pain and numbness. **A.** Sagittal T2-weighted and **B.** Axial T2-weighted image of the lumbar spine demonstrates a large disc extrusion at L4-L5 (*asterisks*). There is severe compression of the cauda equina. Given the appearance of the remainder of the spine, the radiologist can have a high degree of confidence that this finding is the source of the patient's symptoms.

Trauma

Spinal trauma is a common injury. Motor vehicle crashes (MVC) account for most vertebral injuries. Falls from a height of as little as 3 feet are the second most common etiology, particularly in the elderly. Most vertebral injuries could have been prevented by the proper use of seat belts or other restraining devices in motor vehicles. Over the past two decades criteria have been established using clinical and historical data to determine which patients are at high risk or low risk for cervical spinal injury.

High Risk Criteria

Most authorities now agree that if *any* of the following high-risk factors are present imaging should be performed:

- Altered mental status (Glasgow Coma Score <15)
- Multiple fractures
- Drowning or diving accident
- Significant head or facial injury

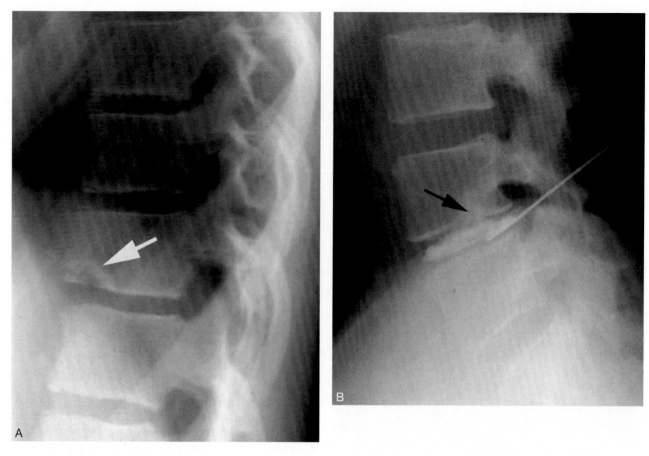

Figure 13.28   Schmorl nodes.   A. Anterior node (*arrow*). **B.** Discogram showing extravasation into a Schmorl node (*arrow*).

- ○ Age >65 years
- ○ "Dangerous mechanism"
  - • Fall >1 m
  - • Axial load to head
  - • High-speed (>100 km/h) MVC
  - • MVC with large vehicle
  - • MVC with rollover or ejection
  - • Pedestrian struck by vehicle
  - • Crash involving motorized recreation vehicle
- ○ Paresthesias in extremities
- ○ Rigid spine disease
  - • Ankylosing spondylitis
  - • DISH.

Low Risk Criteria

A consortium of Canadian traumatologists established low risk criteria to identify patients who did not need imaging. These clinical and historical factors are called the *Canadian C-spine Rule (CCR)*:

- ○ Absence of high-risk factors
- ○ Low-risk factors that allow safe assessment of active range of motion (flexion, extension, 45° right and left rotation)
  - • "Simple" rear-end MVC (none of high-risk factors above)
  - • Sitting position in the emergency department
  - • Ambulatory at any time
  - • Delayed onset of neck pain
  - • Absence of midline cervical tenderness
- ○ Ability to actively flex and extend the neck and rotate 45° left and right.

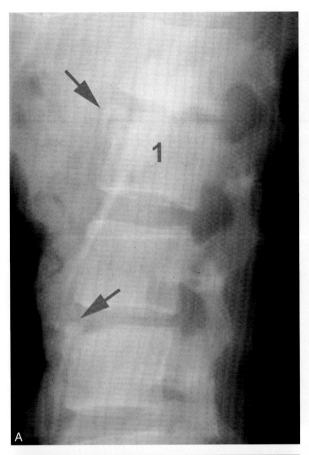

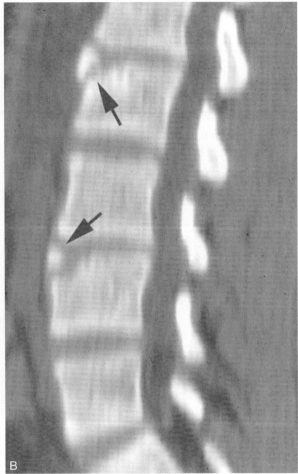

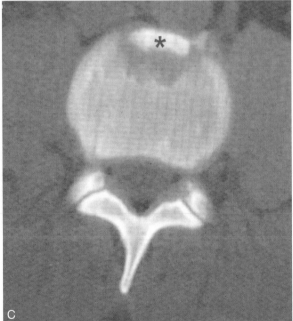

Figure 13.29   Limbus deformities at L1 and L3 from anterior disc herniations.   A. Lateral radiograph and **B.** Sagittal reconstructed CT image shows the limbus fragments (*arrows*). Note the narrow disc spaces at the affected levels. These may be distinguished from fractures by virtue of their sclerotic margins and the absence of the "jigsaw puzzle sign." **C.** Axial CT image at L1 shows the limbus fragment (*asterisk*) and its associated sclerotic margin, representing a Schmorl node.

In the United States, another set of low risk criteria, the *National Emergency X-radiography Utilization Study (NEXUS)* rules are also followed:

- ◌ *No* midline cervical tenderness
- ◌ *No* focal neurologic deficits
- ◌ *No* intoxication or indication of brain injury
- ◌ *No* painful distracting injuries
- ◌ *Normal* alertness

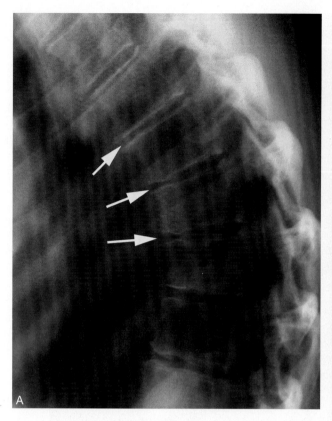
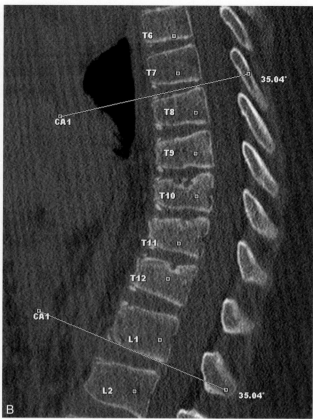

Figure 13.30   Scheuermann disease.   A. Lateral radiograph shows anterior wedging of several vertebral bodies with irregularity along the disc margins (*arrows*) and narrowing of the involved disc spaces. These changes have resulted in kyphotic angulation. **B.** Sagittal reconstructed CT image in another patient shows anterior wedging, irregular disc margins, and multiple Schmorl nodes. The kyphotic curve measures 35° between T8 and L1. (Reproduced with permission from Daffner RH. Imaging of Vertebral Trauma. 3rd Ed. Cambridge, UK: Cambridge University Press, 2011.)

We refer to these as the "Five Nos." There are two indications for thoracic and lumbar imaging. The first is a known cervical injury. The reason for this is that in our experience and that of other investigators, the incidence of multilevel noncontiguous vertebral fractures is 25%. The second indication is a history of rigid spine disease (ankylosing spondylitis or DISH).

Spinal injuries, historically, have produced great anxiety in health care workers. Following some basic principles of interpretation, however, can allow you to determine whether a significant abnormality is present and whether or not additional imaging studies are necessary. Radiography used to be the mainstay for the evaluation of any patient with suspected vertebral injury. However, radiographic studies are not only time consuming, but frequently fail to adequately demonstrate all injuries. For these reasons, in the United States, radiography has been supplanted by CT because of its increased sensitivity for detection of fractures and its rapid acquisition time. In our level I trauma center, the cervical CT scan is reconstructed from data obtained during the cranial scan. We do not perform radiography for the thoracic or lumber regions. Thoracic and lumbar CT images are obtained most commonly from data gathered by the thoracic, abdominal, and pelvic scan (TAP) or, on occasion, as a freestanding study. All studies undergo multiplanar reformation (MPR) to produce sagittal and coronal images. In addition, the workstations in our picture archiving and communications system (PACS) allow additional MPR if necessary.

The interpretation of those studies demands that a logical system be followed in their interpretation. We prefer the *ABCS* system, introduced in Chapter 11:

- ◌ Alignment abnormalities
- ◌ Bony integrity abnormalities
- ◌ Cartilage (joint space) abnormalities
- ◌ Soft tissue abnormalities

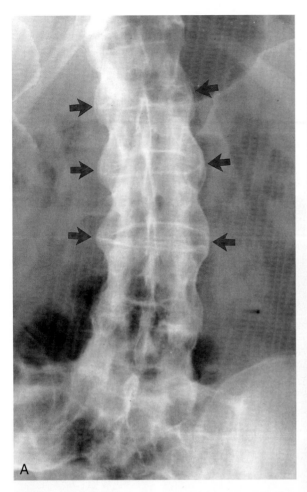

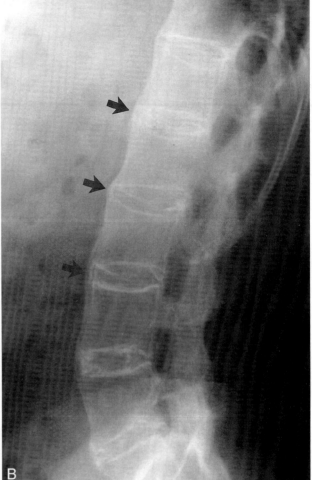

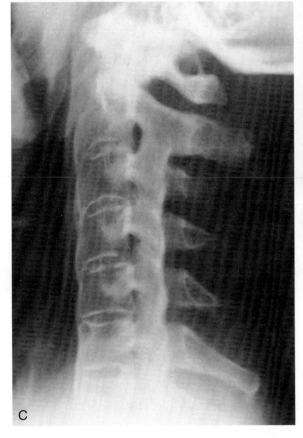

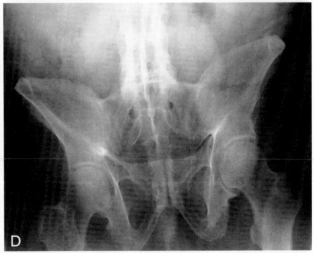

Figure 13.31   Ankylosing spondylitis.   A. Frontal lumbar radiograph shows typical syndesmophytes bridging the intervertebral disc spaces (*arrows*). This gives the vertebral column a distinct "bamboo" appearance. **B.** Lateral lumbar radiograph shows the delicate anterior syndesmophytes (*arrows*). Note the squaring of the disc margins of the vertebral bodies. **C.** Lateral cervical radiograph shows complete ankylosis anteriorly as well as of the facet joints posteriorly. **D.** Pelvic radiograph shows ankylosis of the sacroiliac joints in a symmetric manner, typical of this disease.

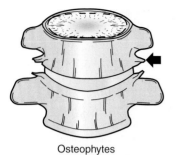
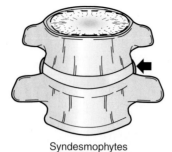

Osteophytes   Syndesmophytes

Figure 13.32   Osteophytes versus Syndesmophytes.   Osteophytes initially extend horizontally from the affected disc (*arrow*). Later, vertical bridging occurs. The syndesmophyte extends vertically across the disc space (*arrow*).

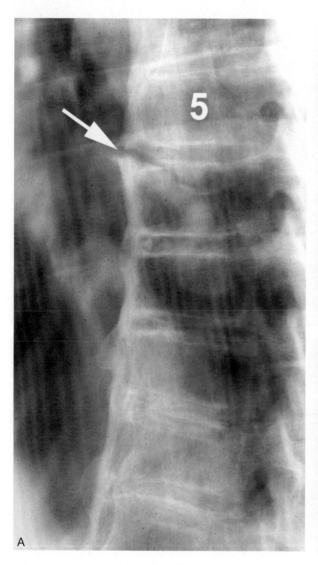

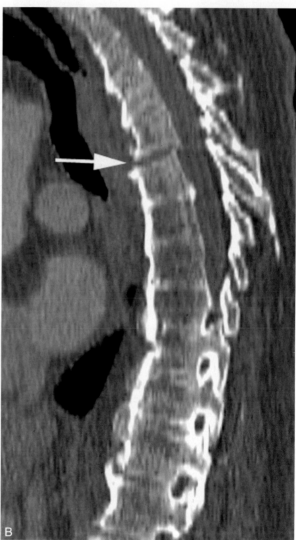

Figure 13.33   Diffuse idiopathic skeletal hyperostosis (DISH).   A. Lateral radiograph shows bony ankylosis along the anterior vertebral margin due to thick syndesmophytes. There is an extension fracture ("broken DISH") at T5-T6 (*arrow*). **B.** Sagittal CT image in another patient shows similar findings, as well as an extension fracture (*arrow*).

Abnormalities of Alignment

The normal anatomic relations were listed in the previous section. The principles discussed here apply to CT studies as well as to radiographs. *Abnormalities of alignment* that may indicate fracture are listed below:

- ⟳ Disruption of the anterior or posterior vertebral body lines (Fig. 13.34)
- ⟳ Disruption of the spinolaminar line

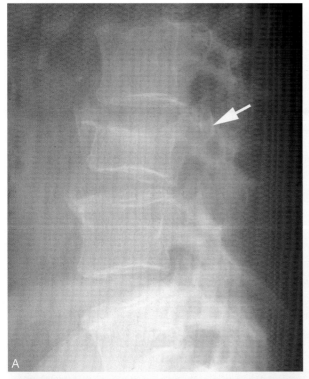

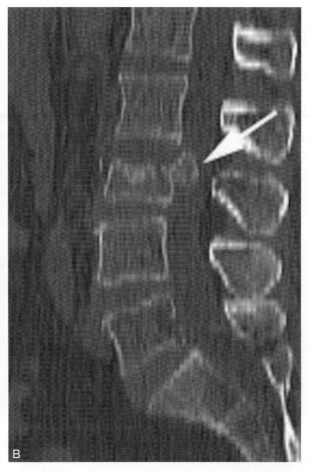

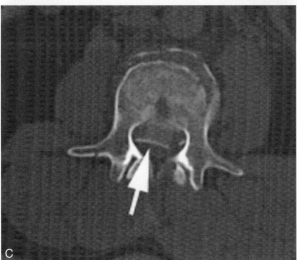

Figure 13.34 Burst fracture of L3. A. Lateral radiograph shows compression of the body of L3 with retropulsion of a bone fragment (*arrow*) from the posterior vertebral body line. **B.** Sagittal reconstructed and **C.** Axial CT images show the fragment displaced into the vertebral canal (*arrows*) as well as fragmentation of the vertebral body.

○ Jumped and locked facets (Fig. 13.35)
○ Rotation of spinous processes
○ Widening of the interpedicle distance
○ Widening of the predental space
○ Kyphotic angulation

Numerous minor variations and discrepancies of alignment measurements occur between various vertebral structures. As a rule, 2 mm is the normal upper limit of the

○ difference for the following measurements:
  • interspinous or interlaminar space,
  • interpedicle distance (transverse or vertical),
  • unilateral or bilateral atlantoaxial offset,
  • anterolisthesis or retrolisthesis with flexion or extension,
  • facet joint width;
○ difference in the height of the anterior and posterior thoracic and lumbar vertebral bodies.

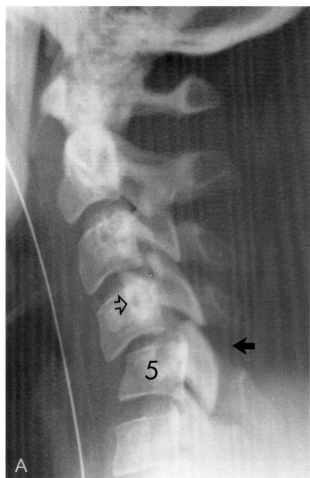

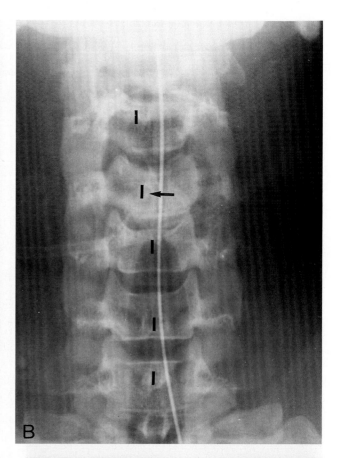

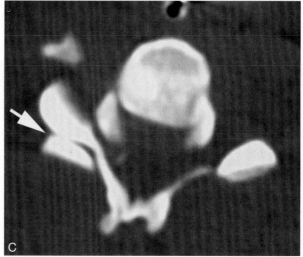

Figure 13.35   Unilateral facet lock.   A. Lateral radiograph shows anterolisthesis of C4 on C5. Note the widening of one facet joint (*solid arrow*). The rotated pillar of C4 (*open arrow*) may be seen through the body of C4 as part of a "bow tie." **B.** Frontal radiograph shows malalignment of the spinous processes (*solid vertical lines*). The spinous processes of C3 and C4 are displaced to the right (*arrow*), indicating that it is the right facet that is locked. **C.** Axial CT image shows the locked facet (*arrow*) on the right. Note the resemblance to a reversed hamburger bun.

As a rule, 2 mm is the normal upper limit of the
⟩ difference for the following measurements:
   • interspinous or interlaminar space,
   • interpedicle distance (transverse or vertical),
   • unilateral or bilateral atlantoaxial offset,
   • anterolisthesis or retrolisthesis with flexion or extension,
   • facet joint width;
⟩ difference in the height of the anterior and posterior thoracic and lumbar vertebral bodies.

This important *rule of 2s* will hold you in good stead in most instances.

Abnormalities of Bony Integrity

Abnormalities of bony integrity include

○ Any obvious fracture (Fig. 13.36)
○ Disruption of the "ring" of C2
○ Widening of C2 (the so-called fat C2 sign; Fig. 13.37)
○ Widening of the interpedicle distance
○ Disruption of the posterior vertebral body line

Cartilage or Joint Space Abnormalities

Cartilage or joint space abnormalities include

○ Widening of the predental space (more than 3 mm in an adult and 5 mm in a child)
○ Abnormally wide intervertebral disc space (Fig. 13.38)
○ Widening of the facet joints (or "naked" facets; Fig. 13.39)
○ Widening of the interlaminar or interspinous distance
○ Abnormal dens-basion line

Soft Tissue Abnormalities

Soft tissue abnormalities play a less important role since CT is used as the primary imaging tool for suspected spine injuries. However, these abnormalities are encountered primarily with cervical injuries. These signs are seen on both radiographs and CT and include

○ Wide cervical prevertebral soft tissues (Fig. 13.40)
○ Soft tissue mass at the craniocervical junction
○ Deviation of the trachea or larynx
○ Paraspinal soft tissue mass (Fig. 13.41)
○ Loss of the psoas stripe

It should go without saying, however, that a patient with known neurologic deficit should undergo MR examination as soon as possible to determine the full extent of spinal

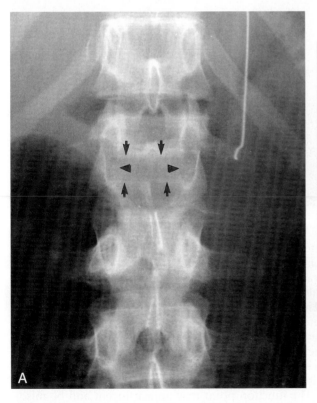
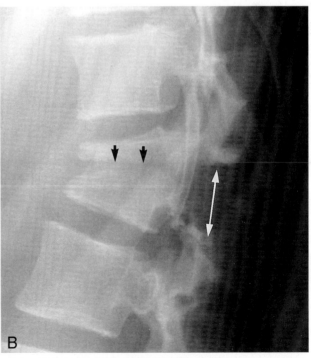

Figure 13.36 Chance fracture of L1. **A.** Frontal radiograph demonstrates a horizontal fracture that involves the lamina (*arrows*) as well as the pedicles (*arrowheads*) of L1. **B.** Lateral radiograph demonstrates the horizontal fracture line (*short arrows*) as well as the posterior distraction (*double arrow*) that occurs with this injury.

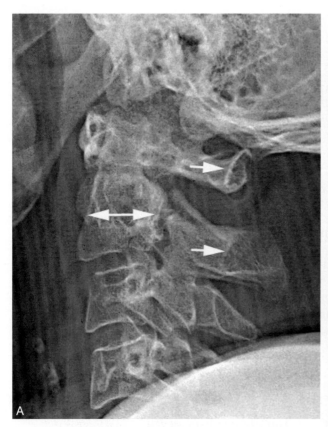

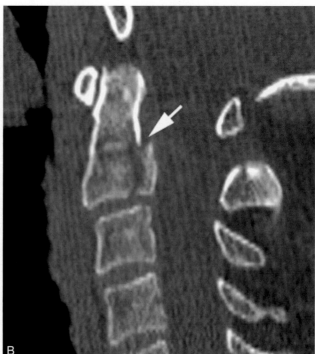

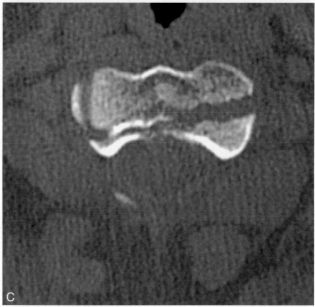

Figure 13.37   Subtle C2 fracture.   A. Lateral radiograph shows widening of the body of C2 (*double arrow*) in relation to C3. This is due to the fact that the posterior vertebral body line remains in its anatomic position and the remainder of the vertebral body is displaced anteriorly. Note the disruption of the spinolaminar line (*single arrows*). **B.** Sagittal reconstructed CT image shows the coronal fracture (*arrow*) in the posterior body of C2. The spinolaminar line of C1 is slightly anterior, as in **A. C.** Axial CT image shows the extent of the fracture.

cord injury and/or epidural hematoma (Figs. 13.42 and 13.43). MRI is also utilized to assess for presence and extent of ligamentous injury (Fig. 13.44).

In addition, CT and MR angiographic techniques should be utilized if there is concern for vascular injury. Most commonly, this occurs when there is a cervical spine fracture involving the transverse foramen (Fig. 13.45). CT is also invaluable in the characterization of injuries to the craniovertebral junction (Fig. 13.46).

Is it still necessary to obtain radiographs if CT is both easier to obtain and more sensitive in identifying fractures? Yes, there are several reasons to do so. First, limited radiography (single lateral view) may be needed to find some horizontal fractures, particularly at C2. Second, partial-volume averaging, a physical phenomenon in CT scanning, produces images with data from two levels. The junction point may appear lucent and be misdiagnosed as a fracture. Radiographs can clarify the problem. Finally, motion artifacts may produce a bizarre reconstructed image that has the appearance of a fracture (Fig. 13.47). In this situation, radiographs will also clarify the problem.

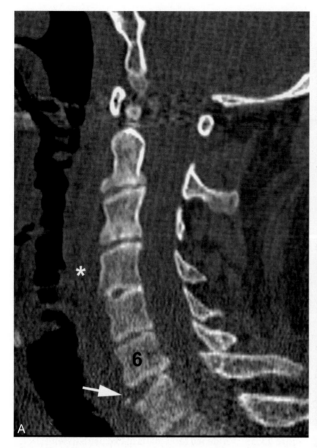

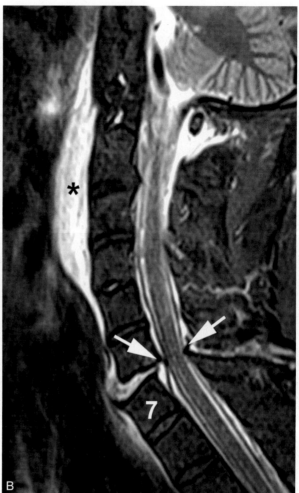

Figure 13.38   Wide disc space (arrows) in a patient with an extension injury.   A. Sagittal reconstructed CT image shows that the C6 disc space (*arrow*) is wider than its mates. There is also retrolisthesis of C6 on C7. Note the massive prevertebral hematoma (*asterisk*). **B.** Sagittal T2-weighted MRI shows the wide disc space as well as impingement of the spinal cord by osteophytes anteriorly and posteriorly (*arrows*). The anterior and posterior longitudinal ligaments are ruptured. Note the massive prevertebral hematoma (*asterisk*). The patient was quadriplegic.

Spinal Fractures without Trauma

When a spine fracture is found in the setting of minimal, or perhaps, absent trauma, particularly in elderly osteoporotic patients, the radiologist is often asked to determine if the fracture could be pathologic—a fracture related to weakening of the underlying bone from an osseous malignancy, usually metastatic disease, or perhaps infection. Obviously, making this determination has important therapeutic and prognostic implications. CT findings suggesting pathologic etiology include a spotty porotic pattern to the bone or perhaps gross bony destruction. MR findings suggestive of pathologic fracture include frank destruction, bowing of the posterior cortex, abnormal marrow signal involving the entire vertebra (separate from fracture-associated edema), abnormal marrow signal involving the posterior elements, extraosseous soft tissue, and additional metastatic lesions elsewhere in the spine. Osteoporotic fractures, on the other hand, have some edema but otherwise normal marrow signal.

Neoplasms

The vertebral column has not only a rich vascular supply but it is also rich in red marrow. As such, it is one of the most frequent sites for metastases to occur. The evaluation of patients for suspected metastases of the vertebral column usually includes radiographs, radionuclide bone scanning, MRI, and CT. MRI is most sensitive because it shows changes

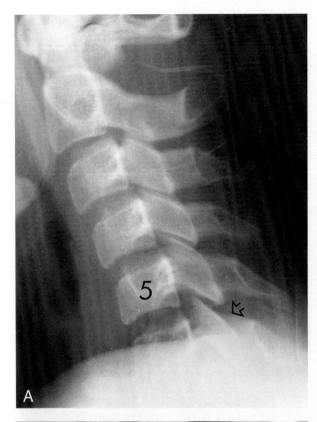

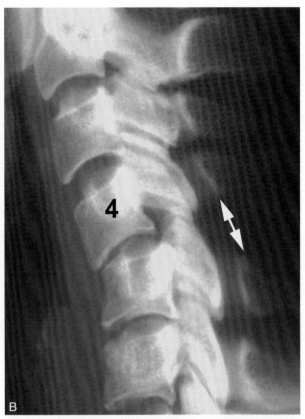

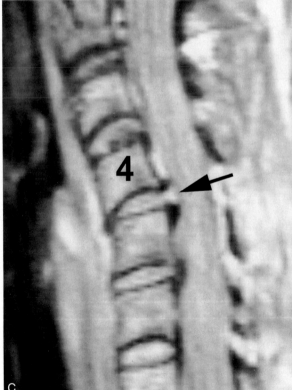

Figure 13.39   Widened facet joints in two patients with flexion sprains.   A. Lateral radiograph in a patient with a mild flexion sprain shows the wide facet joint at C5 (*arrow*). **B.** Patient with a severe flexion sprain. Lateral radiograph shows, in addition to the wide facet joint at C4, widening of the interspinous space (*double arrow*). **C.** Sagittal gradient echo MRI demonstrates rupture of the posterior longitudinal ligament (*arrow*).

in the water content of the marrow that occur as the result of metastases (Fig. 13.48). Often these abnormalities will be detected on MRI and not by radionuclide bone scan, particularly in patients with myeloma. In addition, MRI has the distinct advantage of delineating areas of extension of osseous disease into the spinal canal. This can lead to spinal canal

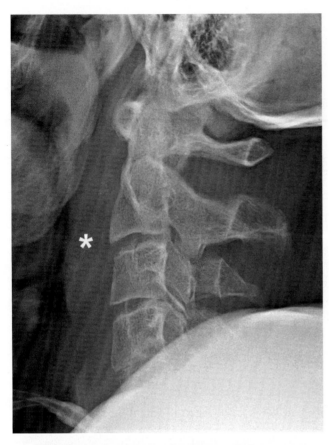

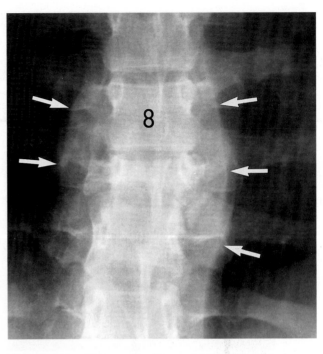

Figure 13.41 **Wide paraspinal line.** Frontal radiograph shows widening of the paraspinal lines (*arrows*) bilaterally in this patient with a T9 fracture-dislocation.

Figure 13.40 **Wide retropharyngeal space.** Lateral radiograph of the same patient as in Figure 13.38 demonstrates massive increase in the retropharyngeal soft tissues (*asterisk*). Now that CT is becoming the screening modality of choice, soft tissue changes play less of a role in diagnosing injuries.

stenosis with associated spinal cord or cauda equina compression (Fig. 13.49). Radiographs are not as sensitive as MR or radionuclide bone scanning. It has been estimated that up to 50% of cancellous bone must be destroyed before the lesion is visible on plain films. In this regard, CT has some advantages. In addition to metastatic disease, there is a wide range of benign and malignant primary tumors of the osseous spine (Table 13.1).

Less commonly, neoplastic masses may be observed within the spinal canal. In order to accurately diagnose these lesions, the radiologist must first localize the disease process to one of three compartments. If the lesion is arising from the spinal cord, it is termed *intramedullary* (Fig. 13.50). If the mass appears to be arising from outside of the spinal cord, but within the thecal sac, it is termed *extramedullary/intradural* (Fig. 13.51). Finally, an *extradural* mass is one that arises from outside of the thecal sac (Fig. 13.52). Table 13.2 lists the differential diagnosis for disease processes than can occur in each of these three compartments.

Infections

Infections often affect the vertebral column either as a direct consequence of surgery or from hematogenous seeding and are most commonly seen in the lumbar region. Early findings of vertebral osteomyelitis include endplate edema and endplate destruction. If untreated, the edema and osseous destruction can extend beyond the endplate to the entire vertebral body, leading to vertebral body collapse. There can also be extension beyond the confines to the vertebral body, most commonly leading to psoas and epidural abscesses. Discitis is often seen in association with vertebral osteomyelitis, and many prefer the term *discitis/osteomyelitis*. Loss of expected disc height and fluid within the disc space are suggestive of discitis. MRI is the preferred imaging modality because of its increased sensitivity

Text continues on page 524.

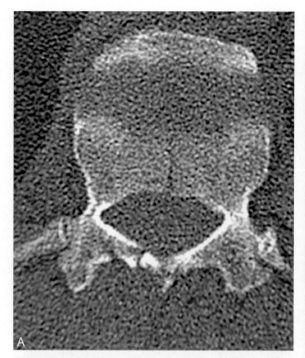

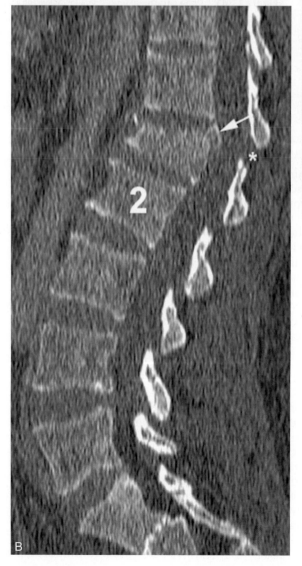

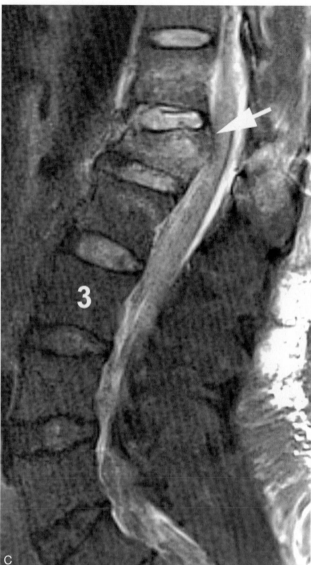

Figure 13.42   Birst fracture of L1.   A. Axial CT image shows fractures of the vertebral body and posterior elements. **B.** Sagittal-reformatted CT image shows anterior wedging and retropulsion of a fracture fragment (*arrow*). Note posterior distraction (*asterisk*). **C.** Sagittal STIR image shows the acute fracture with retropulsed fragment (*arrow*). There is associated spinal canal stenosis and mild compression of the conus medullaris. Note the edema in the T12 and L2 vertebrae, indicative of fractures that were not shown on CT. There are also probable injuries of the anterior longitudinal, posterior longitudinal, and interspinous ligaments.

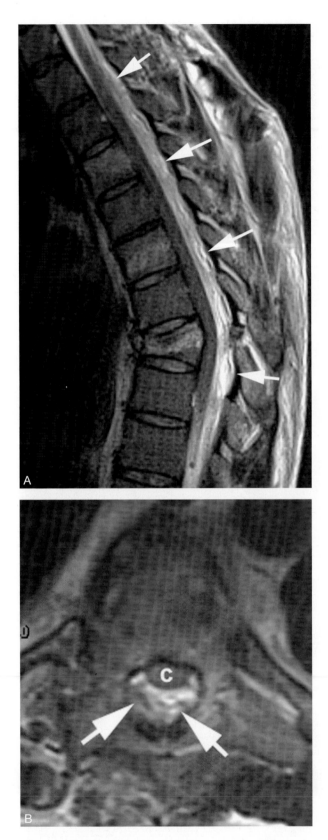

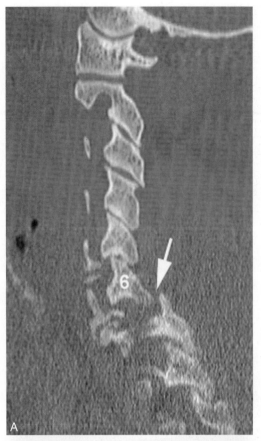

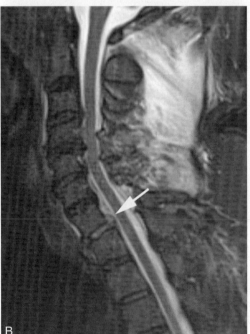

Figure 13.43 **Epidural hematoma.** **A.** Sagittal T2-weighted image shows a Chance fracture at T8. Note the heterogeneous signal in the dorsal epidural space (*arrows*) with associated anterior displacement of the spinal cord. **B.** Axial T2-weighted image at the level of the fracture confirms heterogeneous signal in dorsal epidural space (*arrows*). Spinal cord (*c*) is anteriorly displaced and mildly compressed.

Figure 13.44 **Posttraumatic ligamentous injury.** **A.** Sagittal-reformatted CT image shows a C6-C7 jumped and locked facet (*arrow*) and pedicle fracture. **B.** Sagittal STIR image demonstrates extensive signal hyperintensity consistent with edema related to acute injury of the paraspinal musculature and ligaments. Injured ligaments include the nuchal ligament, interspinous ligaments, and anterior longitudinal ligament. Note the herniated disc at C7-T1 (*arrow*).

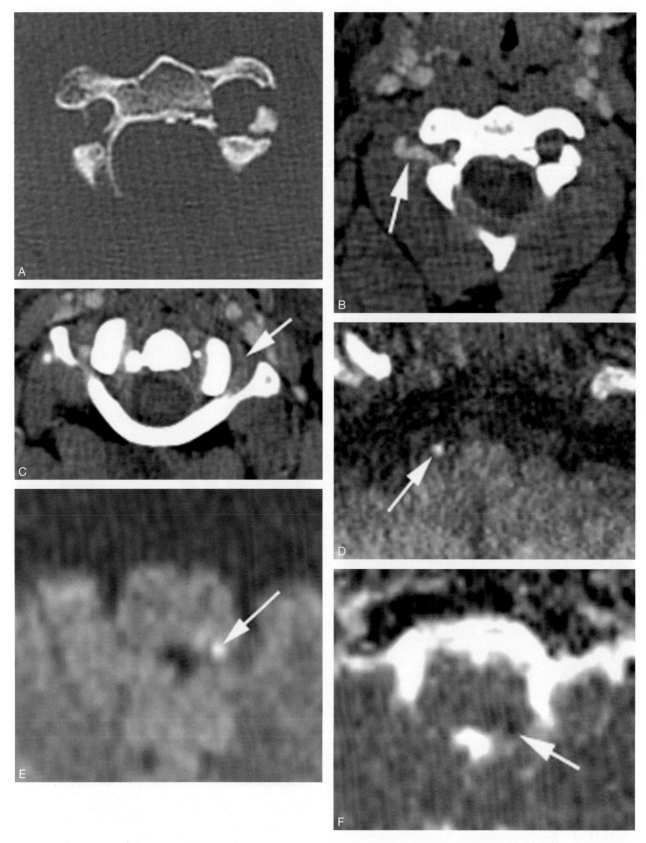

Figure 13.45   Fracture-related vascular injury.   A. Axial CT reveals a comminuted fracture of C2 with involvement of the bilateral transverse foramen, left worse than right. **B.** CT angiogram at the level of C2 reveals atretic flow within the left vertebral artery. Normal flow is seen in the right vertebral artery as it exits the right transverse foramen (*arrow*). **C.** CTA image at the level of C1 shows absence of flow within the left vertebral artery (*arrow*). **D.** 3D time-of-flight MRA reveals absence of flow in the left vertebral artery. Normal flow (*arrow*) identified on the right. Findings are consistent with an acute dissection. **E.** DWI and **F.** ADC images reveal a tiny acute infarct in the left dorsolateral medulla (*arrows*) secondary to the left vertebral artery dissection.

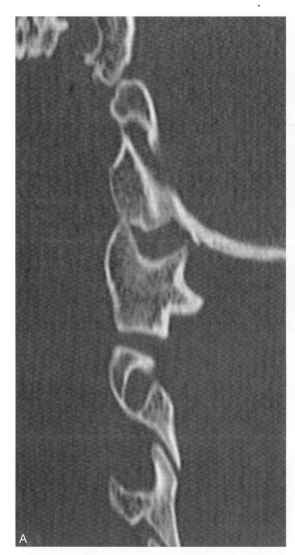

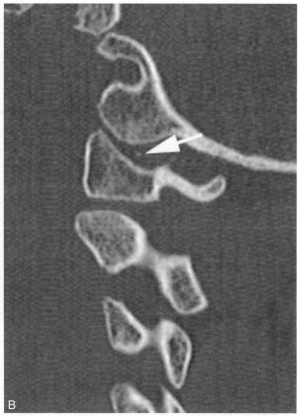

Figure 13.46   Occipitoatlantal dissociation. Pedestrian struck by a train.   A. Right and **B.** Left parasagittal CT images of the craniocervical junction show anterior subluxation of the occipital condyles. Note the abnormally widened space between the condyles and the lateral masses of C1. Note the small osseous fragment (*arrow* in **B**), likely an avulsion fracture.

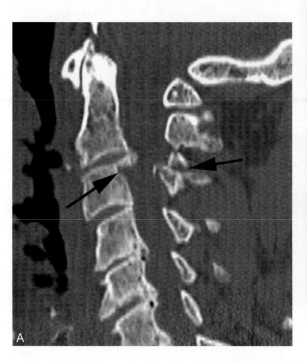

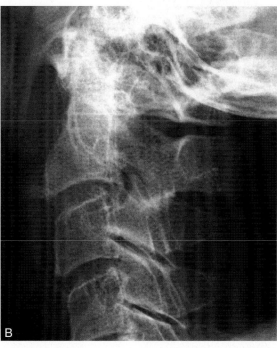

Figure 13.47   (Continued)

Figure 13.47   Motion artifact.   A. Sagittal reconstructed image shows an apparent fracture through C3 (*arrows*). **B.** Lateral radiograph shows no fracture. **C.** CT image shows the motion causing the artifact.

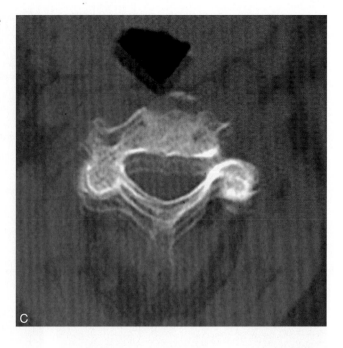

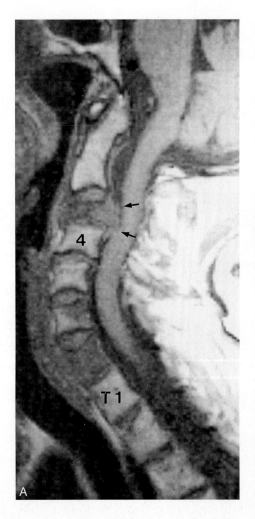

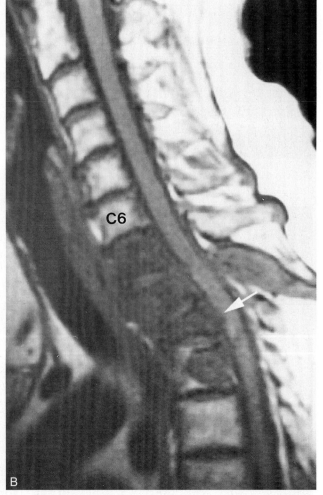

Figure 13.48   (Continued)

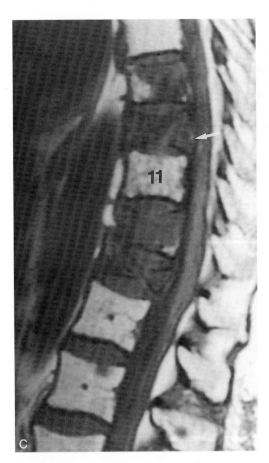

C

Figure 13.48 **Metastases invading the vertebral canal.** **A.** Sagittal T1-weighted MRI shows a destructive process involving C3. There is extradural compression of the spinal cord (*arrows*). Additional metastatic lesions are present at C6 and C7, as evidenced by the low signal (darkness) in those vertebrae. **B.** Sagittal T1-weighted MRI in another patient shows extensive involvement of C7 through T3. Note the canal involvement at T2 (*arrow*) and the spinous process involvement at T1. **C.** Thoracolumbar metastases in another patient. T1-weighted sagittal MRI shows pathologic collapse at T12 and L1. There is posterior breakthrough of tumor at T10 (*arrow*).

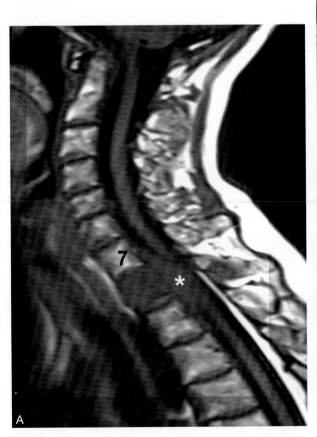

A

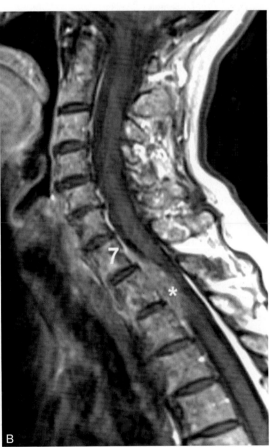

B

Figure 13.49 (Continued)

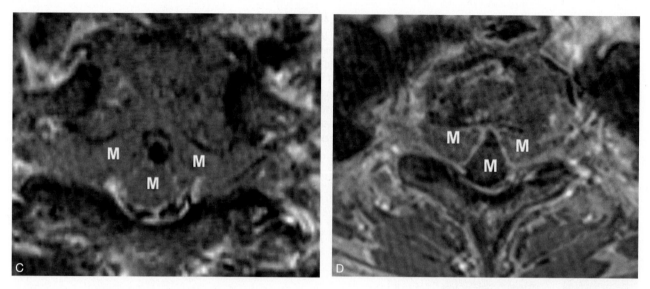

**Figure 13.49	Metastases invading the spinal canal.**	Patient with history of metastatic liver cancer presenting with bilateral hand weakness and paresthesias. Sagittal T1-weighted unenhanced **(A)** and enhanced **(B)** MRI shows abnormal marrow signal and enhancement in the T1 vertebral body and spinous process, consistent with metastasis. Tumor extends into the anterior epidural space (*asterisks*) with resultant spinal cord compression. Axial T1-weighted unenhanced **(C)** and enhanced **(D)** MRI shows mass (*M*) extending from osseous spine into the epidural space partially encasing and compressing the spinal cord. Tumor also extends into both neural foraminae with associated nerve impingement.

Table 13.1 BONY TUMORS OF THE SPINE

Benign
• Osteoid osteoma
• Osteoblastoma
• Aneurysmal bone cyst
• Giant cell tumor
Malignant
• Chordoma
• Chondrosarcoma
• Metastases
• Plasmacytoma/multiple myeloma
• Lymphoma
Tumorlike Conditions
• Fibrous dysplasia
• Langerhans histiocytosis
• Tuberculosis

not only for discitis/osteomyelitis, but also for its complications. Figure 13.53 shows a typical disc space infection.

Postoperative Changes

The most common postoperative change you will encounter is in the patient who has undergone a *laminectomy*. In these patients, segments of lamina of various sizes will be missing at the involved level(s) (Fig. 13.54). Other postoperative changes will include the presence of various types of *stabilizing devices* used to correct abnormalities as the result of trauma (Fig. 13.55) or scoliosis. When reviewing images that have surgical hardware,

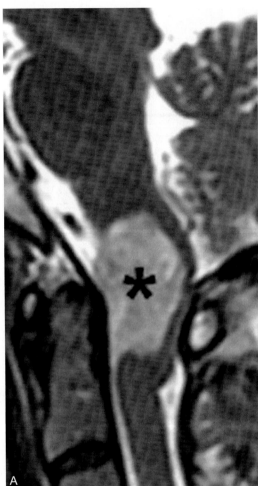

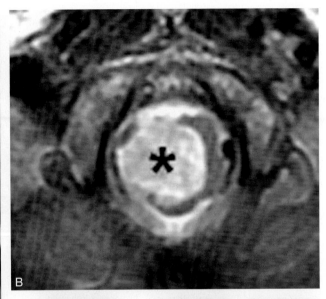

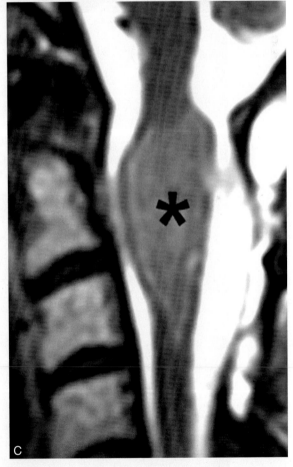

Figure 13.50 Intramedullary masses (asterisks). Sagittal T2-weighted **(A)** and axial T2-weighted **(B)** MRI reveal a hyperintense mass at the level of the cervicomedullary junction. Surgical pathology revealed this to be an astrocytoma. **C.** Another example of a spinal cord astrocytoma in a different patient. Sagittal T2-weighted image at the level of C2 shows a mass arising within the cord.

it is important to compare them with the previous studies to determine whether loosening, fracture, or other complications of the components have occurred (Fig. 13.56). Regardless of the type of surgery, the radiologist should also be vigilant for evidence of postoperative infection (Fig. 13.57).

> When reviewing postoperative images it is important to always compare with previous studies.

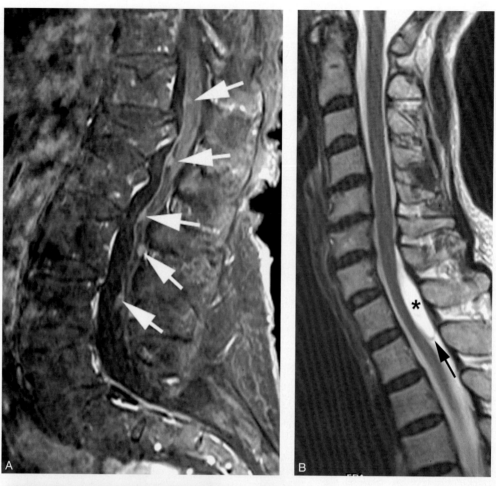

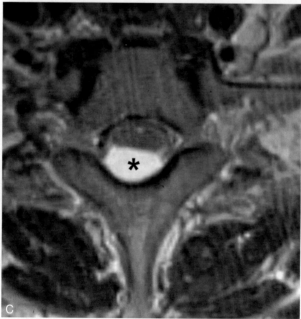

Figure 13.51   Extramedullary/Intradural masses.   A. Leptomeningeal carcinomatosis. Sagittal T1-weighted enhanced image of the lumbar spine demonstrates numerous enhancing nodules (*arrows*) along the cauda equina in this patient with non-small cell lung cancer. **B.** Arachnoid cyst. Sagittal and axial **(C)** T2-weighted image centered at the cervicothoracic junction demonstrates a tapering cystic mass (*asterisks*) with evidence of a thin capsule (*arrow* in **B**), most consistent with an arachnoid cyst. Note the mild cord compression.

In addition, for patients with continued symptoms after surgery, termed *Failed Back Surgery Syndrome* (FBSS), an MRI may be indicated. Contrast should be administered to distinguish between nonenhancing recurrent or residual disc material and enhancing scar tissue (Fig. 13.58). Arachnoiditis can also be a cause of FBSS, and its presence should be assessed on postoperative lumbar spine images (Fig. 13.59).

Text continues on page 533.

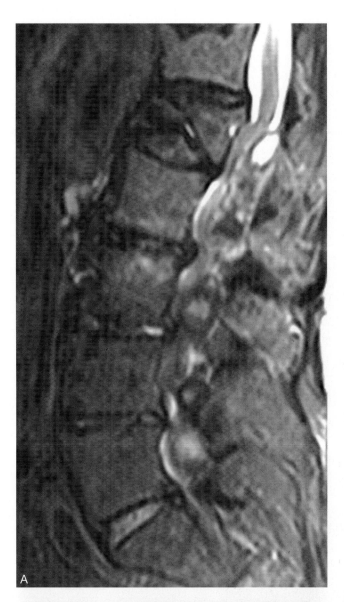

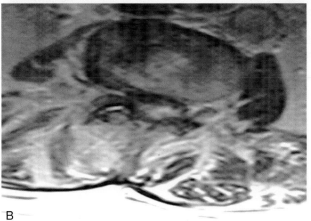

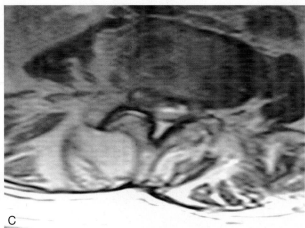

Table 13.2 SOFT TISSUE MASSES OF THE SPINE

Intramedullary

- Astrocytoma
- Ependymoma
- Hemangioblastoma
- Inflammatory lesion (e.g., MS)
- Metastasis
- Vascular malformation

Intradural/Extramedullary

- Schwannoma
- Meningioma
- Neurofibroma
- Leptomeningeal carcinomatosis
- Arachnoid cyst

Extradural

- Epidural hematoma
- Epidural abscess
- Disc bulge or herniation
- Osseous metastasis
- Primary bone tumor
- Arachnoid cyst

Figure 13.52   Epidural hematoma.   A. Sagittal STIR image of the lumbar spine demonstrates a heterogeneous epidural collection. The low signal intensity is suggestive of hemorrhage, and hemorrhage was found at laminectomy and surgical decompression. **B.** and **C.** Axial T2-weighted images of the lumbar spine show heterogeneous epidural collection with a fluid-fluid level. The normal cauda equina is severely compressed and is not well visualized.

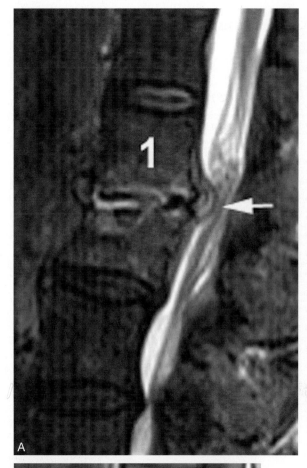

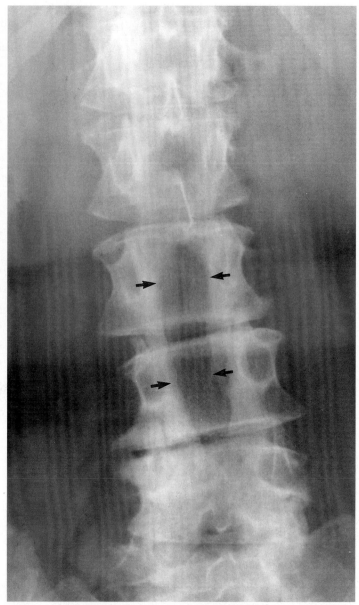

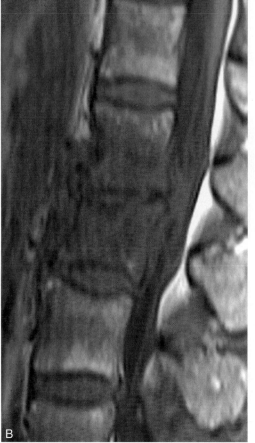

Figure 13.54   Appearance after laminectomy.   Note the absence of the laminae and spinous processes of L3 and L4. The lucency represents the surgical margins (*arrows*).

Figure 13.53   Discitis/osteomyelitis.   A. Sagittal STIR image shows loss of disc height, endplate edema, and abnormal disc space fluid at L1-L2. The L2 vertebral body shows partial collapse. A small epidural abscess (*arrow*) is also present. **B.** Sagittal T1-weighted image confirms abnormal marrow signal. Findings are consistent with infection of both the disc space and adjacent vertebral bodies.

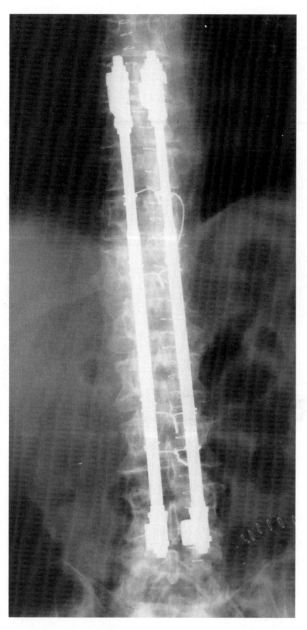

Figure 13.55 Stabilizing rods and hooks for a T12 fracture.
The rods extend from T8 to L4.

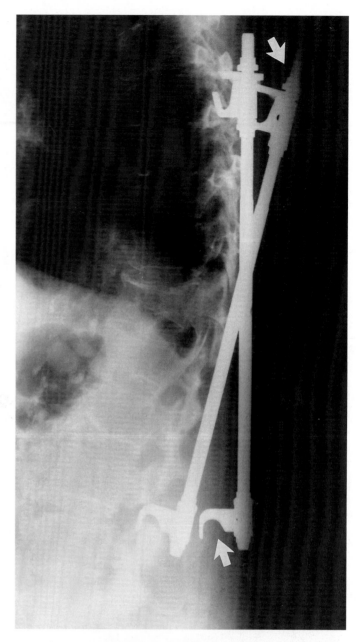

Figure 13.56 Unhooking of stabilizing rods. (This is the same patient as in Fig. 13.55.) One rod has unhooked on top, one on the bottom (*arrows*).

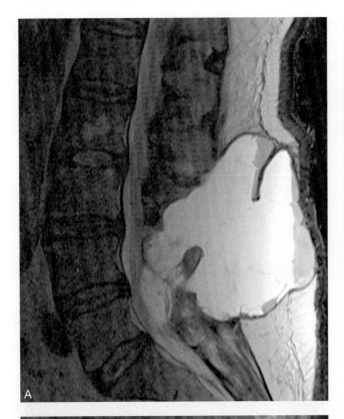

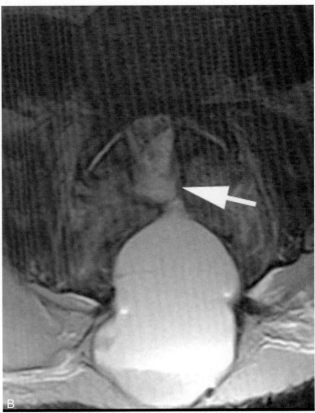

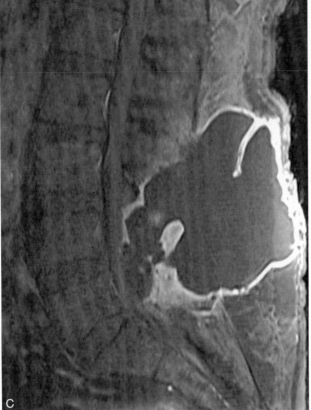

Figure 13.57   Postoperative abscess.   Patient underwent L3-L5 laminectomy 5 weeks prior, now with fever and pain. Sagittal T2-weighted (**A**) and axial T2-weighted (**B**) images of the lumbar spine demonstrate a large fluid collection extending from the laminectomy defect (*arrow* in **B**). Note the fluid-debris level and the mass effect upon the thecal sac as the mass extends into the dorsal epidural space. **C.** Sagittal T1-weighted enhanced image shows enhancement of the walls of this collection. Surgical decompression revealed purulent material that grew Gram-positive cocci. A component of this collection was CSF, and a dural tear was also found at the time of surgery.

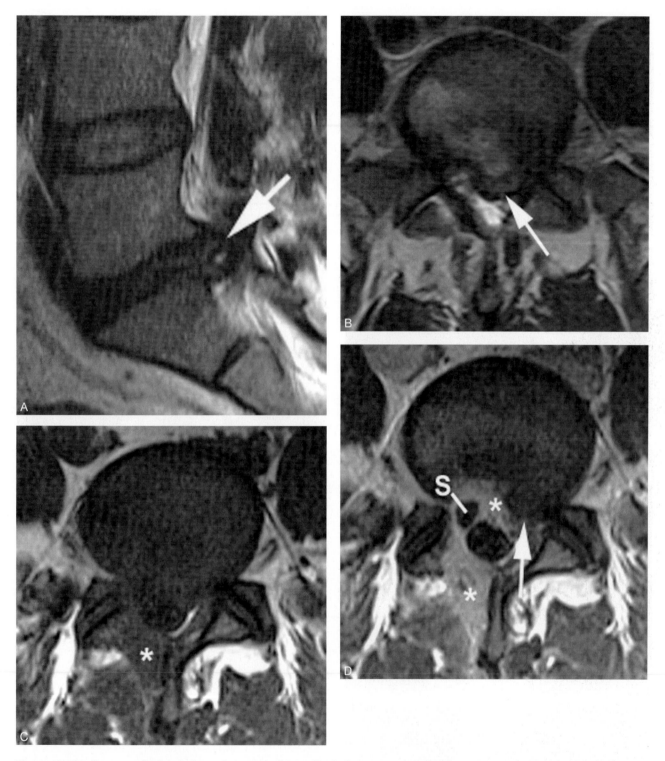

Figure 13.58 Recurrent disc herniation. Patient with a history of L5-S1 discectomy presents for follow-up imaging. Sagittal **(A)** and axial **(B)** T2-weighted images demonstrate a low-signal epidural mass (*arrows*) arising from the L5-S1 disc space. Note the compression of the left S1 nerve root in **B**. Since both scar tissue and disc material exhibit low signal, contrast-enhanced imaging is required for further characterization. Axial unenhanced **(C)** and enhanced **(D)** T1-weighted images at the level of L5-S1. Enhancing scar tissue is present in the right laminectomy defect and in the ventral epidural space (*asterisks*). However, the majority of the epidural mass is nonenhancing and is consistent with recurrent disc herniation (*white arrow*). Note the enlargement of the right S1 nerve root sleeve secondary to scar tissue retraction (*S*).

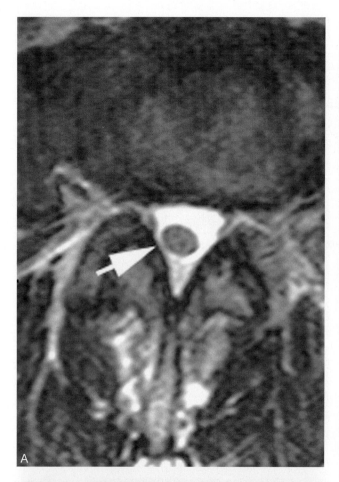

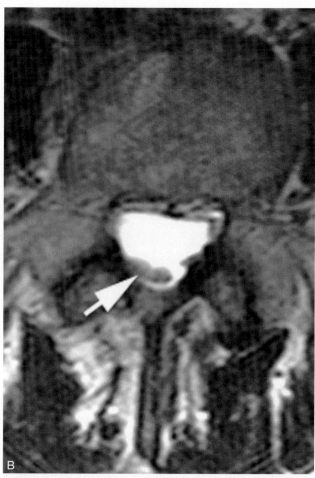

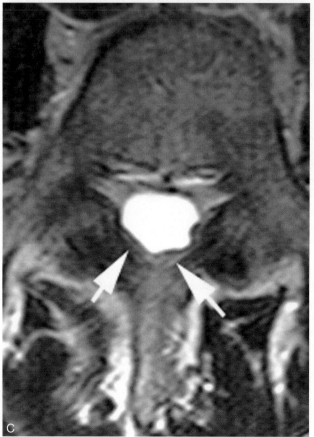

Figure 13.59   Arachnoiditis.   A. Fifty-nine-year-old with lower back pain and incontinence. Past history of two lumbar spine surgeries. Axial T2-weighted images of the lower lumbar spine below the level of the conus. **A** and **B.** There is "clumping" and thickening of the cauda equina nerve roots (*arrows*). **C.** There is adherence of the nerve roots to the walls of the thecal sac (*arrows*), giving the "empty sac" sign.

Summary and Key Points

▶ This chapter reviewed vertebral anatomy and the various techniques for evaluating the vertebral column.

▶ CT is the prime screening method for patients with suspected vertebral trauma.

▶ MRI provides a superior evaluation of the contents of the spinal canal.

▶ Despite the advantages of CT and MRI of the spine, radiography is still necessary.

▶ The assessment of developmental, degenerative and arthritic, traumatic, neoplastic, infectious, and postoperative abnormalities was discussed.

▶ When reviewing postoperative images it is important to always compare with previous studies.

Suggested Additional Reading

American College of Radiology. ACR Appropriateness Criteria® On Suspected Spine Trauma. Reston, VA: American College of Radiology, 2012. Available at http://www.acr.org.

Daffner RH. Cervical radiography for trauma patients: a time-effective technique? AJR Am J Roentgenol 2000;175:1309–1311.

Daffner RH. Helical CT of the cervical spine for trauma patients: a time study. AJR Am J Roentgenol 2001;177:677–679.

Daffner RH. Imaging of Vertebral Trauma. 3rd Ed. Cambridge, UK: Cambridge University Press, 2011.

Fardon DF, Milette PC. Recommendations of the Combined Task Forces of the North American Spine Society, American Society of Spine Radiology, and American Society of Neuroradiology. 2003. Available at http://www.asnr.org/spine_nomenclature/.

Fenton DS, Czervionke LF. Image-Guided Spine Intervention. Philadelphia, PA: WB Saunders, 2003.

Hogan JA, Blackmore CC, Mann FA, Wilson AJ. Cervical spine injury: a clinical decision rule to identify high-risk patients for helical CT scanning. AJR Am J Roentgenol 2000;174:713–717.

Latschaw RE, Kucharczyk J, Moseley M. Imaging of the Nervous System: Diagnostic and Therapeutic Applications. St. Louis, MO: Mosby, 2005.

Renfrew DL. Atlas of Spine Injection. Philadelphia, PA: WB Saunders, 2004.

Ross JS, Moore KR, Bryson B, et al. Diagnostic Imaging: Spine. 2nd Ed. Salt Lake City, UT: Amirsys, 2010.

Stiell IG, Wells GA, Vandemheen KL, et al. The Canadian C-spine rule for radiography in alert and stable trauma patients. JAMA 2001;286:1841–1848.

Vandemark R. Radiology of the cervical spine in trauma patients: practice pitfalls and recommendations for improving efficiency and communication. AJR Am J Roengenol 1990;155:465–472.

Index